Credits

General Editors

Rosalind Fergusson BA
Anne Stibbs BA

Contributors and Advisers

Rajesh Aggarwal BM, MRCP, FRCS, FRCOphth
David Ahearne MB, ChB
W. Leslie Alexander FRCS, FRCOphth
J. A. D. Anderson MA, MD, FRCP, FFPHM, FFOM, FRCGP
J. H. Angel MD, FRCP
Dr Andrea Atherton MA, MSc, MRCP(UK)
John R. Bennett MD, FRCP
Stuart Anthony Bentley MB, BS
Dr J. N. Bowles BSc, MRCP, FRCR
Dr Peter Bradbury FRCP
Bruce M. Bryant MB, ChB, MRCP
Phillip Chan MA, MChir, FRCS
Robert E. Coleman
Patrick Collins MD, MRCP
J. A. Cullen BSc, MSc
W. J. Dinning FRCS, MRCP
Ivan T. Draper MB, ChB, FRCPEd
J. C. Gingell MB, BCh, FRCSEd, FRCS
John M. Goldman DM, FRCP, FRCPath
Helen K. Gordon FRCOG, iFFP
J. Gordon MD, FRCS(G), FRCOG
. Howes MA, MB, BS, MD, CP(I)

Dr Craig Job FRCS, FRCR
Michael Klab
Marc E. Lani
Alexander J. MRCPsych
D. J. McFerr
Gordon Mac
Charles V. N
J. E. Nicholl
Heather E. I
T. R. Pitt Fo
D. L. Phillip
Helen Phill DCH, DRCC
Amin Rahe
Dr John R.
Dr Mary S DTM&H
B. F. Sizer
Dr Tony S
Dr Steve S ChB, MRC
Eric Tayl CPsych
Paul Wat MPH, FF
William I CPath
Robert M DRM&H

Minidictionary for Nurses

Fifth Edition

Minidictionary for
Nurses

Fifth Edition

Consultant

Tanya A. McFerran MA, SRN, RSCN, Cert. Ed.

Senior Lecturer in Childhood Studies
School of Community Health and Social Services
Anglia Polytechnic University, Chelmsford

Editor

Elizabeth A. Martin MA

Market House Books Ltd

Oxford   New York

OXFORD UNIVERSITY PRESS

OXFORD

UNIVERSITY PRESS

Great Clarendon Street, Oxford OX2 6DP

Oxford University Press is a department of the University of Oxford.
It furthers the University's objective of excellence in research, scholarship,
and education by publishing worldwide in

Oxford New York
Auckland Cape Town Dar es Salaam Hong Kong Karachi Kuala Lumpur
Madrid Melbourne Mexico City Nairobi New Delhi Taipei Toronto
Shanghai

With offices in
Argentina Austria Brazil Chile Czech Republic France Greece
Guatemala Hungary Italy Japan South Korea Poland Portugal
Singapore Switzerland Thailand Turkey Ukraine Vietnam

Oxford is a registered trade mark of Oxford University Press
in the UK and in certain other countries

British Library Cataloguing in Publication Data

Data available

ISBN-13:978-0-19-860692-5
ISBN-10:0-19-860692-3

10 9 8 7

Typeset by Market House Books Ltd
Printed and bound in Italy by
Legoprint S.p.A.

Preface

This new edition of the *Minidictionary for Nurses*, first published as the *Pocket Dictionary for Nurses*, provides, in some 11,000 entries, explanations of the terms and concepts likely to be encountered by nurses, therapists, radiographers, and those in similar professions during the course of their work. In addition to terms relating specifically to the nursing profession and the nursing process, there are many entries in the fields of medicine, surgery, anatomy and physiology, endocrinology, psychiatry, and pharmacology. For this edition, many new terms have been added, including those from advanced life-support systems, paediatrics, the theory and practice of nursing, and the reorganization of the NHS. Entries for many new drugs have been included, and drug names have been revised in accordance with the recently implemented EC directive on the use of recommended International Non-proprietary Names (rINNs).

Each entry contains a pronunciation guide, the part of speech, and a concisely written definition. The pronunciation guide, which is described in detail on page viii, follows that used in the *Oxford Paperback Dictionary* and provides an easy and accessible guide to correct pronunciation without the use of special symbols. Most definitions comprise a single sentence, but, where necessary, further explanation is given. Many terms in medicine are used in combination (for example *acute abscess*, *apical abscess*, etc.) and each of these phrases is treated as a separate definition within the main entry (*abscess* in this example). Derived terms (for example, adjectives derived from nouns) are not normally included as separate entries except where their meanings cannot be deduced from the words from which they are derived. Instead they are listed at the end of the definition of the parent word together with the part of speech and, where necessary, a pronunciation guide.

The Appendices include a comprehensive selection of tables of reference values for biochemical data, obtained from the *Oxford Textbook of Medicine* (fourth edition, 2003), together with tables of SI units, conversion tables to and from other systems of units, and formulae for calculating drug doses. Several new appendices have been added for this edition, including a comprehensive list of web site addresses for health-care organizations.

In the preparation of this dictionary a range of entries has been adapted from the *Concise Medical Dictionary*, first published by the Oxford University Press in 1980 (sixth edition published 2002).

E. A. M.

2003

Contents

Pronunciation Guide

A pronunciation guide is given in brackets after the entry word and before the part of speech. Words of two or more syllables are broken up into small units, usually of one syllable, separated by hyphens. The stressed syllable in a word of two or more syllables is shown in bold type.

The sounds represented are as follows:

a *as in* back (bak), active (**ak**-tiv)
ă *as in* abduct (ăb-**dukt**), gamma (**gam**-ă)
ah *as in* after (**ahf**-ter), palm (pahm)
air *as in* aerosol (**air**-ŏ-sol), care (kair)
ar *as in* tar (tar), heart (hart)
aw *as in* jaw (jaw), gall (gawl)
ay *as in* mania (**may**-nia), grey (gray)
b *as in* bed (bed)
ch *as in* chin (chin)
d *as in* day (day)
e *as in* red (red)
ĕ *as in* bowel (**bow**-ĕl)
ee *as in* see (see), haem (heem), caffeine (**kaf**-een)
eer *as in* fear (feer), serum (**seer**-ŭm)
er *as in* dermal (**der**-măl), labour (**lay**-ber)
ew *as in* dew (dew), nucleus (**new**-kli-ŭs)
ewr *as in* pure (pewr), dura (**dewr**-ă)
f *as in* fat (fat), phobia (**foh**-biă), cough (kof)
g *as in* gag (gag)
h *as in* hip (hip)
i *as in* fit (fit), acne (**ak**-ni), reduction (ri-**duk**-shŏn)
I *as in* eye (I), angiitis (an-ji-**I**-tis)
j *as in* jaw (jaw), gene (jeen), ridge (rij)
k *as in* kidney (**kid**-ni), chlorine (**klor**-een)
ks *as in* toxic (**toks**-ik)
kw *as in* quadrate (**kwod**-rayt)
l *as in* liver (**liv**-er)

m *as in* milk (milk)
n *as in* nit (nit)
ng *as in* sing (sing)
nk *as in* rank (rank), bronchus (**bronk**-ŭs)
o *as in* pot (pot)
ŏ *as in* buttock (**but**-ŏk)
oh *as in* home (hohm), post (pohst)
oi *as in* boil (boil)
oo *as in* food (food), croup (kroop), fluke (flook)
oor *as in* pruritus (proor-I-tŭs)
or *as in* organ (**or**-găn), wart (wort)
ow *as in* powder (**pow**-der), pouch (powch)
p *as in* pill (pil)
r *as in* rib (rib)
s *as in* skin (skin), cell (sel)
sh *as in* shock (shok), action (**ak**-shŏn)
t *as in* tone (tohn)
th *as in* bath (bahth)
th as in then (*th*en)
u *as in* pulp (pulp), blood (blud)
ŭ *as in* typhus (**ty** fŭs)
uu *as in* hook (huuk)
v *as in* vein (vayn)
w *as in* wind (wind)
y *as in* yeast (yeest)
or, when preceded by a consonant, *as in* bite (byt)
yoo *as in* unit (**yoo**-nit), formula (**form**-yoo-lă)
yoor *as in* ureter (yoor-**ee**-ter)
yr *as in* fire (fyr)
z *as in* zinc (zink), glucose (**gloo**-kohz)
zh as in vision (**vizh**-ŏn)

A consonant is sometimes doubled to prevent accidental mis-pronunciation of a syllable resembling a familiar word; for example **ass**-id (acid), rather than **as**-id; ultră-**sonn**-iks (ultrasonics), rather than ultră-**son**-iks.

An apostrophe is used (i) between two consonants forming a syllable, as in **den**-t'l (dental), and (ii) between two letters when the syllable might otherwise be mispronounced through resembling a familiar word, as in **th'e**-ră-pi (therapy), th'y (thigh), and tal'k (talc).

Aa

a- (an-) *prefix denoting* absence of; lacking; not.

AA *n.* Alcoholics Anonymous.

AAA *n. see* (abdominal aortic) aneurysm.

A and E medicine *n.* accident and emergency medicine: an important specialty dealing with the immediate problems of the acutely ill and injured.

ab- *prefix denoting* away from.

abarticulation (ab-ar-tik yoo-**lay**-shŏn) *n.* **1.** the dislocation of a joint. **2.** a synovial joint (*see* diarthrosis).

abbreviated injury scale (a-**bree**-vi-ay-tid) *n.* a quick method for determining the severity of a case of serious trauma. It can be used for purposes of triage and clinical audit.

abdomen (ab-dŏm-ĕn) *n.* the part of the body cavity below the chest (*see* thorax), from which it is separated by the diaphragm. The abdomen contains the organs of digestion (stomach, liver, intestines, etc.), excretion (kidneys, bladder, etc.), and in women reproduction (ovaries and uterus). It is lined by a membrane, the peritoneum. —**abdominal** (ab-**dom**-i-năl) *adj.*

abdominal thrusts (Heimlich manoeuvre) *pl. n.* a manoeuvre for the treatment of choking in which the patient is held firmly around the midriff just under the ribcage. The hands of the rescuer are held as a fist and short sharp thrusts into the patient's upper abdomen are made in order to dislodge the obstructing article from the airway.

abdominoperineal excision (ăb-dom-in-oh-pe-ri-**nee**-ăl) *n.* an operation for excision of the rectum in which incisions are made in both the abdomen and the perineum.

right hypochondrium — epigastrium — left hypochondrium

right lumbar — umbilical — left lumbar

right inguinal — hypogastrium — left inguinal

Regions of the abdomen

abducens nerve (ăb-dew-sĕnz) *n.* the sixth cranial nerve (VI), which supplies the lateral rectus muscle of each eyeball.

abduct (ăb-dukt) *vb.* to move a limb or any other part away from the midline of the body. —**abduction** *n.*

abductor (ăb-duk-ter) *n.* any muscle that, when it contracts, moves one part of the body away from another or from the midline of the body. Abductors work antagonistically with adductors.

aberrant (ă-b'e-rănt) *adj.* abnormal: usually applied to a blood vessel or nerve that does not follow its normal course.

aberration (ab-er-ay-shŏn) *n.* **1.** deviation from the normal. **2.** a defect in the image formed by a lens. *chromatic a.* a defect in which the image has coloured fringes as a result of the different extent to which light of different colours is refracted. *spherical a.* a defect in which the image is blurred because curvature of the lens causes light rays from the object to come to a focus in slightly different positions.

ABGs *pl. n. see* arterial blood gases.

ablation (ăb-lay-shŏn) *n.* surgical removal of tissue, a part of the body, or an abnormal growth. *See also* endometrial (ablation).

abnormal (ab-nor-măl) *adj.* deviating from the normal in structure, position, occurrence, etc. (e.g. *a. growth*).

abnormality (ab-nor-mal-iti) *n.* **1.** deviation from the normal or expected. **2.** a malformation or deformity (e.g. *developmental a.*).

abort (ă-bort) *vb.* **1.** to terminate a process or disease before its full course has been run. **2.** to remove or expel an embryo or fetus from the uterus before it is capable of independent existence. *See* abortion.

abortifacient (ă-bor-ti-fay-shĕnt) *n.* a drug that induces abortion or miscarriage.

abortion (ă-bor-shŏn) *n.* the expulsion or removal of an embryo or fetus from the uterus at a stage of pregnancy when it is incapable of independent survival (i.e. at any time between conception and the 24th week of pregnancy). *complete a.* premature expulsion of the fetus and all its membranes. *criminal a.* (in Britain) abortion not carried out within the terms of the Abortion Act 1967 and Abortion Regulations 1991. *habitual* (or *recurrent*) *a.* abortion occurring in three or more successive pregnancies before 20 weeks' gestation, with fetuses weighing under 500 g. *incomplete a.* retention by the uterus of part of the fetus or its membranes during an abortion. *induced a.* the deliberate termination of a pregnancy for medical or social reasons. *inevitable a.* abortion that cannot be prevented as the fetus is dead. *missed a.* abortion in which the fetus is dead but not expelled from the uterus. *recurrent a. see* habitual a. *spontaneous a.* miscarriage; naturally occurring abortion. *therapeutic a.* abortion induced to protect the life or health of the mother. *threatened a.* abdominal pain and bleeding from the uterus while the fetus is still alive. —**abortive** *adj.*

abortus (ă-bor-tŭs) *n.* a fetus, weighing less than 500 g, that is expelled from the uterus either dead or incapable of surviving.

ABO system *n. see* blood group.

abrasion (ă-bray-zhŏn) *n.* a minor wound in which the surface of the skin or a mucous membrane is worn away by rubbing or scraping.

abreaction (ab-ree-ak-shŏn) *n.* the release of strong emotion associated with a buried memory. Abreaction may be induced as a treatment for conversion disorder, anxiety state, and other neurotic conditions.

abruptio placentae (ă-brup-ti-oh plă-sent-i) *n.* bleeding from the placenta causing its complete or partial detachment from the uterine wall after the 24th week of gestation. Abruptio placentae is often associated with hypertension and pre-eclampsia.

abscess (ab-sis) *n.* a collection of pus enclosed by damaged and inflamed tissues. *acute a.* an abscess associated with pain, inflammation, and some fever. *apical a.* an abscess in the bone around the tip of the root of a tooth. *Brodie's a.* a chronic abscess of bone that develops from acute bacterial osteomyelitis. *cerebral a.* an abscess resulting from infection of the brain or meninges. *cold* or *chronic a.* an abscess, usually due to tuberculosis organisms, in which there is little pain or inflammation. *psoas a.* a cold abscess in the psoas muscle (in the groin), which has spread from diseased vertebrae in the lower part of the spine. *subphrenic a.* an abscess in the space below the diaphragm, usually resulting from a spread of infection from the abdomen. *tropical* (or *amoebic*) *a.* an abscess of the liver caused by infection with *Entamoeba histolytica. See also* ischiorectal abscess.

absence (ab-sĕns) *n.* (in neurology) *see* epilepsy.

absorption (ăb-sorp-shŏn) *n.* the uptake of digested food from the intestine into the blood and lymphatic systems. *See also* assimilation, digestion

abulia (ă-boo-liă) *n.* absence or impairment of will power, commonly a symptom of schizophrenia.

a.c. (**ante cibum**) Latin: before food, used as a direction in prescriptions.

acanthosis (ak-ăn-thoh-sis) *n.* an increase in the number of prickle cells in the innermost layer of the epidermis, leading to thickening of the epidermis. *a. nigricans* acanthosis characterized by papillomatous growths, mainly in the armpits, which give the skin a pigmented appearance and a velvety texture. It may be benign or malignant.

acapnia (**hypocapnia**) (ă-kap-niă) *n.* a condition in which there is an abnormally low concentration of carbon dioxide in the blood.

acarbose (ass-ar-bohz) *n.* an oral hypoglycaemic drug that reduces the breakdown and absorption of carbohydrates in the intestine by blocking the action of an important enzyme (α-glucosidase) in this process. Trade name: **Glucobay**.

acardia (ay-kar-diă) *n.* congenital absence of the heart. The condition may occur in conjoined twins; the twin with the heart controls the circulation for both.

acariasis (akă-ry-ă-sis) *n.* an infestation of mites and ticks.

acaricide (ă-ka-ri-syd) *n.* any chemical agent used for destroying mites and ticks.

acatalasia (ă-kat-ă-lay-ziă) *n.* an

inborn lack of the enzyme catalase, leading to recurrent infections of the gums (gingivitis) and mouth.

accessory nerve (spinal accessory nerve) (ăk-sess-er-i) *n.* the eleventh cranial nerve (XI), which arises from two roots, cranial and spinal. Fibres from the cranial root form the recurrent laryngeal nerve, which supplies the internal laryngeal muscles; fibres from the spinal root supply the sternocleidomastoid and trapezius muscles, in the neck region.

accident (ak-sid-ĕnt) *n.* a traumatic incident involving any part of the body. *Accident and emergency (A and E) medicine* is evolving as a specialized area of patient care.

accommodation (ă-kom-ŏ-day-shŏn) *n.* adjustment of the shape of the lens to change the focus of the eye. When the ciliary muscle (*see* ciliary body) is relaxed, the lens is flattened and the eye is then able to focus on distant objects. To focus the eye on near objects the ciliary muscles contract and the lens becomes more spherical. *a. reflex* the constriction of the pupils and inward turning of the eyes that occur when an individual focuses on a near object.

accouchement (ă-koosh-mahnt) *n.* delivery of a baby. *hydrostatic a.* the management of normal labour with the mother partially immersed in a water bath.

accountability (ă-kownt-ă-bil-iti) *n.* (in nursing) the obligation of being answerable for one's own judgments and actions to an appropriate person or authority recognized as having the right to demand information and explanation, according to the terms of reference of the Code of Professional Conduct (*see* Appendix 12). A registered practitioner (nurse, midwife, health visitor) is accountable for her actions as a professional at all times, on or off duty, whether engaged in current practice or not.

accreditation (ă-kred-i-tay-shŏn) *n.* **1.** formal recognition by an organization of an individual as an approved and acknowledged representative, e.g. of a union or staff organization. **2.** (in the USA, Australasia, and some European countries) the licensing of a hospital by government agencies, subject to its meeting certain prerequisite conditions.

Accreditation of Prior (Experiential) Learning *n. see* APEL.

accretion (ă-kree-shŏn) *n.* the accumulation of deposits in an organ or cavity. Calculi may be formed by accretion.

acebutolol (ass-i-bew-toh-lol) *n.* a beta blocker drug commonly used to treat high blood pressure, angina pectoris, and irregular heart rhythms. It is administered by mouth. Trade name: **Sectral**.

ACE inhibitor (ayss) *n.* angiotensin-converting enzyme inhibitor: any one of a group of drugs used in the treatment of raised blood pressure and heart failure. ACE inhibitors act by interfering with the action of the enzyme that converts the inactive angiotensin I to the powerful artery constrictor angiotensin II. ACE inhibitors are administered by mouth; they include *perindopril* (Coversyl) and *ramipril* (Tritace). *See also* captopril, enalapril.

acephalus (ă-sef-ă-lŭs) *n.* a fetus without a head. —**acephalous** *adj.*

acetabuloplasty (ass-i-tab-yoo-loh-plas-ti) *n.* an operation in which the shape of the acetabulum is modified to correct congenital dislocation of the hip or to treat osteoarthritis.

acetabulum (cotyloid cavity) (ass-i-**tab**-yoo-lŭm) *n.* (*pl.* **acetabula**) either of the two deep sockets, one on each side of the hip bone, into which the head of the thigh bone (femur) fits at the hip joint.

acetaminophen (ass-ee-tă-**min**-ŏ-fen) *n. see* paracetamol.

acetate (ass-it-ayt) *n.* any salt or ester of acetic acid.

acetazolamide (ass-ee-tă-zol-ă-myd) *n.* a carbonic anhydrase inhibitor used mainly in the treatment of glaucoma to reduce the pressure inside the eyeball and also as a preventative for epileptic seizures and altitude sickness. Trade name: **Diamox**.

acetic acid (ă **see**-tik) *n.* the acid that is present in vinegar. It is used in the preparation of astringent and antiseptic medicines and in urine testing. Formula: CH_3COOH.

acetoacetic acid (ass-i-toh-ă-**see**-tik) *n.* an organic acid produced in large amounts by the liver in such conditions as starvation. Formula: CH_3COCH_2COOH. *See also* ketone.

acetonaemia (ass-i-toh-nee-miă) *n.* the presence of ketone bodies in the blood. *See* ketone.

acetone (ass-i-tohn) *n.* an organic compound that is produced by the liver in such conditions as starvation. Acetone is of great value as a solvent. Formula: CH_3COCH_3. *a. body see* ketone.

acetonuria (ass-i-toh-**newr**-iă) *n. see* ketonuria.

acetylcholine (ass-i-tyl-koh-leen) *n.* the acetic acid ester of the organic base choline: the neurotransmitter released at the synapses of parasympathetic nerves and at neuromuscular junctions. *See also* cholinesterase.

acetylcholinesterase inhibitor (ass-i-tyl-koh-lin-**est**-er-ayz) *n.* a drug that blocks the action of acetylcholinesterase (*see* cholinesterase). Acetylcholinesterase inhibitors are used to slow down the rate of cognitive decline in the early stages of Alzheimer's disease, which is associated with a reduction in acetylcholine levels. The group includes *donepezil* (Aricept), *galantamine* (Reminyl), and *rivastigmine* (Exelon).

acetylcoenzyme A (ass-i-tyl-koh-en-zym) *n.* a compound formed by the combination of an acetate molecule with coenzyme A. Acetylcoenzyme A has an important role in the Krebs cycle.

acetylcysteine (ass-i-tyl-**sis**-ti-een) *n.* a drug that is administered as eye drops for the treatment of dry eyes, as in Sjögren's syndrome; as an intravenous infusion, it is used to prevent liver damage in paracetamol overdosage. Trade name: **Ilube**.

acetylsalicylic acid (ass-i-tyl-sali-**sil**-ik) *n. see* aspirin.

achalasia (cardiospasm) (ak-ă-**lay**-ziă) *n.* a condition in which the normal muscular activity of the oesophagus (gullet) is disturbed, especially failure of an abnormally strong sphincter at the lower end, which delays the passage of swallowed material.

Achilles tendon (ă-kil-eez) *n*. the tendon of the muscles of the calf of the leg (the gastrocnemius and soleus muscles), situated at the back of the ankle and attached to the calcaneus (heel bone).

achillorrhaphy (ak-i-lo-răfi) *n*. surgical repair of the Achilles tendon.

achillotomy (ak-i-lot-ōmi) *n*. surgical division of the Achilles tendon.

achlorhydria (ay-klor-hy-driă) *n*. absence of hydrochloric acid in the stomach. It is sometimes associated with pernicious anaemia.

acholia (ă-koh-liă) *n*. absence or deficiency of bile secretion or failure of the bile to enter the alimentary canal.

acholuria (ak-oh-lewr-iă) *n*. absence of the bile pigments from the urine, which occurs in some forms of jaundice (*acholuric jaundice*). —**acholuric** *adj*.

achondroplasia (ă-kon-droh-play-ziă) *n*. a disorder, inherited as a dominant characteristic, in which the bones of the arms and legs fail to grow to normal size. It results in a type of dwarfism characterized by short limbs, a normal-sized head and body, and normal intelligence. —**achondroplastic** (ă-kon-droh-plas-tik) *adj*.

achromatic (ak-roh-mat-ik) *adj*. without colour. —**achromasia** (ak-roh-may-ziă) *n*.

achromatopsia (ă-kroh-mă-top-siă) *n*. the inability to perceive colour. Such complete colour blindness is very rare and is usually determined by hereditary factors.

achylia (ă-ky-liă) *n*. absence of secretion. *a. gastrica* a nonsecreting

stomach whose lining (mucosa) is atrophied.

aciclovir (acyclovir) *n*. (ay-sy-klō-veer) an antiviral drug that inhibits DNA synthesis in cells infected by herpesviruses. Aciclovir is administered topically, by mouth, or intravenously; it is useful in patients whose immune systems are disturbed and also in the treatment of herpes zoster, genital herpes, and herpes encephalitis. Trade name: Zovirax.

acid (ass-id) *n*. a substance that releases hydrogen ions when dissolved in water, has a pH below 7 and turns litmus paper red, and reacts with a base to form a salt and water only. *Compare* base.

acidaemia (asid-ee-miă) *n*. a condition of abnormally high blood acidity. *See also* acidosis. *Compare* alkalaemia.

acid-base balance *n*. the balance between the amount of carbonic acid and bicarbonate in the blood, which must be maintained at a constant ratio of 1:20 in order to keep the hydrogen ion concentration of the plasma at a constant value (pH 7.4).

acid-fast *adj*. **1.** describing bacteria that have been stained and continue to hold the stain after treatment with an acidic solution (*a.-f. bacilli*, AFB). **2.** describing a stain that is not removed from a specimen by washing with an acidic solution.

acidity (ă-sid-iti) *n*. the state of being acid. The degree of acidity of a solution is measured on the pH scale (*see* pH).

acidosis (asid-oh-sis) *n*. a condition in which the acidity of body fluids and tissues is abnormally high. This arises because of a failure of the mechanisms responsible for maintaining a balance between acids and alkalis in the blood (*see* acid–base balance). *See also* ketoacidosis, lactic acidosis. —**acidotic** (asid-ot-ik) *adj*.

acid phosphatase *n*. an enzyme secreted in the seminal fluid by the prostate gland.

acinus (ass-in-ŭs) *n*. (*pl*. **acini**) **1.** a small sac or cavity surrounded by the secretory cells of a gland. **2.** (in the lung) the tissue supplied with air by one terminal bronchiole. —**acinous** *adj*.

aclarubicin (ak-lǎ-roo-bi-sin) *n*. an antimitotic drug administered by injection in the treatment of leukaemia and other cancers. It is an anthracycline antibiotic. Trade name: **Aclacin**.

acne (acne vulgaris) (ak-ni vul-gar-iss) *n*. a common inflammatory disorder of the sebaceous glands. It involves the face, back, and chest and is characterized by the presence of blackheads with papules, pustules, and – in more severe cases – cysts and scars. Mild cases respond to topical therapy with benzoyl peroxide, while more refractory conditions require treatment with long-term antibiotics or isotretinoin.

acoustic (ǎ-koo-stik) *adj*. of or relating to sound or the sense of hearing. *a. nerve see* vestibulocochlear nerve.

acquired (ǎ-kwyrd) *adj*. describing a condition or disorder contracted after birth and not attributable to hereditary causes. *Compare* congenital.

acquired immune deficiency syndrome *n*. *see* AIDS.

acrivastine (ak-ri-vas-teen) *n*. an antihistamine drug used to treat hay fever and urticaria (nettle rash). It is administered by mouth. Trade name: **Semprex**.

acro- *prefix denoting* **1.** extremity; tip. **2.** height; promontory. **3.** extreme; intense.

acrocentric (ak-roh-sen-trik) *n*. a chromosome in which the centromere is situated at or very near one end. —**acrocentric** *adj*.

acrocyanosis (ak-roh-sy-ǎ-noh-sis) *n*. bluish-purple discoloration of the hands and feet due to slow circulation of the blood through the small vessels in the skin.

acrodermatitis enteropathica (ak-roh-der-mǎ-ty-tis en-ter-oh-path-ikǎ) *n*. an inherited inability to absorb sufficient zinc, which causes poor growth, patchy sparse hair, a generalized skin rash, and chronic diarrhoea.

acrodynia (ak-roh-din-iǎ) *n*. *see* pink disease.

acromegaly (ak-roh-meg-ǎli) *n*. increase in size of the hands, feet, and the face due to excessive production of growth hormone by a tumour of the anterior pituitary gland. *See also* gigantism.

acromion (ǎ-kroh-mi-ǒn) *n*. an oblong process at the top of the spine of the scapula, part of which articulates with the clavicle (collar bone) to form the *acromioclavicular joint*. —**acromial** *adj*.

acronyx (ak-rŏ-niks) *n*. an ingrowing toenail or fingernail. *See* ingrowing toenail.

acroparaesthesiae (ak-roh-paris-**theez**-i-ee) *pl. n.* tingling sensations in the hands and feet.

acrophobia (ak-rŏ-**foh**-biă) *n.* a morbid dread of heights.

acrosclerosis (ak-roh-skleer-**oh**-sis) *n.* a skin disease thought to be a type of generalized scleroderma, mainly affecting the hands, face, and feet.

acrosome (ak-rŏ-sohm) *n.* the cap-like structure on the front end of a spermatozoon.

ACTH (adrenocorticotrophic hormone, adrenocorticotrophin, corticotrophin) *n.* a hormone synthesized and stored in the anterior pituitary gland, controlling the secretion of corticosteroid hormones from the adrenal gland. Its release is stimulated by corticotrophin-releasing hormone.

actin (ak-tin) *n.* a protein, found in muscle, that plays an important role in the process of contraction. *See* striated muscle.

Actinomyces (ak-ti-noh-**my**-seez) *n.* a genus of Gram-positive nonmotile fungus-like bacteria that cause disease in animals and humans. *A. israelii* the causative organism of human actinomycosis.

actinomycin D (ak-ti-noh-**my**-sin) *n. see* dactinomycin.

actinomycosis (ak-ti-noh-my-**koh**-sis) *n.* a noncontagious disease caused by the bacterium *Actinomyces israelii* and resulting in the formation of multiple sinuses that open onto the skin. Actinomycosis most commonly affects the jaw but may also affect the lungs, brain, or intestines.

actinotherapy (ak-ti-noh-**th'e**-ră-pi) *n.* the treatment of disorders

with infrared or ultraviolet radiation.

action potential (ak-shŏn) *n.* the change in voltage that occurs across the membrane of a nerve or muscle cell when a nerve impulse is triggered.

activator (ak-ti-vay-ter) *n.* a substance that stimulates a chemical change or reaction.

active movement (ak-tiv) *n.* movement brought about by a patient's own efforts. *Compare* passive movement.

active principle *n.* an ingredient of a drug that is actively involved in its therapeutic effect.

activities of daily living (activities of living, ADLs, ALs) (ak-tiv-it-iz) *pl. n.* the routine activities that an individual does for himself during the course of the day, such as eating, drinking, and washing. *See* Roper, Logan, and Tierney model.

actomyosin (ak-toh-my-oh-sin) *n.* a protein complex formed in muscle between actin and myosin during the process of contraction. *See* striated muscle.

acuity (ă-kew-iti) *n. see* visual acuity.

acupuncture (ak-yoo-punk-cher) *n.* a complementary therapy, developed by Eastern physicians, in which thin metal needles are inserted into selected points beneath the skin, usually to relieve chronic pain.

acute (ă-kewt) *adj.* **1.** describing a disease of rapid onset, severe symptoms, and brief duration. *Compare* chronic. **2.** describing any intense symptom, such as severe pain.

acute abdomen *n.* an emergency

surgical condition caused by damage to one or more abdominal organs following injury or disease.

acute rheumatism *n. see* rheumatic fever.

acyclovir *n. see* aciclovir.

acystia (ă-sis-tiă) *n.* congenital absence of the bladder.

ad- *prefix denoting* towards or near.

ADA deficiency *n. see* adenosine deaminase deficiency.

Adam's apple (laryngeal prominence) (ad-ămz) *n.* a projection, lying just under the skin, of the thyroid cartilage of the larynx.

adaptation (ad-ăp-tay-shŏn) *n.* the phenomenon in which a sense organ shows a gradually diminishing response to continuous or repetitive stimulation.

addiction (ă-dik-shŏn) *n.* a state of dependence produced by the habitual taking of drugs. *See also* alcoholism, tolerance.

Addisonian crisis (ad-i-soh-niăn) *n.* an acute medical emergency due to a lack of corticosteroid production by the body, caused by disease of the adrenal glands or long-term suppression of production by steroid medication. It manifests as low blood pressure and collapse, biochemical abnormalities, hypoglycaemia, and (if untreated) coma and death. [T. Addison (1793–1860), British physician]

Addison's disease (ad-i-sŏnz) *n.* a syndrome due to inadequate secretion of corticosteroid hormones by the adrenal glands. Symptoms include weakness, loss of energy, low blood pressure, and dark pigmentation of the skin. [T. Addison]

adduct (ă-dukt) *vb.* to move a limb or any other part towards the midline of the body. —**adduction** *n.*

adductor (ă-duk-ter) *n.* any muscle that moves one part of the body towards another or towards the midline of the body.

aden- (adeno-) *prefix denoting* a gland or glands.

adenine (ad-ĕ-neen) *n.* one of the nitrogen-containing bases (*see* purine) that occurs in the nucleic acids DNA and RNA. *See also* ATP.

adenitis (ad-ĕ-ny-tis) *n.* inflammation of one or more glands or lymph nodes.

adenocarcinoma (ad-in-oh-kar-si-noh-mă) *n.* (*pl.* **adenocarcinomata**) a malignant epithelial tumour arising from glandular tissue. The term is also applied to tumours showing a glandular growth pattern.

adenohypophysis (ad-in-oh-hy-pof-i-sis) *n. see* pituitary gland.

adenoidectomy (ad-in-oid-ek-tŏmi) *n.* surgical removal of the adenoids.

adenoids (nasopharyngeal tonsil) (ad-in-oidz) *n.* the collection of lymphatic tissue at the rear of the nose. Enlargement of the adenoids can cause obstruction to breathing through the nose and can block the Eustachian tubes, causing glue ear.

adenolymphoma (ad-in-oh-lim-foh-mă) *n. see* Warthin's tumour.

adenoma (ad-in-oh-mă) *n.* (*pl.* **adenomata**) a benign tumour of epithelial origin that is derived from glandular tissue or exhibits clearly defined glandular structures. Adenomas may become malignant (*see* adenocarcinoma).

adenomyoma (ad-in-oh-my-oh-mă) *n.* a benign tumour derived from glandular and muscular tissue. Adenomyomas frequently occur in the uterus.

adenomyosis (ad-in-oh-my-oh-sis) *n.* the infiltration of tissue resembling endometrium into the wall of the uterus. *See* endometriosis.

adenopathy (ad-in-op-áthi) *n.* disease of a gland or glandlike structure, especially a lymph node.

adenosclerosis (ad-in-oh-skleer-oh-sis) *n.* hardening of a gland, usually due to calcification.

adenosine (ă-den-ŏ-seen) *n.* a compound containing adenine and the sugar ribose: it occurs in ATP (*see also* nucleoside). It is also injected as an anti-arrhythmic drug to stop supraventricular tachycardias and restore a normal heart rhythm.

adenosine deaminase deficiency (ADA deficiency) (dee-am-in-ayz) *n.* a genetic disorder characterized by a defect in the enzyme *adenosine deaminase* (*ADA*), which is involved in purine metabolism. Deficiency of this enzyme results in damage to the antibody-producing lymphocytes, which leads to severe combined immune deficiency (SCID).

adenosine diphosphate *n. see* ADP.

adenosine monophosphate *n. see* AMP.

adenosine triphosphate *n. see* ATP.

adenosis (ad-in-oh-sis) *n.* (*pl.* **adenoses**) **1.** excessive growth or development of glands. **2.** any disease of a gland or gland-like structure, especially a lymph node.

adenovirus (ad-in-oh-vy-rŭs) *n.* one of a group of DNA-containing viruses causing infections of the upper respiratory tract that produce symptoms resembling those of the common cold.

ADH *n.* antidiuretic hormone (*see* vasopressin).

ADHD *n. see* attention-deficit/ hyperactivity disorder.

adhesion (ăd-hee-*zh*ŏn) *n.* **1.** the union of two normally separate surfaces by fibrous connective tissue developing in an inflamed or damaged region. (The fibrous tissue itself is also called an adhesion.) Adhesions between loops of intestine often occur following abdominal surgery but only rarely cause symptoms, such as intestinal obstruction. **2.** a healing process in which the edges of a wound fit together.

adiadochokinesis (ă-dy-ă-doh-koh-ki-nee-sis) *n. see* dysdiadochokinesis.

adiaphoresis (ă-dy-ă-fŏ-ree-sis) *n.* deficient or reduced secretion of sweat. —**adiaphoretic** (ă-dy-ă-fŏ-ret-ik) *adj.*

Adie's pupil (ay-diz) *n. see* tonic (pupil). [W. J. Adie (1886–1935), British physician]

adipose tissue (ad-i-pohs) *n.* fibrous connective tissue packed with masses of fat cells. It forms a thick layer under the skin and occurs around the kidneys and in the buttocks.

adiposis (liposis) (ad-i-poh-sis) *n.* the presence of abnormally large accumulations of fat in the body. The condition may arise from overeating, hormone irregularities, or a metabolic disorder. *See also* obesity.

adiposuria (ad-i-poh-sewr-iă) *n. see* lipuria.

aditus (ad-i-tŭs) *n.* an anatomical opening or passage; for example, the opening of the tympanic cavity (middle ear) to the air spaces of the mastoid process.

adjuvant (aj-oo-vǎnt) *n.* any substance used in conjunction with another to enhance its activity.

adjuvant therapy *n.* treatment given to cancer patients, usually after surgical removal of their primary tumour when there is known to be a high risk of future tumour recurrence. *Compare* neoadjuvant chemotherapy.

ADLs *pl. n. see* activities of daily living.

admission rate (ǎd-mish-ǒn) *n.* the number of cases of a specified disease or condition admitted to hospitals, related to the population of a given geographical area.

adnexa (ad-neks-ǎ) *pl. n.* adjoining parts. *uterine a.* the Fallopian tubes and ovaries.

adolescence (ad-ŏ-less-ěns) *n.* the period of development between childhood and adulthood. It begins with the start of puberty. —**adolescent** *n., adj.*

ADP (adenosine diphosphate) *n.* a compound containing adenine, ribose, and two phosphate groups. ADP occurs in cells and is involved in processes requiring the transfer of energy (*see* ATP).

adrenalectomy (ǎ-dree-nǎl-ek-tŏmi) *n.* surgical removal of an adrenal gland, usually performed because of cancer.

adrenal glands (suprarenal glands) (ǎ-dree-nǎl) *pl. n.* two triangular endocrine glands, each of which covers the superior surface of a kidney. The *medulla* forms the grey core of the gland and produces adrenaline and noradrenaline. The

cortex is a yellowish tissue surrounding the medulla; it produces corticosteroid hormones.

adrenaline (epinephrine) (ǎ-dren-ǎ-lin) *n.* an important hormone secreted by the medulla of the adrenal gland. It has widespread effects on circulation, the muscles, and sugar metabolism. The action of the heart is increased, the rate and depth of breathing are increased, and the metabolic rate is raised; the force of muscular contraction improves and the onset of muscular fatigue is delayed. At the same time the blood supply to the bladder and intestines is reduced, their muscular walls relax, and the sphincters contract. Adrenaline is administered by injection for the emergency treatment of anaphylaxis and cardiac arrest. It is also included in some local anaesthetic solutions, particularly those used in dentistry, to prolong anaesthesia, and is used as eye drops in treating glaucoma.

adrenarche (ad-ren-ar-ki) *n.* the start of secretion of androgens by the adrenal glands, occurring at around 6–7 years of age in girls and 7–8 in boys. Adrenal androgens are dehydroepiandrosterone (DHEA), DHEA sulphate, and androstenedione. *Compare* gonadarche.

adrenergic (ad-rě-ner-jik) *adj.* describing or relating to nerve fibres that release noradrenaline as a neurotransmitter. *a. receptor* a receptor at which noradrenaline acts to pass on messages from sympathetic nerves. *Compare* cholinergic.

adrenocorticotrophic hormone (adrenocorticotrophin)

(ă-dree-noh-kor-ti-koh-**trof**-ik) *n. see* ACTH.

adrenogenital syndrome (ă-dree-noh-**jen**-it-ăl) *n.* a hormonal disorder resulting from abnormal steroid production by the adrenal cortex, due to a genetic fault. It may cause masculinization in girls, precocious puberty in boys, and adrenocortical failure (*see* Addison's disease) in both sexes. Treatment is by lifelong steroid replacement.

adrenoleukodystrophy (ALD) (ă-dree-noh-loo-koh-**dis**-trŏ-fi) *n.* a genetically determined condition of neurological degeneration with childhood and adult forms. It is characterized by abnormal fatty-acid metabolism with progressive spastic paralysis of the legs and sensory loss, associated with adrenal gland insufficiency and small gonads.

adrenolytic (ă-dree-noh-**lit**-ik) *adj.* inhibiting the activity of adrenergic nerves. Adrenolytic activity is opposite to that of noradrenaline.

ADRs *pl. n.* adverse drug reactions. *See* side-effect.

adsorbent (ăd-**sor**-bĕnt) *n.* a substance that attracts other substances to its surface to form a film. Charcoal and kaolin are adsorbents.

adsorption (ăd-**sorp**-shŏn) *n.* the formation of a layer of atoms or molecules of one substance on the surface of a solid or liquid of different substance. *See* adsorbent.

adult respiratory distress syndrome (ARDS) (ad-ult) *n.* a form of acute respiratory failure that occurs after a precipitating event, such as trauma, aspiration, or inhalation of a toxic substance; it is particularly associated with septic shock.

advance directive (ăd-vahns di-**rek**-tiv) *n. see* living will.

advanced life support (ALS) (ăd-**vahnst**) *n.* a structured and algorithm-driven method of life support for use in the severest of medical emergencies, especially cardiac arrest. Personnel involved in ALS receive special training in the use of equipment (e.g. defibrillators and appropriate drugs). *Compare* basic life support.

advanced trauma life support *n. see* ATLS.

advancement (ăd-**vahns**-mĕnt) *n.* the detachment by surgery of a muscle, musculocutaneous flap, or tendon and its reattachment at a more advanced (anterior) point while preserving its previous nerve and blood supply. The technique is used, for example, in the treatment of squint, and extensively in plastic surgery.

adventitia (tunica adventitia) (ad-ven-ti-shă) *n.* **1.** the outer coat of the wall of a vein or artery. **2.** the outer covering of various other organs or parts.

adventitious (ad-ven-ti-shŭs) *adj.* **1.** occurring in a place other than the usual one. **2.** relating to the adventitia.

advocate (ad-vŏ-kăt) *n.* (in health care) a practitioner, usually a nurse, who utilizes this role to promote and safeguard the wellbeing and interests of his or her patients or clients by ensuring they are aware of their rights and have access to information to make informed decisions. Advocacy in health care is an integral part of professional practice. —**advocacy** (ad-vŏ-kă-si) *n.*

Aëdes (ay-ee-deez) *n.* a genus of widely distributed mosquitoes occurring throughout the tropics and subtropics. *A. aegypti* the principal vector of dengue and yellow fever.

aegophony (e-gof-ŏni) *n. see* vocal resonance.

-aemia *suffix denoting* a specified condition of the blood.

aer- (aero-) *prefix denoting* air or gas.

aerobe (air ohb) *n.* any organism, especially a microbe, that requires the presence of free oxygen for life and growth. *Compare* anaerobe. —**aerobic** (air-oh-bik) *adj.*

aerobic exercise *n. see* exercise.

aerobic respiration *n.* a type of cellular respiration in which foodstuffs (carbohydrates) are completely oxidized by atmospheric oxygen, with the production of maximum chemical energy from the foodstuffs.

aerogenous (air-oj-in-ŭs) *adj.* producing gas. The term is applied to bacteria such as *Clostridium perfringens*, which causes gas gangrene.

aerophagy (air-off-ăji) *n.* the swallowing of air. Voluntary aerophagy is used to permit oesophageal speech after surgical removal of the larynx (usually for cancer).

aerosol (air-ŏ-sol) *n.* a suspension of extremely small liquid or solid particles in the air. Drugs in aerosol form may be administered by inhalation.

aetiology (etiology) (ee-ti-ol-ŏji) *n.* **1.** the study or science of the causes of disease. **2.** the cause of a specific disease.

AF *n. see* (atrial) fibrillation.

AFB *pl. n. see* acid-fast (bacilli).

afebrile (ay-feb-ryl) *adj.* without, or not showing any signs of, a fever.

affect (af-ekt) *n.* (in psychiatry) **1.** the predominant emotion in a person's mental state. **2.** the emotion associated with a particular idea. —**affective** (ă-fek-tiv) *adj.*

affective disorder (dis-or-der) *n.* any psychiatric disorder featuring abnormalities of mood or emotion (affect). The most serious of these are depression and mania. Other affective disorders include SAD (seasonal affective disorder).

afferent (af-er-ĕnt) *adj.* **1.** designating nerves or neurones that convey impulses to the brain or spinal cord. **2.** designating blood vessels that feed a capillary network in an organ or part. **3.** designating lymphatic vessels that enter a lymph node. *Compare* efferent.

affinity (ă-fin-iti) *n.* the chemical attraction of one substance to another or others.

aflatoxin (af-lă-toks-in) *n.* a poisonous substance produced in the spores of the fungus *Aspergillus flavus*, which infects peanuts. It is known to produce cancer in certain animals.

afp (AFP) *n. see* alpha-fetoprotein.

afterbirth (ahf-ter-berth) *n.* the placenta, umbilical cord, and ruptured membranes associated with the fetus, which normally become detached from the uterus and expelled within a few hours of birth.

aftercare (ahf-ter-kair) *n.* **1.** long-term surveillance or rehabilitation as an adjunct or supplement to formal medical treatment of those who are chronically sick or disabled. Aftercare includes the provision of special aids and the adaptation of homes to improve daily living. **2.** surveillance of convalescents.

after-image (ahf-ter-im-ij) *n.* an impression of an image that is registered by the brain for a brief moment after an object is removed from in front of the eye, or after the eye is closed.

afterpains (ahf-ter-paynz) *pl. n.* pains caused by uterine contractions after childbirth, especially during breast feeding, due to release of the hormone oxytocin.

AGA *adj.* appropriate for gestational age.

agammaglobulinaemia (ă-gam-ă-glob-yoo-lin-ee-miă) *n.* a total deficiency of the plasma protein gammaglobulin. *Compare* hypogammaglobulinaemia.

agar (ay-ger) *n.* an extract of certain seaweeds that forms a gel suitable for the solidification of liquid bacteriological culture media. Agar may also be used as a laxative.

agenesis (ă-jen-ĕsis) *n.* absence of an organ, usually due to total failure of its development in the embryo.

age-related macular degeneration (ayj-ri-lay-tid) *n. see* macular degeneration.

agglutination (clumping) (ă-gloo-tin-ay-shŏn) *n.* the sticking together of such microscopic antigenic particles as red blood cells or bacteria so that they form visible clumps. —**agglutinative** *adj.*

agglutinin (ă-gloo-tin-in) *n.* an antibody that brings about the agglutination of bacteria, blood cells, or other antigenic particles.

agglutinogen (ă-gloo-tin-oh-jĕn) *n.* any antigen that provokes formation of an agglutinin in the serum

and is therefore likely to be involved in agglutination.

aglossia (ă-gloss-iă) *n.* congenital absence of the tongue.

aglutition (a-gloo-ti-shŏn) *n.* inability to swallow. *See also* dysphagia.

agnosia (ag-noh-ziă) *n.* a disorder of the brain whereby the patient cannot interpret sensations correctly although the sense organs and nerves conducting sensation to the brain are functioning normally.

agonist (ag-ŏ-nist) *n.* **1. (prime mover)** a muscle whose active contraction causes movement of a part of the body. Contraction of an agonist is associated with relaxation of its antagonist. **2.** a drug or other substance that acts at a cell-receptor site to produce an effect that is the same as, or similar to, that of the body's normal chemical messenger. Cholinergic drugs (*see* parasympathomimetic) are examples.

agoraphobia (ag-er-ă-foh-biă) *n.* a morbid fear of public places and/or of open spaces. *See also* phobia.

agranulocytosis (ă-gran-yoo-loh-sy-toh-sis) *n.* a disorder in which there is a severe acute deficiency of certain blood cells (neutrophils) as a result of damage to the bone marrow by toxic drugs or chemicals. It is characterized by fever, with ulceration of the mouth and throat, and may lead rapidly to prostration and death.

agraphia (dysgraphia) (ă-graf-iă) *n.* an acquired inability to write, although the strength and coordination of the hand remain normal.

ague (ay-gew) *n. see* malaria.

AHF *n.* antihaemophilic factor (*see* Factor VIII).

AIDS (acquired immune deficiency syndrome) (aydz) *n.* a syndrome caused by the human immunodeficiency virus (HIV), which destroys a subgroup of lymphocytes, resulting in suppression of the body's immune response (*see* (helper) T-cell). AIDS is essentially a sexually transmitted disease, either homosexually or heterosexually, but it can also be spread via infected blood or blood products and from an infected mother to her child in the uterus, during parturition, or in breast milk.

Acute infection following exposure to the virus results in the production of antibodies (seroconversion), but not all those who seroconvert progress to chronic infection. The chronic stage may include persistent generalized involvement of the lymph nodes; *AIDS-related complex (ARC)*, including intermittent fever, weight loss, diarrhoea, fatigue, and night sweats; and AIDS itself, presenting as opportunistic infections (especially pneumonia caused by the protozoan *Pneumocystis carinii*) and/or tumours, such as Kaposi's sarcoma.

Ordinary social contact with HIV-positive subjects involves no risk of infection. However, high standards of clinical practice are required by all health workers in order to avoid inadvertent infection via blood, blood products, or body fluids from HIV-positive people. Staff who become HIV-positive are expected to declare their status and will be counselled.

AIH *n. see* artificial insemination (by husband).

air bed (air) *n.* a bed with a mattress whose upper surface is perforated with thousands of holes through which air is forced under pressure, so that the patient is supported on a cushion of air. Air beds are invaluable for the treatment of patients with large areas of burns.

air embolism *n.* an air lock that obstructs the outflow of blood from the right ventricle of the heart. Tipping the patient head down, lying on the left side, may move the air lock.

air hunger *n.* difficulty in breathing characterized by sighing and gasping. It is caused by anoxia.

air sickness *n. see* motion sickness.

akathisia (ak-ă-thiz-iă) *n.* a pattern of involuntary movements induced by antipsychotic drugs, such as phenothiazines. An affected person is driven to restless overactivity, which can be confused with the agitation for which the drug was originally prescribed.

akinesia (ak-in-ee-ziă) *n.* a loss of normal muscular tonicity or responsiveness. *akinetic epilepsy* a form of epilepsy in which there is a sudden loss of muscular tonicity, making the patient fall with momentary loss of consciousness. *akinetic mutism* a state of complete physical unresponsiveness although the patient's eyes remain open and appear to follow movements. It is a consequence of damage to the base of the brain. *akinetic rigid syndrome* a condition, such as parkinsonism or progressive supranuclear palsy, characterized by akinesia. —**akinetic** (a-kin-et-ik) *adj.*

ala (al-ă) *n.* (*pl.* **alae**) (in anatomy) a winglike structure.

alanine (al-ă-neen) *n. see* amino acid.

alanine aminotransferase (ALT) (ă-mee-noh-trans-fer-ayz) *n.* an enzyme involved in the transamination of amino acids. Measurement of ALT in the serum is of use in the diagnosis and study of acute liver disease. It was formerly called *serum glutamic pyruvic transaminase (SGPT)*.

alastrim (ă-las-trim) *n.* a mild form of smallpox, causing only a sparse rash and low-grade fever. Medical name: **variola minor**.

Albee's operation (awl-beez) *n.* **1.** an operation to produce ankylosis of the hip. The upper surface of the femur and the corresponding part of the acetabulum are removed and the two exposed surfaces allowed to remain in contact. **2.** an operation to immobilize part of the spinal column, using a bone graft from the tibia. [F. H. Albee (1876–1945), US surgeon]

albendazole (al-ben-dă-zohl) *n.* an anthelmintic drug used for treating hydatid disease, strongyloidiasis, and creeping eruption. It is administered by mouth. Trade name: **Zentel**.

Albers-Schönberg disease (albers shern-berg) *n. see* osteopetrosis. [H. E. Albers-Schönberg (1865–1921), German radiologist]

Alberti regime (GIK regime) (al-ber-ti ray-zheem) *n.* a method for controlling blood-sugar levels in diabetic patients being fasted. It involves infusing a solution of glucose (G), insulin (I), and potassium (K) chloride intravenously over a standard period. [K. G. M. M. Alberti (1937–), British physician]

albinism (al-bin-izm) *n.* the inherited absence of pigmentation in the skin, hair, and eyes (*see* albino).

albino (al-bee-noh) *n.* an individual lacking the normal body pigment (melanin). Albinos have white hair, pink skin and eyes, reduced visual acuity, and sensitivity to light (*see* photophobia).

Albright's hereditary osteodystrophy (awl-bryts) *n.* the skeletal abnormalities, collectively, of pseudohypoparathyroidism type 1. These include short stature, abnormally short fingers and toes (particularly involving the fourth and fifth metacarpals and metatarsals), and soft-tissue calcification. [F. Albright (1900–69), US physician]

albumin (al-bew-min) *n.* a protein that is soluble in water and coagulated by heat. *serum a.* a protein found in blood plasma that is important for the maintenance of plasma volume.

albuminuria (proteinuria) (albew-min-yoor-iă) *n.* the presence of serum albumin, serum globulin, or other serum proteins in the urine, which may be associated with kidney or heart disease. *orthostatic a.* albuminuria not associated with disease, occurring after strenuous exercise or after a long period of standing.

albumose (al-bew-mohz) *n.* a substance, intermediate between albumin and peptones, produced during the digestion of proteins by pepsin and other endopeptidases (*see* peptidase).

alcaptonuria (alkaptonuria) (alkap-tŏn-yoor-iă) *n.* accumulation in the tissues and excretion in the urine of homogentisic acid due to congenital absence of homogentisic acid oxidase, an enzyme essential for the normal breakdown of the amino acids tyrosine and phenylalanine.

alclometazone (al-kloh-met-ă-zohn) *n.* a corticosteroid drug administered externally as a cream or ointment to treat inflammatory skin disorders. Trade name: **Modrasone**.

alcohol (al-kŏ-hol) *n.* any of a class of organic compounds formed when a hydroxyl group (–OH) is substituted for a hydrogen atom in a hydrocarbon. *ethyl a.* (*ethanol*) the alcohol in alcoholic drinks, produced by the fermentation of sugar by yeast. Formula: C_2H_5OH. 'Pure' alcohol contains not less than 94.9% by volume of ethyl alcohol. A solution of 70% alcohol can be used as a preservative or antiseptic. *See also* alcoholism. —**alcoholic** (al-kŏ-hol-ik) *adj.*, *n.*

alcohol-fast *adj.* describing bacteria that have been stained and continue to hold the stain after treatment with alcohol.

Alcoholics Anonymous (AA) *n.* a voluntary agency of self-help that is organized and operated locally among those with alcoholic dependency.

alcoholism (al-kŏ-hol-izm) *n.* the syndrome due to physical dependence on alcohol, such that sudden deprivation may cause withdrawal symptoms – tremor, anxiety, hallucinations, and delusions (*see* delirium (tremens)). Alcoholism impairs intellectual function, physical skills, memory, and judgment.

Heavy consumption of alcohol also causes cardiomyopathy, peripheral neuritis, cirrhosis of the liver, and enteritis.

alcoholuria (al-kŏ-hol-**yoor**-iă) *n.* the presence of alcohol in the urine.

ALD *n. see* adrenoleukodystrophy.

aldesleukin (al-des-**loo**-kin) *n. see* interleukin.

Aldomet (al-dŏ-met) *n. see* methyldopa.

aldosterone (al-dos-ter-ohn) *n.* a steroid hormone (*see* corticosteroid) that is synthesized and released by the adrenal cortex and acts on the kidney to regulate salt (potassium and sodium) and water balance.

aldosteronism (al-dos-tě-rŏ-nizm) *n.* overproduction of aldosterone, causing electrolyte imbalance and raised blood pressure (hypertension). *See also* Conn's syndrome.

alendronate (ă-len-drŏ-nayt) *n. see* bisphosphonates.

Aleppo boil (ă-lep-oh) *n. see* oriental sore.

alexia (ă-leks-iă) *n.* an acquired inability to read due to disease in the left hemisphere of the brain in a right-handed person. *agnostic a.* (*word blindness*) inability to identify letters and words not affecting the patient's ability to write. *See also* dyslexia.

alfacalcidol (al-fă-**kal**-sid-ol) *n.* a synthetic form of vitamin D used to raise blood-calcium levels in osteomalacia and bone disorders caused by kidney disease. It is administered by mouth or by injection. Trade names: **AlfaD**, **One-alpha**.

alfentanil hydrochloride (al-fen-tă-nil) *n.* a narcotic analgesic drug used to relieve severe pain. It is administered by injection. Trade name: **Rapifen**.

alfuzosin (al-few-zoh-sin) *n.* an alpha blocker commonly used in the treatment of men with lower urinary tract symptoms thought to be due to benign prostatic hyperplasia (*see* prostate gland). Trade name: **Xatral**.

ALG *n.* antilymphocyte globulin. *See* antilymphocyte serum.

algesimeter (al-jĕ-sim-it-er) *n.* a piece of equipment for determining the sensitivity of the skin to various touch stimuli, especially those causing pain.

-algia *suffix denoting* pain.

algid (al-jid) *adj.* cold: usually describing the cold clammy skin associated with certain forms of malaria.

alginic acid (al-gin-ik) *n.* an antacid drug used to treat heartburn caused by acid reflux into the gullet and hiatus hernia. It is administered by mouth, often in the form of alginates and in combination with other drugs. Trade names: **Gastrocote**, **Gaviscon**, etc.

algorithm (al-gŏ-rith-ĕm) *n.* a sequential set of instructions used in calculations or problem solving, such as a stepwise series of instructions with branching pathways to be followed to assist a physician in coming to a diagnosis (*diagnostic a.*) or deciding on a treatment strategy (*therapeutic a.*).

alienation (ay-li-ĕn-ay-shŏn) *n.* (in psychiatry) **1.** the experience that one's thoughts are under the control of somebody else, or that other people participate in one's thinking. **2.** insanity.

alimemazine (trimeprazine)

(ali-**mem**-ă-zeen) *n.* an antihistamine drug (a phenothiazine derivative) that also possesses sedative properties. Given by mouth, it is mainly used in the treatment of pruritus and urticaria (nettle rash). Trade name: **Vallergan**.

alimentary canal (ali-ment-er-i) *n.* the long passage, extending from the mouth to the anus, through which food passes to be digested and absorbed.

aliquot (al-i-kwot) *n.* one of a known number of equal parts of a compound or solution.

alkalaemia (al-kă-lee-miă) *n.* abnormally high blood alkalinity. *See also* alkalosis. *Compare* acidaemia.

alkali (al-kă-ly) *n.* a base that is soluble in water. Alkaline solutions turn litmus paper blue. *See* base.

alkaloid (al-kă-loid) *n.* one of a diverse group of nitrogen-containing substances that are produced by plants and have potent effects on body function. Many alkaloids are important drugs, including morphine, quinine, atropine, and codeine.

alkalosis (al-kă-loh-sis) *n.* a condition in which the alkalinity of body fluids and tissues is abnormally high. This arises because of a failure of the mechanisms that usually maintain a balance between alkalis and acids in the arterial blood (*see* acid-base balance).

alkaptonuria *n. see* alcaptonuria.

alkylating agent (al-ki-lay-ting) *n.* a drug, such as cyclophosphamide, that disrupts the growth of a malignant tumour by damaging the DNA in the tumour cell nuclei.

ALL *n.* acute lymphoblastic leu-salivary gland

soft palate (uvula)

buccal cavity

tongue

hard palate

mouth

epiglottis

salivary glands

larynx

oesophagus

diaphragm

gall bladder

bile duct

liver

duodenum

stomach

pancreas

colon

ileum

caecum

appendix

rectum

anus

The alimentary canal

kaemia. *See* leukaemia, lympho-blast.

allantois (al-ăn-toh-iss) *n.* the membranous sac that develops as an outgrowth of the embryonic hindgut. Its outer (mesodermal) layer carries blood vessels to the placenta and so forms part of the umbilical cord. —**allantoic** *adj.*

allele (allelomorph) (ă-leel) *n.* one of two or more alternative forms of a gene, only one of which can be present in a chromosome. *See also* dominant, recessive. —**allelic** *adj.*

allelomorph (ă-leel-oh-morf) *n. see* allele.

allergen (al-er-jĕn) *n.* any antigen that causes allergy in a hypersensitive person. —**allergenic** *adj.*

allergy (al-er-ji) *n.* a disorder in which the body becomes hypersensitive to particular antigens (called allergens), which provoke characteristic symptoms whenever they are subsequently encountered. Different allergies afflict different tissues and may have either local or general effects, varying from asthma and hay fever to severe dermatitis or gastroenteritis or extremely serious shock (*see* anaphylaxis). —**allergic** *adj.*

allocheiria (al-oh-**keer**-iă) *n.* a condition in which the sensation aroused by a stimulus applied to one side of the body is referred to the opposite side.

allogeneic (al-oh-jě-**nay**-ik) *adj.* describing grafted tissue derived from a donor of the same species as the recipient but with different histocompatibility.

allograft (**al**-oh-grahft) *n.* a living tissue or organ graft between two members of the same species. Unless the graft is from an identical twin, it will not survive unless the recipient is treated to suppress the body's immune response to the foreign tissue.

allopathy (ă-**lop**-ă-thi) *n.* (in homeopathic medicine) the orthodox system of medicine, in which the use of drugs is directed to producing effects in the body that will directly oppose and so alleviate the symptoms of a disease. *Compare* homeopathy.

allopurinol (al-oh-**pewr**-i-nol) *n.* a drug administered by mouth in the treatment of chronic gout. It acts by reducing the level of uric acid in tissues and blood. Trade name: **Zyloric**.

all-or-none law *n.* the principle that tissue, such as nerve fibres, can produce only one of two reactions to a stimulus. Regardless of the intensity of the stimulus, such tissue will show either a total response or no response at all.

almotriptan (al-moh-**trip**-tan) *n. see* 5HT₁ agonist.

alopecia (baldness) (al-ŏ-**pee**-shiă) *n.* absence of hair from areas where it normally grows. *a. areata* a condition characterized by bald patches that may regrow; it is an example of an organ-specific autoimmune disease. *a. totalis* total hair loss, due to an autoimmune condition. *androgenetic a.* hair loss in women, which is associated with increasing age. *scarring* (or *cicatricial*) *a.* alopecia in which the hair does not regrow, as occurs in lichen planus and discoid lupus erythematosus.

alpha agonist (al-fă) *n. see* sympathomimetic.

alpha blocker (alpha-adrenergic blocker) *n.* a drug that prevents the stimulation of alpha-adrenergic receptors at the nerve endings of the sympathetic nervous system by noradrenaline and adrenaline: it therefore causes widening of arteries (vasodilatation) and a drop in blood pressure. Alpha blockers include alfuzosin, doxazosin, phentolamine, phenoxybenzamine, moxisylyte, indoramin, prazosin, and tamsulosin.

alpha cells *pl. n.* the cells in the islets of Langerhans that produce glucagon. *Compare* beta cells, delta cells.

alpha-fetoprotein (afp) (al-fă-fee-toh-**proh**-teen) *n.* a protein that is formed in the liver and yolk sac of the fetus and is present in the amniotic fluid and secondarily in maternal blood. The level of afp is elevated in spina bifida, twin and triplet pregnancies, and certain other conditions and decreased in Down's syndrome. This can be detected by a maternal blood test performed between the 16th and 18th weeks of pregnancy to aid prenatal diagnosis of these conditions.

Alport's syndrome (awl-ports) *n.*

a hereditary disease that causes nephritis accompanied by deafness. Affected males usually develop end-stage renal failure and, unless treated with a kidney transplant, die before the age of 40. Females have a better prognosis. [A. C. Alport (1880–1959), South African physician]

alprazolam *n.* a benzodiazepine used to relieve anxiety and as a sedative. It is administered by mouth. Trade name: **Xanax**.

alprostadil (al pros-tă-dil) *n.* a prostaglandin drug administered by infusion to improve lung blood flow in newborn babies with congenital heart defects who are awaiting surgery and by injection into the corpora cavernosa of the penis or by application into the urethra to treat erectile impotence in men. Trade names: **Prostin VR**, **Caverject**, **MUSE**.

ALS *n.* **1.** *see* advanced life support. **2.** *see* antilymphocyte serum. **3.** *see* (amyotrophic lateral) sclerosis.

ALT *n.* *see* alanine aminotransferase.

alteplase (al-tě-playz) *n.* a tissue-type plasminogen activator made by genetic engineering. Administered by injection, it is used to dissolve blood clots (*see* fibrinolytic), especially in the coronary arteries of the heart. Trade name: **Actilyse**.

alternative medicine (awl-tern-ă-tiv) *n.* *see* complementary medicine.

altitude sickness (mountain sickness) (al-ti-tewd) *n.* the condition that results from unaccustomed exposure to a high altitude (4500 m or more above sea level). Reduced atmospheric pressure and

shortage of oxygen cause deep rapid breathing, which lowers the concentration of carbon dioxide in the blood.

aluminium chloride hexahydrate (al-yoo-min-iŭm) *n.* a powerful antiperspirant used in the treatment of conditions associated with excessive sweating (*see* hyperhidrosis). It is applied to the skin in the form of a solution. Trade names: **Anhydrol Forte**, **Driclor**.

aluminium hydroxide *n.* a safe slow-acting antacid. It is administered by mouth, alone or in combination with other antacids, in the treatment of indigestion, gastric and duodenal ulcers, and reflux oesophagitis. Trade names: **Alu-Cap**, **Aludrox**.

alveolitis (al-vee-oh-ly-tis) *n.* inflammation of an alveolus or alveoli. Chronic inflammation of the walls of the alveoli of the lungs is usually caused by inhaled organic dusts (*extrinsic allergic a.*; *see* bird-fancier's lung, farmer's lung) but may occur spontaneously (*cryptogenic fibrosing a.*).

alveolus (al-vee-oh-lŭs) *n.* (*pl.* **alveoli**) **1.** (in the lung) a blind-ended air sac of microscopic size. **2.** the part of the upper or lower jawbone that supports the roots of the teeth (*see also* mandible, maxilla). **3.** the sac of a racemose gland (*see also* acinus). **4.** any other small cavity, depression, or sac. —**alveolar** *adj.*

alverine citrate (al-vě-reen) *n.* a bulking agent and antispasmodic drug used to treat the irritable bowel syndrome and other colonic disorders. It is administered by mouth. Trade name: **Spasmonal**.

Alzheimer's disease (alts-hymerz) *n.* a progressive form of dementia occurring in middle age or later, characterized by loss of short-term memory, deterioration in both behaviour and intellectual performance, and slowness of thought. It is associated with damage to cholinergic pathways in the brain and the presence of excess amyloid protein in brain tissue. [A. Alzheimer (1864–1915), German physician]

amalgam (ă-mal-găm) *n.* any of a group of alloys containing mercury. In dentistry amalgam fillings are made by mixing a silver-tin alloy with mercury in a machine known as an *amalgamator*.

amantadine (ă-man-tă-deen) *n.* an antiviral drug used in the prevention and treatment of influenza infections. Because it increases the action of dopamine in the brain, it is also used to treat Parkinson's disease. Trade name: **Symmetrel**.

amaurosis (am-aw-roh-sis) *n.* partial or complete blindness. *a. fugax* a condition in which loss of vision is transient. —**amaurotic** (am-aw-rot-ik) *adj.*

amaurotic familial idiocy *n. see* Tay-Sachs disease.

ambivalence (am-biv-ălěns) *n.* (in psychology) the condition of holding opposite feelings (such as love and hate) for the same person or object.

amblyopia (am-blee-oh-piă) *n.* poor sight, not due to any detectable disease of the eyeball or visual system, known colloquially as *lazy eye*. *a. ex anopsia* a condition in which factors such as squint (*see* strabismus), cataract, and other abnormalities of the optics of the eye (*see* refraction) impair its normal use in early child-hood by preventing the formation of a clear image on the retina.

amblyoscope (orthoptoscope, synoptophore) (am-blee-ŏ-skohp) *n.* an instrument for measuring the angle of a squint and assessing the degree to which a person uses both eyes together.

ambulant (am-bew-lănt) *adj.* able to walk.

ambulatory (am-bew-layt-er-i) *adj.* relating to walking. *a. treatment* treatment that enables a patient to remain on his or her feet.

AMD *n. see* (age-related) macular degeneration.

amelia (ă-mee-liă) *n.* congenital total absence of the arms or legs due to a developmental defect. It is one of the fetal abnormalities induced by the drug thalidomide taken early in pregnancy. *See also* phocomelia.

amelioration (ă-mee-li-er-ay-shŏn) *n.* general improvement in the condition of a patient; reduction in severity of the symptoms of a disease.

ameloblastoma (ă-mee-loh-blas-toh-mă) *n.* a locally malignant tumour of the jaw that develops from enamel-forming cells (*ameloblasts*) but does not contain enamel.

amenorrhoea (am-en-ŏ-ree-ă) *n.* the absence or stopping of the menstrual periods. *primary a.* the non-appearance of menstrual periods at puberty. This may be due to absence of the uterus or ovaries, a genetic disorder, or hormonal imbalance. *secondary a.* the stopping of menstrual periods after establishment at puberty, for reasons such as pituitary or thyroid hormone deficiency or anorexia nervosa.

amentia (ă-men-shă) *n.* failure of

development of the intellectual faculties. *See* mental retardation.

amethocaine (ă-meth-ŏ-kayn) *n.* *see* tetracaine.

ametropia (am-ĕ-troh-piă) *n.* any abnormality of refraction of the eye, resulting in blurring of the image formed on the retina.

amiloride (ă-mil-ŏ-ryd) *n.* a potassium-sparing diuretic that causes the increased excretion of sodium and chloride; it is often combined with a thiazide or loop diuretic to reduce the potassium loss that occurs with these drugs. Trade name: **Amilamont**.

amino acid (ă-mee-noh) *n.* an organic compound that contains an amino group (–NH₂) and a carboxyl group (–COOH). Amino acids are fundamental constituents of all proteins (see table). Some can be synthesized by the body; others (*see* essential amino acid) must be obtained from protein in the diet.

aminoacidopathy (ă-mee-noh-asid-op-ă-thi) *n.* *see* maple syrup urine disease.

aminoglutethimide (ă-mee-noh-gloo-teth-i-myd) *n.* a drug used in the treatment of advanced breast and prostate cancer and Cushing's disease due to a malignant tumour. Because it inhibits synthesis of adrenal steroids, it is usually given with corticosteroid replacement therapy. Trade name: **Orimeten**. *See also* aromatase inhibitor.

aminoglycosides (ă-mee-noh-gly-koh-sydz) *pl. n.* a group of antibiotics active against a wide range of bacteria. Included in the group are gentamicin, neomycin, and streptomycin. Because of their toxicity, they are used only when less toxic antibacterials are ineffective or contraindicated. They are usually administered by injection.

aminopeptidase (ă-mee-noh-pep-ti-dayz) *n.* any one of several en-

Amino acid	Abbreviation	Amino acid	Abbreviation
alanine	ala	*leucine	leu
arginine	arg	*lysine	lys
asparagine	asn	*methionine	met
aspartic acid	asp	*phenylalanine	phe
cysteine	cys	proline	pro
glutamic acid	glu	serine	ser
glutamine	gln	*threonine	thr
glycine	gly	*tryptophan	trp
histidine	his	tyrosine	tyr
*isoleucine	ile	*valine	val

* an essential amino acid

The amino acids occurring in proteins

zymes in the intestine that cause the breakdown of a peptide, removing an amino acid.

aminophylline (ami-nof-il-een) *n.* a drug that relaxes smooth muscle and stimulates respiration. Administered by mouth or injection, it is used in the treatment of asthma and chronic bronchitis. Trade name: **Phyllocontin Continus**.

amiodarone (ami-oh-dă-rohn) *n.* an anti-arrhythmic drug used to control a variety of abnormal heart rhythms, including atrial fibrillation and abnormally rapid heartbeat. It is administered by mouth or by injection. Trade name: **Cordarone X**.

amitosis (ami-toh-sis) *n.* division of the nucleus of a cell by a process, not involving mitosis, in which the nucleus is constricted into two.

amitriptyline (ami-trip-til-een) *n.* a tricyclic antidepressant drug that has a mild tranquillizing action. Trade names: **Elavil, Lentizol**.

AML *n.* acute myeloid leukaemia. *See* myeloid (leukaemia).

amlodipine (am-loh-dy-peen) *n.* a calcium antagonist used to treat hypertension and angina pectoris. It is administered by mouth. Trade name: **Istin**.

ammonia (ă-moh-niă) *n.* a colourless gas with a pungent odour that can be cooled and compressed to form a liquid. Ammonium salts are used as expectorants and ammonia itself (in very dilute form) is used as a reflex stimulant. Formula: NH_3.

amnesia (am-nee-ziă) *n.* total or partial loss of memory following physical injury, disease, drugs, or psychological trauma. *anterograde a.* loss of memory for events following the trauma. *retrograde a.* loss of

memory for events preceding the trauma.

amnihook (am-ni-huuk) *n.* a small plastic hooked instrument for performing amniotomy. The hook is introduced through the cervix.

amniocentesis (am-ni-oh-sen-tee-sis) *n.* withdrawal of a sample of amniotic fluid surrounding an embryo in the uterus, by means of a syringe inserted through the abdominal wall, to enable prenatal diagnosis of chromosomal abnormalities (such as Down's syndrome) and metabolic and other congenital disorders (such as spina bifida).

amnion (am-ni-ŏn) *n.* the membrane that forms initially over the dorsal part of the embryo but soon expands to enclose it completely within the amniotic cavity. —**amniotic** (am-ni-ot-ik) *adj.*

amnioscopy (am-ni-oss-kŏ-pi) *n.* examination of the inside of the amniotic sac by means of an instrument (*amnioscope*) that is passed through the abdominal wall. *cervical a.* examination of the amniotic sac through the cervix (neck) of the uterus.

amniotic cavity *n.* the fluid-filled cavity between the embryo and the amnion. *See also* amniotic fluid.

amniotic fluid *n.* the fluid contained within the amniotic cavity. It surrounds the growing fetus, protecting it from external pressure. *See also* amniocentesis.

amniotomy (artificial rupture of membranes, ARM) (am-ni-ot-ŏmi) *n.* a method of surgically inducing labour by puncturing the amnion surrounding the baby in the uterus using an amnihook or similar instrument.

amobarbital (amylobarbitone) (am-oh-**bar**-bi-tal) *n.* an intermediate-acting barbiturate used to treat severe insomnia in patients already taking barbiturates. Trade names: **Amytal**, **Sodium Amytal**.

amoeba (ă-**mee**-bă) *n.* (*pl.* **amoebae**) any protozoan of jelly-like consistency and irregular and constantly changing shape. Some amoebae cause disease in humans (*see* Entamoeba). —**amoebic** *adj.* —**amoeboid** *adj.*

amoebiasis (ami-by-ă-sis) *n. see* dysentery.

amoebicide (ă-**mee**-bi-syd) *n.* an agent that kills amoebae.

amorolfine (am-oh-**rol**-feen) *n.* an antifungal drug used to treat ringworm, candidosis, and other fungal infections of the skin and nails. It is applied externally as a cream or nail lacquer. Trade name: **Loceryl**.

amoxapine (ă-**moks**-ă-peen) *n.* a tricyclic antidepressant drug similar to imipramine. It is administered by mouth. Trade name: **Asendis**.

amoxicillin (ă-mok-si-**sil**-in) *n.* an antibiotic used to treat infections caused by a wide range of bacteria and other microorganisms. It is administered by mouth; sensitivity to penicillin prohibits its use. Trade name: **Amoxil**.

AMP (adenosine monophosphate) *n.* a compound containing adenine, ribose, and one phosphate group. AMP occurs in cells and is involved in processes requiring the transfer of energy (*see* ATP).

ampere (am-pair) *n.* the basic SI unit of electric current. It is equal to the current flowing through a conductor of resistance 1 ohm when a potential difference of 1 volt is applied between its ends. Symbol: A.

amphetamines (am-fet-ăminz) *pl. n.* a group of sympathomimetic drugs that have a marked stimulant action on the central nervous system. *Dexamfetamine* (*dexamfetamine*; Dexedrine), administered by mouth, is used in the treatment of narcolepsy and attention-deficit/hyperactivity disorder. Tolerance to amphetamines develops rapidly, and prolonged use may lead to dependence. *See also* methylphenidate.

amphiarthrosis (am-fi-arth-**roh**-sis) *n.* a slightly movable joint in which the bony surfaces are separated by fibrocartilage (*see* symphysis) or hyaline cartilage (*see* synchondrosis).

amphoric breath sounds (am-**fo**-rik) *pl. n. see* cavernous breath sounds.

amphotericin (am-foh-**te**-ri-sin) *n.* an antifungal drug used to treat deep-seated fungal infections. It can be administered by mouth, but is usually given by intravenous infusion. Trade names: **Abelcet**, **AmBisome**, **Amphocil**, **Fungilin**, **Fungizone**.

ampicillin (am-pi-**sil**-in) *n.* an antibiotic administered by mouth or injection in the treatment of a variety of infections, including those of the urinary, respiratory, biliary, and intestinal tracts. Trade names: **Penbritin**, **Rimacillin**.

ampoule (ampule) (am-pool) *n.* a sealed glass or plastic capsule containing one dose of a drug in the form of a sterile solution for injection.

ampulla (am-puul-ă) *n.* (*pl.* **ampul-**

lae) an enlarged or dilated ending of a tube or canal. *a. of Vater* the dilated part of the common bile duct where it is joined by the pancreatic duct. [A. Vater (1684–1751), German anatomist]

amputation (am-pew-**tay**-shŏn) *n.* the removal of a limb, part of a limb, or any other portion of the body (such as a breast).

amsacrine (am-să-kreen) *n.* a cytotoxic drug administered by injection to treat acute myeloid leukaemia. Trade name: **Amsidine**.

amylase (am-i-layz) *n.* an enzyme that occurs in saliva and pancreatic juice and aids the digestion of starch, which it breaks down into glucose, maltose, and dextrins.

amylobarbitone (ami-loh-bar-bi-tohn) *n.* see amobarbital.

amyloid (am-i-loid) *n.* a glycoprotein, resembling starch, that is deposited in the internal organs in amyloidosis. β-amyloid protein has been found in the brains of Alzheimer's patients.

amyloidosis (ami-loid-oh-sis) *n.* infiltration of the liver, kidneys, spleen, and other tissues with amyloid. *primary a.* amyloidosis without any apparent cause. *secondary a.* a late complication of such chronic infections as tuberculosis or leprosy.

amylopectin (ami-loh-pek-tin) *n.* see starch.

amylopsin (ami-lop-sin) *n.* an amylase found in the pancreatic juice.

amylose (am-i-lohz) *n.* see starch.

amyotonia congenita (floppy baby syndrome) (ay-my-ŏ-toh-niă kon-jen-ită) *n.* a former diagnosis for various conditions, present at birth, in which the baby's muscles are weak and floppy (i.e. hypotonic). The term is becoming obsolete as more specific diagnoses are discovered to explain the cause of floppiness in babies.

amyotrophy (ami-ot-rŏfi) *n.* a progressive loss of muscle bulk associated with weakness, caused by disease of the nerve that supplies the affected muscle. *diabetic a.* wasting of the quadriceps muscle and loss of the knee jerk due to disease of the femoral nerve, associated with poor diabetic control.

an- *prefix. see* a-.

anabolic (ană-bol-ik) *adj.* promoting tissue growth by increasing the metabolic processes that are involved in protein synthesis. Anabolic steroids are synthetic forms of male sex hormones. *See* nandrolone, stanozolol.

anabolism (ă-nab-ŏl-izm) *n.* the synthesis of complex molecules, such as proteins and fats, from simpler ones by living organisms. *See also* anabolic, metabolism.

anacidity (ană-sid-iti) *n.* a deficiency or abnormal absence of acid in the body fluids.

anacrotism (ăn-ak-rŏt-izm) *n.* the condition in which there is an abnormal curve in the ascending line of a pulse tracing. It may be seen in cases of aortic stenosis. —**anacrotic** *adj.*

anaemia (ă-nee-miă) *n.* a reduction in the quantity of the oxygen-carrying pigment haemoglobin in the blood. The main symptoms are excessive tiredness and fatigability, breathlessness on exertion, pallor, and poor resistance to infection. The many causes of anaemia include loss of blood (*haemorrhagic* *a*.); lack of iron (*iron-deficiency a*.); the increased destruction of red blood cells (*haemolytic a*.); and the impaired production of red blood cells (*see also* aplastic anaemia, leukaemia, pernicious (anaemia)). Anaemias can be classified on the basis of the size of the red cells, which may be large (*macrocytic a*.), small (*microcytic a*.), or normal-sized (*normocytic a*.). —**anaemic** *adj*.

anaerobe (an-air-rohb) *n*. any organism, especially a microbe, that is able to live and grow in the absence of free oxygen. Compare aerobe. —**anaerobic** (an-air-roh-bik) *adj*.

anaerobic respiration *n*. a type of cellular respiration in which foodstuffs (usually carbohydrates) are never completely oxidized because molecular oxygen is not used.

anaesthesia (anis-theez-iǎ) *n*. loss of feeling or sensation in a part or all of the body, especially when induced by drugs. *general a*. total unconsciousness, usually achieved by administering a combination of injections and gases. *local a*. loss of feeling in a limited area of the body, induced for minor operations, particularly many dental procedures. It may be achieved by injections of substances such as lidocaine close to a local nerve, which deadens the tissues supplied by that nerve. *regional a*. anaesthesia (usually of a limb) achieved by encircling local anaesthetic solutions or by direct application of anaesthetic to one or more peripheral nerves. *See also* epidural, spinal anaesthesia.

anaesthetic (anis-thet-ik) **1**. *n*. an agent that reduces or abolishes sen-

sation. *general a*. an anaesthetic, such as halothane, that affects the whole body. *local a*. an anaesthetic, such as lidocaine, that affects a particular area or region of the body. **2**. *adj*. reducing or abolishing sensation.

anaesthetist (ăn-ees-thĕt-ist) *n*. a medically qualified doctor who administers an anaesthetic to induce unconsciousness in a patient before a surgical operation.

anagen (an-ǎ-jěn) *n*. the growth phase of a hair follicle, lasting two to three years. It is followed by a transitional stage, called *catagen*, which lasts for about two weeks, and then a resting phase, *telogen*. On average about 85% of hairs are in anagen and hence growing actively.

anal (ay-nǎl) *adj*. of, relating to, or affecting the anus. *a. canal* the terminal portion of the large intestine, which is surrounded by the muscles of defecation (*a. sphincters*). The canal ends on the surface at the anal orifice (*see* anus). *a. fissure see* fissure.

analeptic (anǎ-lep-tik) *n*. a drug that restores consciousness to a patient in a coma. Analeptics act on the central nervous system to stimulate the muscles involved in breathing.

analgesia (an-ăl-jeez-iǎ) *n*. reduced sensibility to pain, without loss of consciousness and without the sense of touch necessarily being affected.

analgesic (an-ăl-jee-sik) **1**. *n*. a drug that relieves pain. Aspirin and paracetamol are mild analgesics; morphine and pethidine (*narcotic* or *opioid analgesics*) are more potent.

See also narcotic. **2.** *adj.* relieving pain.

analogous (ă-nal-ŏ-gŭs) *adj.* describing organs or parts that have similar functions in different organisms although they do not have the same evolutionary origin or development. *Compare* homologous.

analogue (an-ă-log) **1.** *n.* a drug that differs in minor ways in molecular structure from its parent compound. Useful analogues of existing drugs are either more potent or cause fewer side-effects. Carboplatin, for example, is a less toxic analogue of cisplatin. *a. insulin see* insulin. *See also* LHRH analogue. **2.** *adj.* relating to or designating information that can be represented by a continuously varying quantity. *a. hearing aid see* hearing aid. *a. image* a traditional X-ray image on film in shades ranging smoothly from black to white. It can be converted to digital format. *Compare* digital.

analysis (ă-nal-isis) *n.* (in psychology) any means of understanding complex mental processes or experiences. *See also* psychoanalysis.

analyst (an-ă-list) *n.* a person who performs analysis.

anaphase (an-ă-fayz) *n.* the third stage of mitosis and of each division of meiosis.

anaphylaxis (ană-fil-aks-iss) *n.* an emergency condition resulting from an abnormal and immediate allergic response to a substance to which the body has become intensely sensitized. It results in flushing, itching, nausea and vomiting, swelling of the mouth and tongue and airway enough to often cause obstruction, wheezing, a sudden drop in blood pressure, and even sudden death. In this extreme form it is called *anaphylactic shock*. Treatment, which must be given immediately, consists of adrenaline (epinephrine) injection, oxygen with possible advanced support of the airway, intravenous fluids, intravenous corticosteroids, and antihistamines. —**anaphylactic** *adj.*

anaplasia (ană-play-ziă) *n.* a loss of normal cell characteristics or differentiation. Anaplasia is typical of rapidly growing malignant tumours (called *anaplastic tumours*).

anasarca (ană-sar-kă) *n.* massive swelling of the legs, trunk, and genitalia due to retention of fluid (oedema): found in congestive heart failure and some forms of renal failure.

anastomosis (ă-nass-tŏ-moh-sis) *n.* **1.** (in anatomy) a communication between two blood vessels without any intervening capillary network. *arteriovenous a.* a thick-walled blood vessel that connects an arteriole directly with a venule, found in the skin of the lips, nose, ears, hands, and feet. **2.** (in surgery) an artificial connection between two tubular organs or parts, especially between two normally separate parts of the intestine or two blood vessels. *See also* shunt.

anastrozole (an-ass-tră-zohl) *n. see* aromatase inhibitor.

anatomy (ă-nat-ŏmi) *n.* the study of the structure of living organisms. In medicine it refers to the study of the form and gross structure of the various parts of the human body. *See also* cytology, histology, physiology. —**anatomical** (ană-tom-i-k'l) *adj.* —**anatomist** *n.*

anconeus (an-koh-niŭs) *n.* a muscle behind the elbow that assists in extending the forearm.

Ancylostoma (Ankylostoma) (an-si-loh-**stoh**-mă) *n.* a genus of small parasitic nematodes that inhabit the small intestine (*see* hookworm). *A. duodenale* the species that most commonly infests humans.

ancylostomiasis (an-si-loh-stoh-my-ăsis) *n.* an infestation of the small intestine by the *parasitic* hookworm *Ancylostoma duodenale*. *See* hookworm (disease).

ANDI (an-di) *n.* an acronym for *ab*normal *d*evelopment and *i*nvolution, used to tabulate benign disorders of the breast.

andr- (andro-) *prefix denoting* man or the male sex.

androgen (an-drŏ-jĕn) *n.* one of a group of steroid hormones, including testosterone, androsterone, and dihydrotestosterone, that stimulate the development of male sex organs and male secondary sexual characteristics. The principal source of these hormones is the testis but they are also secreted by the adrenal cortex and ovaries in small amounts. In women excessive production of androgens gives rise to masculinization. Naturally occurring and synthetic androgens are used in replacement therapy and as anabolic agents. *See also* dehydroepiandrosterone. —**androgenic** *adj.*

androgen insensitivity syndrome *n.* a form of pseudohermaphroditism in which an individual who is genetically male (XY) has female external genitalia and secondary sexual characteristics but lacks female reproductive organs; testes are present internally. The syndrome is an X-linked (*see* sex-linked) recessive condition, in which the body does not react to androgens because androgen receptors do not function.

androgenization (an-droj-ĕn-I-zay-shŏn) *n.* the final effects of the exposure of sensitive tissues to androgens, i.e. the development of secondary male sexual characteristics. Androgenization can occur abnormally in females, who may develop excessive body hair, male-pattern baldness, and clitoromegaly.

andrology (an-drol-ŏji) *n.* **1.** the study of male infertility and impotence. It includes seminal analysis and other investigation procedures to determine the causes of infertility, which determine the treatment undertaken. **2.** the study of androgen production and the relationship of plasma androgen to androgen action. —**andrologist** *n.*

androstenedione (an-drŏ-steen-dy-ohn) *n. see* adrenarche, dehydroepiandrosterone.

androsterone (an-drost-er-ohn) *n.* a steroid hormone (*see* androgen) that is synthesized and released by the testes and is responsible for controlling male sexual development.

anencephaly (an-en-**sef**-ăli) *n.* partial or complete absence of the bones of the rear of the skull, the meninges, and the cerebral hemispheres of the brain. It occurs as a developmental defect and most affected infants are stillborn; if born live they do not survive for more than a few hours. *See also* alphafetoprotein. —**anencephalic** *adj.*

anergy (an-er-ji) *n.* **1.** lack of response to a specific antigen or allergen. **2.** lack of energy. —**anergic** *adj.*

aneurine (vitamin B₁) (an-yoor-in) *n.* see vitamin B.

aneurysm (an-yoor-izm) *n.* a balloon-like swelling in the wall of an artery, due to disease or congenital deficiency. *aortic a.* an aneurysm that most frequently occurs in the abdominal aorta, below the level of the renal arteries (*abdominal aortic a.*, *AAA*). Beyond a certain size it is prone to rupture: an acute surgical emergency. *arteriovenous a.* a direct communication between an artery and vein, without an intervening capillary bed. *berry a.* a small saccular aneurysm commonly affecting branches of the circle of Willis in the brain. Usually associated with congenital weakness of the vessels, they are a cause of cerebral haemorrhage in young adults. *Charcot-Bouchard a.* a small aneurysm found within the brain of elderly and hypertensive subjects. Such aneurysms may rupture, causing cerebral haemorrhage. *dissecting a.* a condition in which a tear occurs in the lining of (usually) the first part of the aorta, which allows blood to enter the wall and track along (dissect) the muscular coat. A dissecting aneurysm may rupture or it may compress the blood vessels arising from the aorta and produce infarction (localized necrosis) in the organs they supply. *ventricular a.* a condition that may develop in the wall of the left ventricle after myocardial infarction. Heart failure may result or thrombosis within the aneurysm may act as a source of embolism. —**aneurysmal** *adj.*

Angelman syndrome (happy puppet syndrome) (ayn-jěl-măn) *n.* a disorder of development characterized by severe learning difficulties, absence of speech, seizures, jerky movements, a characteristic facial expression, and a happy social disposition. It is caused by a genetic abnormality on chromosome 15. [H. Angelman (1915–96), British paediatrician]

angi- (angio-) *prefix denoting* blood or lymph vessels.

angiectasis (an-ji-ek-tă-sis) *n.* abnormal dilation of blood vessels.

angiitis (vasculitis) (an-ji-I-tis) *n.* a patchy inflammation of the walls of small blood vessels.

angina (an-jy-nă) *n.* a sense of suffocation or suffocating pain. *a. pectoris* pain in the centre of the chest, which is induced by exercise and relieved by rest and may spread to the jaws and arms. Angina pectoris occurs when the demand for blood by the heart exceeds the supply of the coronary arteries and it usually results from coronary artery atheroma. It may be prevented or relieved by such drugs as glyceryl trinitrate and propranolol or by surgery (see angioplasty, coronary artery bypass graft). See also Ludwig's angina.

angiocardiography (an-ji-oh-kar-di-og-răfi) *n.* X-ray examination of the chambers of the heart after introducing a radiopaque contrast medium into the atria, ventricles, or great vessels by cardiac catheterization. Video images are recorded on film or electronic media, often using digital subtraction techniques.

angiodysplasia (an-ji-oh-dis-play-ziă) *n.* an abnormal collection of small blood vessels in the wall of the bowel, which may bleed.

angiogenesis (an-ji-oh-jen-i-sis) *n.* the formation of new blood vessels. This process is essential for the development of a tumour and is promoted by growth factors.

angiography (an-ji-og-răfi) *n.* imaging of blood vessels. *computerized tomographic a.* angiography in which a contrast agent, usually injected into a vein, enhances the density of the blood, which can then be seen on two- or three-dimensional images, with surrounding tissues hidden by the computer. *coronary a.* an X-ray technique for examining the coronary arteries and chambers of the heart in which video images are recorded during contrast-medium injection. *See* arteriography. *fluorescein a.* a technique for visualizing blood flow in the retina, in which the dye fluorescein sodium, injected into the blood stream, causes the retinal blood vessels to fluoresce. *fluoroscopic a.* angiography in which the contrast medium is injected during X-ray fluoroscopy. Positive (radiopaque) contrast medium containing iodine or negative (radiolucent) gas (carbon dioxide) may be used. *indocyanine green a.* a technique for visualizing blood flow in the choroid layer of the eye after the injection of the dye indocyanine green. *magnetic resonance a.* magnetic resonance imaging of blood vessels, either after injection of magnetic resonance contrast agent, which gives an increased signal from the blood, or relying on the movement of blood to give a lack of signal in the plane being examined.

angiology (an-ji-ol-ŏji) *n.* the branch of medicine concerned with the structure, function, and diseases of blood vessels.

angioma (an-ji-oh-mǎ) *n.* (*pl.* **angiomata**) a benign tumour composed of blood vessels or lymph vessels. *arteriovenous a.* (*arteriovenous malformation, AVM*) a knot of distended blood vessels that may occur in many parts of the body. When overlying and compressing the surface of the brain, it may cause epilepsy or subdural haemorrhage. *cherry a.* (*Campbell de Morgan spot*) a small red spot, consisting of a minor vascular malformation, occurring on the trunk in middle-aged and elderly people. *See also* haemangioma, lymphangioma.

angio-oedema (angioneurotic oedema) (an-ji-oh-ee-dee-mǎ) *n. see* urticaria.

angioplasty (an-ji-oh-plasti) *n.* repair or reconstruction of narrowed or completely obstructed blood vessels. *balloon a.* (*percutaneous transluminal a., PTA*) enlargement of the lumen of a blood vessel by means of an inflatable balloon, mounted on the tip of a flexible catheter, under X-ray screening control. *coronary a.* balloon angioplasty of a section of coronary artery narrowed by atheroma.

angiosarcoma (an-ji-oh-sar-koh-mǎ) *n.* a sarcoma arising in the blood vessels.

angiospasm (an-ji-oh-spazm) *n. see* Raynaud's disease.

angiotensin (an-ji-oh-ten-sin) *n.* either of two peptides. *a. I* peptide derived, by the action of renin, from a protein secreted by the liver into the bloodstream. *a. II* a peptide, formed from angiotensin I by enzyme action, that causes constriction of blood vessels and stimulates the release of vasopressin and aldosterone, which increase blood pressure. *See also* ACE inhibitor.

angiotensin II antagonist *n.* a drug that blocks the action of the hormone angiotensin II, which constricts blood vessels, and is therefore useful in treating hypertension. Such drugs include *candesartan* (Amias), *irbesartan* (Aprovel), *losartan* (Cozaar), *telmisartan* (Micardis), and *valsartan* (Diovan). They are taken by mouth.

angstrom (ang-strŏm) *n.* a unit of length equal to one ten millionth of a millimetre (10^{-10} m), sometimes used to express wavelengths and interatomic distances. Symbol Å.

anhedonia (an-hee-doh-niă) *n.* total loss of the feeling of pleasure in acts that normally give pleasure.

anhidrosis (an-hy-droh-sis) *n.* the absence of sweating in the presence of an appropriate stimulus for sweating, such as heat, which may accompany disease or occur as a congenital defect. *See also* hypohidrosis.

anhidrotic (an-hy-drot-ik) **1.** *n.* any drug that inhibits the secretion of sweat, such as an anticholinergic drug. **2.** *adj.* inhibiting sweating.

anhydraemia (an-hy-dree-miă) *n.* a decrease in the proportion of water, and therefore plasma, in the blood.

anhydrous (an-hy-drŭs) *adj.* containing no water.

aniline (an-il-een) *n.* an oily compound obtained from coal tar and widely used in the preparation of dyes.

anion (an-I-ŏn) *n.* a negatively charged ion, which moves towards the anode (positive electrode) when an electric current is passed through the solution containing it. *Compare* cation. **a. gap** the difference between the concentrations of cations (positively charged ions) and anions, calculated from the formula $(Na^+ + K^+) - (HCO_3^- + Cl^-)$: it is used to estimate the unaccounted-for anions in the blood in cases of metabolic disturbance.

aniridia (ani-rid-iă) *n.* congenital absence of the iris (of the eye).

anisocytosis (an-I-soh-sy-toh-sis) *n.* an excessive variation in size between individual red blood cells.

anisomelia (an-I-soh-mee-liă) *n.* a difference in size or shape between the arms or the legs.

anisometropia (an-I-soh-mě-troh-piă) *n.* the condition in which the power of refraction in one eye differs markedly from that in the other.

ankle (an-k'l) *n.* **1.** the hinge joint between the leg and the foot. It consists of the talus (ankle bone), which projects into a socket formed by the lower ends of the tibia and fibula. **2.** the whole region of the ankle joint, including the tarsus and the lower parts of the tibia and fibula.

ankyloblepharon (anki-loh-blef-er-on) *n.* abnormal fusion (partial or complete) of the upper and lower eyelid margins.

ankylosing spondylitis (anki-loh-zing) *n. see* spondylitis.

ankylosis (anki-loh-sis) *n.* pathological fusion of the bones across a joint space, either by bony tissue (*bony a.*) or by shortening of connecting fibrous tissue (*fibrous a.*).

Ankylostoma (anki-loh-**stoh**-mǎ) *n. see* Ancylostoma.

annulus (an-yoo-lǔs) *n.* (in anatomy) a circular opening or ring-shaped structure. —**annular** *adj.*

ano- *prefix denoting* the anus.

anodyne (an-ŏ-dyn) *n.* any treatment or drug that soothes and eases pain.

anomaly (ǎ-nom-ǎli) *n.* any deviation from the normal, especially a congenital or developmental defect. —**anomalous** *adj.*

anomia (ǎ-noh-miǎ) *n.* a form of aphasia in which the patient is unable to give the names of objects, but retains the ability to put words together into speech.

anomie (an-oh-mi) *n.* a condition in which a person is no longer able to identify with or relate to others, resulting in apathy, loneliness, and distress.

anonychia (anŏ-nik-iǎ) *n.* congenital absence of one or more nails.

Anopheles (ǎ-nof-i-leez) *n.* a genus of widely distributed mosquitoes. The malarial parasite (*see* Plasmodium) is transmitted to humans solely through the bite of female *Anopheles* mosquitoes.

anophthalmos (an-off-thal-mŏs) *n.* congenital absence of the eye.

anoplasty (ay-noh-plasti) *n.* a surgical technique used to repair a weak or injured anal sphincter.

anorchism (an-or-kizm) *n.* congenital absence of one or both testes.

anorexia (an-er-eks-iǎ) *n.* loss of appetite. *a. nervosa* a psychological illness, most common in female adolescents, in which the patients starve themselves or use other techniques, such as vomiting or taking laxatives, to induce weight loss. The result is severe loss of weight, often with amenorrhoea, and sometimes even death from starvation. The problem often starts with an obsessive desire to lose weight but the underlying cause of the illness is more complicated. Patients must be persuaded to eat enough to maintain a normal body weight and their emotional disturbance is usually treated with psychotherapy. *See also* bulimia.

anosmia (an-oz-miǎ) *n.* absence of the sense of smell. Permanent anosmia may follow certain viral infections, head injuries, and tumours affecting the olfactory nerve.

anovular (anovulatory) (an-ov-yoo-ler) *adj.* not associated with the development and release of a female germ cell (ovum) in the ovary, as in *anovular menstruation*.

anoxaemia (an-oks-ee-miǎ) *n.* a condition in which there is less than the normal concentration of oxygen in the blood. *See also* hypoxaemia.

anoxia (an-oks-iǎ) *n.* a condition in which the tissues of the body receive inadequate amounts of oxygen. *See also* hypoxia. —**anoxic** *adj.*

ant- (anti-) *prefix denoting* opposed to; counteracting; relieving.

Antabuse (ant-ǎ-bews) *n. see* disulfiram.

antacid (ant-ass-id) *n.* a drug, such as aluminium or magnesium hydroxide, sodium bicarbonate, or calcium carbonate, that neutralizes the hydrochloric acid secreted in the digestive juices of the stomach. Antacids are used to relieve discomfort in disorders of the digestive system.

antagonist (an-tag-ŏn-ist) *n.* **1.** a muscle whose action (contraction) opposes that of another muscle (*see* agonist). **2.** a drug or other substance with opposite action to that of another drug or natural body chemical. —**antagonism** *n*.

ante- *prefix denoting* before.

anteflexion (anti-flek-shŏn) *n*. the bending forward of an organ. A mild degree of anteflexion of the uterus is considered to be normal.

ante mortem (an-ti mor-těm) *adj*. before death. *Compare* post mortem.

antenatal (anti-nay-t'l) *adj*. of or relating to the period of pregnancy; before birth. *a. diagnosis see* prenatal diagnosis.

antepartum (anti-par-tŭm) *adj*. occurring before the onset of labour. *a. haemorrhage* bleeding from the genital tract after the 24th week of pregnancy until the birth of the baby.

anterior (an-teer-i-er) *adj*. **1.** describing or relating to the front (ventral) portion of the body or limbs. **2.** describing the front part of any organ. *a. chamber* the part of the eye between the cornea and lens, which is filled with aqueous humour.

anteversion (anti-ver-shŏn) *n*. the forward inclination of an organ, especially the normal forward inclination of the uterus.

anthelmintic (an-thel-min-tik) **1.** *n*. any drug, such as piperazine, or chemical agent used to destroy parasitic worms (helminths) and/or remove them from the body. **2.** *adj*. having the power to destroy or eliminate helminths.

anthracosis (an-thră-koh-sis) *n*. *see* coal-worker's pneumoconiosis.

anthracycline (an-thră-sy-kleen) *n*. any of numerous antibiotics synthesized or isolated from species of

Streptomyces. Doxorubicin is the most important member of this group of compounds, which have wide activity against tumours.

anthrax (an-thraks) *n*. an acute infectious disease of farm animals caused by the bacterium *Bacillus anthracis*. In humans the disease attacks either the lungs, causing pneumonia, or the skin, producing severe ulceration (*malignant pustule*). Woolsorter's disease is a serious infection of the skin or lungs by *B. anthracis*, affecting those handling wool or pelts (*see* occupational disease). Anthrax can be treated with penicillin or tetracycline.

anthrop- (anthropo-) *prefix denoting* the human race.

anti-androgen (anti-an-drŏ-jĕn) *n*. any one of a group of drugs that block the cellular uptake of testosterone by the prostate gland and are therefore used in the treatment of prostate cancer, which is an androgen-dependent tumour, and various sexual disorders in men. *See* bicalutamide, cyproterone, finasteride, flutamide.

anti-arrhythmic (anti-ă-rith-mik) *n*. any of a group of drugs used to correct irregularities in the heartbeat (*see* arrhythmia). They include adenosine, amiodarone, quinidine, verapamil, disopyramide, and lidocaine.

antibacterial (anti-bak-teer-iăl) *adj*. describing an antibiotic that is active against bacteria.

antibiotic (anti-by-ot-ik) *n*. a substance, produced by or derived from a microorganism, that destroys or inhibits the growth of other microorganisms. Antibiotics are used to treat infections caused by organisms that are sensitive to them, usually bacteria or fungi. *See also* aminoglycosides, antifungal, antiviral drug, cephalosporin, chloramphenicol, penicillin, quinolone, streptomycin, tetracycline.

antibody (an-ti-bodi) *n.* a special kind of blood protein that is synthesized in lymphoid tissue in response to the presence of a particular antigen and circulates in the plasma to attack the antigen and render it harmless. Antibody formation is the basis of both immunity and allergy.

anticholinergic (anti-koli-ner-jik) *adj.* inhibiting the action of acetylcholine, a neurotransmitter in the parasympathetic nervous system. Anticholinergic drugs relax smooth muscle, decrease the secretion of saliva, sweat, and digestive juice, and dilate the pupil of the eye.

anticholinesterase (anti-kolines-ter-ayz) *n.* any drug or other substance that inhibits the action of cholinesterase and therefore allows acetylcholine to continue transmitting nerve impulses.

anticoagulant (anti-koh-ag-yoo-lănt) *n.* an agent, such as heparin or warfarin, that prevents the clotting of blood and is used in the treatment of such conditions as thrombosis and embolism. Incorrect dosage may result in haemorrhage.

anticonvulsant (anti-kŏn-vul-sănt) *n.* a drug, such as sodium valproate or phenytoin, that prevents or reduces the severity of seizures in various types of epilepsy. Anticonvulsants are also known as *antiepileptic drugs*.

anti D *n.* the rhesus-factor antibody, formed by rhesus-negative individuals following exposure to rhesus-positive blood. *See* haemolytic disease of the newborn.

antidepressant (anti-di-press-ănt) *n.* a drug that alleviates the symptoms of depression. The most widely prescribed group are the *tricyclic antidepressants* (*TCAs*), such as amitriptyline and imipramine. *See also* MAO inhibitor, SSRI.

antidiabetic drugs (anti-dy-ă-bet-ik) *pl. n.* drugs used to control diabetes mellitus. Type 1 diabetes is treated with the wide range of formulations of insulin. Type 2 diabetes is treated mainly with oral hypoglycaemic drugs but in some cases insulin may be required.

antidiuretic hormone (ADH) (anti-dy-yoor-et-ik) *n. see* vasopressin.

antidote (an-ti-doht) *n.* a drug that counteracts the effects of a poison.

antiemetic (anti-i-met-ik) *n.* a drug that prevents vomiting, used to treat such conditions as motion sickness and vertigo and to counteract nausea and vomiting caused by other drugs.

antiepileptic drug (anti-epi-lep-tik) *n. see* anticonvulsant.

antifibrinolytic (anti-fib-rin-ŏ-lit-ik) *adj.* describing an agent that inhibits the dissolution of blood clots (*see* fibrinolysis). Antifibrinolytic drugs include aprotinin and tranexamic acid.

antifungal (antimycotic) (anti-fung-ăl) *adj.* describing a drug that kills or inactivates fungi and is used to treat fungal (including yeast) infections. Antifungal drugs include amphotericin, griseofulvin, the imidazoles, nystatin, terbinafine, and tolnaftate.

antigen (an-ti-jĕn) *n.* any substance

that may be specifically bound by an antibody molecule. —**antigenic** *adj.*

antihaemophilic factor (anti-heem-ŏ-fil-ik) *n. see* Factor VIII.

anti HBc *n.* antibody against hepatitis B core antigen.

anti HBs *n.* antibody against hepatitis B surface antigen.

antihistamine (anti-hist-ă-meen) *n.* a drug that inhibits the action of histamine in the body by blocking the receptors for histamine, of which there are two types: H_1 and H_2. When stimulated by histamine, H_1 receptors may produce such allergic reactions as hay fever, pruritus (itching), and urticaria (nettle rash). Antihistamines that block H_1 receptors (*H_1-receptor antagonists*), such as acrivastine, astemizole, and chlorphenamine, are used to relieve these conditions. Many H_1-receptor antagonists (e.g. cyclizine, promethazine) also have strong antiemetic activity and are used to prevent motion sickness. The most common side-effect of these drugs, especially the older ones (e.g. azatadine, diphenhydramine, promethazine), is drowsiness and because of this they are sometimes used to promote sleep. H_2 receptors are found mainly in the stomach, where stimulation by histamine causes secretion of acid gastric juice. *H_2-receptor antagonists* (e.g. cimetidine, famotidine, nizatidine, ranitidine) block these receptors and so reduce gastric acid secretion; they are used in the treatment of peptic ulcers and gastro-oesophageal reflux disease.

anti-inflammatory (anti-in-flam-ă-tŏ-ri) **1.** *adj.* describing a drug that reduces inflammation. The various groups of anti-inflammatory drugs act against one or more of the mediators that initiate or maintain inflammation. They include antihistamines, glucocorticoids (*see* corticosteroid), and nonsteroidal anti-inflammatory drugs (*see* NSAID). **2.** *n.* an anti-inflammatory drug.

antilymphocyte serum (antilymphocyte globulin, ALS, ALG) (anti-lim-foh-syt) *n.* an antiserum containing antibodies that suppress lymphocytic activity. ALS may be given to prevent the immune reaction that causes tissue rejection following transplantation of organs (e.g. kidneys) or bone marrow.

antimetabolite (anti-mi-tab-ŏ-lyt) *n.* a drug that interferes with the normal metabolic processes within cells by combining with the enzymes responsible for them. Some drugs used in the treatment of cancer (fluorouracil, methotrexate, and mercaptopurine, are antimetabolites. Side-effects can be severe, involving blood cell disorders and digestive disturbances. *See also* cytotoxic drug.

antimitotic (anti-my-tot-ik) *n.* a drug that inhibits cell division and growth. The drugs used to treat cancer are mainly antimitotics. *See also* antimetabolite, cytotoxic drug.

antimycotic (anti-my-kot-ik) *adj. see* antifungal.

anti-oestrogen (anti-ees-trŏ-jĕn) *n.* one of a group of drugs that oppose the action of oestrogen. It includes tamoxifen, which is used in the treatment of breast cancers dependent on oestrogen. Because they stimulate the production of pituitary gonadotrophins, some anti-oestrogens (e.g. clomifene) are used to induce or stimulate ovulation in infertility treatment (*see* super-ovulation). Side-effects of anti-oestrogens include hot flushes, itching of the vulva, nausea, vomiting, and fluid retention.

antioxidant (anti-**oks**-i-dănt) *n.* a substance capable of neutralizing oxygen free radicals, the highly active and damaging atoms and chemical groups produced by various disease processes and by poisons, radiation, smoking, and other agencies. Antioxidants include vitamin C (ascorbic acid), vitamin E (tocopherols), and beta carotene. Evidence is accumulating that administration of these substances can reduce the incidence of a number of serious diseases.

antiperistalsis (anti-pe-ri-**stal**-sis) *n.* a wave of contraction in the alimentary canal that passes in an oral (i.e. upward or backwards) direction. *Compare* peristalsis.

antiphospholipid antibody syndrome (anti-fos-foh-**lip**-id) *n.* an autoimmune disease in which the presence of antibody against phospholipid is associated with a tendency to thrombosis and – in women of childbearing age – recurrent (three or more) miscarriages. In pregnant women blood clots form in the placenta, resulting in the fetus being deprived of nourishment. Treatment is by low-dose aspirin or heparin.

antipruritic (anti-proor-**it**-ik) *n.* an agent, such as calamine or crotamiton, that relieves itching.

antipsychotic (anti-sy-**kot**-ik) *adj.* describing one of a group of drugs

used to treat severe mental disorders (psychoses), including schizophrenia and mania; some are administered in small doses to relieve anxiety. Formerly known as *major tranquillizers*, antipsychotic drugs include the phenothiazines (e.g. chlorpromazine), butyrophenones (e.g. haloperidol) and thioxanthenes (e.g. flupentixol). *atypical a.* one of a group of antipsychotics, including clozapine and risperidone, that are used in treating patients unresponsive to conventional antipsychotics. Side-effects of many antipsychotics at high doses include abnormal involuntary movements.

antipyretic (anti-py-**ret**-ik) *n.* a drug that reduces fever by lowering the body temperature.

antisecretory drug (anti-si-**kree**-tŏri) *n.* any drug that reduces the normal rate of secretion of a body fluid, usually one that reduces acid secretion into the stomach. Such drugs include anticholinergic drugs, H_2-receptor antagonists (*see* antihistamine), and proton-pump inhibitors.

antisepsis (anti-**sep**-sis) *n.* the elimination of bacteria, fungi, viruses, and other microorganisms that cause disease by the use of chemical or physical methods.

antiseptic (anti-**sep**-tik) *n.* a chemical, such as methenamine or cetrimide, that destroys or inhibits the growth of disease-causing bacteria and other microorganisms. Antiseptics are used externally to cleanse wounds and internally to treat infections of the intestine and bladder.

antiserum (anti-**seer**-ŭm) *n.* (*pl.* **antisera**) a serum that contains antibodies against particular antigens; it may be injected to treat, or give temporary protection against, specific diseases. Antisera are prepared in large quantities in such animals as horses.

antisocial (anti-soh-shăl) *adj.* contrary to the accepted standards of behaviour in society.

antisocial personality disorder *n.* a personality disorder characterized by callous unconcern for others, irresponsibility, violence, disregard for social rules, and an incapacity for maintaining enduring relationships. It was formerly known as *dyssocial personality, psychopathy,* or *sociopathy.*

antispasmodic (anti-spaz-mod-ik) *n.* a drug, such as alverine citrate or mebeverine, that relieves spasm of smooth muscle in the gut.

antispastic (anti-spas-tik) *n.* a drug that relieves spasm of skeletal muscle. *See also* muscle relaxant.

antistatic (anti-stat-ik) *adj.* preventing the accumulation of static electricity.

antithrombin (anti-throm-bin) *n.* a substance or effect that inhibits the action of thrombin in the circulation, preventing unwanted clotting.

antitoxin (anti-toks-in) *n.* an antibody produced by the body to counteract a toxin formed by invading bacteria or from any other source.

antitragus (anti-tray-gŭs) *n.* a small projection of cartilage above the lobe of the ear, opposite the tragus. *See* pinna.

antitussive (anti-tuss-iv) *n.* a drug, such as pholcodine, that suppresses coughing.

antivenene (antivenin) (anti-ven-een) *n.* an antiserum containing antibodies against specific poisons in the venom of such an animal as a snake, spider, or scorpion.

antiviral drug (anti-vy-răl) *n.* a drug effective against viruses that cause disease. Antiviral drugs include aciclovir, ganciclovir, foscarnet, zidovudine, amantadine, and ribavirin. They are used for treating herpes, cytomegalovirus, HIV, and respiratory syncytial virus infections (among others).

antrectomy (an-trek-tŏmi) *n.* **1.** surgical removal of the bony walls of an antrum. *See* antrostomy. **2.** a surgical operation in which a part of the stomach (the antrum) is removed, used in the treatment of some peptic ulcers.

antroscopy (an-tros-kŏpi) *n.* inspection of the inside of the maxillary sinus (*see* paranasal sinuses) using an endoscope (called an *antroscope*).

antrostomy (an-trost-ŏmi) *n.* a surgical operation to produce an artificial opening to an antrum in a bone, so providing drainage for any fluid. The operation is sometimes carried out to treat infection of the paranasal sinuses.

antrum (an-trŭm) *n.* **1.** a cavity, especially a cavity in a bone. *a. of Highmore* the maxillary sinus (*see* paranasal sinuses). [N. Highmore (1613–85), English physician] *mastoid* (or *tympanic*) *a.* the space connecting the air cells of the mastoid process with the chamber of the inner ear. **2.** the part of the stomach adjoining the pylorus.

anuria (ă-newr-iă) *n.* failure of the kidneys to produce urine.

anus (ay-nŭs) *n.* the opening at the lower end of the alimentary canal, through which the faeces are discharged. It opens out from the anal canal and is guarded by two sphincters. —**anal** *adj.*

anvil (an-vil) *n.* (in anatomy) *see* incus.

anxiety (ang-zy-iti) *n.* generalized pervasive fear. *a. disorder* any one of a group of mental or behavioural disorders in which anxiety is the most prominent feature. *See* generalized anxiety disorder, neurosis, panic disorder, post-traumatic stress disorder. *a. state* a condition in which anxiety dominates the patient's life.

anxiolytic (angk-si-oh-lit-ik) *adj.* describing a group of drugs used to treat anxiety of various causes. Formerly known as *minor tranquillizers*, they include the benzodiazepines, buspirone, and meprobamate. Prolonged use may result in dependence.

aorta (ay-ort-ă) *n.* (*pl.* **aortae** or **aortas**) the main artery of the body, from which all others derive. *abdominal a.* the part of the descending aorta below the diaphragm. *arch of the a.* the part of the aorta that arches over the heart. *ascending a.* the part of the aorta that arises from the left ventricle. *descending a.* the part of the aorta that descends in front of the backbone. *thoracic a.* the part of the descending aorta from the arch of the aorta to the diaphragm. —**aortic** (ay-or-tik) *adj.*

aortic aneurysm *n. see* aneurysm.

aortic regurgitation *n.* reflux of blood from the aorta into the left ventricle during diastole. Aortic regurgitation most commonly follows scarring of the aortic valve as a result of previous acute rheumatic fever, but it may also result from other conditions, such as syphilis or dissecting aneurysm.

aortic replacement *n.* a surgical technique used to replace a diseased length of aorta, most often the abdominal aorta. It usually involves inserting into the aorta a flexible tube of artificial material, which functions as a substitute for the diseased section.

aortic stenosis *n.* narrowing of the opening of the aortic valve due to fusion of the cusps that comprise the valve. It may result from previous rheumatic fever, or from calcification and scarring in a valve that has two cusps instead of the normal three, or it may be congenital.

aortic valve *n. see* semilunar valve.

aortitis (ay-or-ty-tis) *n.* inflammation of the aorta, which is often associated with a variety of poorly understood autoimmune conditions, such as Behçet's syndrome and Takayasu's disease.

aortography (ay-or-tog-răfi) *n.* X-ray examination of the aorta in which a series of images is taken during the injection of a radiopaque contrast medium. It has now largely been replaced by other cross-sectional imaging techniques.

apathetic hyperthyroidism (apă-thet-ik) *n. see* hyperthyroidism.

APEL (APL) *n.* Accreditation of Prior (Experiential) Learning: a system in which previous experience and learning are acknowledged by educational establishments and are given academic value. Evidence for the learning and experience must be provided for scrutiny. The level at which learning and experience is valued varies between educational establishments. *See also* CATS.

aperient (ă-**peer**-iĕnt) *n.* a mild laxative.

aperistalsis (ay-pe-ri-stal-sis) *n.* the absence of peristaltic movement in the intestines.

apex (ay-peks) *n.* the tip or summit of an organ; for example the heart or lung. The apex of a tooth is the tip of the root. *See also* apical.

apex beat *n.* the impact of the heart against the chest wall during systole. It can be felt or heard to the left of the breastbone, in the space between the fifth and sixth ribs.

Apgar score (ap-gar) *n.* a method of rapidly assessing the general state of a baby immediately after birth. A maximum of 2 points is given for each of the following signs, usually measured at one minute and five minutes after delivery: type of breathing, heart rate, colour, muscle tone, and response to stimuli. [V. Apgar (1909–74), US anaesthetist]

aphagia (ă-**fay**-jiă) *n.* loss of the ability to swallow.

aphakia (ă-**fay**-kiă) *n.* absence of the lens of the eye: the state of the eye after a cataract has been removed and no intraocular lens has been inserted. —**aphakic** *adj.*

aphasia (dysphasia) (ă-**fay**-ziă) *n.* a disorder of language affecting the generation and content of speech and its understanding. It is caused by disease in the left half of the brain (the dominant hemisphere) in a right-handed person. —**aphasic** *adj.*

aphonia (ă-**foh**-niă) *n.* absence or loss of the voice caused by disease of the larynx or mouth or disease of

the nerves and muscles involved in the generation and articulation of speech.

aphrodisiac (afrŏ-**diz**-iak) *n.* an agent that stimulates sexual excitement.

aphthous ulcer (af-thŭs) *n.* a small ulcer, occurring singly or in groups in the mouth as white or red spots.

apical (ay-pi-k'l) *adj.* of or relating to the apex of an organ or tooth. *a. abscess see* abscess.

apicectomy (ay-pi-sek-tŏmi) *n.* (in dentistry) surgical removal of the apex of the root of a tooth, now often called *root end resection*.

APL *n. see* APEL.

aplasia (ă-**play**-ziă) *n.* total or partial failure of development of an organ or tissue. *See also* agenesis. —**aplastic** (ay-**plas**-tik) *adj.*

aplastic anaemia *n.* a severe form of anaemia, resistant to therapy, in which the bone marrow fails to produce new blood cells (*see* pancytopenia). There are several causes, including a reaction to toxic drugs.

apnoea (ap-**nee**-ă) *n.* temporary cessation of breathing from any cause, formally defined as a reduction in nasal air flow to less than 30% of normal for more than 10 seconds. *a. index* the number of apnoea episodes per hour of sleep. *a. monitor* an electronic alarm, responding to a baby's breathing movements, that can monitor babies at risk from cot death. *See also* sleep apnoea. —**apnoeic** *adj.*

apocrine (ap-ŏ-kryn) *adj.* **1.** describing sweat glands that occur only in hairy parts of the body, especially the armpit and groin. These glands develop in the hair follicles and appear after puberty has been reached. Compare eccrine. **2.** describing a type of gland that loses part of its protoplasm when secreting. See secretion.

apolipoprotein (apoprotein) (apŏ-lip-oh-**proh**-teen) *n.* any one of a family of proteins found in lipoproteins. Apolipoproteins have a variety of functions, which include acting as ligands for the binding of enzymes (apolipoprotein B) and as cofactors for the action of other enzymes (apolipoproteins A and C).

apomorphine (apŏ-**mor**-feen) *n.* a drug used mainly in the treatment of parkinsonism that is poorly controlled by levodopa. It is administered by subcutaneous injection or infusion. Trade names: **APO-go, Britaject.**

aponeurosis (apŏ-newr-**oh**-sis) *n.* a thin but strong fibrous sheet of tissue that replaces a tendon in muscles that are flat and sheetlike and have a wide area of attachment (e.g. to bones). —**aponeurotic** (apŏ-newr-**ot**-ik) *adj.*

apophysis (ă-**pof**-i-sis) *n.* a protuberance of bone to which a tendon is attached. *a. cerebri* the pineal gland. —**apophyseal** *adj.*

apophysitis (ă-pof-i-**sy**-tis) *n.* inflammation of any apophysis caused by excessive pull of a tendon to which it is attached. See Osgood-Schlatter disease, Sever's disease.

apoplexy (**ap**-ŏ-plek-si) *n.* see stroke.

apoprotein (apŏ-**proh**-teen) *n.* see apolipoprotein.

apoptosis (ă-**pop**-tŏ-sis) *n.* programmed cell death, which results in the ordered removal of cells and occurs naturally as part of the normal development, maintenance, and renewal of cells, tissues, and organs. Failure of apoptosis has been implicated in the uncontrolled cell division that occurs in cancer.

appendectomy (ap-ĕn-**dek**-tŏmi) *n. US* appendicectomy.

appendicectomy (ă-pen-di-**sek**-tŏmi) *n.* surgical removal of the vermiform appendix. See also appendicitis.

appendicitis (ă-pen-di-**sy**-tis) *n.* inflammation of the vermiform appendix. *acute a.* the most common form of the condition, usually affecting young people. The chief symptom is abdominal pain, first central and later in the right lower abdomen, over the appendix. If not treated by surgical removal (appendicectomy) the condition usually progresses to cause an abscess or generalized peritonitis. *chronic a.* a formerly popular diagnosis to explain recurrent pains in the lower abdomen. It is rare, and appendicectomy will not usually cure such pains.

appendicular (ap-ĕn-**dik**-yoo-ler) *adj.* **1.** relating to or affecting the vermiform appendix. **2.** relating to the limbs.

appendix (vermiform appendix) (ă-**pen**-diks) *n.* the short thin blind-ended tube, 7–10 cm long, that is attached to the end of the caecum. It has no known function in humans and is liable to become infected and inflamed (see appendicitis).

apperception (ap-er-sep-shŏn) *n.* (in psychology) the process by which the qualities of an object, situation, etc., perceived by an individual are correlated with his/her preexisting knowledge.

appestat (ap-ĕs-tat) *n.* a region in the brain that controls the amount of food intake. Appetite suppressants probably decrease hunger by changing the chemical characteristics of this centre.

applanation (ap-lă-nay-shŏn) *n.* flattening of the cornea. It is used to determine intraocular pressure (*a. tonometry*). *See* tonometer.

applicator (ap-li-kay-ter) *n.* any device used to apply medication or treatment to a particular part of the body.

apposition (apŏ-zish-ŏn) *n.* the state of two structures, such as parts of the body, being in close contact. For example, the fingers are brought into apposition when the fist is clenched.

appraisal (ă-pray-z'l) *n.* the evaluation of an individual's performance, usually by an immediate line manager. Appraisals are performed on a regular basis for National Health Service employees.

apraclonidine (ap-ră-kloh-ni-deen) *n.* a sympathomimetic drug administered in the form of eye drops to reduce or prevent raised intraocular pressure after laser surgery. Trade name: **Iopidine**.

apraxia (dyspraxia) (ă-praks-iă) *n.* an inability to make skilled movements with accuracy. This is a disorder of the cerebral cortex most often caused by disease of the parietal lobes of the brain.

aprotinin (ă-proh-tin-in) *n.* a drug that prevents the breakdown of blood clots (fibrinolysis) by blocking the action of the enzyme plasmin, i.e. it is an antifibrinolytic drug. It is administered by injection to control the severe bleeding that may occur in certain cancers, with fibrinolytic treatments, and during open-heart surgery. Trade name: **Trasylol**.

APT *n.* alum precipitated toxoid: a preparation used for immunization against diphtheria.

APTT *n.* activated partial thromboplastin time (*see* PTTK).

APUD cells *pl. n.* cells that share the metabolic property of *amine*-precursor *u*ptake and *d*ecarboxylation. They are widely distributed, especially in the mucosa of the gastrointestinal tract and pancreas, and are able to form a large variety of peptide substances.

apudoma (apuud-oh-mă) *n.* a tumour that contains APUD cells and may give rise to symptoms caused by excessive production of the hormones and other peptides that these cells produce. Argentaffinomas, gastrinomas, and VIPomas are examples.

apyrexia (ap-I-reks-iă) *n.* the absence of fever.

aqua (ak-wă) *n.* water. *a. destillata* distilled water. *a. fortis* nitric acid.

aqueduct (ak-wi-dukt) *n.* (in anatomy) a canal containing fluid. *a. of the midbrain* (*cerebral a.*, *a. of Sylvius*) a canal connecting the third and fourth ventricles. [F. Sylvius de la Boe (1614–72), French anatomist]

aqueous humour (ay-kwi-ŭs) *n.* the watery fluid that fills the chamber of the eye immediately behind the cornea and in front of the lens.

arachidonic acid (ă-rak-i-don-ik) *n. see* essential fatty acid.

arachnodactyly (ă-rak-noh-dak-tili) *n. see* Marfan's syndrome.

arachnoid (arachnoid mater) (ă-rak-noid) *n.* the middle of the three membranes covering the brain and spinal cord (*see* meninges), which has a fine, almost cobweb-like, texture. *a. villi* thin-walled projections of the arachnoid into the blood-filled sinuses of the dura, through which cerebrospinal fluid flows from the subarachnoid space into the bloodstream. Large villi (*Pacchionian bodies*) are found in the region of the superior sagittal sinus.

arachnoiditis (ă-rak-noid-I-tis) *n.* an inflammatory process causing thickening and scarring (fibrosis) of the membranous linings (meninges) of the spinal canal. The resulting entrapment of nerve roots may result in weakness, pain, and numbness in the affected area. Arachnoiditis may result from infection of the meninges, surgery, or as a response to the oil-based dyes formerly used in myelography.

arbor (ar-ber) *n.* (in anatomy) a tree-like structure. *a. vitae* **1.** the tree-like outline of white matter seen in sections of the cerebellum. **2.** the treelike appearance of the inner folds of the cervix (neck) of the uterus.

arborization (ar-ber-I-zay-shŏn) *n.* the branching termination of certain neurone processes.

arbovirus (ar-boh-vy-rŭs) *n.* one of a group of RNA-containing viruses that are transmitted by arthropods (hence *arthropod-borne* viruses) and cause diseases resulting in encephalitis or serious fever, such as dengue and yellow fever.

ARC *n.* AIDS-related complex: *see* AIDS.

arch- (arche-, archi-, archo-) *prefix denoting* first; beginning; primitive; ancestral.

arcus (ar-kŭs) *n.* (in anatomy) an arch. *a. senilis* a greyish line in the periphery of the cornea, common in the elderly. It begins above and below the cornea but may become a continuous ring.

ARDS *n. see* adult respiratory distress syndrome.

areola (ă-ree-ŏlă) *n.* **1.** the brownish or pink ring of tissue surrounding the nipple of the breast. **2.** the part of the iris that surrounds the pupil of the eye. **3.** a small space in a tissue. —**areolar** (ă-ree-ŏler) *adj.*

areolar tissue *n.* loose connective tissue consisting of a meshwork of collagen, elastic tissue, and reticular fibres interspersed with numerous connective tissue cells.

ARF *n.* **1.** acute renal failure. **2.** acute respiratory failure.

argentaffin cells (ar-jen-tă-fin) *pl. n.* cells that stain readily with silver salts. Such cells occur, for example, in the crypts of Lieberkühn in the intestine.

argentaffinoma (carcinoid) (ar-jen-tafi-**noh**-mă) *n.* a tumour of the argentaffin cells in the glands of the intestine (*see* apudoma). Argentaffinomas typically occur in the tip of the appendix and are among the commonest tumours of the small intestine.

arginine (ar-ji-neen) *n.* an amino acid that plays an important role in the formation of urea by the liver.

argon laser (ar-gŏn) *n. see* laser.

Argyll Robertson pupil (ar-gyl rob-ert-sŏn) *n.* a disorder of the eyes, common to several diseases of the central nervous system (such as syphilis), in which the pupillary (light) reflex is absent. Although the pupils contract normally for near vision, they fail to contract in bright light. [D. Argyll Robertson (1837–1909), Scottish ophthalmologist]

ariboflavinosis (ă-ry-boh-flay-vin-oh-sis) *n.* the group of symptoms caused by deficiency of riboflavin (vitamin B₂). These symptoms include inflammation of the tongue and lips and sores in the corners of the mouth.

ARM *n.* artificial rupture of membranes: *see* amniotomy.

ARMD *n. see* (age-related) macular degeneration.

Arnold-Chiari malformation (ar-nʹld ki-ar-i) *n.* a congenital disorder in which there is distortion of the base of the skull with protrusion of the lower brainstem and parts of the cerebellum. [J. Arnold (1835–1915) and H. Chiari (1851–1916), German pathologists]

aromatase inhibitor (ă-roh-mă-tayz) *n.* any of a class of drugs used in the treatment of advanced breast cancer in postmenopausal women. By inhibiting the action of aromatase, an enzyme that promotes the conversion of testosterone to oestradiol, they reduce oestrogen levels, which helps in the control of oestrogen-dependent tumours. Aromatase inhibitors include *anastrazole* (Arimidex), *exemestane* (Aromasin), *formestan* (Lentaron), and *letrozole* (Femara). *See also* aminoglutethimide.

aromatherapy (ă-roh-mă-th'e-ră-pi) *n.* the therapeutic use of fragrances derived from essential oils. These can be inhaled through an infusion of the essential oils that pro-

duce them, or the oils can be combined with a base oil and massaged into the skin.

arrector pili (ă-rek-tor py-ly) *n.* (*pl.* **arrectores pilorum**) a small erector muscle attached to the hair follicle. Contraction of the arrectores pilorum causes goose flesh.

arrhythmia (ă-rith-miă) *n.* any deviation from the normal rhythm (sinus rhythm) of the heart. Arrhythmias include ectopic beats, ectopic tachycardias, fibrillation, and heart block. *sinus* (SA) a normal variation in the heart rate, which accelerates slightly on inspiration and slows on expiration.

arsenic (ar-sĕn-ik) *n.* a poisonous greyish metallic element producing the symptoms of nausea, vomiting, diarrhoea, cramps, convulsions, and coma when ingested in large doses. Arsenic was formerly used in medicine, the most important arsenical drugs being *arsphenamine* (*Salvarsan*) and *neoarsphenamine*, used in the treatment of syphilis and dangerous parasitic diseases. Symbol: As.

arter- (arteri-, arterio-) *prefix denoting* an artery.

arterial blood gases (ABGs) (ar-teer-iăl) *pl. n.* gases present in arterial blood, normally including oxygen, carbon dioxide, and nitrogen. Measurements of the partial pressures of oxygen and carbon dioxide, together with the blood's pH, give information on the oxygen saturation of the haemoglobin and the acid-base state of the blood, which is relevant in critical care situations and for those requiring respiratory support.

arteriectomy (ar-teer-i-ek-tŏmi) *n.*

surgical excision of an artery or part of an artery.

arteriogram (ar-teer-i-oh-gram) *n.* the image produced during arteriography, which is usually stored on photographic film or electronic media.

arteriography (ar-teer-i-og-răfi) *n.* imaging of arteries (*see* angiography). The major roles of arteriography are to demonstrate the site and extent of atheroma, especially in the coronary arteries (*see* coronary angiography) and leg arteries (*peripheral a.*), and to demonstrate the anatomy of aneurysms within the skull (*carotid* and *vertebral a.*).

arteriole (ar-teer-i-ohl) *n.* a small branch of an artery, leading into many smaller vessels – the capillaries. By their constriction and dilation, under the regulation of the sympathetic nervous system, arterioles are the principal controllers of blood flow and pressure.

arteriopathy (ar-teer-i-op-ăthi) *n.* disease of an artery.

arterioplasty (ar-teer-i-oh-plas-ti) *n.* surgical reconstruction of an artery; for example, in the treatment of aneurysms.

arteriorrhaphy (ar-teer-i-o-răfi) *n.* suture of an artery.

arteriosclerosis (ar-teer-i-oh-skleer-**oh**-sis) *n.* any of several conditions affecting the arteries, especially atherosclerosis.

arteriotomy (ar-teer-i-ot-ŏmi) *n.* an incision into, or a needle puncture of, the wall of an artery.

arteriovenous (ar-teer-i-oh-vee-nŭs) *adj.* relating to or affecting an artery and a vein. *a. anastomosis see* anastomosis. *a. fistula see* fistula. *a. malformation see* angioma.

arteritis (ar-ter-**I**-tis) *n.* an inflammatory disease affecting the muscular walls of the arteries. The affected vessels are swollen and tender and may become blocked. *temporal* (or *giant-cell*) *a.* a condition that occurs in the elderly. It most commonly affects the arteries of the scalp and blindness may result from thrombosis of the arteries to the eyes.

artery (ar-ter-i) *n.* a blood vessel carrying blood away from the heart. The walls of arteries contain smooth muscle fibres, which contract or relax under the control of the sympathetic nervous system. See illustration. *See also* aorta, arteriole. —**arterial** *adj.*

arthr- (arthro-) *prefix denoting* a joint.

arthralgia (arthrodynia) (arth-ral-jă) *n.* severe pain in a joint, without swelling or other signs of arthritis. *Compare* arthritis.

arthrectomy (arth-rek-tŏmi) *n.* surgical excision of a joint.

arthritis (arth-ry-tis) *n.* inflammation of one or more joints, characterized by swelling, warmth, redness of the overlying skin, pain, and restriction of motion. Any disease involving the synovial membranes or resulting in the degeneration of cartilage may cause arthritis. Treatment of arthritis depends on the cause, but aspirin and similar analgesics are often used to suppress inflammation, and hence reduce pain and swelling. *See also* juvenile chronic arthritis, osteoarthritis, psoriasis, rheumatoid arthritis, septic (arthritis), haemarthrosis, pyarthrosis, hydrarthrosis. —**arthritic** (arth-rit-ik) *adj.*

The principal arteries of the body

arthrocentesis (arth-roh-sen-tee-sis) *n.* aspiration of fluid from a joint through a puncture needle.

arthroclasia (arth-roh-klay-ziă) *n.* the surgical breaking down of ankylosis in a joint to permit freer movement.

arthrodesis (arth-roh-dee-sis) *n.* artificial ankylosis: the fusion of bones across a joint space by surgery, which eliminates movement.

arthrodynia (arth-roh-din-iă) *n. see* arthralgia.

arthrography (arth-rog-răfi) *n.* an X-ray imaging technique for examining joints. A contrast medium (either radiolucent gas or radiopaque material) is injected into the joint space, outlining its contents and extent accurately.

arthrogryposis (arth-roh-gri-poh-sis) *n.* congenital defects of limbs characterized by contractures (both flexion and extension) causing fixed deformities of the joints if untreated. *a. multiplex congenita* a congenital disease with multiple causes in which there are contractures, stiff joints, and absent skin creases, as a result of the muscles being replaced by fibrous tissue.

arthropathy (arth-rop-ăthi) *n.* any disease or disorder involving a joint.

arthroplasty (arth-roh-plasti) *n.* surgical remodelling of a diseased joint. To prevent the ends of the bones fusing after the operation, a large gap may be created between them (*gap* or *excision a.*), a barrier of artificial material may be inserted (*interposition a.*), or one or both bone ends may be replaced by a prosthesis of metal or plastic (*replacement a.*). *McKee-Farrar a.* replacement arthroplasty of the hip joint. Both the head of the femur and the acetabulum are replaced by metal prostheses; the replacement acetabulum is cemented into the bone. *total a.* replacement arthroplasty in which both joint surfaces are replaced. *See also* hemiarthroplasty.

arthroscope (arth-roh-skohp) *n.* a telescope that is inserted into a joint through a small incision in order to inspect its contents (*see* arthroscopy).

arthroscopy (ar-thros-kŏpi) *n.* inspection of a joint cavity with an arthroscope, enabling percutaneous surgery (such as meniscectomy) and biopsy to be performed.

arthrostomy (ar-thros-tŏmi) *n.* a procedure to enable a temporary opening to be made into a joint cavity.

arthrotomy (arth-rot-ŏmi) *n.* a surgical incision to open a joint in order to inspect the contents or to drain pus (in septic arthritis).

articulation (ar-tik-yoo-lay-shŏn) *n.* (in anatomy) the point or type of contact between two bones. *See* joint.

artificial heart (ar-ti-fish-ăl) *n.* a titanium pump that is implanted into the body to take over the function of a failing left ventricle in patients with heart disease. This allows the diseased ventricle time to recover its function. The pump is powered by an external battery, strapped to the patient's body, to which it is connected by wires passed through the patient's skin. The most recent devices are small enough to fit into the heart itself.

artificial insemination *n.* instrumental introduction of semen into the vagina in order that a woman may conceive. The semen specimen may be provided by the husband (*AIH – artificial insemination by husband*) in cases of impotence or by an anonymous donor (*DI – donor insemination*), usually in cases where the husband is sterile.

artificial kidney (dialyser) *n.* see haemodialysis.

artificial respiration *n.* an emergency procedure for maintaining a flow of air into and out of a patient's lungs when the natural breathing reflexes are absent or insufficient. The simplest and most efficient method is mouth-to-mouth respiration.

artificial rupture of membranes (ARM) *n.* see amniotomy.

artificial sphincter *n.* an apparatus designed to replace or support a sphincter that is either absent or ineffective. *See also* neosphincter.

arytenoid cartilage (a-ri-tee-noid) *n.* either of the two pyramid-shaped cartilages that lie at the back of the larynx next to the upper edges of the cricoid cartilage.

arytenoidectomy (a-ri-tee-noid-ek-tŏmi) *n.* surgical excision of the arytenoid cartilage of the larynx in the treatment of paralysis of the vocal folds.

asbestos (ass-best-os) *n.* a fibrous mineral that is incombustible and does not conduct heat. It is used in the form of fabric or boards for its heat-resistant properties.

asbestosis (ass-best-oh-sis) *n.* a lung disease – a form of pneumoconiosis – caused by fibres of asbestos inhaled by those who are exposed to the mineral. *See also* mesothelioma.

ascariasis (askă-ry-ăsis) *n.* a disease caused by an infestation with the parasitic worm *Ascaris lumbricoides*. Adult worms in the intestine can cause abdominal pain, vomiting, constipation, diarrhoea, appendicitis, and peritonitis; migrating larvae in the lungs can provoke pneumonia.

Ascaris (ass-kă-ris) *n.* a genus of parasitic nematode worms. *A. lumbricoides* the largest of the human intestinal nematodes. Larvae hatch out in the intestine and then migrate via the hepatic portal vein, liver, heart, lungs, windpipe, and pharynx, before returning to the intestine where they later develop into adult worms (*see also* ascariasis).

Aschoff nodules (ash-off) *pl. n.* nodules that occur in the muscular and connective tissue of the heart in rheumatic myocarditis. [K. A. L. Aschoff (1866–1942), German pathologist]

ascites (hydroperitoneum) (ă-sy-teez) *n.* the accumulation of fluid in the peritoneal cavity, causing abdominal swelling. *chylous a.* ascites that occurs when the drainage of lymph from the abdomen is obstructed. *See also* oedema.

ascorbic acid (ă-skor-bik) *n.* see vitamin C.

ASD *n.* see (atrial) septal defect.

-ase *suffix denoting* an enzyme.

asepsis (ay-sep-sis) *n.* the complete absence of bacteria, fungi, viruses, or other microorganisms that could cause disease. Asepsis is the ideal state for the performance of surgical operations and is achieved by using sterilization techniques. —**aseptic** *adj.*

Asherman syndrome (ash-er-măn) n. a condition in which amenorrhoea and infertility follow a major haemorrhage in pregnancy. It may result from overvigorous curettage of the uterus in an attempt to control the bleeding. This removes the lining, the walls adhere, and the cavity is obliterated to a greater or lesser degree. *Compare* Sheehan's syndrome. [J. G. Asherman (20th century), Czechoslovakian gynaecologist]

asparaginase (ă-spa-ră-jin-ayz) n. an enzyme that inhibits the growth of certain tumours and is used (in the form of *crisantaspase*) in the treatment of acute lymphoblastic leukaemia. Trade name: **Erwinase**.

asparagine (ă-spa-ră-jeen) n. *see* amino acid.

aspartate aminotransferase (AST) (ass-par-tayt) n. an enzyme involved in the transamination of amino acids. Measurement of AST in the serum may be used in the diagnosis of acute myocardial infarction and acute liver disease. It was formerly called *serum glutamic oxaloacetic transaminase* (*SGOT*).

aspartic acid (aspartate) (ă-spar-tik) n. *see* amino acid.

Asperger's syndrome (ass-pergerz) n. a mild form of autism characterized by aloofness, lack of interest in other people, stilted and pedantic styles of speech, and an excessive preoccupation with a very specialized interest (such as timetables). [H. Asperger (1906–80), Austrian paediatrician]

aspergillosis (ass-per-jil-oh-sis) n. a group of conditions caused by fungi of the genus *Aspergillus*, usually *Aspergillus fumigatus*. These conditions nearly always arise in patients with pre-existing lung disease and fall into three categories. The allergic form most commonly affects asthmatic patients and may cause collapse of segments or lobes of a lung. The colonizing form leads to formation of a fungus ball (*aspergilloma*), usually within a pre-existing cavity in the lung. In the third category the fungus spreads throughout the lungs and may even disseminate throughout the body; this form is rare but potentially fatal.

Aspergillus (ass-per-jil-ŭs) n. a genus of fungi, including many common moulds, some of which cause infections of the respiratory system in humans. *A. fumigatus* the cause of aspergillosis.

aspermia (ă-sperm-iă) n. strictly, a lack or failure of formation of semen. More usually, however, the term is used to mean the total absence of sperm from the semen (*see* azoospermia).

asphyxia (ă-sfiks-iă) n. suffocation: a life-threatening condition in which oxygen is prevented from reaching the tissues by obstruction of or damage to any part of the respiratory system.

aspiration (ass-per-ay-shŏn) n. the withdrawal of fluid from the body by means of suction. **vacuum a.** a method of terminating pregnancy by suction of the products of conception through an intrauterine cannula. *See also* (aspiration) cytology, endometrial (aspiration).

aspirator (ass-per-ay-ter) n. any of various instruments used for aspiration. Some employ hollow needles for removing fluid from cysts, inflamed joint cavities, etc.; another kind is used to suck debris and water from the patient's mouth during dental treatment.

aspirin (acetylsalicylic acid) (*ass*-prin) *n.* a widely used drug that relieves pain and also reduces inflammation and fever. It is taken by mouth for the relief of headache, toothache, neuralgias, etc. It is also taken to reduce fever in influenza and the common cold, and daily doses are used in the prevention of coronary thrombosis and strokes in those at risk. Aspirin works by inhibiting the production of prostaglandins; it may irritate the lining of the stomach, causing nausea, vomiting, pain, and bleeding. It has been implicated as a cause of Reye's syndrome and should therefore not be given to children below the age of 15 unless specifically indicated.

assertion (ă-ser-shŏn) *n.* the skill to communicate positively in order to press one's own claims, rights, or opinions.

assessment (ă-ses-mĕnt) *n.* **1.** the first stage of the nursing process, in which data about the patient's health status is collected and from which a nursing care plan may be devised. **2.** an examination set by an examining body to test a candidate's theoretical and practical nursing skills.

assimilation (ă-simi-lay-shŏn) *n.* the process by which food substances are taken into the cells of the body after they have been digested and absorbed.

assistive listening device (ă-sis-tiv) *n. see* hearing aid.

associate nurse (ă-soh-si-ăt) *n.* a nurse who provides care for a patient on the instructions of the patient's primary nurse or in her absence. *See* primary nursing.

association area (ă-soh-si-ay-shŏn) *n.* an area of cerebral cortex that lies away from the main areas that are concerned with the reception of sensory impulses and the start of motor impulses but is linked to them by many neurones (*association fibres*).

association of ideas *n.* (in psychology) linkage of one idea to another in a regular way according to their meaning. *See also* free association.

AST *n. see* aspartate aminotransferase.

astereognosis (ă-ste-ri-ŏg-noh-sis) *n. see* agnosia.

asteroid hyalosis (ass-tĕ-roid hy-ă-loh-sis) *n.* a degenerative condition, formerly known as *asteroid hyalitis*, in which tiny deposits of calcium are suspended in the vitreous humour. Vision is usually not affected.

asthenia (ass-theen-iă) *n.* weakness or loss of strength.

asthenic (ass-th'en-ik) *adj.* describing a personality disorder characterized by low energy, susceptibility to physical and emotional stress, and a diminished capacity for pleasure.

asthenopia (ass-thi-noh-piă) *n. see* eyestrain.

asthenospermia (ass-thi-noh-sper-miă) *n.* the presence in the semen of spermatozoa with poor motility, revealed by seminal analysis.

asthma (ass-mă) *n.* the condition of subjects with widespread narrowing of the bronchial airways, which changes in severity over short periods of time and leads to coughing, wheezing, and difficulty in breathing. *bronchial a.* asthma that may be precipitated by exposure to one or more of a wide range of stimuli, including allergens, drugs (such as aspirin), exertion, emotion, infections, and air pollution. Treatment is with bronchodilators, with or without corticosteroids, usually administered via aerosol or dry-powder inhalers, or – if the condition is more severe – via a nebulizer. Severe asthmatic attacks may need large doses or oral corticosteroids (*see* status asthmaticus). *cardiac a.* asthma that occurs in left ventricular heart failure and must be distinguished from bronchial asthma, as the treatment is quite different. —**asthmatic** (ass-mat-ik) *adj.*

astigmatism (ă-stig-mă-tizm) *n.* a defect of vision in which the image of an object is distorted because not all the light rays come to a focus on the retina. This is usually due to abnormal curvature of the cornea and/or lens, whose surface resembles part of the surface of an egg (rather than a sphere). —**astigmatic** (ass-tig-mat-ik) *adj.*

astragalus (ass-trag-ălŭs) *n. see* talus.

astringent (ă-strin-jĕnt) *n.* a drug that causes cells to shrink by precipitating proteins from their surfaces. Astringents are used in lotions to harden and protect the skin and to reduce bleeding from minor abrasions.

astrocytoma (ass-troh-sy-toh-mă) *n.* any brain tumour derived from non-nervous supporting cells (glia), which may be benign or malignant.

In adults astrocytomas are usually found in the cerebral hemispheres but in children they also occur in the cerebellum.

asymmetric tonic neck reflex *n.* a primitive reflex that is present from birth but should disappear by six months of age. If the infant is lying on its back and the head is turned to one side, the arm and leg on the side to which the head is turned should straighten, and the arm and leg on the opposite side should bend (the 'fencer' position). Persistence of the reflex beyond six months is suggestive of cerebral palsy.

asymmetry (ay-sim-it-ri) *n.* (in anatomy) the state in which opposite parts of an organ or parts at opposite sides of the body do not correspond with each other. —**asymmetric** (ay-si-met-rik) *adj.*

asymptomatic (ay-simp-tŏm-at-ik) *adj.* not showing any symptoms of disease, whether disease is present or not.

asynclitism (ă-sin-klit-izm) *n.* tilting of the fetal skull towards one or other shoulder causing the top of the skull to be either nearer to the sacrum (*anterior a.* or *Naegele's obliquity*) or nearer to the pubis (*posterior a.* or *Litzmann's obliquity*). These mechanisms enable the fetal head to pass more easily through the maternal pelvis.

asynergia (a-sin-er-jiă) *n. see* dyssynergia.

asystole (ă-sis-tŏ-li) *n.* a condition in which the heart no longer beats, accompanied by the absence of complexes in the electrocardiogram. —**asystolic** (a-sis-tol-ik) *adj.*

ataraxia (at-ă-raks-iă) *n.* a state of

calmness and freedom from anxiety, especially the state produced by tranquillizing drugs.

atavism (at-ă-vizm) *n.* the phenomenon in which an individual has a character or disease known to have occurred in a remote ancestor but not in his parents.

ataxia (ă-taks-iă) *n.* the shaky movements and unsteady gait that result from the brain's failure to regulate the body's posture and the strength and direction of limb movements. **cerebellar a.** a condition in which the patient staggers when walking, cannot pronounce words properly, and may have nystagmus. **Friedreich's a.** an inherited disorder appearing first in adolescence. It has the features of cerebellar ataxia, together with spasticity of the limbs. **sensory a.** ataxia that is exaggerated when the patient closes his eyes (*see* Romberg's sign). *See also* ataxia telangiectasia, tabes dorsalis (locomotor ataxia). **—ataxic** *adj.*

ataxia telangiectasia (til-an-ji-ek-**tay**-ziă) *n.* an inherited (autosomal recessive) neurological disorder. Ataxia is usually noted early in life. Prominent blood vessels are visible in the sclerae of the eyes, and mental retardation, growth retardation, abnormal eye movements, skin lesions, and immune deficiency may be found.

atel- (atelo-) *prefix denoting* imperfect or incomplete development.

atelectasis (at-ĕ-**lek**-tă-sis) *n.* failure of part of the lung to expand. This occurs when the cells lining the alveoli are immature, as in premature babies; it also occurs when the larger bronchial tubes are blocked by retained secretions, in-

haled foreign bodies, bronchial cancers, or enlarged lymph nodes.

atenolol *n.* a drug (*see* beta blocker) used to treat angina and high blood pressure. It is administered by mouth or intravenous injection. Trade name: **Tenormin**.

atherogenic (ath-er-oh-**jen**-ik) *adj.* denoting a factor that may cause atheroma. Such factors include cigarette smoking, excessive consumption of animal fats and refined sugar, obesity, and inactivity.

atheroma (ath-er-**oh**-ma) *n.* degeneration of the walls of the arteries due to the formation in them of fatty plaques and scar tissue. This limits blood circulation and predisposes to thrombosis. **—atheromatous** *adj.*

atherosclerosis (ath-er-oh-skleer-**oh**-sis) *n.* a disease of the arteries in which fatty plaques develop on their inner walls, with eventual obstruction of blood flow. *See* atheroma.

athetosis (ath-ĕ-**toh**-sis) *n.* a writhing involuntary movement especially affecting the hands, face, and tongue. It is usually a form of cerebral palsy but can be caused by drugs used to treat parkinsonism or by the withdrawal of phenothiazines. **—athetotic** *adj.*

athlete's foot (ath-leets) *n.* a fungus infection of the skin between the toes: a type of ringworm. Medical name: **tinea pedis**.

atlas (at-lăs) *n.* the first cervical vertebra, by means of which the skull is articulated to the backbone.

ATLS *n.* advanced trauma life support, which comprises the treatment programmes for patients who have been subjected to major trauma (e.g. serious road traffic accidents, missile injuries). Doctors, nurses, and paramedical personnel involved in ATLS receive special training for dealing with such emergencies.

ATN *n. see* (acute) tubular necrosis.

atom (at-ŏm) *n.* the smallest constituent of an element that can take part in a chemical reaction. An atom consists of a positively charged nucleus with negatively charged electrons orbiting around it.

atomizer (at-ŏ-my-zer) *n.* an instrument that reduces liquids to a fine spray of minute droplets.

atony (at-ŏni) *n.* a state in which muscles are floppy, lacking their normal elasticity. —**atonic** (ă-ton-ik) *adj.*

atopen (at-oh-pĕn) *n. see* atopy.

atopy (at-oh-pi) *n.* a form of allergy in which there is a hereditary or constitutional tendency to develop hypersensitivity reactions (e.g. hay fever, allergic asthma, atopic eczema) in response to allergens (*atopens*). Individuals with this predisposition – and the conditions provoked in them by contact with allergens – are described as *atopic*.

atorvastatin (at-or-vas-tă-tin) *n.* a drug used to reduce abnormally high levels of cholesterol and other lipids in the blood (*see* statin). It is administered by mouth. Trade name: **Lipitor**.

ATP (adenosine triphosphate) *n.* a compound that contains adenine, ribose, and three phosphate groups and occurs in cells. The chemical bonds of the phosphate groups store energy needed by the cell, for muscle contraction; this energy is released when ATP is split into ADP or AMP. ATP is formed from ADP or AMP using energy produced by the breakdown of carbohydrates or other food substances. *See also* mitochondrion.

atracurium besilate (at-ră-kewr-iŭm bes-il-ayt) *n.* a muscle relaxant administered by injection during anaesthesia. Trade name: **Tracrium**.

atresia (ă-tree-ziă) *n.* **1.** congenital absence or abnormal narrowing of a body opening. *biliary a.* narrowing of the bile ducts, which fail to drain, causing jaundice in affected babies. *duodenal a.* narrowing of the duodenum, causing complete obstruction of its lumen. *tricuspid a.* absence of the tricuspid valve, with resultant lack of communication between the right atrium and right ventricle of the heart. **2.** the degenerative process that affects the majority of ovarian follicles. Usually only one Graafian follicle will ovulate in each menstrual cycle. —**atretic** (ă-tret-ik) *adj.*

atri- (atrio-) *prefix denoting* an atrium, especially the atrium of the heart.

atrial (ay-tri-ăl) *adj.* of or relating to the atrium or atria. *a. fibrillation see* fibrillation. *a. septal defect see* septal defect.

atrioventricular (AV) (ay-tri-oh-ven-trik-yoo-ler) *adj.* relating to the atria and ventricles of the heart.

atrioventricular bundle (AV bundle, bundle of His) *n.* a bundle of modified heart muscle fibres (*Purkinje fibres*) passing from the atrioventricular (AV) node forward to the septum between the ventricles, where it divides into right and left bundles, one for each ventricle. The fibres transmit contraction waves from the atria, via the AV node, to the ventricles.

atrioventricular node (AV node) *n.* a mass of modified heart muscle situated in the lower middle part of the right atrium. It receives the impulse to contract from the sinoatrial node, via the atria, and transmits it through the atrioventricular bundle to the ventricles.

atrium (ay-tri-ŭm) *n.* (*pl.* **atria**) **1.** either of the two upper chambers of the heart. The left atrium receives arterial blood from the lungs via the pulmonary artery; the right atrium receives venous blood from the venae cavae. *See also* auricle. **2.** any of various anatomical chambers into which one or more cavities open. —**atrial** *adj.*

atrophy (at-rŏ-fi) *n.* the wasting away of a normally developed organ or tissue due to degeneration of cells. This may occur through undernourishment, disuse, or ageing. **muscular a.** atrophy of muscular tissue associated with various diseases, such as poliomyelitis. *See also* multiple system atrophy, spinal muscular atrophy, Sudek's atrophy.

atropine (at-rŏ-peen) *n.* an anticholinergic drug extracted from belladonna. Atropine relaxes smooth muscle and is used to treat biliary colic and renal colic. It also reduces secretions of the bronchial tubes, salivary glands, stomach, and intestines and is used before general anaesthesia and to relieve peptic ulcers. It is also used to dilate the pupil of the eye. Trade name: **Minims Atropine**.

ATT *n.* antitetanus toxoid. *See* DPT vaccine.

attachment (ă-tach-mĕnt) *n.* **1.** (in

psychology) the process of developing the first close selective relationship of a child's life, most commonly with the mother. **a. disorder** a psychiatric disorder in infants and young children resulting from institutionalization, emotional neglect, or child abuse. Affected children are either withdrawn, aggressive, and fearful or attention-seeking and indiscriminately friendly. **2.** (in Britain) working arrangements in the National Health Service by which district nurses, social workers, etc., are engaged in association with specific general practitioners, caring for their registered patients rather than working solely on a geographical or district basis.

attention-deficit/hyperactivity disorder (ADHD, hyperkinetic disorder) (ă-ten-shŏn def-i-sit dis-or-der) *n.* a mental disorder, usually of children, characterized by a grossly excessive level of activity and a marked impairment of the ability to attend, resulting in aggressive disruptive behaviour. Treatment usually involves drugs (such as methylphenidate) and behaviour therapy.

attenuation (ă-ten-yoo-ay-shŏn) *n.* reduction of the disease-producing ability (virulence) of a bacterium or virus so that it may be used for immunization.

atticotomy (at-i-kot-ŏmi) *n.* a surgical operation to remove cholesteatoma from the ear. It is a form of limited mastoidectomy.

atypical (ay-tip-ik-ăl) *adj.* not conforming to type. **a. antipsychotic** *see* antipsychotic. **a. facial pain** neuralgia typified by pain in the face that does not fit the distribution of nerves. *a. pneumonia* pneumonia, caused by such organisms as *Mycoplasma pneumoniae*, that does not respond to penicillin but does respond to such antibiotics as tetracycline and erythromycin.

audi- (audio-) *prefix denoting* hearing or sound.

audiogram (aw-dioh-gram) *n*. the graphic record of a test of hearing carried out on an audiometer.

audiology (awdi-ol-ŏji) *n*. the study of disorders of hearing.

audiometer (awdi-om-it-er) *n*. an apparatus for measuring hearing at different sound frequencies, so helping in the diagnosis of deafness. —**audiometry** *n*.

audit (aw-dit) *n*. *see* clinical audit, nursing audit.

auditory (aw-dit-er-i) *adj*. relating to the ear or to the sense of hearing. *a. canal* the canal leading from the pinna to the eardrum. *a. nerve see* vestibulocochlear nerve.

auditory verbal therapy (AVT) *n*. a technique for teaching deaf children to communicate that focuses on speech and residual hearing rather than sign language.

Auerbach's plexus (myenteric plexus) (ow-er-bahks) *n*. a collection of nerve fibres – fine branches of the vagus nerve – within the walls of the intestine. It supplies the muscle layers and controls the movements of peristalsis. [L. Auerbach (1828–97), German anatomist]

AUR *n*. *see* (acute urinary) retention.

aura (or-ă) *n*. the forewarning of an attack, as occurs in epilepsy (e.g. as an odd smell or taste) and migraine (e.g. as flickering lights, blurring of vision, pins and needles).

aural (or-ăl) *adj*. relating to the ear.

auranofin (or-an-oh-fin) *n*. a gold preparation administered by mouth to treat rheumatoid arthritis. Side-effects include nausea, abdominal pain, diarrhoea, and mouth ulcers. Trade name: **Ridaura**.

Aureomycin (or-i-oh-my-sin) *n*. *see* chlortetracycline.

auricle (or-i-k'l) *n*. **1.** a small pouch in the wall of each atrium of the heart: the term is also used incorrectly as a synonym for atrium. **2.** *see* pinna.

auriscope (otoscope) (or-i-skohp) *n*. an apparatus for examining the eardrum and the external meatus.

light
lens and viewing aperture
speculum
switch
battery case and handle

An auriscope

auscultation (aw-skŭl-tay-shŏn) *n*. the process of listening, usually with a stethoscope, to sounds produced by movement of gas or liquid within the body, as an aid to diagnosis. —**auscultatory** *adj*.

Australia antigen (oss-tray-liă) *n*. another name for the hepatitis B antigen, first found in the blood of an Australian aborigine.

aut- (auto-) *prefix denoting* self.

autism (aw-tizm) *n.* **1. (Kanner's syndrome, infantile autism)** a psychiatric disorder of childhood marked by severe difficulties in communicating and forming relationships with other people, in developing language, and in using abstract concepts; repetitive and limited patterns of behaviour; and obsessive resistance to tiny changes in familiar surroundings. About 50% of autistic children have learning disabilities, but some are gifted in specific areas. **2.** the condition of retreating from realistic thinking to self-centred fantasy thinking: a symptom of personality disorder and schizophrenia. —**autistic** *adj.*

autoantibody (aw-toh-an-ti-bodi) *n.* an antibody formed against one of the body's own components in an autoimmune disease.

autoclave (aw-tŏ-klayv) **1.** *n.* a piece of sterilizing equipment in which surgical instruments, dressings, etc., are treated with steam at high pressure. **2.** *vb.* to sterilize in an autoclave.

autogenous (aw-toj-in-ŭs) *adj.* originating within the body of the patient. *a. vein graft* a graft to bypass a blocked artery, made from material derived from the body of the patient receiving the graft.

autograft (aw-tŏ-grahft) *n.* a tissue graft taken from one part of the body and transferred to another part of the same individual. Unlike allografts, autografts are not rejected by the body's immunity defences. *See also* skin (graft).

autoimmune disease (aw-toh-i-mewn) *n.* one of a group of otherwise unrelated disorders caused by inflammation and destruction of tissues by the body's own immune response. These disorders include pernicious anaemia, rheumatic fever, rheumatoid arthritis, glomerulonephritis, myasthenia gravis, and Hashimoto's disease.

autoimmunity (aw-toh-i-mewn-iti) *n.* a disorder of the body's defence mechanisms in which an immune response is generated against components or products of its own tissues, treating them as foreign material and attacking them. *See* autoimmune disease, immunity.

autoinfection (aw-toh-in-fek-shŏn) *n.* **1.** infection by an organism that is already present in the body. **2.** infection transferred from one part of the body to another via the fingers, towels, etc.

autointoxication (aw-toh-in-toks-i-kay-shŏn) *n.* poisoning by a toxin formed within the body.

autologous (aw-tol-ŏ-gŭs) *adj.* denoting a graft that is derived from the recipient of the graft.

autolysis (aw-tol-i-sis) *n.* the destruction of tissues or cells brought about by the actions of their own enzymes. *See* lysosome.

automatism (aw-tom-ă-tizm) *n.* behaviour that may be associated with epilepsy, in which the patient performs well-organized movements or tasks while unaware of doing so.

autonomic nervous system (aw-tŏ-nom-ik) *n.* the part of the peripheral nervous system responsible for the control of involuntary muscles (e.g. heart, bladder, bowels) and hence bodily functions that are not consciously directed. *See* parasympathetic nervous system, sympathetic nervous system.

autonomy (aw-tonn-ŏmi) *n.* the right of personal freedom of action, said to be one of the characteristics of a profession.

autopsy (necropsy, post mortem) (aw-top-si) *n.* dissection and examination of a body after death to determine the cause of death or the presence of disease.

autoradiography (radioautography) (aw-toh-ray-di-og-răfi) *n.* a technique for examining the distribution of a radioactive tracer in the tissues of an experimental animal.

autoscopy (aw-tos-kŏpi) *n.* the experience of seeing one's whole body as though from a vantage point some distance away. It can be a symptom in epilepsy. *See also* out-of-the-body experience.

autosomal (aw-tŏ-soh-măl) *adj.* relating to an autosome. *a.* **dominant** denoting hereditary diseases in which the defective gene is dominant and will therefore tend to be inherited by (and be expressed in) 50% of the offspring (of either sex) of the person with the disease. *a.* **recessive** denoting inherited diseases in which the defective gene is recessive but not sex-linked. *See also* recessive.

autosome (aw-tŏ-sohm) *n.* any chromosome that is not a sex chromosome and that occurs in pairs in diploid cells.

autosuggestion (aw-toh-sŭ-jes-chŏn) *n.* self-suggestion or self-conditioning that involves repeating ideas to oneself in order to change psychological or physiological states. *See* suggestion.

autotransfusion (aw-toh-transfew-zhŏn) *n.* reintroduction into a patient of his or her own blood, which has either been previously drawn and stored in a blood bank or lost and then collected from the patient's circulation during surgical operation.

aux- (auxo-) *prefix denoting* increase; growth.

AV *adj. see* atrioventricular.

avascular (ă-vas-kew-ler) *adj.* lacking blood vessels or having a poor blood supply.

aversion therapy (ă-ver-shŏn) *n.* a form of behaviour therapy that is used (now rarely) to reduce the occurrence of undesirable behaviour. The patient is conditioned by repeated pairing of some unpleasant stimulus with a stimulus related to the undesirable behaviour. *See also* sensitization.

avitaminosis (avi-tami-noh-sis) *n.* the condition caused by lack of a vitamin. *See also* deficiency disease.

AVM *n.* arteriovenous malformation (*see* angioma).

avoidant (ă-void-ănt) *adj.* describing a personality type characterized by self-consciousness, hypersensitivity to rejection and criticism, avoidance of normal situations because of their potential risk, high levels of tension and anxiety, and consequently a restricted life.

AVPU *n.* a system for assessing the depth of unconsciousness: A = alert; V = voice responses present; P = pain responses present; U = unresponsive. It is useful for judging the severity of head injury and the need for specialized neurosurgical assistance before formal evaluation using the Glasgow scoring system.

AVT *n. see* auditory verbal therapy.

avulsion (ă-vul-shŏn) *n.* the tearing

or forcible separation of part of a structure.

axilla (ak-sil-ă) *n.* (*pl.* **axillae**) the armpit. —**axillary** *adj.*

axis (aks-is) *n.* **1.** a real or imaginary line through the centre of the body or one of its parts or a line about which the body or a part rotates. **2.** the second cervical vertebra, which articulates with the atlas vertebra above and allows rotational movement of the head.

axon (aks-on) *n.* a nerve fibre: a single process extending from the cell body of a neurone and carrying nerve impulses away from it.

axonotmesis (aks-on-ŏt-mee-sis) *n.* rupture of nerve fibres (axons) within an intact nerve sheath. This may result from prolonged pressure or crushing and it is followed by peripheral degeneration of the nerve beyond the point of rupture. The prognosis for regeneration is good.

azapropazone (ază-proh-pă-zohn) *n.* an anti-inflammatory drug (*see* NSAID) taken by mouth to treat rheumatoid arthritis, osteoarthritis, ankylosing spondylitis, and gout. Trade name: **Rheumox**.

azatadine (ay-zat-ă-deen) *n.* an antihistamine used to treat hay fever, urticaria, itching, and stings. It is administered by mouth. Trade name: **Optimine**.

azathioprine (ază-th'y-ŏ-preen) *n.* an immunosuppressant drug, used mainly to aid the survival of organ or tissue transplants. Trade name: **Imuran**.

azelaic acid (az-ĕ-lay-ik) *n.* an antibacterial drug applied externally as a cream in the treatment of acne. Trade name: **Skinoren**.

azelastine (ay-zel-ă-steen) *n.* an antihistamine drug that is administered in a metered-dose nasal spray for the treatment of hay fever and as eye drops to treat allergic conjunctivitis. Trade names: **Optilast**, **Rhinolast**.

azithromycin (ă-zith-roh-my-sin) *n.* an antibiotic used to treat respiratory, skin, soft-tissue, and other infections, especially those caused by the organism *Chlamydia trachomatis*. It is administered by mouth. Trade name: **Zithromax**.

azo- (**azoto-**) *prefix denoting* a nitrogenous compound, such as urea.

azoospermia (aspermia) (ay-zoh-ŏ-sperm-iă) *n.* the absence of sperm from the seminal fluid.

azotaemia (azŏ-tee-miă) *n.* a former name for uraemia.

azoturia (azŏ-tewr-iă) *n.* the presence in the urine of an abnormally high concentration of nitrogenous compounds, especially urea.

aztreonam (az-tree-ŏ-nam) *n.* an antibiotic administered by injection to treat infections caused by Gram-negative organisms. It is especially useful for treating lung infections in children with cystic fibrosis. Trade name: **Azactam**.

azygos vein (az-i-gos) *n.* an unpaired vein that arises from the inferior vena cava and drains into the superior vena cava, returning blood from the thorax and abdomen.

Babinski reflex (extensor response) (ba-**bin**-ski) *n.* an upward movement of the big toe that is an abnormal plantar reflex indicating damage to the pyramidal system in the brain or spinal cord in those over the age of 18 months. [J. F. F. Babinski (1857–1932), French neurologist]

baby blues (bay-bi) *n. see* postnatal (depression).

bacillaemia (ba-si-lee-miă) *n.* the presence of bacilli in the blood, resulting from infection.

bacille Calmette-Guérin (ba-seel kal-met gay-**ran**) *n. see* BCG. [A. L. C. Calmette (1863–1933) and C. Guérin (1872–1961), French bacteriologists]

bacilluria (ba-sil-**yoor**-iă) *n.* the presence of bacilli in the urine, resulting from a bladder or kidney infection. *See* cystitis.

bacillus (bă-**sil**-ŭs) *n.* (*pl.* **bacilli**) any rod-shaped bacterium. *See also* Bacillus, Lactobacillus, Streptobacillus.

Bacillus *n.* a large genus of Gram-positive spore-bearing rodlike bacteria. They are widely distributed in soil and air (usually as spores). *B. anthracis* a nonmotile species that causes anthrax. *B. polymyxa* the source of the polymyxin group of antibiotics. *B. subtilis* a species that may cause conjunctivitis; it also produces the antibiotic bacitracin.

bacitracin (ba-si-**tray**-sin) *n.* an antibiotic produced by certain strains of bacteria and effective against a number of microorganisms. Combined with other antibiotics, it is applied externally to treat infections of the skin and eyes.

backbone (spinal column, spine, vertebral column) (bak-bohn) *n.* the flexible bony column, extending from the base of the skull to the small of the back, that encloses and protects the spinal cord. It is made up of individual bones (*see* vertebra) connected by discs of fibrocartilage (*see* intervertebral disc). The backbone of a newborn baby contains 33 vertebrae: seven cervical, 12 thoracic, five lumbar, five sacral, and four coccygeal. In the adult the sacral and coccygeal vertebrae become fused into two single bones (sacrum and coccyx, respectively). See illustration. Anatomical name: **rachis**.

back slaps (bak) *pl. n.* a manoeuvre for the treatment of a choking patient. Firm slaps are given to the patient's back in an attempt to dislodge the obstructing article from the upper airway.

baclofen (bak-lō-fen) *n.* a skeletal muscle relaxant drug administered orally to relieve spasm resulting from injury or disease of the brain or spinal cord, including cerebral palsy and multiple sclerosis. Trade names: **Baclospas, Lioresal**.

cervical vertebrae (7)

thoracic vertebrae (12)

lumbar vertebrae (5)

sacrum (5 fused)

coccyx (4 fused)

A   B

The backbone, seen from the back (A) and left side (B)

bacteraemia (bak-ter-ee-miă) *n.* the presence of bacteria in the blood: a sign of infection.

bacteri- (bacterio-) *prefix denoting* bacteria.

bacteria (bak-teer-iă) *pl. n.* (*sing.* **bacterium**) a group of microorganisms all of which lack a distinct nuclear membrane and most of which have a cell wall of unique composition. Most bacteria are unicellular; the cells may be spherical (see coccus), rodlike (see bacillus), spiral (see Spirillum), comma-shaped (see Vibrio) or corkscrew-shaped (see spirochaete). Generally, they range in size between 0.5 and 5 μm. Motile species bear one or more fine hairs (flagella) arising from their surface. Bacteria reproduce asexually by simple division of cells. They live in soil, water, or air or as parasites of humans, animals, and plants. Some parasitic bacteria cause diseases by producing poisons (see endotoxin, exotoxin). —**bacterial** adj.

bactericidal (bak-teer-i-sy-dǎl) adj. capable of killing bacteria. Substances with this property include antibiotics, antiseptics, and disinfectants. Compare bacteriostatic. —**bactericide** n.

bacteriology (bak-teer-i-ol-ŏji) n. the science concerned with the study of bacteria. See also microbiology. —**bacteriological** adj. —**bacteriologist** n.

bacteriolysin (bak-teer-i-ol-i-sin) n. see lysin.

bacteriolysis (bak-teer-i-ol-i-sis) n. the destruction of bacteria by lysis. —**bacteriolytic** adj.

bacteriophage (phage) (bak-teer-i-oh-fayj) n. a virus that attacks bacteria. The phage grows and replicates in the bacterial cell, which is eventually destroyed with the release of new phages. Each phage acts specifically against a particular species of bacterium. This is utilized in phage typing, a technique of identifying bacteria by the action of known phages on them.

bacteriostatic (bak-teer-i-oh-stat-ik) adj. capable of inhibiting or re-

tarding the growth and multiplication of bacteria. Compare bactericidal.

bacterium (bak-teer-iŭm) n. see bacteria.

bacteriuria (bak-teer-i-yoor-iǎ) n. the presence of bacteria in the urine.

bagassosis (bag-ǎ-soh-sis) n. a form of external allergic alveolitis caused by exposure to the dust of mouldy bagasse, the residue of sugar cane after the sugar has been extracted. Symptoms include fever, malaise, irritant cough, and respiratory distress.

Baghdad boil (bag-dad) n. see oriental sore.

BAHA n. see (bone-anchored) hearing aid.

BAI n. see Beck Anxiety Inventory.

Baker's cyst (bay-kerz) n. a cyst behind the knee resulting from rupture or herniation of the synovial membrane from a knee joint affected by osteoarthritis. [W. M. Baker (1839–96), British surgeon]

BAL n. **1.** see bronchoalveolar lavage. **2.** British Anti-Lewisite (see dimercaprol).

balanced salt solution (BSS) (bal-ǎnst) n. a solution made to a physiological pH and having physiological concentrations of salts, including sodium, potassium, calcium, magnesium, and chloride. Such fluids are used during intraocular surgery and to replace intraocular fluids.

balanitis (bal-ǎ-ny-tis) n. inflammation of the glans penis, usually associated with tightness of the foreskin (phimosis). b. xerotica obliterans (BXO) an autoimmune condition characterized by ivory-white patches on the glans.

balanoposthitis (bal-ă-noh-pos-th'y-tis) *n.* inflammation of the foreskin and the surface of the underlying glans penis. It usually occurs as a consequence of phimosis and represents a more extensive local reaction than simple balanitis.

balantidiasis (bal-ăn-ti-dy-ă-sis) *n.* an infestation of the large intestine of humans with the parasitic protozoan *Balantidium coli*. The parasite invades and destroys the intestinal wall, causing ulceration and necrosis, and the patient may experience diarrhoea and dysentery.

baldness (bawld-nis) *n.* see alopecia.

Balkan beam (Balkan frame) (bawl-kăn) *n.* a rectangular frame attached over a bed, used for the support of splints, pulleys, or slings for an immobilized limb.

ball-and-cage valve (bawl-ănd-kayj) *n.* a form of prosthesis commonly used for replacing damaged heart valves.

ball-and-socket joint (bawl-ănd-sok-it) *n.* see enarthrosis.

balloon (bă-loon) *n.* an inflatable plastic cylinder of variable size that is mounted on a thin tube and used for dilating narrow areas in blood vessels or in the alimentary tract (strictures). *b. angioplasty see* angioplasty.

ballottement (bă-lot-měnt) *n.* the technique of examining a fluid-filled part of the body to detect a floating object. During pregnancy, a sharp tap with the fingers, applied to the uterus through the abdominal wall or the vagina, causes the fetus to move away and then return, with an answering tap, to its original position.

balneotherapy (bal-ni-oh-th'e-ră-pi) *n.* the treatment of disease by bathing, originally in the mineral-containing waters of hot springs. Today, specialized remedial treatment in baths is used to alleviate pain and improve blood circulation and limb mobility in conditions such as arthritis.

balsam (bawl-săm) *n.* an aromatic resinous substance of plant origin. *b. of Peru* a South American balsam used in skin preparations as a mild antiseptic. *See* friar's balsam.

bandage (band-ij) *n.* a piece of material, in the form of a pad or strip, applied to a wound or bound around an injured or diseased part of the body.

Bandl's ring (ban-d'lz) *n.* an abnormal retraction ring (*see* retraction) that occurs in obstructed labour. It is a sign of impending rupture of the lower segment of the uterus, which becomes progressively thinner as Bandl's ring rises upwards. Immediate action to relieve the obstruction is then necessary, usually in the form of Caesarean section. [L. Bandl (1842–92), German obstetrician]

Bankart's operation (bank-arts) *n.* an operation to repair a defect in the glenoid cavity in cases of recurrent dislocation of the shoulder. [A. S. B. Bankart (1879–1951), British orthopaedic surgeon]

Banti's syndrome (ban-teez) *n.* a disorder in which enlargement and overactivity of the spleen occurs as a result of increased pressure within the splenic vein. The commonest cause is cirrhosis of the liver. [G. Banti (1852–1925), Italian pathologist]

barbiturate (bar-bit-yoor-ăt) n. any of a group of drugs, derived from barbituric acid, that depress activity of the central nervous system. Because barbiturates produce psychological and physical dependence and have serious toxic side-effects (*see* barbiturism), their use as sleeping pills has declined. *See* amobarbital, butobarbital, phenobarbital, thiopental.

barbiturism (bar-bit-yoor-izm) n. addiction to drugs of the barbiturate group. Signs of intoxication include slurring of speech, sleepiness, and loss of balance. Withdrawal of the drugs must be undertaken slowly.

barbotage (bar-bŏ-tahzh) n. a method of spinal anaesthesia in which a small amount of anaesthetic is injected into the subarachnoid space followed by withdrawal of cerebrospinal fluid into the syringe. This process is repeated until all the anaesthetic has been injected.

barium enema (bair-ium) n. *see* enema.

barium follow-through n. *see* small bowel (meal).

barium meal n. a technique for examining the oesophagus, stomach, and duodenum. The patient swallows barium sulphate to coat the lining of the organs, and a series of X-rays is taken. Granules that produce gas to distend the stomach may be given to produce a double-contrast effect.

barium sulphate n. a barium salt, insoluble in water, that is opaque to X-rays and is used as a contrast medium in radiography of the gastrointestinal tract. *See* (barium) enema, barium meal, small bowel (meal).

Barlow's disease (bar-lohz) n. infantile scurvy: scurvy occurring in young children due to dietary deficiency of vitamin C. [Sir T. Barlow (1845–1945), British physician]

Barlow's manoeuvre (mă-noo-ver) n. a test for congenital dislocation of the hip. A clunk felt and sometimes heard when the hip is gently adducted and backward pressure is applied to the head of the femur indicates instability of the joint. [Sir T. Barlow]

baroreceptor (baroceptor) (ba-roh-ri-sep-ter) n. a collection of sensory nerve endings specialized to monitor changes in blood pressure. The main receptors lie in the carotid sinuses and the aortic arch.

Barr body (bar) n. *see* sex chromatin. [M. L. Barr (1908–95), Canadian anatomist]

Barrett's oesophagus (ba-rěts) n. a condition in which the normal squamous epithelium lining the oesophagus is replaced by columnar epithelium because of damage caused by gastro-oesophageal reflux or (rarely) by corrosive oesophagitis. The condition may be associated with an ulcer (*Barrett's ulcer*). [N. R. Barrett (1903–79), British surgeon]

barrier cream (ba-ri-er) n. a preparation used to protect the skin against water-soluble irritants (e.g. detergents, breakdown products of urine). Usually applied in the form of a cream or ointment and often containing a silicone (e.g. dimeticone), barrier creams are useful in the alleviation of various skin disorders, including napkin rash and bedsores.

barrier nursing *n.* the nursing care of an infectious patient in isolation from other patients, to prevent the spread of infection.

bartholinitis (vulvovaginitis) (bar-thŏ-li-**ny**-tis) *n.* inflammation of Bartholin's glands. *acute b.* bartholinitis in which abscess formation may occur (*Bartholin's abscess*). *chronic b.* bartholinitis in which cysts may form in the glands as a result of blockage of their ducts.

Bartholin's glands (greater vestibular glands) (bar-thŏ-linz) *pl. n.* a pair of glands that open at the junction of the vagina and the vulva. Their secretions lubricate the vulva and so assist penetration by the penis during coitus. [C. Bartholin (1655–1748), Danish anatomist]

Bartter syndrome (bar-tĕr) *n.* an inherited condition of the kidney, which causes abnormalities in the excretion and reabsorption of salts from the blood. This results in lowered levels of potassium and chloride and an increased level of calcium. The baby fails to grow properly and becomes progressively weaker and dehydrated. [F. C. Bartter (1914–83), US physician]

basal cell carcinoma (BCC) (bay-săl) *n.* the commonest form of skin cancer: a slow-growing tumour that usually occurs on the central area of the face, especially in fair-skinned people. The prevalence increases greatly with exposure to sunlight. Treatment involves curettage and cautery, surgical excision, cryotherapy, or radiotherapy. If neglected for decades, a BCC eventu-

ally becomes a *rodent ulcer* and destroys the surrounding tissue. The term 'rodent ulcer' is sometimes used to mean any basal cell carcinoma.

basal ganglia *pl. n.* several large masses of grey matter embedded deep within the white matter of the cerebrum. They include the *caudate* and *lenticular nuclei* (together known as the *corpus striatum*) and the *amygdaloid nucleus*. The lenticular nucleus consists of the *putamen* and *globus pallidus*. The basal ganglia are involved with the regulation of voluntary movements at a subconscious level.

basal metabolism *n.* the minimum amount of energy expended by the body to maintain vital processes, e.g. respiration, circulation, and digestion. It is expressed in terms of heat production per unit of body surface area per day (*basal metabolic rate – BMR*). BMR is normally determined indirectly, by measuring the respiratory quotient. Measurements are best taken during a period of least activity, i.e. during sleep and 12–18 hours after a meal, under controlled temperature conditions.

basal narcosis *n.* preliminary unconsciousness induced in a patient by administration of a narcotic drug prior to administration of a general anaesthetic by inhalation.

base (bayss) *n.* **1.** the main ingredient of an ointment or other medicinal preparation. **2.** a substance that releases hydroxyl ions when dissolved in water, has a pH greater than 7 and turns litmus paper blue, and reacts with an acid to form a salt and water only. *Compare* acid.

basement membrane (bayss-mĕnt) n. the thin delicate membrane that lies at the base of an epithelium.

basic life support (BLS) (bay-sik) n. the provision of treatment designed to maintain adequate circulation and ventilation to a patient in cardiac arrest, without the use of drugs or specialist equipment. *See also* cardiopulmonary resuscitation. *Compare* advanced life support.

basilar artery (ba-si-ler) n. an artery in the base of the brain, formed by the union of the two vertebral arteries.

basilic vein (bă-zil-ik) n. a large vein in the arm, extending from the hand along the back of the forearm, then passing forward to the inner side of the arm at the elbow.

basophil (bay-sŏ-fil) n. a variety of white blood cell distinguished by the presence in its cytoplasm of coarse granules that stain purple-black with Romanowsky stains. Basophils are capable of ingesting foreign particles and contain histamine and heparin.

basophilia (bay-sŏ-fil-iă) n. 1. a property of a microscopic structure whereby it shows an affinity for basic dyes. 2. an increase in the number of basophils in the blood. —**basophilic** *adj.*

Batchelor plaster (ba-chě-ler) n. a type of plaster that keeps both legs abducted and medially rotated, used to correct congenital dislocation of the hip. [J. S. Batchelor (1905–), British orthopaedic surgeon]

bat ears (bat) *pl.* n. protuberant external ears as a result of the absence of the antihelical fold in the pinna. It can be surgically corrected using an otoplasty operation.

Batten's disease (bat-t'nz) n. a rare hereditary disorder of lipid metabolism. Fatty substances accumulate in the cells of the nervous system, causing progressive dementia, epilepsy, spasticity, and visual failure. The condition starts in late infancy or childhood. [F. E. Batten (1865–1918), British neurologist]

battered baby syndrome (bat-erd) n. *see* nonaccidental injury.

battledore placenta (bat-t'l-dor) n. a placenta to which the umbilical cord is attached at the margin (rather than at the centre).

Bazin's disease (ba-zanz) n. a rare disease of young women in which tender nodules develop under the skin in the calves; it is a tuberculide. The nodules may break down and ulcerate though they may clear up spontaneously. Medical name: **erythema induratum**. [A. P. E. Bazin (1807–78), French dermatologist]

BBB n. 1. *see* bundle branch block. 2. *see* blood-brain barrier.

BBV n. blood-borne virus.

BCC n. *see* basal cell carcinoma.

B-cell n. *see* lymphocyte.

BCG (bacille Calmette-Guérin) n. a strain of tubercle bacillus that has lost the power to cause tuberculosis but retains its antigenic activity; it is therefore used to prepare a vaccine against the disease.

b.d. (**bis die**) Latin: twice daily, used as a direction in prescriptions.

bearing down (bair-ing down) n. 1. the expulsive uterine contractions of a woman in the second stage of labour. 2. a sensation of heaviness and descent in the pelvis associated with pelvic tumours and certain other disorders.

Beck Anxiety Inventory (BAI) (bek) *n.* a questionnaire that assesses levels of anxiety experienced by patients. It consists of an evaluation of the cognitive and physical manifestations of anxiety, which are rated on a scale from 0 to 3. [A. T. Beck (1921–), US psychiatrist]

Becker muscular dystrophy (bek-er) *n.* a sex-linked (X-linked) disorder in which affected males develop an increase in muscle size followed by weakness and wasting. It usually starts between the ages of 5 and 15, and 25 years after onset most patients are wheelchair-bound. Although most men become severely disabled, life expectancy is close to normal. The disorder is similar to Duchenne muscular dystrophy but less severe. [P. E. Becker (1908–), German geneticist]

Beck Scale for Suicide Ideation (BSS) *n.* an assessment tool designed to identify vulnerability to and risk of suicide in patients. [A. T. Beck]

Beck's triad *n.* the classical diagnostic features of cardiac tamponade: dilated neck veins, a fall in blood pressure, and muffled heart sounds. [C. S. Beck (1894–1971), US surgeon]

beclometasone (bek-loh-met-a-zohn) *n.* a corticosteroid drug that is administered by inhaler to treat hay fever and asthma and is applied externally in the treatment of inflammatory skin disorders. Trade names: **Beconase**, **Becotide**, **Propaderm**.

becquerel (bek-er-el) *n.* the SI unit of activity of a radioactive source, being the activity of a radionuclide decaying at a rate of one spontaneous nuclear transition per second. It has replaced the curie. Symbol: Bq.

bed bug (bed bug) *n.* a bloodsucking insect of the genus *Cimex*, especially *C. lectularius*. They live and lay their eggs in the crevices of walls and furniture and emerge at night to suck blood; their bites leave a route for bacterial infection.

bed occupancy *n.* the number of hospital beds occupied by patients expressed as a percentage of the total beds available in the ward, specialty, hospital, area, or region. It is used to assess the demands for hospital beds and hence to gauge an appropriate balance between health needs and beds.

bedsore (decubitus ulcer, pressure sore) (bed-sor) *n.* an ulcerated area of skin caused by continuous pressure on part of the body in a bedridden patient. Careful nursing is necessary to prevent local gangrene. The patient's position should be changed frequently, and the buttocks, heels, elbows, and other regions at risk kept dry and clean.

bedwetting (bed-wet-ing) *n. see* enuresis.

behavioural objective (bi-hayv-yer-ăl) *n.* the goal of a particular nursing intervention or a specific lesson, in terms of what a person is expected to be able to do as a result of it.

behaviourism (bi-hayv-yer-izm) *n.* an approach to psychology postulating that only observable behaviour need be studied, thus denying any importance to unconscious processes. —**behaviourist** n.

behaviour therapy (bi-hayv-yer) n. treatment based on the belief that psychological problems are the products of faulty learning and not the symptoms of an underlying disease. See also aversion therapy, conditioning, desensitization, exposure.

Behçet's syndrome (bay-setz) n. a recurrent disease, involving many body systems, characterized by oral and genital ulceration and inflammation of the iris; skin lesions occur in most cases. It may also involve the joints and cause inflammation of the veins. The condition, whose cause is unknown, occurs more often in men. [H. Behçet (1889–1948), Turkish dermatologist]

bejel (endemic syphilis) (bej-ĕl) n. a long-lasting nonvenereal form of syphilis, particularly prevalent where standards of personal hygiene are low. The disease is spread among children and adults by direct body contact.

belladonna (bel-ă-don-ă) n. **1.** deadly nightshade (Atropa belladonna). **2.** the alkaloid derived from deadly nightshade, from which atropine is extracted. Preparations containing belladonna are used for treating diarrhoea. Trade names: **Alophen, Bellocarb**.

belle indifférence (bel an-di-fay-rahns) n. a symptom of conversion disorder in which an apparently grave physical affliction (which has no physical cause) is accepted in a calm and smiling fashion.

Bellocq's cannula (Bellocq's sound) (bel-oks) n. a curved hollow tube used for inserting a plug into the nose to arrest nosebleeding. [J. J. Bellocq (1732–1807), French surgeon]

Bell's palsy (belz) n. paralysis of the facial nerve causing weakness of the muscles of one side of the face and an inability to close the eye. The cause is usually a viral infection. [Sir C. Bell (1774–1842), Scottish physiologist]

Bell's phenomenon n. the normal outward and upward rotation of the eyes that occurs when the lids are closed. [Sir C. Bell]

belly (bel-i) n. **1.** the abdomen or abdominal cavity. **2.** the central fleshy portion of a muscle.

Bence-Jones protein (benss-joh'nz) n. a protein of low molecular weight found in the urine of patients with multiple myeloma and rarely in patients with lymphoma, leukaemia, and Hodgkin's disease. [H. Bence-Jones (1814–73), British physician]

benchmarking (bench-mark-ing) n. a process by which best practice is identified and continuous improvement is generated through the sharing of evidence and the comparison of practice.

bendroflumethiazide (bendrofluazide) (ben-droh-floo-mi-th'y-ă-zyd) n. a potent thiazide diuretic used in the treatment of conditions involving retention of fluid, such as hypertension and oedema. Trade names: **Aprinox, Berkozide**.

bends (bendz) n. see compressed air illness.

Benedict's test (ben-i-dikts) n. a test for the presence of sugar in urine or other liquids, using a solution of sodium or potassium citrate, sodium carbonate, and copper sulphate (*Benedict's solution*). [S. R. Benedict (1884–1936), US chemist]

beneficence (bi-**nef**-i-sĕns) *n*. (in health care) the duty to do good and avoid doing harm to other people, which includes acting to promote their interests and protecting the weak and vulnerable. It includes the duty of advocacy (*see* advocate).

benign (bi-**nyn**) *adj*. **1.** describing a tumour that is not cancerous. **2.** describing any disorder or condition that does not produce harmful effects. *Compare* malignant.

benign paroxysmal positional vertigo (BPPV) *n*. brief episodes of rotary vertigo precipitated by sudden head movements: a common cause of vertigo. It is thought to be due to microscopic debris in the posterior semicircular canal and is treated by a predetermined set of head movements to move the debris.

benign prostatic hyperplasia (BPH) *n*. *see* prostate gland.

benorilate (ben-**or**-i-layt) *n*. a compound of aspirin and paracetamol that relieves pain, inflammation, and fever. It is an alternative to aspirin, particularly in the treatment of rheumatoid arthritis. Trade name: **Benoral**.

benperidol (ben-**pe**-ri-dol) *n*. a butyrophenone antipsychotic drug used mainly to treat deviant and antisocial sexual behaviour. It is administered by mouth. Trade name: **Anquil**.

benserazide (ben-**ser**-ă-zyd) *n*. a drug administered by mouth in combination with levodopa (as *Madopar*) to treat Parkinson's disease.

benzalkonium (ben-zăl-**koh**-niŭm) *n*. an antiseptic used in prepara-

tions for treating mouth and throat infections and skin conditions.

benzatropine (benztropine) (benz-**at**-trŏ-peen) *n*. a drug similar to trihexyphenidyl (benzhexol), used mainly in the treatment of parkinsonism to reduce rigidity and muscle cramps. Trade name: **Cogentin**.

benzene (ben-zeen) *n*. a toxic liquid hydrocarbon. Continued inhalation of benzene vapour may result in aplastic anaemia or a form of leukaemia. Formula: C_6H_6.

benzhexol (benz-**heks**-ol) *n*. *see* trihexyphenidyl.

benzocaine (ben-zoh-kayn) *n*. a local anaesthetic applied externally to relieve painful conditions of the skin and mucous membranes. Virtually nontoxic, it can also be administered orally to treat mouth lacerations or gastric ulcers.

benzodiazepines (ben-zoh-dy-az-ĕ-peenz) *pl. n*. a group of anxiolytics and hypnotics, including bromazepam, diazepam, and oxazepam.

benzoic acid (ben-zoh-ik) *n*. an antiseptic used as a preservative and to treat fungal infections of the skin.

benzoin (ben-zoh-in) *n*. a fragrant gum resin used as a constituent of friar's balsam.

benzoyl peroxide (ben-zoh-il pĕ-rok-syd) *n*. a preparation administered as a cream, lotion, or gel in the treatment of acne and fungal skin conditions. It removes the surface layers of the epidermis, unblocks skin pores, and has an antiseptic effect. Trade names: **Acnecide, Brevoxyl, PanOxyl, Quinoped**.

benzthiazide (benz-**th'**y-ă-zyd) *n*. a thiazide diuretic used in the treatment of conditions involving fluid retention.

benzydamine hydrochloride (ben-zy-dă-meen hy-droh-**klor**-ryd) *n.* an anti-inflammatory drug (*see* NSAID) administered as a cream, mouthwash, or throat spray. Trade name: **Difflam**.

benzyl benzoate (ben-zyl ben-zoh-ayt) *n.* an oily aromatic liquid that is applied externally for the treatment of scabies. Trade name: **Ascabiol**.

benzylpenicillin (ben-zyl-pen-i-**sil**-in) *n. see* penicillin.

bereavement (bi-reev-měnt) *n.* the feelings that arise as the result of being deprived, especially of a relation, friend, or other loved one through death but also of previous good health. No time limit can be put on the period of bereavement.

beriberi (b'e-ri-**b'e**-ri) *n.* a nutritional disorder due to deficiency of vitamin B_1 (thiamin). It is widespread in communities in which the diet is based on polished rice. *dry b.* a form of beriberi in which there is extreme emaciation. *wet b.* a form of beriberi in which there is an accumulation of tissue fluid (oedema). There is nervous degeneration in both forms of the disease and death from heart failure is often the outcome.

berry aneurysm (b'e-ri) *n. see* aneurysm.

berylliosis (b'e-ri-li-oh-**ohs**-is) *n.* poisoning by beryllium or its compounds, either by inhalation or by skin contamination. Inhalation of fumes from molten beryllium causes an acute alveolitis and is usually fatal. Subacute and chronic forms can result from exposure to

the powder and can produce granulomata in the skin or lungs. In the lungs, these can lead to fibrosis unless prevented by prompt use of oral corticosteroids.

Best's disease (bests) *n. see* vitelliform degeneration. [F. Best (1878–1920), German physician]

beta agonist (bee-tă) *n. see* sympathomimetic.

beta blocker *n.* a drug that prevents stimulation of the beta-adrenergic receptors at the nerve endings of the sympathetic nervous system. Beta blockers decrease the activity of the heart and some reduce the production of aqueous humour (and therefore pressure) inside the eye. They include propranolol, oxprenolol, sotalol, levobunolol, and timolol.

beta cells *pl. n.* the cells of the islets of Langerhans that produce insulin. *Compare* alpha cells, delta cells.

betahistine (bee-tă-**hist**-een) *n.* a drug that is an analogue of histamine and increases blood flow through the inner ear. It is administered by mouth to treat Ménière's disease. Trade name: **Serc**.

betamethasone (bee-tă-**meth**-ă-sohn) *n.* a synthetic corticosteroid drug with effects and uses similar to those of prednisolone. The side-effects are those of cortisone. Trade names: **Betnelan, Betnesol, Betnovate**.

betatron (bee-tă-tron) *n.* a device used to accelerate a stream of electrons (*beta particles*) into a beam of radiation that can be used in radiotherapy.

betaxolol (bet-**aks**-oh-lol) *n.* a beta blocker drug used to treat high blood pressure and chronic simple glaucoma. It is administered by mouth and as eye drops. Trade names: **Kerlone**, **Betoptic**.

bethanechol (beth-an-ē-kol) *n.* a cholinergic drug (*see* parasympathomimetic) that acts mainly on the bowel and bladder, stimulating these organs to empty. It is administered by mouth. Trade name: **Myotonine**.

bezafibrate (bee-ză-fy-brayt) *n.* a drug used to treat hyperlipidaemia that fails to respond to diet (*see* fibrate). It is administered by mouth. Trade name: **Bezalip**.

bezoar (bee-zor) *n.* a mass of swallowed foreign material within the stomach.

bi- *prefix denoting* two; double.

bicalutamide (bi-kă-loot-ă-myd) *n.* an anti-androgen commonly used to treat prostate cancer because in men it blocks androgen receptors without reducing levels of testosterone in the blood, preserving libido and general energy levels. Trade name: **Casodex**.

bicarbonate (by-kar-bŏ-nit) *n.* a salt containing the ion HCO_3^-. *b. of soda see* sodium bicarbonate.

biceps (by-seps) *n.* a muscle with two heads. *b. brachii* a muscle that extends from the shoulder to the elbow and is responsible for flexing the arm and forearm. *b. femoris* a muscle at the back of the thigh, responsible for flexing the knee.

biconcave (by-kon-kayv) *adj.* having a hollowed surface on both sides. Biconcave lenses are used to correct short-sightedness. *Compare* biconvex.

biconvex (by-kon-veks) *adj.* having a surface on each side that

curves outwards. Biconvex lenses are used to correct long-sightedness. *Compare* biconcave.

bicornuate (by-kor-new-it) *adj.* having two hornlike processes or projections. The term is applied to an abnormal uterus that is divided into two separate halves at the upper end.

bicuspid (by-kus-pid) *adj.* having two cusps, as in the premolar teeth and the mitral valve of the heart. *b. valve see* mitral valve.

bifid (by-fid) *adj.* split or cleft into two parts.

bifocal lens (by-foh-kăl) *n.* a lens with two principal focal lengths: the upper part of the lens gives a sharp image of distant objects and the lower part is for near vision, such as reading. *See also* multifocal lens.

bifurcation (by-fer-kay-shŏn) *n.* (in anatomy) the point at which division into two branches occurs; for example in blood vessels or in the trachea.

bigeminy (by-jem-ini) *n.* the condi-

The biceps muscle of the arm

tion in which alternate ectopic beats of the heart are transmitted to the pulse and felt as a double pulse beat (*pulsus bigeminus*).

biguanide (by-gwah-nyd) *n.* any of a class of drugs that increase glucose uptake by the muscles and reduce glucose release by the liver. These drugs, which include metformin, are taken by mouth in the treatment of type 2 diabetes mellitus.

bilateral (by-lat-er-ăl) *adj.* (in anatomy) relating to or affecting both sides of the body or of a tissue or organ or both of a pair of organs.

bile (byl) *n.* a thick alkaline fluid that is secreted by the liver and stored in the gall bladder. It is ejected intermittently into the duodenum, where it helps to emulsify fats so that they can be more easily digested. Bile may be yellow, green, or brown; its constituents include bile pigments and salts, lecithin, and cholesterol.

bile acids *pl. n.* the organic acids in bile; mostly occurring as bile salts. They are cholic acid, deoxycholic acid, glycocholic acid, and taurocholic acid.

bile-acid sequestrant (si-kwes-trănt) *n.* a drug that binds to bile acids, forming a complex that is excreted in the faeces. The reduction in bile acids causes cholesterol to be oxidized to bile acids, decreases low-density lipoprotein serum levels, and decreases serum cholesterol levels. See colestipol, colestyramine.

bile duct *n.* any of the ducts that convey bile from the liver. Many small ducts unite to form the main bile duct, the *hepatic duct*. This joins the *cystic duct*, which leads from the

gall bladder, to form the *common bile duct*, which drains into the duodenum.

bile pigments *pl. n.* coloured compounds – breakdown products of the blood pigment haemoglobin – that are excreted in bile. The two most important bile pigments are *bilirubin*, which is orange or yellow, and its oxidized form *biliverdin*, which is green. Mixed with the intestinal contents, they give the brown colour to the faeces (*see* urobilinogen).

bile salts *pl. n.* sodium glycocholate and sodium taurocholate – the alkaline salts of bile – necessary for the emulsification of fats.

Bilharzia (bil-harts-iă) *n. see* Schistosoma.

bilharziasis (bil-harts-I-ă-sis) *n. see* schistosomiasis.

bili- *prefix denoting* bile.

biliary (bil-yer-i) *adj.* relating to or affecting the bile duct or bile. *b. colic* severe steady pain in the upper abdomen (in the mid-line or to the right) resulting from obstruction of the gall bladder or common bile duct, usually by a stone. Vomiting often occurs simultaneously. *b. fistula see* fistula.

bilious (bil-yŭs) *adj.* **1.** containing bile. **2.** a lay term used to describe attacks of nausea or vomiting.

bilirubin (bili-roo-bin) *n. see* bile pigments.

biliuria (choluria) (bili-yoor-iă) *n.* the presence of bile in the urine: a feature of certain forms of jaundice.

biliverdin (bili-ver-din) *n. see* bile pigments.

Billings method (bil-ingz) *n.* a method of planning pregnancy involving the daily examination of cervical mucus, which varies in consistency and colour throughout the menstrual cycle. [J. and E. Billings (20th century), Australian physicians]

Billroth's operation (bil-rohts) *n.* an operation in which the lower part of the stomach is removed and the remaining portion joined to the duodenum (*B. o. I*) or the lower stomach and duodenum are removed, with attachment of the remaining stomach to the jejunum (*B. o. II*). See gastrectomy. [C. A. T. Billroth (1829–94), Austrian surgeon]

bimanual (by-man-yoo-ăl) *adj.* using two hands to perform an activity, such as a gynaecological examination.

binaural (byn-or-ăl) *adj.* relating to or involving the use of both ears.

binder (byn-der) *n.* a bandage that is wound around a part of the body, usually the abdomen, to apply pressure or to give support or protection.

binge–purge syndrome (binj-perj) *n. see* bulimia.

binocular (bin-ok-yoo-ler) *adj.* relating to or involving the use of both eyes. *b. vision* the acquired ability to focus both eyes on an object at the same time, so that only one image is seen.

binovular (bin-ov-yoo-ler) *adj.* derived from two separate ova, as are fraternal twins. *Compare* uniovular.

bio- *prefix denoting* life or living organisms.

bioassay (by-oh-ass-ay) *n.* estimation of the activity or potency of a drug or other substance by comparing its effects on living organisms with effects of a preparation of known strength.

bioavailability (by-oh-ă-vayl-ă-bil-iti) *n.* the proportion of a drug that is delivered to its site of action in the body. This is usually the amount entering the circulation and may be low when the drugs are given by mouth.

biochemistry (by-oh-kem-istri) *n.* the study of the chemical processes and substances occurring in living things. —**biochemical** *adj.* —**biochemist** *n.*

bioengineering (by-oh-en-ji-neer-ing) *n.* the application of biological and engineering principles to the development and manufacture of equipment and devices for use in biological systems. Examples of such products include orthopaedic prostheses and heart pacemakers.

biogenesis (by-oh-jen-i-sis) *n.* the theory that living organisms can arise only from other living organisms and not from nonliving matter.

biology (by-ol-ŏji) *n.* the study of living organisms including their structure and function and their relationships with one another and with the inanimate world. —**biological** (by-ŏ-loj-ik-ăl) *adj.* —**biologist** *n.*

bionics (by-on-iks) *n.* the science of mechanical or electronic systems that function in the same way as, or have characteristics of, living systems. *Compare* cybernetics. —**bionic** *adj.*

bionomics (by-ŏ-nom-iks) *n. see* ecology.

biophysical profile (by-oh-fiz-ikăl proh-fyl) *n.* a physiological assessment of fetal wellbeing, including ultrasound scans, cardiotocograms, and fetal movements.

biopsy (by-op-si) *n.* the removal of a

small piece of living tissue from an organ or part of the body for microscopic examination.

biostatistics (by-oh-stă-**tist**-iks) *n.* statistical information and techniques used with special reference to studies of health and social problems. *See also* demography, vital statistics.

biotin (by-ŏ-tin) *n.* a vitamin of the B complex that is essential for the metabolism of fat, being involved in fatty acid synthesis and gluconeogenesis. Rich sources of the vitamin are egg yolk, yeast, and liver.

bipolar (by-**poh**-ler) *adj.* (in neurology) describing a neurone (nerve cell) that has two processes extending in different directions from its cell body.

bipolar disorder *n.* see manic-depressive psychosis.

bird-fancier's lung (berd-fan-si-erz) *n.* a form of extrinsic allergic alveolitis caused by the inhalation of avian proteins present in the droppings and feathers of certain birds, especially pigeons and caged birds (such as budgerigars). There is an acute and a chronic form. *See also* alveolitis.

birth (berth) *n.* (in obstetrics) *see* labour.

birth control *n.* the use of contraception or sterilization (male or female) to prevent unwanted pregnancies.

birthing chair (berth-ing) *n.* a chair specially adapted to allow childbirth to take place in a sitting position. Its recent introduction in the Western world followed the increasing demand by women for greater mobility during labour. The chair is electronically powered and

can be tilted back quickly and easily should the need arise.

birthmark (berth-mark) *n.* a skin blemish or mark present at birth.

birth rate (live birth rate) *n.* the number of live births occurring in a year per 1000 total population. *See also* fertility rate.

bisacodyl (bis-**ak**-oh-dil) *n.* a laxative that acts on the large intestine to cause reflex movement and bowel evacuation. It is administered by mouth or in a suppository. Trade name: **Dulco-lax.**

bisexual (by-seks-yoo-ăl) *adj.* **1.** describing an individual who is sexually attracted to both men and women. **2.** describing an individual who possesses the qualities of both sexes.

bismuth (biz-mŭth) *n.* a white metallic element. Its salts are used in some antacid mixtures and as protective agents in skin powders and pastes. They were formerly widely used in the treatment of syphilis. Symbol: Bi.

bisoprolol (hy-soh-**proh**-lol) *n.* a beta blocker drug used to treat angina pectoris. It is administered by mouth. Trade names: **Emcor, Monocor.**

bisphosphonates (bis-fos-fŏ-nayts) *pl. n.* a group of drugs that inhibit the resorption of bone by blocking the action of osteoclasts. Bisphosphonates are used in the treatment of Paget's disea... percalcaemia due t... the treatment a... postmenopaus... include etidr... midronate (... (Fosamax), an...

bistoury (bis-te...

gical knife, with a straight or curved blade. See illustration.

Types of bistoury

bite-wing (byt-wing) *n.* a dental X-ray film that provides a view of the crowns of the teeth in part of both upper and lower jaws.

Bitot's spots (bee-tohz) *pl. n.* cheesy foamy greyish spots that form on the surface of dry patches of conjunctiva at the sides of the eyes. They consist of fragments of keratinized epithelium. A common cause is vitamin A deficiency. [P. A. Bitot (1822–88), French physician]

bivalve (by-valv) *adj.* consisting of or possessing two valves or sections. *b. cast* a plaster cast that is cut into anterior and posterior sections to monitor pressure beneath the cast. *b. speculum* a vaginal speculum that has two blades.

black eye (blak) *n.* bruising of the eyelids.

blackhead (blak-hed) *n.* a plug formed of fatty material (sebum and keratin) in the outlet of a sebaceous gland in the skin. *See also* acne. Medical name: **comedo.**

black heel *n.* a black area, usually [over] the Achilles tendon, resulting [from] the rupture of capillaries in [ski]n in those who play basketball, [squa]sh, etc. It may be mistaken [for malign]ant melanoma.

blackwater fever (blak-waw-ter) *n.* a rare and serious complication of malignant tertian (falciparum) malaria in which there is massive destruction of the red blood cells, leading to the presence of the blood pigment haemoglobin in the urine.

bladder (blad-er) *n.* **1. (urinary bladder)** a sac-shaped organ that has a wall of smooth muscle and stores the urine produced by the kidneys. *b. neck incision see* incision. *b. outflow obstruction see* BOO. **2.** any of several other hollow organs containing fluid, such as the gall bladder.

bladder pressure study *n.* a combined X-ray and manometry examination of the bladder to look for abnormal function. The bladder is filled slowly with contrast medium using a small urinary catheter and the pressure is monitored during filling and voiding (micturition).

bladderworm (blad-er-werm) *n. see* cysticercus.

Blalock-Taussig operation (blay-lok taw-sig) *n.* an operation in which the pulmonary artery is anastomosed to the subclavian artery, performed on patients with tetralogy of Fallot. [A. Blalock (1899–1964), US surgeon; H. B. Taussig (20th century), US paediatrician]

bland (bland) *adj.* nonirritating; mild; soothing: applied to foods and diets.

blast (blahst) *n.* an important cause of serious soft-tissue injury that is associated with explosions or high-velocity missiles. The eardrums, lungs, and gastrointestinal tract are especially vulnerable to the indirect effects of the blast wave.

-blast *suffix denoting* a formative cell.

blasto- *prefix denoting* a germ cell or embryo.

blastocyst (blast-oh-sist) *n.* an early stage of embryonic development that consists of a hollow ball of cells with a localized thickening (the *inner cell mass*) that will develop into the actual embryo. *See also* implantation.

blastomycosis (blast-oh-my-**koh**-sis) *n.* any disease caused by parasitic fungi of the genus *Blastomyces*, which may affect the skin (forming wartlike ulcers and tumours) or involve various internal tissues.

blastula (blast-yoo-lǎ) *n.* an early stage of the embryonic development of many animals. The equivalent stage in mammals (including humans) is the blastocyst.

bleb (bleb) *n.* a blister or large vesicle. *filtering b.* a blister-like cyst underneath the conjunctiva resulting from trabeculectomy, a surgical procedure commonly used in the treatment of glaucoma.

bleeding (bleed-ing) *n. see* haemorrhage.

bleeding time *n.* the time taken for bleeding to cease from a small wound, such as a puncture in a finger or ear lobe. It is used as a test of platelet function.

blenn- (**blenno-**) *prefix denoting* mucus.

blennorrhagia (blen-ŏ-ray-jiǎ) *n.* a copious discharge of mucus, particularly from the urethra.

blennorrhoea (blen-ŏ-ree-ǎ) *n.* a profuse watery discharge from the urethra.

bleomycin (bli-oh-**my**-sin) *n.* an antibiotic with action against can-

cer cells (*see* cytotoxic drug), administered by injection in the treatment of Hodgkin's disease and other lymphomas and in squamous cell carcinoma.

blephar- (**blepharo-**) *prefix denoting* the eyelid.

blepharitis (blef-ǎ-ry-tis) *n.* inflammation of the eyelids.

blepharochalasis (blef-er-oh-kǎ-lay-sis) *n.* excessive eyelid skin resulting from recurrent episodes of oedema and inflammation of the eyelid. It occurs in young people, causing drooping of the lid. *Compare* dermatochalasis.

blepharoconjunctivitis (blef-er-oh-kŏn-junk-ti-vy-tis) *n.* inflammation involving the eyelid margins and conjunctiva.

blepharon (blef-er-ŏn) *n. see* eyelid.

blepharoptosis (blef-er-op-tŏ-sis) *n. see* ptosis.

blepharospasm (blef-er-oh-spazm) *n.* involuntary tight contraction of the eyelids, either in response to painful conditions of the eye or as a form of dystonia.

blind loop syndrome (stagnant loop syndrome) (blynd) *n.* a condition of stasis of the small intestine allowing the overgrowth of bacteria, which causes malabsorption and the passage of fatty stools (*see* steatorrhoea). It is usually the result of chronic obstruction, surgical bypass operations producing a stagnant length of bowel, or conditions in which a segment of intestine is out of continuity with the rest...

blindness (blynd-nis) *n.* ...ability to see. For ad...purposes, the term a...of partial blindness (s...

ter). The commonest causes of blindness worldwide are trachoma, onchocerciasis, and vitamin A deficiency, and in Great Britain age-related macular degeneration, glaucoma, cataract, myopic retinal degeneration, and diabetic retinopathy. *See also* colour blindness, day blindness, night blindness, snow blindness.

blind register *n.* (in Britain) a list of persons maintained by local social service departments who are technically blind due to reduced visual acuity or who have severely restricted fields of vision.

blind spot *n.* the small area of the retina of the eye where the nerve fibres from the light-sensitive cells lead into the optic nerve. There are no rods or cones in this area and hence it does not register light. Anatomical name: **punctum caecum**.

blister (blis-ter) *n.* a swelling containing watery fluid (serum) and sometimes also blood (*blood b.*) or pus, within or just beneath the skin.

block (blok) *n.* any interruption of physiological or mental function, brought about intentionally (as part of a therapeutic procedure) or by disease. *See also* heart block, nerve block.

blood (blud) *n.* a fluid that circulates throughout the body, via the arteries and veins, providing a vehicle by which an immense variety of different substances are transported between the various organs and tissues. It is composed of cells (*see* blood cell), which are suspended in liquid medium (*see* plasma).

bank *n.* a department within spital or blood transfusion centre in which blood collected from donors is stored prior to transfusion.

blood-brain barrier (BBB) *n.* the mechanism that controls the passage of molecules from the blood into the cerebrospinal fluid and the tissue spaces surrounding the cells of the brain and thus protects the brain from the effects of substances harmful to it. The endothelial cells lining the walls of the brain capillaries are more tightly joined together at their edges than those lining capillaries supplying other parts of the body, which allows the passage of solutions and fat-soluble compounds but excludes particles and large molecules.

blood casts *pl. n.* fragments of cellular material (*see* cast) to which blood cells are attached, which are derived from the kidney tubules and are excreted in the urine in certain kidney diseases.

blood cell (blood corpuscle) *n.* any of the cells that are present in the blood in health or disease. The cells may be subclassified into three major categories: red cells (*see* erythrocyte), white cells (*see* leucocyte), and platelets. See illustration.

blood clot *n.* a solid mass formed as the result of blood coagulation, either within the blood vessels and heart or elsewhere. *See also* thrombosis.

blood clotting *n. see* blood coagulation.

blood coagulation (blood clotting) *n.* the process whereby blood is converted from a liquid to a solid state. The process involves the interaction of a variety of substances (*see* coagulation factors) and leads

small lymphocyte

erythrocyte

large lymphocyte

neutrophil

monocyte

eosinophil

granulocytes

platelets

basophil

Types of blood cells

to the production of the enzyme thrombin, which converts the soluble blood protein fibrinogen to the insoluble protein fibrin. Blood coagulation is an essential mechanism for the arrest of bleeding (haemostasis).

blood corpuscle *n. see* blood cell.

blood count *n.* the numbers of different blood cells in a known volume of blood, usually expressed as the number of cells per litre. *full b. c.* (*FBC*) a blood count that includes measures of the amount of haemoglobin and size of red cells, as well as counts of red cells, white cells, and platelets. *See also* differential leucocyte count.

blood donor *n.* a person who gives blood for storage in a blood bank.

blood group *n.* any one of the many types into which a person's blood may be classified, based on the presence or absence of certain inherited antigens on the surface of the red blood cells. Blood of one group contains antibodies in the serum that react against the cells of other groups. One of the most important blood group systems is the *ABO system*. It is based on the presence or absence of antigens A and B: blood of groups A and B contains antigens A and B, respectively;

Donor's blood group	Blood group of people donor can receive blood from	Blood group of people donor can give blood to
A	A, O	A, AB
B	B, O	B, AB
AB	A, B, AB, O	AB
O	O	A, B, AB, O

group AB contains both antigens and group O neither. Blood of group A contains antibodies to antigen B; group B blood contains anti-A antibodies or isoagglutinins; group AB has neither antibody and group O has both. The table illustrates which blood groups can be used in transfusion for each of the four groups. *See also* rhesus factor.

blood plasma *n. see* plasma.

blood poisoning *n.* the presence of either bacterial toxins or large numbers of bacteria in the bloodstream causing serious illness. *See* pyaemia, septicaemia, toxaemia.

blood pressure (BP) *n.* the pressure of blood against the walls of the main arteries. Pressure is highest during systole, when the ventricles are contracting (*systolic pressure*), and lowest during diastole, when the ventricles are relaxing and refilling (*diastolic pressure*). Blood pressure is measured – in millimetres of mercury – by means of a sphygmomanometer at the brachial artery of the arm. A young adult would be expected to have a systolic pressure of around 120 mm and a diastolic pressure of 80 mm. These are recorded as 120/80. *See also* hypertension, hypotension.

blood serum *n. see* serum.

blood sugar *n.* the concentration of glucose in the blood, normally expressed in millimoles per litre. The normal range is 3.5–5.5 mmol/l. Blood-sugar estimation is an important investigation in a variety of diseases, most notably in diabetes mellitus. *fasting b. s. (FBS)* the concentration of glucose in the blood after an overnight fast. *See also* hyperglycaemia, hypoglycaemia.

blood test *n.* any test designed to discover abnormalities in a sample of a person's blood or to determine the blood group.

blood transfusion *n. see* transfusion.

blood vessel *n.* a tube carrying blood away from or towards the heart. *See* artery, arteriole, vein, venule, capillary.

Bloom's syndrome (bloomz) *n.* a specific abnormality of chromosome 15 in which the individual suffers from recurrent infections, blistering areas of the hands and lips, and poor growth. Such children have a much higher than normal risk of developing cancer. [D. Bloom (20th century), US dermatologist]

Blount disease (blownt) *n.* a condition causing bow-legs as a result of abnormal growth at the epiphysis at the top of the tibia. It is more common in Africans and is most noticeable in childhood. [W. P. Blount (1900–92), US orthopaedic surgeon]

BLS *n. see* basic life support.

blue baby (bloo) *n.* an infant suffering from congenital heart disease in which the circulation is misdirected. This results in the presence of partially deoxygenated blood (which is blue in colour) in the peripheral circulation, which gives the skin and lips a characteristic purple colour (*see* cyanosis).

B-lymphocyte *n. see* lymphocyte.

BMI *n. see* body mass index.

BMR *n.* basal metabolic rate (*see* basal metabolism).

BMT *n.* bone-marrow transplant. *See* transplantation.

Boari flap (boh-ah-ri) *n.* a tube of bladder tissue constructed to replace the lower third of the ureter when this has been destroyed or damaged or has to be removed because of the presence of a tumour. *See also* ureteroplasty. [A. Boari (19th century), Italian surgeon]

body (bod-i) *n.* **1.** an entire animal organism. **2.** the trunk of an individual, excluding the limbs. **3.** the main or largest part of an organ. **4.** a solid discrete mass of tissue; e.g. the carotid body. *See also* corpus.

body image (body schema) *n.* the individual's concept of the disposition of his limbs and the identity of the different parts of his body.

body mass index (BMI) *n.* the weight of a person (in kilograms) divided by the square of the height of that person (in metres): used as an indicator of whether or not a person is over- or underweight. A BMI of between 20 and 25 is considered normal, between 25 and 30 is overweight, and greater than 30 indicates clinical obesity.

body temperature *n.* the temperature of the body, as measured by a thermometer. In most normal individuals body temperature is maintained at about 37°C (98.4°F). A rise in body temperature occurs in fever.

Boeck's disease (beeks) *n. see* sarcoidosis. [C. P. M. Boeck (1845–1913), Norwegian dermatologist]

boil (boil) *n.* a tender inflamed area of the skin containing pus. The infection is usually caused by the bacterium *Staphylococcus aureus*, which enters through a hair follicle or a break in the skin. Boils usually heal when the pus is released or with antibiotic treatment, though occasionally they may cause more widespread infection. Medical name: **furuncle**.

bolus (boh-lǔs) *n.* **1.** a soft mass of chewed food. **2.** a tablet or pill containing a large dose of a drug.

bonding (bond-ing) *n.* **1.** (in psychology) the development of a close and selective relationship, such as that of attachment. **2.** (in dentistry) the attachment of dental restorations, sealants, and orthodontic brackets to teeth.

bone (bohn) *n.* the hard extremely dense connective tissue that forms the skeleton of the body. It is composed of a matrix of collagen fibres impregnated with bone salts, chiefly calcium carbonate and calcium phosphate (hydroxyapatite), in which bone cells (osteocytes) are embedded. *compact* (or *cortical*) *b.* the outer shell of bones, consisting of a hard virtually solid mass made up of bony tissue arranged in concentric layers (*Haversian systems*). *spongy* (or *cancellous*) *b.* bone found beneath the outer shell; it consists of a meshwork of bony bars (*trabeculae*) with many interconnecting spaces containing marrow. See illustrations.

bone graft *n. see* graft.

bone marrow (marrow) *n.* the tissue contained within the internal cavities of the bones. At birth, these cavities are filled entirely with blood-forming *myeloid tissue* (*red marrow*) but in later life the marrow in the limb bones is replaced by fat (*yellow marrow*).

Bonney's blue (bon-iz) *n.* a dye consisting of a mixture of crystal violet and brilliant green. It is used as a skin disinfectant and to demonstrate the presence of a fistula, by instilling it via a cannula and trac-

Haversian systems

periosteum

compact bone

spongy bone

canaliculi

lymphatic vessel

Volkmann canal

vein

Haversian canal

two lamellae of matrix

artery

lacunae containing bone cells

Section of the shaft of a long bone (above) with detail of a single Haversian system (below)

ing its path. [W. F. V. Bonney (1872–1953), British gynaecologist]

bony labyrinth (boh-ni) *n. see* labyrinth.

BOO *n.* bladder outflow obstruction, usually by an enlarged prostate gland but also by a high bladder neck or uncoordinated contraction of the urinary sphincters and detrusor muscle of the bladder.

BOOP *n. see* bronchiolitis (obliterans organizing pneumonia).

borborygmus (bor-ber-**ig**-mǔs) *n.* (*pl.* **borborygmi**) an abdominal gurgle due to movement of fluid and gas in the intestine.

borderline (**bor**-der-lyn) *adj.* describing a personality disorder characterized by unstable and intense relationships, exploiting and manipulating other people, rapidly changing moods, recurrent suicidal or self-injuring acts, and a pervasive inner feeling of emptiness and boredom.

Bordetella (bor-dě-**tel**-ǎ) *n.* a genus of tiny Gram-negative aerobic bacteria. *B. pertussis* the cause of whooping cough.

borneol (**bor**-nee-ol) *n.* an essential oil used, in preparations with other essential oils, such as menthol, menthone, and camphene, to disperse gallstones and kidney stones. It is administered by mouth. Trade names: **Rowachol, Rowatinex**.

Bornholm disease (devil's grip, epidemic myalgia, epidemic pleurodynia) (**born**-holm) *n.* a disease caused by Coxsackie viruses. It is spread by contact; symptoms include fever, headache, and attacks of severe pain in the lower chest. The illness lasts about a week and is rarely fatal.

bottom shuffling (bot-ŏm **shuf**-ling) *n.* a normal variant of crawling in which babies sit upright and move on their bottoms, usually by pulling forward on their heels. Babies who bottom-shuffle tend to walk slightly later. There is often a family history of bottom shuffling.

botulinum toxin (bot-yoo-ly-nŭm) *n.* a powerful nerve toxin, produced by the bacterium *Clostridium botulinum*, that is injected, in minute dosage, for the treatment of various conditions of muscle overaction, such as strabismus (squint) and dystonia (including blepharospasm), achalasia, and spastic paralysis associated with cerebral palsy. Trade names: **Botox, Dysport**.

botulism (bot-yoo-lizm) *n.* a serious form of food poisoning from foods containing the toxin produced by the bacterium *Clostridium botulinum*, which thrives in improperly preserved foods. The toxin selectively affects the central nervous system; some cases are fatal.

Bouchard's node (boo-shahdz) *n.* a bony thickening arising at the proximal interphalangeal joint of a finger in osteoarthritis. It is often found together with Heberden's nodes. [J. C. Bouchard (1837–1915), French physician]

bougie (boo-zhee) *n.* a hollow or solid cylindrical instrument, usually flexible, that is inserted into a tubular passage, such as the oesophagus (gullet), rectum, or urethra. Bougies are used in diagnosis and treatment, particularly by enlarging strictures.

Bourneville's disease (born-ĕ-veez) *n. see* tuberous (sclerosis). [D.-M. Bourneville (1840–1909), French neurologist]

bowel (bow-ĕl) *n. see* intestine.

Bowen's disease (boh-ĕnz) *n.* a type of in-situ carcinoma of the squamous epidermal cells of the skin that does not spread to the basal layers. [J. T. Bowen (1857–1941), US dermatologist]

bow-legs (boh-legz) *pl. n.* abnormal out-curving of the legs at the knees, resulting in a gap between the knees on standing. Medical name: **genu varum**.

Bowman's capsule (boh-mănz) *n. see* glomerulus. [Sir W. P. Bowman (1816–92), British physician]

BP *n. see* blood pressure.

BPD *n. see* bronchopulmonary (dysplasia).

BPH *n.* benign prostatic hyperplasia. *See* prostate gland.

BPPV *n. see* benign paroxysmal positional vertigo.

BPRS *n. see* Brief Psychiatric Rating Scale.

brachi- (brachio-) *prefix denoting* the arm.

brachial (brayk-iăl) *adj.* relating to or affecting the arm.

brachial artery *n.* an artery that extends from the axillary artery at the armpit, down the side and inner surface of the upper arm to the elbow, where it divides into the radial and ulnar arteries.

brachial plexus *n.* a network of nerves, arising from the spine at the base of the neck, from which arise the nerves supplying the arm, forearm and hand, and parts of the shoulder girdle. *See also* radial (nerve).

brachiocephalic artery (brayki-oh-si-fal-ik) *n. see* innominate artery.

brachium (brayk-iŭm) *n.* (*pl.* **brachia**) the arm, especially the part of the arm between the shoulder and the elbow.

central sulcus

choroid plexus of third ventricle

pineal body

corpus callosum

thalamus

hypothalamus

optic chiasma

cerebral aqueduct

fourth ventricle

infundibulum

vermis

pituitary body

white matter of cerebellum

mamillary body

pons Varolii

medulla oblongata

The brain (midsagittal section)

brachy- *prefix denoting* shortness.

brachycephaly (brak-i-sef-ăli) *n.* shortness of the skull, with a cephalic index of about 80. —**brachycephalic** *adj.*

brachytherapy (brak-i-th'e-răpi) *n.* radiotherapy administered by implanting radioactive wires or grains into or close to a tumour. This technique is used in the treatment of many accessible tumours (e.g. breast cancer and localized prostate cancer). *intravascular b.* the insertion into arteries of radioactive metallic stents to delay or prevent restenosis.

Bradford's frame (brad-ferdz) *n.* a rectangular metal frame with canvas slings attached, used to support and immobilize a patient in a prone or supine position. [E. H. Bradford (1848–1926), US orthopaedic surgeon]

brady- *prefix denoting* slowness.

bradycardia (brad-i-kar-diă) *n.*

slowing of the heart rate to less than 50 beats per minute.

bradykinin (brad-i-ky-nin) *n.* a naturally occurring polypeptide consisting of nine amino acids; it is a very powerful vasodilator and causes contraction of smooth muscle.

brain (brayn) *n.* the enlarged and highly developed mass of nervous tissue that forms the upper end of the central nervous system. It is invested by three connective tissue membranes (*see* meninges) and floats in cerebrospinal fluid within the rigid casing formed by the bones of the skull. See illustration. *See also* forebrain, hindbrain, midbrain. Anatomical name: **encephalon**.

brain death *n. see* death.

brainstem (brayn-stem) *n.* the enlarged extension upwards within the skull of the spinal cord, consisting of the medulla oblongata, the pons, and the midbrain.

branchial cyst (brank-iăl) *n.* a

cyst that arises at the site of one of the embryonic pharyngeal pouches due to a developmental anomaly.

branchial pouch n. see pharyngeal (pouch).

Brandt Andrews method (brant an-drooz) n. a technique for expelling the placenta from the uterus. Upward pressure is applied to the uterus through the abdominal wall while holding the umbilical cord taut. When the uterus is elevated in this way, the placenta will be in the cervix or upper vagina and is then expelled by applying pressure below the base of the uterus. [T. Brandt (1819–95), Swedish obstetrician; H. R. Andrews (1872–1942), British gynaecologist]

Braun's splint (brawnz) n. a metal splint with attachments for pulleys, used to support or apply traction to a fractured lower limb. [H. F. W. Braun (1862–1934), German surgeon]

tractions of the uterus that occur intermittently during pregnancy and become stronger towards term. [J. Braxton Hicks (1825–97), British obstetrician]

breakbone fever (brayk-bohn) n. see dengue.

breast (brest) n. **1.** the mammary gland of a woman: one of two compound glands that produce milk. Each breast consists of glandular lobules – the milk-secreting areas – embedded in fatty tissue. The milk passes from the lobules into *lactiferous ducts*, each of which discharges through a separate orifice in the nipple. *See also* lactation. Anatomical name: **mamma. 2.** the front part of the chest (thorax).

Longitudinal section through a breast

Braun's splint

Braxton Hicks contractions (braks-tŏn hiks) pl. n. painless con-

Position of the diaphragm (from the side) during breathing

breastbone (brest-bohn) *n. see* sternum.

breast cancer *n.* a malignant tumour of the breast, usually a carcinoma, rarely a sarcoma. It is unusual in men but is the commonest form of cancer in women, in some cases involving both breasts.

breast implant *n. see* implant.

breast-milk jaundice *n.* prolonged jaundice lasting several weeks after birth in breast-fed babies for which no other cause can be found. It improves with time and is not an indication to stop breast-feeding.

breath-holding attacks (breth-hohld-ing) *pl. n.* episodes in which a young child cries, holds its breath, and goes blue, which may result in loss of consciousness. The attacks cease spontaneously.

breathing (breeth-ing) *n.* the alternation of active inhalation of air into the lungs through the mouth or nose with the passive exhalation of the air. Breathing is part of respiration and is sometimes called *external respiration*.

breathlessness (breth-lis-nis) *n. see* dyspnoea.

breath sounds (breth) *pl. n.* the sounds heard through a stethoscope placed over the lungs during breathing. *See* bronchial breath sounds, cavernous breath sounds, vesicular breath sounds.

breech presentation (breech) *n.* the position of a baby in the uterus such that it would be delivered buttocks first (instead of the normal head-first position).

bregma (breg-mǎ) *n.* the point on the top of the skull at which the coronal and sagittal sutures meet. In a young infant this is an opening, the anterior fontanelle.

Breslow's thickness (brez-lohz) *n.* the distance (in millimetres) between the surface and the deepest extent of a malignant melanoma. The measurement correlates with prognosis; tumours that are less than 0.76 mm thick have a good prognosis. [A. Breslow (1928–80), US pathologist]

bretylium tosylate (bre-til-iŭm to-sy-layt) *n.* an anti-arrhythmic drug used in patients with cardiac arrest to reverse ventricular fibrillation that has failed to respond to electrical defibrillation. It is administered by intravenous injection. Trade name: **Bretylate**.

Brief Psychiatric Rating Scale (BPRS) *n.* a measure of general psychiatric symptoms based on patients' verbal responses and observation of patients at the time of interview.

Bright's disease (bryts) *n. see* nephritis. [R. Bright (1789–1858), British physician]

brilliant green (bril-yănt) *n.* an aniline dye used as an antiseptic.

brimonidine (bri-mon-i-deen) *n.* an alpha agonist (*see* sympathomimetic) used in the form of eye drops in the treatment of glaucoma. Trade name: **Alphagan**.

brinzolamide (brin-zol-ă-myd) *n.* a carbonic anhydrase inhibitor used in the form of eye drops to reduce intraocular pressure in the treatment of glaucoma. Trade name: **Azopt**.

Briquet's syndrome (bree-kayz) *n. see* somatization disorder. [P. Briquet (1796–1881), French psychiatrist]

British Anti-Lewisite (BAL) (brit-ish anti-loo-i-syt) *n. see* dimercaprol.

brittle diabetes (brit'l) *n.* type 1 diabetes mellitus that constantly causes disruption of lifestyle due to recurrent attacks of hypo- or hyperglycaemia.

Broadbent's sign (brawd-bents) *n.* retraction of the left side and back near the 11th and 12th ribs with every heartbeat, indicating adhesions between the pericardium and the diaphragm. [Sir W. H. Broadbent (1835–1907), British physician]

broad ligaments (brawd) *pl. n.* folds of peritoneum extending from each side of the uterus to the lateral walls of the pelvis, supporting the uterus and Fallopian tubes, and forming a partition across the pelvic cavity.

Broca's area (broh-kăz) *n.* the area of cerebral motor cortex responsible for the initiation of speech. It is situated in the left frontal lobe in most (but not all) right-handed people. [P. P. Broca (1824–80), French surgeon]

Brodie's abscess (broh-diz) *n. see* abscess. [Sir B. C. Brodie (1783–1862), British surgeon]

bromazepam (broh-maz-ĕ-pam) *n.* a long-acting benzodiazepine drug used in the short-term treatment of disabling anxiety. It is administered by mouth. Trade name: **Lexotan**.

bromism (broh-mizm) *n.* a group of symptoms, including drowsiness, loss of sensation, and slurred speech, caused by excessive intake of bromides.

bromocriptine (broh-moh-krip-teen) *n.* a drug, derived from ergot, that is administered by mouth in the treatment of parkinsonism, acromegaly, and disorders associated with excessive secretion of prolactin and to prevent lactation. Trade name: **Parlodel**.

Brompton cocktail (bromp-tŏn

kok-tayl) *n.* a mixture of alcohol, morphine, and cocaine sometimes given to control severe pain in terminally ill people, especially those dying of cancer. The mixture was first tried at the Brompton Hospital, London.

bromsulphthalein (brom-sulf-thă-lin) *n.* a blue dye used in tests of liver function.

bronch- (broncho-) *prefix denoting* the bronchial tree.

bronchial breath sounds (bronk-iăl) *pl. n.* breath sounds transmitted through consolidated lungs in pneumonia; they are similar to the sounds heard normally over the larger bronchi and are louder and harsher than vesicular breath sounds.

bronchial carcinoma *n.* cancer of the bronchus, a common cause of death in smokers. *See also* lung cancer, oat-cell carcinoma.

bronchial tree *n.* a branching system of tubes conducting air from the trachea to the lungs: includes the bronchi and their subdivisions and the bronchioles.

bronchiectasis (bronk-i-ek-tă-sis) *n.* widening of the bronchi or their branches. It may be congenital or it may result from infection or obstruction. Pus may form in the widened bronchus so that the patient coughs up purulent sputum, which may contain blood. Treatment consists of antibiotic drugs to control the infection and physiotherapy to drain the sputum. Surgery may be used if only a few segments of the bronchi are affected.

bronchiole (bronk-i-ohl) *n.* a subdivision of the bronchial tree that does not contain cartilage or mucous glands in its wall. The smallest bronchioles open into the alveoli. —**bronchiolar** *adj.*

bronchiolitis (bronk-i-oh-ly-titis) *n.* inflammation of the small airways in the lungs (*see* bronchiole) due to infection by viruses, usually the respiratory syncytial virus, and occurring most commonly in infants of less than one year. *b. obliterans organizing pneumonia* (BOOP) a flu-like illness with cough, fever, and shortness of breath; there are patchy infiltrates on X-ray. It may result from a viral infection, be caused by certain drugs, or be associated with connective tissue disease.

bronchitis (brong-ky-tis) *n.* inflammation of the bronchi. *acute b.* bronchitis caused by viruses or bacteria. It is characterized by coughing, the production of mucopurulent sputum, and bronchospasm. *chronic b.* bronchitis in which the patient coughs up excessive mucus secreted by enlarged bronchial mucous glands; the bronchospasm cannot be relieved by bronchodilator drugs. The disease is particularly prevalent in Britain in association with cigarette smoking, air pollution, and emphysema.

bronchoalveolar lavage (BAL) (brong-koh-al-vee-oh-ler) *n.* a method of obtaining cellular material from the lungs that is used particularly in the investigation and monitoring of interstitial lung disease and in the investigation of pulmonary infiltrates in immunosuppressed patients.

bronchoconstrictor (brong-koh-kŏn-strik-ter) *n.* a drug that causes narrowing of the air passages by producing spasm of bronchial smooth muscle.

bronchodilator (brong-koh-dy-**lay**-ter) *n.* an agent, such as ephedrine, salbutamol, ipratropium, or theophylline, that causes widening of the air passages by relaxing bronchial smooth muscle.

bronchography (brong-**kog**-răfi) *n.* X-ray examination of the bronchial tree after it has been made visible by the injection of radiopaque dye or contrast medium. It has been largely superseded by CT scanning.

bronchomycosis (brong-koh-my-**koh**-sis) *n.* any of various fungal infections of the bronchi, such as candidosis of the lungs.

bronchophony (brong-**kof**-ŏni) *n.* *see* vocal resonance.

bronchopleural (brong-koh-**ploor**-ăl) *adj.* relating to a bronchus and the pleura. *b. fistula* an abnormal communication (*see* fistula) between a bronchus and the pleural cavity.

bronchopneumonia (brong-koh-new-**moh**-niă) *n.* *see* pneumonia.

bronchopulmonary (brong-koh-**pul**-mŏn-er-i) *adj.* relating to the lungs and the bronchial tree. *b. dysplasia (BPD)* a condition seen usually in premature babies as a result of respiratory distress syndrome, requiring prolonged treatment with oxygen beyond the age of 28 days.

bronchoscope (**bronk**-ŏ-skohp) *n.* an instrument used to look into the trachea and bronchi. With the aid of a bronchoscope the bronchial tree can be washed out (*see* bronchoalveolar lavage) and samples of tissue and foreign bodies can be re-

moved with long forceps. —**bronchoscopy** (brong-**kos**-kŏ-pi) *n.*

bronchospasm (**brong**-koh-spazm) *n.* narrowing of bronchi by muscular contraction in response to some stimulus, as in asthma and bronchitis. Some types of bronchospasm can usually be relieved by bronchodilator drugs; others, such as chronic bronchitis, usually cannot.

bronchus (**bronk**-ŭs) *n.* (*pl.* **bronchi**) any of the air passages beyond the trachea that has cartilage and mucous glands in its wall. *See also* bronchiole. —**bronchial** *adj.*

bronze diabetes (bronz) *n.* *see* haemochromatosis.

brown fat (brown) *n.* a form of fat in adipose tissue that is a rich source of energy and can be converted rapidly to heat. There is speculation that a rapid turnover of brown fat occurs to balance excessive intake of food and unnecessary production of white fat (making up the bulk of adipose tissue). Some forms of obesity may be linked to lack of – or inability to synthesize – brown fat.

Brown-Séquard syndrome (brown say-**kar**) *n.* the neurological condition resulting when the spinal cord has been damaged. Below the lesion there is a spastic paralysis on the same side and a loss of pain and temperature sensation on the opposite side. [C. E. Brown-Séquard (1818–94), French physiologist]

Brucella (broo-**sel**-ă) *n.* a genus of Gram-negative aerobic spherical or rodlike parasitic bacteria responsible for brucellosis (undulant fever) in humans and contagious abortion in cattle, pigs, sheep, and goats. The principal species are *B. abortus* and *B. melitensis*.

brucellosis (Malta fever, Mediterranean fever, undulant fever) (broo-si-loh-sis) *n*. a chronic disease of farm animals caused by bacteria of the genus *Brucella*, which can be transmitted to humans either by contact with an infected animal or by drinking nonpasteurized contaminated milk. Symptoms include headache, fever, aches and pains, and sickness; occasionally a chronic form develops with recurrent symptoms.

Bruch's membrane (bruuks) *n*. the transparent innermost layer of the choroid, which is in contact with the retinal pigment epithelium (*see* retina). [K. W. L. Bruch (1819–84), German anatomist]

Brudzinski sign (bruud-zin-ski) *n*. a sign present when there is irritation of the meninges (the membranes covering the brain), for example in meningitis. As the neck is pulled forward, the hips and the knees bend involuntarily. [J. von Brudzinski (1874–1917), Polish physician]

Brufen (broo-fen) *n*. *see* ibuprofen.

bruise (contusion) (brooz) *n*. an area of skin discoloration caused by the escape of blood from ruptured underlying vessels following injury.

bruit (broot) *n*. a sharp or harsh systolic sound, heard on auscultation, that is due to turbulent blood flow in a peripheral artery, usually the carotid or iliofemoral artery. Bruits can also be heard over arteriovenous fistulae or malformations.

Brunner's glands (brun-erz) *pl. n*. compound glands of the small intestine, found in the duodenum and the upper part of the jejunum. They are embedded in the submucosa and secrete mucus. [J. C. Brunner (1653–1727), Swiss anatomist]

Brushfield spots (brush-feeld) *pl. n*. greyish-brown spots seen in the iris of the eye. They can be found in normal individuals but are usually associated with Down's syndrome. [T. Brushfield (1858–1937), British physician]

BSA *n*. body surface area.

BSE *n*. bovine spongiform encephalopathy. *See* Creutzfeldt-Jakob disease, spongiform encephalopathy.

BSS *n*. **1.** *see* balanced salt solution. **2.** *see* Beck Scale for Suicide Ideation.

bubo (bew-boh) *n*. a swollen inflamed lymph node in the armpit or groin, commonly developing in soft sexually transmitted diseases (e.g. soft sore), bubonic plague, and leishmaniasis.

bubonic plague (bew-bon-ik) *n*. *see* plague.

buccal (buk-ăl) *adj*. relating to the mouth or the hollow part of the cheek.

buccinator (buks-i-nay-ter) *n*. a muscle of the cheek that has its origin in the maxilla and mandible. It is responsible for compressing the cheek and is important in mastication.

Budd-Chiari syndrome (bud-ki-ah-ri) *n*. a rare condition that follows obstruction of the hepatic vein by a blood clot or tumour. It is characterized by ascites and cirrhosis of the liver. [G. Budd (1808–82), British physician; H. Chiari (1851–1916), German pathologist]

budesonide (bew-dess-ŏ-nyd) *n*. a corticosteroid drug used in a nasal spray to treat hay fever or as an inhalant for asthma. It is also administered by mouth or enema for the treatment of Crohn's disease and ulcerative colitis. Trade names: **Budenofalk**, **Entocort**, **Pulmicort**.

Buerger's disease (ber-gerz) *n.* an inflammatory condition affecting the arteries, especially the arteries of the legs. The condition may lead to gangrene of the limbs and venous or coronary thrombosis. Medical name: **thromboangiitis obliterans**. [L. Buerger (1879–1943), US physician]

bufexamac (bew-feks-ă-mak) *n.* an anti-inflammatory drug (*see* NSAID) administered externally in the form of a cream for the treatment of skin inflammation and to relieve itching.

buffer (buf-er) *n.* a solution whose hydrogen ion concentration (pH) remains virtually unchanged by dilution or by the addition of acid or alkali. *See also* acid-base balance.

bulb (bulb) *n.* (in anatomy) any rounded structure or a rounded expansion at the end of an organ or part.

bulbar (bul-ber) *adj.* **1.** relating to or affecting the medulla oblongata. **2.** relating to a bulb. **3.** relating to the eyeball.

bulbourethral glands (bul-bo-yoor-ee-thrăl) *n.* *see* Cowper's glands.

bulimia (bew-lim-iă) *n.* insatiable overeating. This symptom may be psychogenic, as in anorexia nervosa (*b. nervosa* or the *binge-purge syndrome*); or it may be due to neurological causes, such as a lesion of the hypothalamus.

bulla (buul-ă) *n.* (*pl.* **bullae**) **1.** a large blister, containing serous

fluid. **2.** (in anatomy) a rounded bony prominence. **3.** a thin-walled air-filled space within the lung, arising congenitally or in emphysema. —**bullous** *adj.*

Buller's shield (buul-erz) *n.* a protective shield placed over one eye when the other is infected. It consists of a watch glass taped in position with adhesive tape. [F. Buller (1844–1905), Canadian ophthalmologist]

bullous pemphigoid (buul-ŭs) *n.* *see* pemphigoid.

bumetanide (bew-met-ă-nyd) *n.* a quick-acting loop diuretic used to relieve the fluid retention (oedema) occurring in heart failure, kidney disease, and cirrhosis of the liver. It is administered by mouth or by injection. Trade name: **Burinex**.

bundle (bun-d'l) *n.* a group of muscles or nerve fibres situated close together and running in the same direction.

bundle branch block (BBB) *n.* a defect in the specialized conducting tissue of the heart that is recognized as an electrocardiographic abnormality.

bundle of His (hiss) *n.* *see* atrioventricular bundle. [W. His (1863–1934), Swiss anatomist]

bunion (bun-yŏn) *n.* a swelling of the joint between the great toe and the first metatarsal bone. A bursa often develops over the site and the great toe becomes displaced towards the others. Bunions are usually caused by ill-fitting shoes and may require surgical treatment.

buphthalmos (**hydrophthalmos**) (buf-thal-mŏs) *n.* infantile or congenital glaucoma: increased pressure within the eye due to a defect in the development of the tissues through which fluid drains from the eye.

bupivacaine (bew-piv-ă-kayn) *n.* a potent local anaesthetic, used mainly for regional nerve block. Trade name: **Marcain**.

buprenorphine (bew-pren-or-feen) *n.* a powerful synthetic opiate painkilling drug; it acts for 6–8 hours and is administered by mouth. Trade name: **Temgesic**.

bur (ber) *n.* **1.** a cutting drill that fits in a dentist's handpiece. Burs are mainly used for cutting cavities in teeth, removing old restorations, and preparing teeth to receive crowns. **2. (burr)** a surgical drill for cutting through bone. *b. hole* a circular hole drilled through the skull to release pressure inside the skull or to facilitate biopsies and other procedures.

Burkitt's lymphoma (Burkitt's tumour) (ber-kits) *n.* a malignant tumour of the lymphatic system, most commonly affecting children and largely confined to tropical Africa. It is the most rapidly growing malignancy, with a tumour doubling time of about five days. It can arise at various sites, most commonly the facial structures, such as the jaw, and in the abdomen. [D. P. Burkitt (1911–93), Irish surgeon]

burn (bern) *n.* tissue damage caused by such agents as heat, chemicals, electricity, sunlight, or nuclear radiation. Burns cause swelling and blistering; loss of plasma from damaged blood vessels may lead to severe shock. There is also a risk of bacterial infection. *first-degree b.* a burn affecting only the outer layer (epidermis) of the skin. *second-*

degree b. a burn in which both the epidermis and the underlying dermis are damaged. *third-degree b.* a burn that involves damage or destruction of the skin to its full depth and damage to the tissues beneath.

burr (ber) *n. see* bur.

bursa (ber-să) *n.* (*pl.* **bursae**) a small sac of fibrous tissue that is lined with synovial membrane and filled with fluid. Bursae help to reduce friction; they are normally formed round joints and in places where ligaments and tendons pass over bones. —**bursal** *adj.*

bursa of Fabricius (fă-brish-ŭs) *n.* a mass of lymphoid tissue occurring as an outgrowth of the cloaca of young birds. It is an important source of B-lymphocytes. [H. Fabricius (1537–1619), Italian anatomist]

bursitis (bursal synovitis) (ber-sy-tis) *n.* inflammation of a bursa, resulting from injury, infection, or rheumatoid synovitis. It produces pain and sometimes restricts movement at a nearby joint. *See also* housemaid's knee.

buserelin (bew-sĕ-rel-in) *n.* a drug (*see* LHRH analogue) that is administered as a nasal spray for the treatment of endometriosis and to help in the management of advanced cancer of the prostate gland. Trade names: **Suprecur**, **Suprefact**.

buspirone (bew-spy-rohn) *n.* a drug used to relieve the symptoms of anxiety. Trade name: **Buspar**.

busulfan (busulphan) (bew-sulfan) *n.* an alkylating agent that destroys cancer cells by acting on the bone marrow. It is administered by mouth, mainly in the treatment of chronic myeloid leukaemia. Trade name: **Myleran**.

byssinosis

butobarbital (butobarbitone) (bew-toh-**bar**-bi-tal) *n.* an intermediate-acting barbiturate, used for the treatment of insomnia and for sedation. Trade name: **Soneryl**.

butriptyline (bew-**trip**-ti-leen) *n.* a tricyclic antidepressant drug administered by mouth.

buttock (but-ŏk) *n.* either of the two fleshy protuberances at the lower posterior section of the trunk, consisting of muscles (*see* gluteus) and fat. Anatomical name: **natis**.

butyrophenone (bew-ti-roh-**fee**-nohn) *n.* one of a group of chemically related antipsychotic drugs that includes haloperidol, droperidol, benperidol, and trifluperidol.

bypass (by-pahs) *n.* diversion of a flow from its normal channels, usually by means of surgery. *See* anastomosis, cardiopulmonary bypass, coronary artery bypass graft, shunt.

byssinosis (bis-i-**noh**-sis) *n.* an industrial disease of the lungs caused by inhalation of dusts of cotton, flax, hemp, or sisal.

Cc

C 1. *symbol for* carbon. **2.** *symbol for* Celsius *or* centigrade.

Ca *symbol for* calcium.

cabergoline (kă-ber-gŏ-leen) *n.* a drug used in the treatment of parkinsonism. It is administered by mouth. Trade name **Cabaser.**

CABG *n. see* coronary artery bypass graft.

cac- (caco-) *prefix denoting* disease or deformity.

cachet (kash-ay) *n.* a flat capsule containing a drug that has an unpleasant taste. The cachet is swallowed intact by the patient.

cachexia (kă-keks-iă) *n.* a condition of abnormally low weight, weakness, and general bodily decline associated with chronic disease, such as cancer.

cadaver (kă-dav-er) *n.* a dead body, especially one preserved and used for dissection and anatomical study.

caecosigmoidostomy (see-koh-sig-moid-**ost**-ŏmi) *n.* an operation in which the caecum is joined to the sigmoid colon.

caecostomy (see-**kost**-ŏmi) *n.* an operation in which the caecum is brought through the abdominal wall and opened in order to drain or decompress the intestine.

caecum (see-kŭm) *n.* a blind-ended pouch at the junction of the small and large intestines, to which the vermiform appendix is attached. —**caecal** *adj.*

Caesarean section (siz-air-iăn) *n.* a surgical operation for delivering a baby through the abdominal wall, usually by a transverse incision in the lower segment of the uterus (*lower uterine segment C. s.*). It is carried out when there are risks to the baby or to the mother from normal childbirth and may be performed, if necessary, as soon as the child is viable.

caesium-137 (seez-iŭm) *n.* an artificial radioactive isotope of the metallic element caesium, used rarely in radiotherapy. Symbol: ^{137}Cs. *See also* teletherapy.

café au lait spots (kaf-ay-oh-**lay**) *pl. n.* well-defined pale-brown patches on the skin. The presence of six or more in an individual is strongly suggestive of neurofibromatosis.

caffeine (kaf-een) *n.* an alkaloid drug, present in coffee and tea, that has a stimulant action on the central nervous system and is a weak diuretic. It is used in analgesic preparations.

Caffey's disease (kaf-iz) *n. see* hyperostosis. [J. Caffey (1895–1966), US paediatrician]

CAH *n. see* congenital adrenal hyperplasia.

caisson disease (kay-sŏn) *n. see* compressed air illness.

calamine (kal-ă-myn) *n.* a preparation of zinc carbonate used as a mild astringent on the skin in the form of a lotion, cream, or ointment.

calc- (calci-, calco-) *prefix denoting* calcium or calcium salts.

calcaneus (heel bone) (kal-kay-niŭs) *n.* the large bone in the tarsus of the foot that forms the projection of the heel behind the foot.

calcareous (kal-**kair**-iŭs) *adj.* containing calcium, especially calcium carbonate; chalky.

calciferol (kal-**sif**-er-ol) *n. see* vitamin D.

calcification (kal-si-fi-**kay**-shŏn) *n.* the deposition of calcium salts in tissue. This occurs as part of the normal process of bone formation (*see* ossification).

calcinosis (kal-si-**noh**-sis) *n.* the abnormal deposition of calcium salts in the tissues.

calcipotriol (kal-si-**pot**-ri-ol) *n.* a vitamin D analogue administered as an ointment, cream, or scalp solution for the treatment of psoriasis. Trade name: **Dovonex**.

calcitonin (thyrocalcitonin) (kal-si-**toh**-nin) *n.* a hormone, produced by the C cells of the thyroid gland, that lowers the levels of calcium and phosphate in the blood. Calcitonin is given by injection to treat hypercalcaemia and Paget's disease of bones. *Compare* parathyroid hormone.

calcium (kal-siŭm) *n.* a metallic element that is an important constituent of bones, teeth, and blood. It is also essential for many metabolic processes, including nerve function, muscle contraction, and blood clotting. Symbol: Ca.

calcium antagonist *n.* a drug that inhibits the influx of calcium ions into cardiac and smooth-muscle cells; it therefore reduces the strength of heart-muscle contrac-

tion, reduces conduction of impulses in the heart, and causes vasodilatation. Calcium antagonists include amlodipine, diltiazem, nicardipine, nifedipine, and verapamil, which are used to treat angina and high blood pressure.

calcium carbonate (kar-bŏ-nayt) *n.* a salt of calcium that neutralizes acids and is used in many antacid preparations. It is also used as a calcium supplement and to reduce high blood levels of phosphates (which it binds) in patients with renal failure. Formula: $CaCO_3$.

calcium gluconate and lactate (gloo-kŏ-nayt, lak-tayt) *n.* salts of calcium that are used to treat and prevent disorders caused by calcium deficiency, such as tetany and rickets, and to prevent osteoporosis. Formulae: $(CH_2OH(CHOH)_4COO)_2Ca.H_2O$; $(CH_3CHOHCOO)_2Ca.5H_2O$.

calculosis (kal-kew-**loh**-sis) *n.* the presence of multiple calculi in the body.

calculus (kal-kew-lŭs) *n. (pl.* **calculi**) **1.** a stone: a hard pebble-like mass formed within the body, particularly in the gall bladder (*see* gallstone) or anywhere in the urinary tract. Calculi may also occur in the ducts of the salivary glands. **2.** a calcified deposit that forms on the surface of a tooth as it is covered with plaque.

Caldwell-Luc operation (kawld-wel look) *n.* an operation in which the maxillary sinus is drained through an incision above the upper canine tooth. [G. W. Caldwell (1834–1918), US otolaryngologist; H. Luc (1855–1925), French laryngologist]

Calgary Depression Scale

(CDS) (kal-gă-ri) *n.* a structured interview tool that enables the assessment of depression in people suffering from schizophrenia.

calibrator (kal-i-bray-ter) *n.* **1.** an instrument used for measuring the size of a tube or opening. **2.** an instrument used for dilating a tubular part, such as the gullet.

caliectasis (hydrocalycosis) (kal-i-**ek**-tā-sis) *n.* dilatation or distension of the calyces of the kidney, which is mainly associated with hydronephrosis and usually demonstrated by ultrasound or intravenous urogram.

calliper (caliper) (kal-i-per) *n.* **1.** an instrument with two prongs or jaws, used for measuring diameters, particularly of the pelvis in obstetrics. **2. (calliper splint)** a surgical appliance (*see* orthosis) that is used to correct or control deformity of a joint in the leg. It consists of a metal bar that is fixed to the shoe and held to the leg by means of straps.

callosity (callus) (kă-los-iti) *n.* a hard thick area of skin occurring in parts of the body subject to pressure or friction, particularly the soles of the feet and palms of the hands.

callus (kal-ŭs) *n.* **1.** the composite mass of tissue that forms between bone ends when a fracture is healing. It initially consists of blood clot and granulation tissue, which develops into cartilage and eventually new bone, which unites the fracture. **2.** *see* callosity.

calor (kal-er) *n.* heat: one of the four classical signs of inflammation in a tissue. *See also* dolor, rubor, tumor.

calorie (kal-er-i) *n.* a unit of heat equal to the amount of heat required to raise the temperature of 1 gram of

water from 14.5°C to 15.5°C (the 15° calorie). One *Calorie* (*kilocalorie* or *kilogram calorie*) is equal to 1000 calories; this unit is used to indicate the energy value of foods. Both these units have now largely been replaced by the joule and kilojoule respectively (1 calorie = 4.1855 joules).

calorific (kal-er-if-ik) *adj.* producing heat.

calorimeter (kal-er-im-it-er) *n.* any apparatus used to measure the heat lost or gained during various chemical and physical changes. Calorimeters are used to determine the energy value of different foods. —**calorimetry** *n.*

calvaria (kal-vair-iă) *n.* the vault of the skull.

calyx (kay-liks) *n.* (*pl.* **calyces**) a cup-shaped part, especially any of the divisions of the pelvis of the kidney.

camphor (kam-fer) *n.* a crystalline aromatic substance obtained from the tree *Cinnamomum camphora*. It is used in liniments, creams, and sprays as a counterirritant and antipruritic.

Campylobacter (kam-pi-loh-**bak**-ter) *n.* a genus of spiral motile Gram-negative bacteria that are a common cause of food poisoning, producing headache, nausea, diarrhoea, and vomiting. *C. pylori see* Helicobacter.

canal (kă-nal) *n.* a tubular channel or passage; e.g. the alimentary canal.

canaliculitis (ka-nă-lik-yoo-ly-tis) *n.* inflammation of a canaliculus, especially a lacrimal canaliculus (*see* lacrimal (apparatus)).

canaliculus (ka-nă-lik-yoo-lŭs) *n.* (*pl.* **canaliculi**) a small channel or canal. Canaliculi occur, for example, in compact bone, linking lacunae containing bone cells; in the liver, transporting bile to the bile duct; and as part of the lacrimal apparatus of the eye.

cancellous (kan-si-lŭs) *adj.* latticelike. **c. bone** spongy bone, which in a mature bone has a low density and is surrounded by denser cortical bone.

cancer (kan-ser) *n.* any malignant tumour, including carcinoma and sarcoma. It arises from the abnormal and uncontrolled division of cells that then invade and destroy the surrounding tissues. The cancer cells spread (*see* metastasis), setting up secondary tumours (metastases) at sites distant from the original tumour.

There are probably many causative factors, some of which are known; for example, cigarette smoking is associated with lung cancer, radiation with some sarcomas and leukaemia, and several viruses are implicated; genetic factors are involved in the development of many cancers. Treatment of cancer depends on the type of tumour, the site of the primary tumour, and the extent of spread.

cancer phobia *n.* a disorder in which minor symptoms are interpreted as signs of cancer and panic attacks may occur. It leads to compulsively performed rituals, especially repeated hand-washing.

cancrum oris (kank-rŭm or-iss) *n.* ulceration of the lips and mouth. *See also* noma.

candesartan (kan-dess-ar-tan) *n. see* angiotensin II antagonist.

Candida (kan-di-dă) *n.* a genus of yeasts (formerly called *Monilia*) that inhabit the vagina and alimentary tract. *C. albicans* a small oval budding species primarily responsible for candidosis. —**candidal** *adj.*

candidosis (candidiasis) (kan-di-doh-sis) *n.* a common yeast infection of moist areas of the body, usually caused by *Candida albicans*. It is common in the vagina, where it is known as *thrush*, but is also found in the mouth and skin folds. On the skin the lesions are bright red with small satellite pustules, while in the mouth candidosis appears as white patches on the tongue or inside the cheeks. In the vagina it produces itching and sometimes a thick white discharge. Topical, intravaginal, or oral therapy with imidazoles is effective; nystatin, administered by mouth, helps to reduce candidal infection of the bowel.

canine (kay-nyn) *n.* the third tooth from the midline of each jaw. There are thus four canines, two in each jaw. It is known colloquially as the *eye tooth*.

cannabis (kan-ă-bis) *n.* a drug prepared from the Indian hemp plant (*Cannabis sativa*), also known as *pot, marijuana, hashish*, and *bhang*. It produces euphoria and hallucinations and has little therapeutic value; its nonmedical use is illegal. *See also* dependence.

cannula (kan-yoo-lă) *n.* a hollow tube designed for insertion into a body cavity. The tube contains a sharp pointed solid core (*trocar*), which facilitates its insertion and is withdrawn when the cannula is in place.

cantharidin (kan-tha-ri-din) *n.* the active principle of *cantharides* (*see*

Spanish fly). A toxic and irritant chemical, cantharidin causes blistering of the skin and was formerly used in veterinary medicine as a counterirritant and vesicant.

cantholysis (kan-thol-i-sis) *n.* a surgical procedure to divide the attachment of the canthus (corner of the eye) from its underlying bone and tendon. It is performed as part of some operations on the eyelid.

canthoplasty (kan-thoh-plasti) *n.* a surgical procedure to reconstruct the canthus.

canthus (kan-thŭs) *n.* either corner of the eye; the angle at which the upper and lower eyelids meet. —**canthal** *adj.*

cap (kap) *n.* a covering or a cover-like part.

CAPD *n.* continuous ambulatory peritoneal dialysis: a method of treating renal failure on an outpatient basis.

CAPE *n. see* Clifton Assessment Procedures for the Elderly.

capecitabine (kap-i-sit-ă-been) *n.* a drug that is used in treatment of cancers of the rectum, colon, or breast that have spread to other sites. It is taken by mouth. Trade name: **Xeloda**.

capillary (kă-pil-er-i) *n.* an extremely narrow blood vessel. Capillaries form networks in most tissues; they are supplied with blood by arterioles and drained by venules. The vessel wall is only one cell thick, which enables exchange of oxygen, carbon dioxide, water, salts, etc., between the blood and the tissues.

capitate (kap-i-tayt) *adj.* head-shaped; having a rounded extremity. *c. bone* the largest bone of the wrist (*see* carpus). It articulates with the scaphoid and lunate bones behind, with the second, third, and fourth metacarpal bones in front, and with the trapezoid and hamate laterally.

capitellum (kap-i-tel-ŭm) *n. see* capitulum.

capitulum (kă-pit-yoo-lŭm) *n.* the small rounded end of a bone that articulates with another bone. *c. humeri* (or *capitellum*) the round prominence at the elbow end of the humerus that articulates with the radius.

capreomycin (kap-ri-oh-my-sin) *n.* an antibiotic drug, derived from the bacterium *Streptomyces capreolus*, that is administered by intramuscular injection in the treatment of tuberculosis. Trade name: **Capastat**.

capsule (kaps-yool) *n.* **1.** a membrane, sheath, or other structure that encloses a tissue or organ. *joint c.* the fibrous tissue, including the synovial membrane, that surrounds a freely movable joint. **2.** a soluble case, usually made of gelatin, in which certain drugs are administered. **3.** the slimy substance that forms a protective layer around certain bacteria.

capsulitis (kaps-yoo-ly-tis) *n.* inflammation of a joint capsule. *adhesive c. see* frozen shoulder.

capsulorrhexis (kaps-yoo-loh-rek-sis) *n.* a surgical procedure in which a continuous circular tear is made in the lens capsule of the eye. *anterior c.* a tear made in the anterior surface of the lens capsule during cataract surgery, which makes the residual capsule much more resilient to being torn during surgery.

capsulotomy (kaps-yoo-lot-ŏmi) *n.* an incision into the capsule of the lens, made after modern operations for cataract in which the capsule is not removed.

captopril (kap-tŏ-pril) *n.* a drug used in the treatment of heart failure and hypertension; it acts by inhibiting the action of angiotensin (*see* ACE inhibitor). Trade names: **Acepril**, **Capoten**.

caput succedaneum (kap-ŭt suk-si-**day**-niŭm) *n.* a temporary swelling of the soft parts of the head of a newly born infant that occurs during birth, due to compression by the muscles of the cervix (neck) of the uterus.

carbachol (kar-bă-kol) *n.* a parasympathomimetic drug used occasionally in the treatment of urinary retention and (as eye drops) glaucoma.

carbamazepine (kar-bă-**maz**-ĕ-pcen) *n.* an anticonvulsant drug used in the treatment of epilepsy and to relieve the pain of trigeminal neuralgia. Trade name: **Tegretol**.

carbaryl (kar-bă-ril) *n.* a drug administered in the form of a lotion or shampoo to kill head and pubic lice. Trade name: **Carylderm**.

carbenoxolone (kar-bĕ-**noks**-ŏ-lohn) *n.* a drug that reduces inflammation, administered by mouth in the treatment of gastric ulcers or ulcers of the mouth. Trade names: **Biogastrone**, **Bioral**.

carbimazole (kar-bim-ă-zohl) *n.* a drug used to reduce the production of thyroid hormone in cases of overactivity of the gland (thyrotoxicosis). Trade name: **Neo-Mercazole**.

carbohydrate (kar-boh-**hy**-drayt)

n. any one of a large group of compounds, including the sugars and starch, that contain carbon, hydrogen, and oxygen and have the general formula $C_x(H_2O)_y$. Carbohydrates are important as a source of energy: they are manufactured by plants and obtained by animals and humans from the diet, being one of the three main constituents of food. *See also* disaccharide, monosaccharide, polysaccharide.

carbol fuchsin (kar-bol fuuk-sin) *n.* a red stain for bacteria and fungi, consisting of carbolic acid and fuchsin dissolved in alcohol and water.

carbolic acid (kar-bol-ik) *n. see* phenol.

carbon dioxide (kar-bŏn dy-oksyd) *n.* a colourless gas formed in the tissues during metabolism and carried in the blood to the lungs, where it is exhaled (an increase in the concentration of this gas in the blood stimulates respiration). It forms a solid (dry ice) at $-75°C$ (at atmospheric pressure) and in this form is used as a refrigerant. Formula: CO_2.

carbonic anhydrase (kar-bon-ik an-hy-drayz) *n.* an enzyme that catalyses the breakdown of carbonic acid into carbon dioxide and water or the combination of carbon dioxide and water to form carbonic acid. It therefore facilitates the transport of carbon dioxide from the tissues to the lungs.

carbonic anhydrase inhibitor *n.* a drug that blocks the action of carbonic anhydrase, which is present in high concentrations in the eye, kidneys, stomach lining, and pancreas. Carbonic anhydrase inhibitors reduce the production of aqueous humour in the eye and are used mainly in treating glaucoma. See acetazolamide, brinzolamide, dorzolamide.

carbon monoxide (mŏn-ok-syd) *n.* a colourless almost odourless gas that is very poisonous. When breathed in it combines with haemoglobin in the red blood cells (*see* carboxyhaemoglobin). Carbon monoxide is present in coal gas and motor exhaust fumes. Formula: CO.

carbon tetrachloride (tet-ră-klor-ryd) *n.* a pungent volatile fluid used as a dry-cleaner. When inhaled or swallowed it may severely damage the heart, liver, and kidneys. Treatment is by administration of oxygen. Formula: CCl_4.

carboplatin (kar-boh-**plat**-in) *n.* a derivative of platinum that is used in the treatment of certain types of cancer (e.g. ovarian cancer). It is similar to cisplatin but causes less nausea and vomiting. Trade name: **Paraplatin**.

carboxyhaemoglobin (kar-boks-i-heem-ŏ-**gloh**-bin) *n.* a substance formed when carbon monoxide combines with the pigment haemoglobin in the blood. Carboxyhaemoglobin is incapable of transporting oxygen to the tissues and this is the cause of death in carbon monoxide poisoning.

carboxyhaemoglobinaemia (kar-boks-i-heem-ŏ-gloh-bi-**nee**-miă) *n.* the presence of carboxyhaemoglobin in the blood.

carbuncle (kar-bung-kŭl) *n.* a collection of boils with multiple drainage channels. The infection is usually caused by *Staphylococcus*

aureus and may result in an extensive slough of skin.

carcin- (carcino-) *prefix denoting* cancer or carcinoma.

carcinogen (kar-sin-ŏ-jin) *n.* any substance that, when exposed to living tissue, may cause the production of cancer. —**carcinogenic** (kar-sin-ŏ-**jen**-ik) *adj.*

carcinogenesis (kar-sin-oh-jen-ĕ-sis) *n.* the evolution of an invasive cancer cell from a normal cell. Intermediate stages, known as carcinoma in situ, may be recognizable.

carcinoid (kar-sin-oid) *n. see* argentaffinoma.

carcinoma (kar-sin-oh-mă) *n.* cancer that arises in epithelium, the tissue that lines the skin and internal organs of the body. It may occur in any tissue containing epithelial cells. Organs may exhibit more than one type of carcinoma; for example, an adenocarcinoma and a squamous carcinoma may be found in the cervix (but not usually concurrently). —**carcinomatous** *adj.*

carcinoma in situ (CIS) *n.* the earliest stage of cancer spread, in which the tumour is confined to the epithelium and surgical removal of the growth should lead to cure. *ductal c. i. s.* (*DCIS*) the earliest stage of breast cancer, which is confined to the lactiferous (milk) ducts. See also cervical (cancer), CIN (cervical intraepithelial neoplasia).

carcinomatosis (kar-sin-oh-mă-toh-sis) *n.* carcinoma that has spread widely throughout the body.

carcinosarcoma (kar-sin-oh-sar-koh-mă) *n.* a malignant tumour of the cervix, uterus, or vagina containing a mixture of adenocarcinoma, sarcoma cells, and stroma.

cardi- (cardio-) *prefix denoting* the heart.

cardia (kar-diă) *n.* **1.** the opening at the upper end of the stomach that connects with the oesophagus (gullet). **2.** the heart.

cardiac (kar-di-ak) *adj.* **1.** of, relating to, or affecting the heart. **2.** of or relating to the upper part of the stomach (*see* cardia).

cardiac arrest *n.* the cessation of effective pumping action of the heart, which most commonly occurs when the muscle fibres of the ventricles start to beat rapidly without pumping any blood (ventricular fibrillation) or when the heart stops beating completely (asystole). There is abrupt loss of consciousness, absence of the pulse, and breathing stops. Unless it is treated promptly, irreversible brain damage and death follow within minutes. Some patients may be resuscitated by massage of the heart, artificial respiration, and defibrillation.

cardiac-arrest team *n.* a designated team of doctors in a hospital who attend cardiac arrests as they occur and administer appropriate treatment.

cardiac cycle *n.* the sequence of events between one heartbeat and the next, normally occupying less than a second. *See* diastole, systole.

cardiac muscle *n.* the specialized muscle of which the walls of the heart are composed. It consists of a network of branching elongated cells (fibres).

cardiac reflex *n.* reflex control of the heart rate.

cardiac tamponade *n. see* tamponade.

cardinal ligaments (Macken-

rodt's ligaments) (kar-din-ăl) *pl. n.* fan-shaped sheets of fascia that extend from the vagina and the cervix of the uterus to the walls of the pelvis.

cardiology (kar-di-ol-ŏji) *n.* the science concerned with the study of the structure, function, and diseases of the heart. **nuclear c.** the study and diagnosis of heart disease by the intravenous injection of a radionuclide, which emits gamma rays, enabling a gamma camera and computer to form an image of the heart. **—cardiologist** *n.*

cardiomyopathy (kar-di-oh-my-op-ă-thi) *n.* any chronic disorder affecting the muscle of the heart. It may result in enlargement of the heart, heart failure, arrhythmias, and embolism.

cardiomyoplasty (kar-di-oh-my-oh-plasti) *n.* a surgical technique to replace or reinforce damaged cardiac muscle with skeletal muscle.

cardiomyotomy (Heller's operation) (kar-di-oh-my-ot-ŏmi) *n.* surgical splitting of the muscular ring at the junction of the stomach and oesophagus to relieve achalasia.

cardiopathy (kar-di-op-ă-thi) *n.* any disease of the heart. **—cardiopathic** (kar-di-oh-path-ik) *adj.*

cardioplegia (kar-di-oh-plee-jiă) *n.* a technique in which the heart is stopped by injecting it with a solution of salts, by hypothermia, or by an electrical stimulus. This has enabled complex cardiac surgery and transplants to be performed safely.

cardiopulmonary bypass (kar-di-oh-pul-mŏn-er-i) *n.* a method by which the circulation to the body is maintained while the heart is deliberately stopped during heart surgery. The function of the heart and lungs is carried out by a pump-oxygenator (heart-lung machine) until the natural circulation is restored.

cardiopulmonary resuscitation (CPR) *n.* an emergency procedure for life support, consisting of artificial respiration and manual external cardiac massage. It is used in cases of cardiac arrest or apparent sudden death resulting from electric shock, drowning, respiratory arrest, or other causes, to establish effective circulation and ventilation in order to prevent irreversible brain damage.

cardiospasm (kar-di-oh-spazm) *n.* *see* achalasia.

cardiotocograph (kar-di-oh-tok-oh-graf) *n.* the instrument used in cardiotocography to produce a *cardiotocogram*, the graphic printout of the measurements obtained.

cardiotocography (kar-di-oh-tŏ-kog-răfi) *n.* the electronic monitoring of the fetal heart rate and rhythm, either by an external microphone or transducer or by applying an electrode to the fetal scalp, recording the fetal ECG and hence the heart rate. The procedure also includes a measurement of the strength and frequency of uterine contractions by means of an external transducer or an intrauterine catheter.

cardiotomy syndrome (post-cardiotomy syndrome) (kar-di-ot-ŏmi) *n.* a condition that may develop after surgery to the heart and the pericardium and is characterized by fever and pericarditis. Pneu-monia and pleurisy may form part of the syndrome.

cardiovascular system (circulatory system) (kar-di-oh-vas-kew-ler) *n.* the heart together with two networks of blood vessels – the systemic circulation and the pulmonary circulation. The cardiovascular system effects the circulation of blood around the body, which brings about transport of nutrients and oxygen to the tissues and the removal of waste products.

cardioversion (countershock) (kar-di-oh-ver-shŏn) *n.* a method of restoring the normal rhythm of the heart in patients with increased heart rate caused by arrhythmia. A controlled direct-current shock is given through electrodes placed on the chest wall of the anaesthetized patient. The apparatus is called a *cardiovertor*.

care assistant (kair) *n.* a person who assists with the general care of a patient, usually assisting a nurse or social worker with care of the vulnerable elderly in the community.

Caregiver Strain Index (CSI) (kair-giv-er) *n.* an assessment tool used by nurses (predominantly mental health nurses) to assess stress in caregivers.

care plan *n.* *see* planning.

caries (kair-eez) *n.* decay and crumbling of the substance of a bone. *dental c.* tooth decay, caused by the metabolism of the bacteria in plaque attached to the surface of the tooth. Acid formed by bacterial breakdown of sugar in the diet gradually etches and decomposes the enamel of the tooth; if left unrepaired, it spreads in and progressively destroys the tooth completely. —**carious** *adj.*

carina (kǎ-ree-nǎ) *n.* a keel-like structure, such as the keel-shaped cartilage at the bifurcation of the trachea into the two main bronchi.

cariogenic (kair-i-oh-jen-ik) *adj.* causing caries, particularly dental caries.

carminative (kar-min-ǎ-tiv) *n.* a drug that relieves flatulence, used to treat gastric discomfort and colic.

carmustine (kar-mus-teen) *n.* an alkylating agent administered by injection in the treatment of certain cancers, including myeloma, lymphomas, and brain tumours. Trade name: **BiCNU**.

carneous mole (kar-niǔs) *n.* a fleshy mass in the uterus consisting of pieces of placenta and products of conception that have not been expelled after abortion.

Caroli's disease (ka-rŏ-leez) *n.* an inherited condition in which the bile ducts, which drain the liver, are widened, causing an increased risk of infection or cancer in the gall bladder. *Compare* Caroli's syndrome. [J. Caroli (20th century), French physician]

Caroli's syndrome *n.* an inherited condition in which the bile ducts, which drain the liver, are widened and there are fibrous changes in the liver and cysts within the kidneys. *Compare* Caroli's disease. [J. Caroli]

carotenaemia (ka-rŏ-ti-nee-miǎ) *n. see* xanthaema.

carotene (ka-rŏ-teen) *n.* a yellow, orange, red, or brown plant pigment; one of the carotenoids. The most important form, β-carotene, is an antioxidant and can be converted in the body to retinol (vitamin A).

carotenoid (kǎ-rot-in-oid) *n.* any one of a group of about 100 naturally occurring yellow to red pigments found mostly in plants.

carotid artery (kǎ-rot-id) *n.* either of the two main arteries in the neck whose branches supply the head and neck.

The origin and main branches of the carotid arteries

carotid-artery stenosis (carotid stenosis) *n.* narrowing of the carotid artery, which reduces the supply of blood to the brain and is a cause of strokes. Many cases can be treated by surgical excision or bypass of the narrowed segment (*see also* endarterectomy).

carotid body *n.* a small mass of tissue in the carotid sinus containing chemoreceptors that monitor levels of oxygen, carbon dioxide, and hydrogen ions in the blood.

carotid sinus *n.* a pocket in the wall of the carotid artery, at its division in the neck, containing receptors that monitor blood pressure (baroreceptors).

carp- (carpo-) *prefix denoting* the wrist (carpus).

carpal (kar-păl) **1.** *adj.* relating to the wrist. **2.** *n.* any of the bones forming the carpus.

carpal tunnel syndrome *n.* tingling, numbness, and pain affecting all the hand except the little finger and half of the ring finger; there may be weakness of the thumb due to wasting of the thenar eminence. It is caused by pressure on the median nerve as it passes through the wrist, which may result from any continuous repetitive movements of the hand, such as keyboarding.

carphology (floccillation) (kar-fol-ŏji) *n.* plucking at the bedclothes by a delirious patient. This is often a sign of extreme exhaustion and may be the prelude to death.

carpopedal spasm (kar-poh-pee-d'l) *n. see* spasm.

carpus (kar-pŭs) *n.* the eight bones of the wrist (see illustration). The carpus articulates with the metacarpals distally and with the ulna and radius proximally.

carrier (ka-ri-er) *n.* **1.** a person who harbours the microorganisms causing a particular disease without experiencing signs or symptoms of infection and who can transmit the disease to others. **2.** (in genetics) a person who bears a gene for an abnormal trait without showing signs of the disorder. **3.** an animal, usually an insect, that passively transmits infectious organisms from one animal to another or from an animal to a human being. *See also* vector.

carteolol (kar-tee-ŏ-lol) *n.* a beta blocker used as eye drops in the treatment of glaucoma. Trade name: **Teoptic**.

cartilage (kar-til-ij) *n.* a dense connective tissue, consisting chiefly of chondroitin sulphate, that is capable of withstanding considerable pressure. In the fetus and infant cartilage occurs in many parts of the body, but most of this cartilage disappears during development. Cartilage is the precursor of bone following a fracture (*see* callus). *elastic c.* cartilage occurring in the external ear. *fibrocartilage* cartilage occurring in the intervertebral discs and tendons. *hyaline c.* cartilage found in the costal cartilages, larynx, trachea, bronchi, nose, and covering the surface of the bones at joints.

caruncle (ka-rŭng-kŭl) *n.* a small red fleshy swelling. *hymenal c.* a caruncle occurring around the mucous membrane lining the vaginal

Bones of the left wrist and hand
(from the front)

Hyaline cartilage

fibrocytes
perichondrium
chondrocytes
hyaline matrix

Elastic cartilage

chondrocytes
elastic fibres

Fibrocartilage

chondrocytes
collagen fibres

Types of cartilage

opening. *lacrimal c.* the red prominence at the inner angle of the eye.

cascara (cascara sagrada) (kas-**kar**-ă) *n.* the dried bark of an American buckthorn, *Rhamnus purshiana*, used as a laxative.

caseation (kay-si-**ay**-shŏn) *n.* the breakdown of diseased tissue into a dry cheeselike mass: a type of degeneration associated with tubercular lesions.

casein (**kay**-si-in) *n.* a milk protein. Casein is precipitated out of milk in acid conditions or by the action of rennin. It is very easily prepared and is useful as a protein supplement, particularly in the treatment of malnutrition.

caseinogen (kay-si-**in**-ŏ-jin) *n.* a protein, present in milk, that is converted into casein by the action of rennin.

Casey's model (**kay**-siz) *n.* a model of family-centred care for paediatric nursing in which the care of children (well or sick) is regarded as best carried out by their families, with varying degrees of assistance from members of a suitably qualified health-care team as necessary. *See also* nursing models. [A. Casey (1951–   ), British nurse theorist]

cast (kahst) *n.* **1.** a rigid casing designed to immobilize part of the body, usually a fractured limb, until healing has progressed sufficiently. It is made of plastic or with open-woven bandage impregnated with plaster of Paris and applied while wet. **2.** a mass of dead cellular, fatty, and other material that forms within a body cavity and takes its shape. It may then be released and appear elsewhere.

castration (kas-**tray**-shŏn) *n.* removal of the sex glands (the testes or the ovaries).

CAT *n.* computerized axial tomography, now referred to as CT (*see* computerized tomography).

cata- *prefix denoting* downward or against.

catabolism (kă-tab-ŏl-izm) *n.* the chemical decomposition of complex substances by the body to form simpler ones, accompanied by the release of energy. *See also* metabolism. —**catabolic** (kat-ă-bol-ik) *adj.*

catagen (kat-ă-jĕn) *n. see* anagen.

catalase (kat-ă-layz) *n.* an enzyme, present in many cells (including red blood cells and liver cells), that catalyses the breakdown of hydrogen peroxide.

catalepsy (kat-a-lep-si) *n.* the abnormal maintenance of postures or physical attitudes, occurring in catatonia.

catalyst (kat-ă-list) *n.* a substance that alters the rate of a chemical reaction but is itself unchanged at the end of the reaction. The catalysts of biochemical reactions are the enzymes.

cataphoresis (kat-ă-fŏ-ree-sis) *n.* the introduction into the tissues of positively charged ionized substances (cations) by the use of a direct electric current. *See* iontophoresis.

cataplexy (kat-ă-pleks-i) *n.* a sudden onset of muscle weakness that may be precipitated by excitement or emotion. There may be total loss of muscle tone, resulting in collapse, or simply jaw dropping or head nodding. It occurs in 60–90% of patients with narcolepsy.

cataract (kat-ă-rakt) *n.* any opacity in the lens of the eye, resulting in blurred vision. Cataracts most commonly occur in the elderly (*senile c.*), but some are congenital or re-

sult from metabolic disease (such as diabetes) or from injury or exposure of the eye to harmful radiation.

cataract extraction *n.* surgical removal of a cataract from the eye. *extracapsular c. e.* removal of the cataract alone, leaving the lens capsule behind to support the remaining lens tissue. *intracapsular c. e.* removal of the whole lens, including the capsule that surrounds it.

catarrh (kă-tar) *n.* the excessive secretion of thick phlegm or mucus by the mucous membrane of the nose, nasal sinuses, nasopharynx, or air passages.

catatonia (kat-ă-toh-niă) *n.* a state in which a person becomes mute or stuporous or adopts bizarre postures (*see also* flexibilitas cerea). Catatonia was once a noted feature of schizophrenia but is now hardly ever seen in developed countries. It remains common in developing countries. —**catatonic** *adj.*

CATCH-22 *n.* Cardiac abnormalities, Abnormal facies, T-cell deficiency (from absent thymus), Cleft palate, Hypocalcaemia, chromosome 22 (in which the defect lies): another name for di George syndrome.

catchment area (kach-mĕnt) *n.* the geographic area from which a hospital can expect to receive patients and on which in Britain the designated population of the hospital is based.

catecholamines (kat-ĕ-kol-ă-meenz) *pl. n.* a group of physiologically important substances, including adrenaline, noradrenaline, and dopamine, with different roles (mainly as neurotransmitters) in the functioning of the sympathetic and central nervous systems.

catgut (kat-gut) *n.* a natural fibrous material prepared from the tissues of animals, usually from sheep intestines, formerly widely used to sew up wounds and tie off blood vessels during surgery. The catgut gradually dissolves and is absorbed by the tissues, so that the stitches do not have to be removed later.

catharsis (kǎ-thar-sis) *n.* purging or cleansing out of the bowels by giving the patient a laxative (cathartic) to stimulate intestinal activity.

cathartic (kǎ-thar-tik) *n.* see laxative.

catheter (kath-it-er) *n.* a flexible tube for insertion into a narrow opening so that fluids may be introduced or removed. *suprapubic c.* a catheter passed through the abdominal wall above the pubis into the bladder, usually when this is very enlarged to relieve urinary retention. *urinary c.* a catheter passed into the bladder through the urethra to allow drainage of urine in certain disorders and to empty the bladder before abdominal operations.

catheterization (kath-it-er-I-zay-shŏn) *n.* the introduction of a catheter into a hollow organ. *cardiac c.* the introduction of special catheters into the chambers of the heart, usually via the arteries and veins of the arms or legs. It allows the measurement of pressures in the chambers and pressure gradients across the valves and the introduction of contrast medium (*see* angiocardiography). *urethral c.* the introduction of a catheter into the bladder in order to relieve obstruc-

tion to the outflow of urine (*see also* intermittent self-catheterization). *vascular c.* the introduction, via catheters, into the arteries or veins of contrast medium for radiography, drugs to constrict or expand vessels or to dissolve a thrombus, metal coils or other solid materials to block bleeding vessels or to thrombose aneurysms (*see* embolization), or devices for monitoring pressures within important vessels.

cation (kat-I-ŏn) *n.* a positively charged ion, which moves towards the cathode (negative electrode) when an electric current is passed through the solution containing it. *Compare* anion.

CATS *n.* Credit Accumulation Transfer Scheme: a system in educational establishments in which credit ratings are awarded at various levels of achievement (certificate, diploma, and first-degree level). *See also* APEL.

cat-scratch fever (kat-skrach) *n.* an infectious disease, possibly viral in origin, transmitted to humans following injury to the skin by a cat scratch, splinter, or thorn. The injury becomes inflamed and mild fever and swelling of the lymph nodes (usually those closest to the wound) develop about a week after infection.

cauda (kaw-dǎ) *n.* a tail-like structure. *c. equina* a bundle of nerve roots from the lumbar, sacral, and coccygeal spinal nerves that descend from the spinal cord to their respective openings in the vertebral column.

caudal (kaw-d'l) *adj.* relating to the lower part or tail end of the body.

caul (kawl) *n.* **1.** (in obstetrics) the amnion, a piece of which may cover an infant's head at birth. **2.** (in anatomy) *see* omentum.

causal agent (kaw-zăl) *n.* a factor associated with the definitive onset of an illness (or other response, including an accident). Examples of causal agents are bacteria, trauma, and noxious agents.

causalgia (kaw-zal-jiă) *n.* an intensely unpleasant burning pain felt in a limb where there has been partial damage to the sympathetic and somatic sensory nerves.

caustic (kaw-stik) *n.* an agent, such as silver nitrate, that destroys tissue. Caustic agents may be used to remove dead skin, warts, etc.

cauterize (kaw-tě-ryz) *vb.* to destroy tissues by direct application of a heated instrument (known as a *cautery*): used for the removal of small warts or other growths and also to stop bleeding from small vessels. —**cautery** *n.*

cavernosography (kav-er-noh-sog-răfi) *n.* a radiological examination of the erectile tissue of the penis that entails the infusion of radiopaque contrast material into the corpora cavernosa via a small butterfly needle. Radiographs taken during the infusion give information regarding the veins draining the penis.

cavernosometry (kav-er-noh-som-itri) *n.* the measurement of pressure within the corpora cavernosa of the penis during infusion. The flow rate required to produce an erection is recorded and also the flow necessary to maintain the induced erection. The examination is important in the investigation of failure of erection and impotence.

cavernous breath sounds (amphoric breath sounds) (kav-er-nŭs) *pl. n.* hollow breath sounds heard over cavities in the lung.

cavernous sinus *n.* one of the paired cavities within the sphenoid bone, at the base of the skull behind the eye sockets, into which blood drains from the brain, eye, nose, and upper cheek before leaving the skull through connections with the internal jugular and facial veins.

cavity (kav-iti) *n.* **1.** (in anatomy) a hollow enclosed area; for example, the abdominal cavity or the buccal cavity (mouth). **2.** (in dentistry) the hole in a tooth caused by caries or abrasion or formed by a dentist to retain a filling.

CBF *n.* cerebral blood flow.

C cells *pl. n.* parafollicular cells of the thyroid gland, which produce calcitonin.

CCF *n.* congestive cardiac failure. *See* heart failure.

CCU *n. see* coronary care (unit).

CD *n.* controlled drug. *See* Misuse of Drugs Act 1971.

CD4 *n.* a surface antigen on helper T-cells that is particularly important for immune resistance to viruses. It is also a receptor for HIV; progressive reduction of CD4-bearing T-cells reflects the progression of AIDS.

CDH *n. see* congenital dislocation of the hip.

CDS *n. see* Calgary Depression Scale.

cefaclor (sef-ă-klor) *n.* a cephalosporin antibiotic that is administered by mouth for the treatment of otitis media, upper and lower respiratory-tract infections, urinary-tract infections, and skin infections. Trade name: **Distaclor**.

cefadroxil (sef-ă-droks-il) *n.* a cephalosporin antibiotic administered by mouth for the treatment of urinary-tract infections, skin infections, pharyngitis, and tonsillitis. Trade name: **Baxan**.

cefalexin (sef-ă-leks-in) *n.* a cephalosporin antibiotic administered by mouth for the treatment of respiratory-tract and genitourinary-tract infections, bone and skin infections, and otitis media. Trade names: **Ceporex, Keflex**.

cefazolin (sef-ă-zoh-lin) *n.* a cephalosporin antibiotic, given by intramuscular or intravenous injection in the treatment of a number of infections. Trade name: **Kefzol**.

-cele (-coele) *suffix denoting* swelling, hernia, or tumour.

celecoxib (sel-i-koks-ib) *n.* an anti-inflammatory drug (*see* COX-2 inhibitor) that is taken by mouth in the treatment of osteoarthritis and rheumatoid arthritis. Trade name: **Celebrex**.

cell (sel) *n.* the basic unit of all living organisms, which can reproduce itself exactly (*see* mitosis). Cells contain cytoplasm, in which are suspended a nucleus and other structures (organelles) specialized to carry out particular activities in the cell. Complex organisms are built up of millions of cells that are specially adapted to carry out particular functions. See illustration.

cell division *n.* reproduction of cells by division first of the chro-

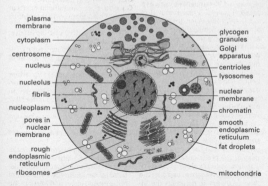

An animal cell (microscopical structure)

mosomes (karyokinesis) and then of the cytoplasm (cytokinesis). Cell division to produce more body (somatic) cells is by mitosis; cell division during the formation of gametes is by meiosis.

cellulitis (sel-yoo-ly-tis) *n.* an infection of the deep dermis of the skin by β-haemolytic streptococci. It is most common on the lower legs and there may be associated lymphangitis and lymphadenitis. It is otherwise similar to erysipelas, but the margins are less clearly defined because the infection is deeper.

cellulose (sel-yoo-lohz) *n.* a carbohydrate consisting of linked glucose units. It is an important constituent of plant cell walls. Cellulose cannot be digested by humans and is a component of dietary fibre (roughage).

Celsius temperature (centigrade temperature) (sel-si-ŭs) *n.* temperature expressed on a scale in which the melting point of ice is assigned a temperature of 0° and the boiling point of water a temperature of 100°. The formula for converting from Celsius (C) to Fahrenheit (F) is: F = 9/5C + 32. *See also* Fahrenheit temperature. [A. Celsius (1701–44), Swedish astronomer]

cement (si-ment) *n.* **1.** any of a group of materials used in dentistry either as fillings or as lutes for crowns. **2.** *see* cementum.

cementum (cement) (si-men-tŭm) *n.* a thin layer of hard tissue on the surface of the root of a tooth. It anchors the fibres of the periodontal membrane to the tooth.

censor (sen-ser) *n.* (in psychology) the mechanism, postulated by Freud, that suppresses or modifies desires that are inappropriate or feared.

-centesis *suffix denoting* puncture or perforation.

centi- *prefix denoting* one hundredth or a hundred.

centigrade temperature (sent-i-grayd) *n. see* Celsius temperature.

centile chart (sen-tyl) *n.* a graph with lines showing average measurements of height, weight, and head circumference compared with age and sex, against which a child's physical development can be assessed. The lines of growth on the graph are called *centiles*, and the number of a centile predicts the percentage of children who are below that measurement at a given age; for example, the 10th centile means that 10% of the age- and sex-matched population will be smaller and 90% will be bigger. Children whose growth lies outside the 97th or 3rd centiles may need to be investigated.

central auditory processing disorder (sen-tral) *n. see* obscure auditory dysfunction.

central nervous system (CNS) *n.* the brain and the spinal cord, as opposed to the peripheral nervous system. The CNS is responsible for the integration of all nervous activities.

central venous catheter *n.* an intravenous catheter for insertion directly into a large vein, most commonly the subclavian under the clavicle or the jugular in the neck, or indirectly via a peripheral vein (e.g. the femoral vein in the groin). It enables intravenous drugs and fluids to be given and intravenous pressures to be measured during operations or in intensive care.

central venous pressure (CVP) *n.* blood pressure in the right atrium, recorded by means of a catheter inserted into the vena cava and attached to a manometer. It is monitored particularly after heart surgery.

centri- *prefix denoting* centre.

centrifugal (sen-tri-few-găl) *adj.* moving away from a centre, as from the brain to the peripheral tissues.

centrifuge (sen-tri-fewj) *n.* a device for separating components of different densities in a liquid, using centrifugal force. The liquid is placed in special containers that are spun at high speed around a central axis.

centriole (sen-tri-ohl) *n.* a small particle found in the cytoplasm of cells, near the nucleus. Centrioles are involved in the formation of the spindle and aster during cell division.

centripetal (sen-trip-it'l) *adj.* moving towards a centre, as from the peripheral tissues to the brain.

centromere (kinetochore) (sen-trŏ-meer) *n.* the part of a chromosome that joins the two chromatids to each other and becomes attached to the spindle during mitosis and meiosis. When chromosome division takes place the centromeres split longitudinally.

centrosome (centrosphere) (sen-trŏ-sohm) *n.* an area of clear cytoplasm, found next to the nucleus in nondividing cells, that contains the centrioles.

centrosphere (sen-trŏ-sfeer) *n.* **1.** an area of clear cytoplasm seen in dividing cells around the poles of the spindle. **2.** *see* centrosome.

cephal- (cephalo-) *prefix denoting* the head.

cephalalgia (sef-ă-lal-jiă) *n.* pain in the head; headache.

cephalhaematoma (sef-ăl-heem-ă-toh-mă) *n.* a swelling on the head caused by a collection of bloody fluid between one or more of the skull bones and its covering membrane (periosteum). It is most commonly seen in newborn infants delivered with the aid of forceps or subjected to pressures during passage through the birth canal. No treatment is necessary and the swelling disappears in a few months. If it is extensive, the blood in the fluid may break down, releasing bilirubin into the bloodstream and causing jaundice.

cephalic (si-fal-ik) *adj.* of or relating to the head.

cephalic index *n.* a measure of the shape of a skull, commonly used in craniometry.

cephalic version *n.* a procedure for turning a fetus that is lying in a breech or transverse position so that its head will enter the birth canal first.

cephalocele (si-fal-ŏ-seel) *n.* protrusion of the contents of the skull through a defect in the bones of the skull. *See* neural tube defects.

cephalogram (sef-ă-loh-gram) *n.* a special standardized X-ray picture that can be used to measure alterations in the growth of skull bones.

cephalometry (sef-ă-lom-itri) *n.* the study of facial growth by examination of standardized lateral radiographs of the head. It is used mainly for diagnosis in orthodontics.

cephalosporin (sef-ă-loh-spor-rin)

n. any one of a group of semisynthetic antibiotics, derived from the mould *Cephalosporium*, which are effective against a wide range of microorganisms and are therefore used to treat a variety of infections (*see* cefaclor, cefadroxil, cefalexin, cefazolin). Cross-sensitivity with penicillin may occur and the principal side-effects are allergic reactions and irritation of the digestive tract.

cerclage (ser-klahzh) *n. see* cervical (cerclage).

cerebellar syndrome (Nonne's syndrome) (se-ri-bel-er) *n. see* (cerebellar) ataxia.

cerebellum (se-ri-bel-ŭm) *n.* the largest part of the hindbrain, bulging back behind the pons and the medulla oblongata and overhung by the occipital lobes of the cerebrum. The cerebellum is essential for the maintenance of muscle tone, balance, and the synchronization of activity in groups of muscles under voluntary control, converting muscular contractions into smooth coordinated movement. —**cerebellar** *adj.*

cerebr- (cerebri-, cerebro-) *prefix denoting* the cerebrum or brain.

cerebral abscess (se-ri-brăl) *n. see* abscess.

cerebral aqueduct *n. see* aqueduct.

cerebral cortex *n.* the intricately folded outer layer of the cerebrum, making up some 40% of the brain by weight. It is directly responsible for consciousness, with essential roles in perception, memory, thought, mental ability, and intellect, and it is responsible for initiating voluntary activity.

cerebral haemorrhage *n.* bleeding from a cerebral blood vessel into the tissue of the brain. It is commonly caused by degenerative disease of the arteries and high blood pressure but may result from bleeding from congenital abnormalities of blood vessels. The symptoms vary from a transient weakness or numbness to profound coma and death. *See also* atheroma, hypertension, stroke.

cerebral hemisphere *n.* one of the two paired halves of the cerebrum.

cerebral palsy *n.* a disorder of movement and/or posture as a result of nonprogressive but permanent damage to the developing brain, which may occur before, during, or immediately after delivery. Causes include an inadequate supply of oxygen to the brain, low levels of glucose in the blood, and infection. Cerebral palsy is often associated with other problems, such as learning difficulties, hearing difficulties, poor speech, and epilepsy. There are three main types: *spastic*, in which the limbs are difficult to control; *ataxic hypotonic*, in which the main problem is poor balance and uncoordinated movements; and *dyskinetic*, in which there is involuntary movement of the limbs.

cerebration (se-ri-bray-shŏn) *n.* **1.** the functioning of the brain as a whole. **2.** the unconscious activities of the brain.

cerebrospinal fever (spotted fever) (se-ri-broh-spy-nǎl) *n.* a former name for meningococcal meningitis.

cerebrospinal fluid (CSF) *n.* the clear watery fluid that surrounds and protects the brain and spinal cord. It is contained in the subarachnoid space and circulates in the ventricles of the brain and in the central canal of the spinal cord.

cerebrovascular accident (CVA) (se-ri-broh-vas-kew-ler) *n.* the clinical syndrome accompanying a sudden and sometimes severe attack of cerebrovascular disease, which leads to a stroke.

cerebrovascular disease *n.* any disorder of the blood vessels of the brain and its covering membranes (meninges). Most cases are due to atheroma and/or hypertension, clinical effects being caused by rupture of diseased blood vessels or inadequacy of the blood supply to the brain, due to cerebral thrombosis or embolism.

cerebrum (telencephalon) (se-ri-brŭm) *n.* the largest and most

parieto-occipital fissure
parietal lobe
central sulcus
frontal lobe
lateral sulcus
temporal lobe
occipital lobe

Lobes of cerebrum
(from right side)

highly developed part of the brain, composed of the two cerebral hemispheres, separated from each other by the longitudinal fissure in the midline and connected at the base by the corpus callosum. The cerebrum is responsible for the initiation and coordination of all voluntary activity in the body and for governing the functioning of lower parts of the nervous system. —**cerebral** *adj.*

cerivastatin (se-ri-va-stă-tin) *n.* a drug used to reduce abnormally high levels of cholesterol and other lipids in the blood (*see* statin). It is taken by mouth. Trade name: **Lipobay.**

cerumen (earwax) (si-roo-men) *n.* the waxy material that is secreted by the sebaceous glands in the external auditory meatus of the outer ear.

cervic- (cervico-) *prefix denoting* **1.** the neck. **2.** the cervix, especially of the uterus.

cervical (ser-vy-kăl) *adj.* **1.** of or relating to the neck. *c. vertebrae* the seven bones making up the neck region of the backbone. *See also* (cervical) fracture, vertebra. **2.** of, relating to, or affecting the cervix of an organ, especially the cervix of the uterus. *c. cancer* cancer of the cervix of the uterus. The growth can be detected at an early stage by periodic microscopical examination of a cervical smear. *c. cerclage* a procedure to help prevent preterm delivery. It involves placing a stitch around the cervix of the uterus to keep it closed and reduce the possibility of preterm cervical dilatation and rupture of membranes. *c. incompetence* unnatural spontaneous dilatation of the cervix of the uterus during the second trimester of pregnancy. The membranes bulge and subsequently rupture, and the fetus is expelled prematurely. *c. intraepithelial neoplasia see* CIN. *c. smear* a specimen of cellular material, scraped from the cervix of the uterus, that is stained and examined under a microscope in order to detect cell changes indicating the presence of cancer.

cervicitis (ser-vi-sy-tis) *n.* inflammation of the cervix of the uterus.

cervix (ser-viks) *n.* a necklike part. *c. uteri* the neck of the uterus, which projects into the vagina and contains the cervical canal.

cestode (ses-tohd) *n. see* tapeworm.

cetirizine (sē-ti-ri-zeen) *n.* a nonsedating antihistamine used to treat such allergic conditions as hay fever and urticaria. It is administered by mouth. Trade name: **Zirtek**.

cetrimide (set-ri-myd) *n.* a detergent disinfectant, used for cleansing skin surfaces and wounds, sterilizing surgical instruments and babies' napkins, and in shampoos.

CF *n. see* cystic fibrosis.

CFS/ME *n.* the approved name for the condition formerly known as *chronic fatigue syndrome, myalgic encephalomyelitis* (or *encephalopathy*), or *postviral fatigue syndrome*. It is characterized by extreme disabling fatigue that has lasted for at least six months, is made worse by physical or mental exertion, does not resolve with bed rest, and cannot be attributed to other disorders. The fatigue is accompanied by at least some of the following: muscle pain or weakness (*see* fibromyalgia), poor coordination, joint pain, recurrent sore throat, slight fever, painful lymph nodes in the neck and armpits, depression, cognitive impairment (especially an inability to concentrate), and general malaise. The cause is unknown, but some viral conditions (especially glandular fever) are known to trigger the disease.

CFTR gene *n.* the gene, lying on chromosome no. 7, that encodes a protein, cystic fibrosis transmembrane regulator (CFTR), enabling the transport of chloride ions across cell membranes. Patients with cystic fibrosis lack CFTR due to a mutation in this gene.

chalazion (meibomian cyst) (kǎ-lay-zi-ŏn) *n.* a swollen sebaceous gland in the eyelid, caused by chronic inflammation following blockage of the gland's duct.

chalcosis (kal-koh-sis) *n.* the deposition of copper in the tissues of the eye, usually resulting from the presence of a copper foreign body within the eye.

chancre (shang-ker) *n.* a painless ulcer that develops at the site where infection enters the body, e.g. on the lips, penis, urethra, or eyelid. It is the primary symptom of such infections as sleeping sickness and syphilis.

chancroid (shank-roid) *n. see* soft sore.

charcoal (char-kohl) *n.* a fine black powder, a form of carbon that is the residue from the partial burning of wood and other organic materials. *activated c.* charcoal that has been treated to increase its properties as an adsorbent, used as an emergency antidote to various poisons.

Charcot-Bouchard aneurysm

(shar-**koh boo**-shard) *n. see* aneurysm. [J. M. Charcot (1825–93), French neurologist; C. J. Bouchard (1837–1915), French physician]

Charcot-Marie-Tooth disease (peroneal muscular atrophy, hereditary sensorimotor neuropathy) (mă-**ree** tooth) *n.* a group of inherited diseases of the peripheral nerves, now more commonly known as *hereditary sensorimotor neuropathy*, causing a gradually progressive weakness and wasting of the muscles of the legs and the lower part of the thighs. The hands and arms are eventually affected. [J. M. Charcot; P. Marie (1853–1940), French physician; H. H. Tooth (1856–1925), British physician]

Charcot's joint *n.* a damaged, swollen, and deformed joint resulting from repeated minor injuries of which the patient is unaware because the nerves that normally register pain are not functioning. The condition may occur in syphilis, diabetes mellitus, and syringomyelia. [J. M. Charcot]

Charcot's triad *n.* the combination of fever, rigors, and jaundice that indicates acute cholangitis. [J. M. Charcot]

Charnley clamps (charn-li) *pl. n.* an apparatus used to encourage arthrodesis between the ends of two bones on either side of a joint. Parallel pins driven through the bone ends are connected on each side of the joint by bolts bearing wing nuts; tightening of the screw arrangements forces the surfaces of the bones together. [Sir J. Charnley (1911–82), British orthopaedic surgeon]

CHC *n. see* Community Health Council.

CHD *n.* coronary heart disease (*see* ischaemic heart disease).

Chediak-Higashi syndrome (ched-i-ak hi-**gash**-i) *n.* a rare fatal hereditary disease in children, inherited as an autosomal recessive condition, causing enlargement of the liver and spleen, albinism, and abnormalities of the eye. The cause is unknown but thought to be due to a disorder of glycolipid metabolism. [A. Chediak (20th century), Cuban physician; O. Higashi (20th century), Japanese paediatrician]

cheil- (cheilo-) *prefix denoting* the lip(s).

cheilitis (ky-ly-tis) *n.* inflammation of the lips. *angular c.* cheilitis that affects the angles of the lips and may be caused by a staphylococcal or candidal infection.

cheiloplasty (ky-loh-plasti) *n. see* labioplasty.

cheiloschisis (ky-losk-i sis) *n. see* cleft lip.

cheilosis (ky-loh-sis) *n.* swollen cracked bright-red lips. This is a common symptom of many nutritional disorders, including aribo-flavinosis (vitamin B_2 deficiency).

cheir- (cheiro-) *prefix denoting* the hand(s).

cheiroarthropathy (ky-roh-arth-rop-ăthi) *n.* the restricted hand movement seen in long-standing diabetes, due to chronic thickening of the skin limiting joint flexibility. *See* diabetic hand syndrome.

cheiropompholyx (ky-roh-pom-fŏ-liks) *n.* a type of eczema affecting the palms and fingers. *See* pompholyx.

chelating agent (kee-layt-ing) *n.*

a chemical compound that forms complexes by binding metal ions. Some chelating agents, including desferrioxamine and penicillamine, are drugs used to treat metal poisoning: the metal is bound to the drug and excreted safely.

chem- (chemo-) *prefix denoting* chemical or chemistry.

chemoreceptor (kee-moh-ri-**sep**-ter) *n.* a cell or group of cells that responds to the presence of specific chemical compounds by initiating an impulse in a sensory nerve. Chemoreceptors are found in the taste buds and in the mucous membranes of the nose. *See also* receptor.

chemosis (ki-**moh**-sis) *n.* swelling (oedema) of the conjunctiva.

chemotaxis (kee-moh-**taks**-iss) *n.* movement of a cell or organism in response to the stimulus of a gradient of chemical concentration.

chemotherapy (kee-moh-**th'e**-ră-pi) *n.* the prevention or treatment of disease by the use of chemical substances. The term is increasingly restricted to the treatment of cancer with antimetabolites and similar drugs (in contrast to radiotherapy). *See also* cytotoxic drug.

cherry angioma (che-ri) *n. see* angioma.

chest (chest) *n. see* thorax.

Cheyne-Stokes respiration (chayn-**stohks**) *n.* a striking form of breathing in which there is a cyclical variation in the rate, which becomes slower until breathing stops for several seconds before speeding up to a peak and then slowing again. It occurs particularly in states of coma. [J. Cheyne (1777–1836), Scottish physician; W. Stokes (1804–78), Irish physician]

CHF *n. see* (congestive) heart failure.

CHI *n. see* Commission for Health Improvement.

chiasma (ky-**az**-mă) *n.* (*pl.* **chiasmata**) *see* optic (chiasma).

chickenpox (**chik**-in-poks) *n.* a highly infectious disease caused by the varicella-zoster virus (a herpesvirus), which is transmitted by airborne droplets. Symptoms are mild fever followed by an itchy rash of red pimples that spread from the trunk to the face, scalp, and limbs. These develop into vesicles and then scabs, which drop off after about 12 days. The patient is infectious from the onset of symptoms until all the spots have gone. Medical name: **varicella**.

Chief Nursing Officer (cheef) *n.* the government's chief nursing adviser, who is responsible for providing an expert professional contribution and advice on nursing, midwifery, and health visiting matters to ministers and senior officials. There are separate officers for England, Scotland, Wales, and Northern Ireland.

chilblains (perniosis) (**chil**-blaynz) *pl. n.* dusky red itchy swellings that develop on the extremities in cold weather. They usually settle in two weeks but treatment with nifedipine is helpful in severe cases.

child abuse (chyld) *n.* the maltreatment of children. It may take the form of *sexual abuse*, when a child is involved in sexual activity by an adult; *physical abuse*, when physical injury is caused by cruelty or undue punishment (*see* nonaccidental injury); *neglect*, when basic physical provision for needs is lacking; and *emotional abuse*, when lack of affection and/or hostility from caregivers damage a child's emotional development.

childbirth (chyld-berth) *n. see* labour.

child health clinic *n.* (in Britain) a special clinic for the routine care of infants and preschool children. The service provides screening tests for such conditions as congenital dislocation of hips, suppressed squint, and impaired speech and/or hearing, education for mothers (especially those having their first child) in feeding techniques and hygiene, and immunizations against infectious diseases.

chir- (chiro-) *prefix denoting* the hand(s). *See also* cheir-.

chiropody (podiatry) (ki-rop-ŏdi) *n.* the study and care of the foot, including its normal structure, its diseases, and their treatment. - **chiropodist** *n.*

chiropractic (ky-rŏ-prak-tik) *n.* a system of treating diseases by manipulation, mainly of the vertebrae of the backbone. It is based on the theory that nearly all disorders can be traced to the incorrect alignment of bones, with consequent malfunctioning of nerves and muscle throughout the body. —**chiropractor** (ky-rŏ-prak-ter) *n.*

Chlamydia (klă-mid-iă) *n.* a genus of Gram-negative bacteria that are obligate intracellular parasites of humans and other animals, in which they cause disease. *C. pneumoniae* a cause of pneumonia. *C. psittaci* the cause of psittacosis. *C. trachomatis* the causative agent of the eye disease trachoma and a common cause of sexually trans-

mitted infections (*see* urethritis). —**chlamydial** *adj.*

chloasma (melasma) (kloh-az-mă) *n.* ill-defined symmetrical brown patches on the cheeks or elsewhere on the face. Chloasma is a photosensitivity reaction in women on combined oral contraceptive pills or who are pregnant; very rarely it occurs in men.

chlor- (chloro-) *prefix denoting* **1.** chlorine or chlorides. **2.** green.

chloracne (klor-ak-ni) *n.* an occupational acne-like skin disorder that occurs after regular contact with chlorinated hydrocarbons.

chloral hydrate (klor-ăl hy-drayt) *n.* a sedative and hypnotic drug administered by mouth as a syrup, mainly in children and the elderly; its derivative *chloral betaine* is formulated as tablets. Trade name: **Welldorm**.

chlorambucil (klor-am-bew-sil) *n.* an alkylating agent used in chemotherapy, mainly in the treatment of chronic leukaemias. It is given by mouth; prolonged large doses may cause damage to the bone marrow. Trade name: **Leukeran**.

chloramphenicol (klor-am-fen-i-kol) *n.* an antibiotic that is effective against a wide variety of microorganisms. However, due to its serious side-effects, especially damage to the bone marrow, it is usually reserved for serious infections (such as typhoid fever) when less toxic drugs are ineffective. It is also used, in the form of eye drops or ointment, to treat bacterial conjunctivitis. Trade names: **Chloromycetin, Kemicetine**.

chlorbutanol (klor-bew-tă-nol) *n.* an antibacterial and antifungal agent used in injection solutions, in eye and nose drops, in powder form for irritational skin conditions, and as a gargle or mouthwash (combined with chlorhexidine).

chlordiazepoxide (klor-dy-az-i-pok-syd) *n.* a benzodiazepine with muscle relaxant properties, administered by mouth or injection. Trade names: **Librium**, **Tropium**.

chlorhexidine (klor-heks-i-deen) *n.* an antiseptic used in solutions, creams, gels, and lozenges as a general disinfectant for skin and mucous membranes, as a preservative (for example, in eye drops), or (in very dilute solution) as a mouthwash to prevent or control mouth infections. Trade name: **Hibitane**.

chlorine (klor-een) *n.* an extremely pungent gaseous element with antiseptic and bleaching properties. It is widely used to sterilize drinking water and purify swimming pools. In high concentrations it is toxic. Symbol: Cl.

chlormethiazole (klor-mi-th'y-ā-zohl) *n. see* clomethiazole.

chlormethine (mustine, nitrogen mustard) (klor-mi-theen) *n.* an alkylating agent now only occasionally used for treating Hodgkin's disease. Administered by injection, it is very toxic, causing severe nausea and vomiting and bone-marrow damage.

chloroform (klo-rŏ-form) *n.* a volatile liquid formerly widely used as a general anaesthetic. Chloroform is now used only in low concentrations as a flavouring agent and preservative, in the treatment of flatulence, and in liniments as a rubefacient.

chlorophenothane (klo-roh-feen-ŏ-thayn) *n. see* DDT.

chlorophyll (klo-rŏ-fil) *n.* one of a group of green pigments, found in all green plants and some bacteria, that absorb light to provide energy for the synthesis of carbohydrates from carbon dioxide and water (photosynthesis).

chloroquine (klo-roh-kween) *n.* a drug used principally in the treatment and prevention of malaria but also used in rheumatoid arthritis and lupus erythematosus. It is administered by mouth or injection; a side-effect of prolonged use in large doses is eye damage. Trade names: **Avloclor**, **Nivaquine**.

chlorphenamine (chlorpheniramine) (klor-fen-ămeen) *n.* a potent antihistamine used to treat such allergies as hay fever, rhinitis, and urticaria. It is administered by mouth or, to relieve severe conditions, by injection. Trade name: **Piriton**.

chlorpromazine (klor-prom-ǎ-zeen) *n.* a phenothiazine antipsychotic drug, administered by mouth or injection or as a rectal suppository. It is used in the treatment of schizophrenia and mania; it is also used to treat severe anxiety and agitation and to control nausea and vomiting. It also enhances the effects of analgesics and is used in terminal illness and preparation for anaesthesia. Trade name: **Largactil**.

chlorpropamide (klor-proh-pǎ-myd) *n.* a drug that reduces blood sugar levels and is administered by mouth to treat noninsulin-dependent diabetes in adults. Trade name: **Diabinese**. *See also* sulphonylurea.

chlortalidone (chlorthalidone) (klor-**tal**-i-dohn) *n.* a thiazide diuretic administered by mouth to treat fluid retention (oedema) and high blood pressure (hypertension). Trade name: **Hygroton**.

chlortetracycline (klor-tet-ră-**sy**-kleen) *n.* an antibiotic active against many bacteria and fungi. It is administered as an ointment for skin and eye infections and, in combination with other tetracyclines, by mouth for systemic infections. Trade names: **Aureomycin**, **Deteclo**.

choana (koh-ă-nă) *n.* (*pl.* **choanae**) a funnel-shaped opening, particularly either of the two openings between the nasal cavity and the pharynx.

chocolate cyst (chok-ŏ-lit) *n.* a cyst filled with dark fluid, occurring in the ovary in endometriosis.

chol- (chole-, cholo-) *prefix denoting* bile.

cholaemia (kol-eem-iă) *n.* the presence of bile or bile pigments in the blood. *See* jaundice.

cholagogue (kol-ă-gog) *n.* a drug that stimulates the flow of bile from the gall bladder and bile ducts into the duodenum.

cholangiocarcinoma (kol-anji-oh-kar-sin-**oh**-mă) *n.* a malignant tumour of the bile ducts. It is particularly likely to occur at the junction of the two main bile ducts within the liver, causing obstructive jaundice.

cholangiography (kol-anji-og-răfi) *n.* X-ray examination of the bile ducts, used to demonstrate the site and nature of any obstruction to the ducts or to show the presence of stones within them. A medium that

is opaque to X-rays is introduced into the ducts by injection into the bloodstream, the liver, the bile ducts themselves, or the duodenal opening of the ducts.

cholangiolitis (kol-anji-ŏ-ly-tis) *n.* inflammation of the smallest bile ducts (*cholangioles*). *See* cholangitis.

cholangiopancreatography (kol-anji-oh-pank-ri-ă-**tog**-răfi) *n.* a method for outlining the bile ducts and pancreatic ducts with radio-opaque dyes. *endoscopic retrograde c. see* ERCP. *percutaneous transhepatic c.* (*PTC*) cholangiopancreatography in which the dyes are introduced by a catheter inserted into the ducts from the surface of the skin.

cholangitis (kol-an-jy-tis) *n.* inflammation of the bile ducts, often caused by an obstruction in the ducts. Initial treatment is by antibiotics, but removal of the obstruction is essential for permanent cure.

cholecalciferol (koli-kal-**sif**-er-ol) *n. see* vitamin D.

cholecyst- *prefix denoting* the gall bladder.

cholecystectomy (koli-sis-tek-tŏmi) *n.* surgical removal of the gall bladder, usually for cholecystitis or gallstones.

cholecystenterostomy (koli-sist-en ter-ost-ŏmi) *n.* a surgical procedure in which the gall bladder is joined to the small intestine. It is performed in order to allow bile to pass from the liver to the intestine when the common bile duct is obstructed by an irremovable cause.

cholecystitis (koli-sis-ty-tis) *n.* inflammation of the gall bladder.

cholecystoduodenostomy (koli-sis-toh-dew-oh-di-**nost**-ŏmi) *n.* a form of cholecystenterostomy in which the gall bladder is joined to the duodenum.

cholecystogastrostomy (koli-sis-toh-gas-**trost**-ŏmi) *n.* a form of cholecystenterostomy in which the gall bladder is joined to the stomach. It is rarely performed.

cholecystography (koli-sis-tog-răfi) *n.* X-ray examination of the gall bladder. A compound opaque to X-rays is administered by mouth and an X-ray photograph (*cholecystogram*) is taken.

cholecystojejunostomy (koli-sis-toh-jĕ-joo-**nost**-ŏmi) *n.* a form of cholecystenterostomy in which the gall bladder is joined to the jejunum.

cholecystokinin (koli-sis-toh-**ky**-nin) *n.* a hormone secreted by cells of the duodenum in response to the presence of partly digested food in the duodenum. It causes contraction of the gall bladder and expulsion of bile into the intestine and stimulates the production of digestive enzymes by the pancreas.

cholecystolithiasis (koli-sis-toh-lith-I-ă-sis) *n. see* cholelithiasis.

cholecystotomy (koli-sis-tot-ŏmi) *n.* a surgical operation in which the gall bladder is opened, usually to remove gallstones.

choledoch- (choledocho-) *prefix denoting* the common bile duct.

choledocholithiasis (koli-dok-oh-lith-I-ă-sis) *n.* stones within the common bile duct. The stones usually form in the gall bladder and pass into the bile duct, but they may develop within the duct after cholecystectomy.

choledochotomy (koli-dŏ-kot-ŏmi) *n.* a surgical operation in which the common bile duct is opened, to search for or to remove stones within it.

cholelithiasis (cholecysto-lithiasis) (koli-lith-I-ă-sis) *n.* the formation of stones in the gall bladder or bile duct (*see* gallstone).

cholelithotomy (koli-lith-**ot**-ŏmi) *n.* the surgical removal of gallstones by cholecystotomy.

cholera (kol-er-ă) *n.* an acute infection of the small intestine by the bacterium *Vibrio cholerae*, which causes severe vomiting and diarrhoea (known as *ricewater stools*) leading to dehydration. The disease is contracted from contaminated food or drinking water and often occurs in epidemics. Initial treatment is concentrated on replacing the fluid loss by oral rehydration therapy; tetracycline eradicates the bacteria and hastens recovery. The mortality rate in untreated cases is over 50%. Vaccination against cholera is effective for only 6–9 months.

choleresis (kol-er-ee-sis) *n.* the production of bile by the liver.

choleretic (kol-er-et-ik) *n.* an agent that stimulates the secretion of bile by the liver thereby increasing the flow of bile.

cholestasis (koli-**stay**-sis) *n.* failure of normal amounts of bile to reach the intestine, resulting in obstructive jaundice. The symptoms are jaundice with dark urine, pale faeces, and usually itching (pruritus).

cholesteatoma (koli-sti-ă-toh-mă) *n.* a skin-lined sac containing debris from dead skin cells that grows from the eardrum into the mastoid bone. Unless treated (by mastoidectomy), it can carry infection to the brain, causing meningitis or a cerebral abscess.

cholesterol (kŏl-est-er-ol) *n.* a fat-like material (a sterol) present in the blood and most tissues, especially nervous tissue. Elevated blood concentration of cholesterol (*hypercholesterolaemia*) is often associated with atheroma, of which cholesterol is a major component. Cholesterol is also a constituent of gallstones.

cholesterosis (kŏl-est-er-oh-sis) *n.* a form of chronic cholecystitis in which small crystals of cholesterol are deposited on the internal wall of the gall bladder. The crystals may enlarge to become gallstones.

cholestyramine *n. see* colestyramine.

cholic acid (cholalic acid) (kol-ik) *n. see* bile acids.

choline (koh-leen) *n.* a basic compound important in the synthesis of phosphatidylcholine (lecithin) and other phospholipids and of acetylcholine. It is also involved in the transport of fat in the body. Choline is sometimes classed as a vitamin but, although it is essential for life, it can be synthesized in the body.

cholinergic (koh-lin-er-jik) *adj.* 1. describing or relating to nerve fibres that release acetylcholine as a neurotransmitter. *c. receptor* a receptor at which acetylcholine acts to pass on messages from cholinergic nerve fibres. *c. urticaria see* urticaria. 2. describing drugs that mimic the actions of acetylcholine (*see* parasympathomimetic). *Compare* adrenergic.

cholinesterase (koh-lin-est-er-ayz) *n.* an enzyme that breaks down a choline ester into its choline and acid components. The term usually refers to *acetylcholinesterase*, which breaks down the neurotransmitter acetylcholine into choline and acetic acid.

choluria (kol-yoor-iă) *n.* bile in the urine, which occurs when the level of bile in the blood is raised, especially in obstructive jaundice.

chondr- (chondro-) *prefix denoting* cartilage.

chondritis (kon-dry-tis) *n.* any inflammatory condition affecting cartilage.

chondroblast (kon-droh-blast) *n.* a cell that produces the matrix of cartilage.

chondroblastoma (kon-droh-blas-toh-mă) *n.* a tumour derived from chondroblasts, having the appearance of a mass of well-differentiated cartilage.

chondroclast (kon-droh-klast) *n.* a cell that is concerned with the absorption of cartilage.

chondrocyte (kon-droh-syt) *n.* a cartilage cell, found embedded in the matrix.

chondroma (kon-droh-mă) *n.* a relatively common benign tumour of cartilage-forming cells, which may occur at the growing end of any bone but is found most commonly in the bones of the feet and hands.

chondromalacia (kon-droh-mă-lay-shiă) *n.* softening, inflammation, and degeneration of cartilage at a joint. *c. patellae* chondromalacia affecting the undersurface of the kneecap, resulting in pain in the front of the knee and grating, which is made worse by kneeling, squatting, or climbing stairs.

chondrosarcoma (kon-droh-sar-koh-ma) *n.* (*pl.* **chondrosarco-**

mata) a malignant tumour of cartilage cells, occurring in a bone. Restricted to the axial skeleton, such tumours are slow-growing but infiltrate adjacent structures.

chord- (chordo-) *prefix denoting* **1.** a cord. **2.** the notochord.

chorda (kor-da) *n.* (*pl.* **chordae**) a cord, tendon, or nerve fibre. *chordae tendineae* stringlike processes in the heart that attach the margins of the mitral and tricuspid valve leaflets to projections of the wall of the ventricle (*papillary muscles*).

chordee (kor-dee) *n.* acute angulation of the penis. It may occur as a result of Peyronie's disease or, in a child, of hypospadias.

chordotomy (kor-dot-ŏmi) *n. see* cordotomy.

chorea (ko-ree-ă) *n.* a jerky involuntary movement particularly affecting the head, face, or limbs. The symptoms are most commonly due to disease of the basal ganglia. *Huntington's c. see* Huntington's disease. *Sydenham's c.* chorea that mainly affects children and typically occurs after an infection caused by β-haemolytic streptococci (such as rheumatic fever or scarlet fever).

chorion (kor-iŏn) *n.* the embryonic membrane that totally surrounds the embryo from the time of implantation. —**chorionic** *adj.*

chorionepithelioma (choriocarcinoma) (kor-i-ŏn-ep-i-theel-i-oh-mă) *n.* a rare form of cancer originating in the chorion. It is a highly malignant tumour usually following a hydatidiform mole, although it may follow abortion or even a normal pregnancy.

chorionic gonadotrophin (kor-i-

on-ik) *n. see* human chorionic gonadotrophin.

chorionic villi *pl. n. see* villus.

chorionic villus sampling (CVS) *n.* a fetal monitoring technique in which a sample of chorionic villus is extracted through the cervix or abdomen under ultrasound visualization. The earliest recommended time for sampling is the ninth week of pregnancy. The cells so obtained are subjected to chromosomal and biochemical studies to determine if any abnormalities are present in the fetus. This enables the prenatal diagnosis of such congenital disorders as Down's syndrome and thalassaemia.

chorioretinopathy (kor-i-oh-ret-in-op-ă-thi) *n.* any eye disease involving both the choroid and the retina. *central serous c.* shallow retinal detachment in the area of the macula due to leakage through the retinal pigment epithelium (*see* retina) into the subretinal space. The cause is unknown. It affects young adult males, causing reduced or distorted vision that usually settles in a few months.

choroid (ko-roid) *n.* the layer of the eyeball between the retina and the sclera. It contains blood vessels and a pigment that absorbs excess light and so prevents blurring of vision. *See* eye. —**choroidal** (kŏ-roid-ăl) *adj.*

choroidal detachment *n.* the separation of the choroid from the sclera of the eye as a result of leakage of fluid from the vessels of the choroid. It occurs when pressure inside the eyeball is very low, usually after trauma or intraocular surgery.

choroiditis (ko-roid-I-tis) *n.* inflammation of the choroid layer of the eye. Vision becomes blurred but the eye is usually painless. *See* uveitis.

choroidocyclitis (ko-roid-oh-sy-**kly**-tis) *n.* inflammation of the choroid layer and the ciliary body of the eye.

choroid plexus *n.* a rich network of blood vessels, derived from those of the pia mater, in each of the brain's ventricles. It is responsible for the production of cerebrospinal fluid.

Christmas disease (haemophilia B) (kris-măs) *n.* a disorder that is identical in its effects to haemophilia A, but is due to a deficiency of a different blood coagulation factor, Factor IX. [S. Christmas (20th century), in whom the factor was first identified]

Christmas factor *n. see* Factor IX.

chrom- (chromo-) *prefix denoting* colour or pigment.

-chromasia *suffix denoting* staining or pigmentation.

chromat- (chromato-) *prefix denoting* colour or pigment.

chromatid (**kroh**-mă-tid) *n.* one of the two threadlike strands formed by longitudinal division of a chromosome during mitosis and meiosis. They remain attached to the centromere.

chromatin (**kroh**-mă-tin) *n.* the material of a cell nucleus that stains with basic dyes and consists of DNA and protein: the substance of which the chromosomes are made.

chromatography (kroh-mă-**tog**-răfi) *n.* any of several techniques for separating the components of a mixture by selective absorption. In two such techniques, widely used in medicine, a sample of the mixture is placed at the edge of a sheet of filter paper (*paper c.*) or a column of a powdered absorbent (*column c.*). The components of the mixture are absorbed to different extents and thus move along the paper or column at different rates.

chromatolysis (kroh-mă-**tol**-i-sis) *n.* the dispersal or disintegration of the microscopic structures within the nerve cells that normally produce proteins. It is part of the cell's response to injury.

chromatophore (kroh-mă-tŏ-for) *n.* a cell containing pigment. In humans chromatophores containing melanin are found in the skin, hair, and eyes.

chromatosis (kroh-mă-toh-sis) *n.* abnormal pigmentation of the skin, as occurs in Addison's disease.

chromic acid (**kroh**-mik) *n.* a compound of chromium used in solution as a caustic for the removal of warts. Formula: CrO_3.

chromosome (**kroh**-mŏ-sohm) *n.* one of the threadlike structures in a cell nucleus that carry the genetic information in the form of genes. It is composed of a long double filament of DNA coiled into a helix together with associated proteins. The nucleus of each human somatic cell contains 46 chromosomes, 23 being of maternal and 23 of paternal origin. *See also* chromatid, centromere, sex chromosome. —**chromosomal** *adj.*

chronic (kron-ik) *adj.* describing a disease of long duration involving very slow changes. Such disease is often of gradual onset. *Compare* acute. —**chronicity** (kron-**iss**-lti) *n.*

chronic fatigue syndrome *n. see* CFS/ME.

chronic obstructive pulmonary disease (COPD, chronic obstructive airways disease, COAD) *n.* a disease of adults, especially those over the age of 45 with a history of smoking or inhalation of airborne pollution. It has features of emphysema and chronic bronchitis and is diagnosed when the forced expiratory volume in 1 second (FEV_1) is less than 60% of the predicted value for the patient's age and height and the patient does not respond to steroid drugs or bronchodilators.

Chronic Sick and Disabled Persons Act 1970 *n.* (in Britain) an Act providing for the identification and care of those suffering from a chronic or degenerative disease for which there is no cure and which can be only partially alleviated by treatment.

Churg-Strauss syndrome (cherg-strows) *n.* a clinical syndrome comprising severe asthma associated with an increased eosinophil count in the peripheral blood and eosinophilic deposits in the small vessels of the lungs. It usually responds to oral corticosteroids. Untreated, it may result in severe and widespread systemic angiitis. [J. Churg (1910–) and L. Strauss (1913–), US pathologists]

Chvostek's sign (vos-teks) *n.* a spasm of the facial muscles elicited by lightly tapping the facial nerve. It is a sign of tetany. [F. Chvostek (1835–84), Austrian surgeon]

chyle (kyl) *n.* an alkaline milky liquid found within the lacteals after a period of absorption. It consists of lymph with a suspension of minute droplets of digested fats, which have been absorbed from the small intestine.

chyluria (kyl-yoor-iă) *n.* the presence of chyle in the urine.

chyme (kym) *n.* the semiliquid acid mass that is the form in which food passes from the stomach to the small intestine. It is produced by the action of gastric juice and the churning of the stomach.

chymotrypsin (ky-moh-**trip**-sin) *n.* a protein-digesting enzyme (*see* peptidase). It is secreted by the pancreas in an inactive form, *chymotrypsinogen*, that is converted into chymotrypsin in the duodenum by the action of trypsin.

chymotrypsinogen (ky-moh-trip-sin-ŏ-jin) *n. see* chymotrypsin.

cicatricial (sik-ă-**trish**-ăl) *adj.* associated with scarring. *c. alopecia see* alopecia.

ciclosporin (cyclosporin) (sik-loh-spo-rin) *n.* an immunosuppressant drug used to prevent and treat rejection of a transplanted organ or bone marrow. It is also used to treat rheumatoid arthritis, psoriasis, and atopic eczema. Ciclosporin is administered orally or by intravenous infusion. Trade names: **Neoral**, **Sandimmun**, **Sang-Cya**.

-cide *suffix* denoting killer or killing.

ciliary body (sil-i-er-i) *n.* the part of the eye that connects the choroid with the iris. It consists of three zones: the *ciliary ring*, which adjoins the choroid; the *ciliary processes*, a series of about 70 radial ridges behind the iris to which the suspensory ligament of the lens is attached; and the *ciliary muscle*, contraction of which alters the curvature of the lens (*see* accommodation).

cilium (sil-iŭm) *n.* (*pl.* **cilia**) **1.** a hairlike process, large numbers of which are found on certain epithelial cells, particularly on the epithelium that lines the upper respiratory tract, and on certain protozoa. **2.** an eyelash or eyelid. —**ciliary** *adj.*

cimetidine (si-met-i-deen) *n.* an H₂-receptor antagonist (*see* antihistamine) that is administered by mouth or injection to treat such digestive disorders as stomach and duodenal ulcers and gastro-oesophageal reflux disease. Trade names: **Dyspamet, Galenamet, Tagamet.**

Cimex (sy-meks) *n. see* bed bug.

CIN (cervical intraepithelial neoplasia) *n.* cellular changes in the cervix of the uterus preceding the invasive stages of cervical cancer. The CIN grading system distinguishes three stages: *CIN 1* (mild dysplasia); *CIN 2* (moderate dysplasia); and *CIN 3* (severe dysplasia, carcinoma in situ).

cinchocaine (sink-ŏ-kayn) *n.* a local anaesthetic administered as an ointment to relieve the pain of haemorrhoids. Trade name: **Nupercainal.**

cinchona (sing-koh-nă) *n.* the dried bark of *Cinchona* trees, formerly used in medicine to stimulate the appetite and to prevent haemorrhage and diarrhoea. Cinchona is the source of quinine.

cinchonism (sink-ŏ-nizm) *n.* poisoning caused by an overdose of cinchona or the alkaloids quinine, quinidine, or cinchonine derived

from it. The symptoms include ringing noises in the ears, dizziness, and blurring of vision.

cine- *prefix denoting* any technique of recording a rapid series of X-ray images on cine film for later analysis. Examples: *cineangiography; cinefluorography.* Cine film is now being replaced by electronic storage media.

cingulectomy (sing-yoo-lek-tŏmi) *n.* surgical excision of the cingulum, occasionally carried out as psychosurgery for intractable mental illness.

cingulum (sing-yoo-lŭm) *n.* (*pl.* **cingula**) a curved bundle of nerve fibres in each cerebral hemisphere, nearly encircling its connection with the corpus callosum. It is the part of the brain controlling anger and depression. *See* cerebrum.

ciprofibrate (sip-roh-fy-brayt) *n.* a drug used for treating hyperlipidaemia (*see* fibrate). It is administered by mouth. Trade name: **Modalim.**

ciprofloxacin (sip-roh-floks ă-sin) *n.* a broad-spectrum quinolone antibiotic that can be given orally and is particularly useful against Gram-negative bacteria, such as *Pseudomonas*, that are resistant to all other oral antibiotics. It is also used as eye drops to treat eye infections. Trade names: **Ciloxan, Ciproxin.**

circadian rhythm (ser-kay-diăn) *n.* the periodic rhythm, synchronized approximately to the 24-hour day/night cycle, seen in various metabolic activities of most living organisms (e.g. sleeping, hormone secretion).

circle of Willis (ser-kŭl ŏv wil-iss)

n. a circle on the undersurface of the brain formed by linked branches of the arteries that supply the brain. [T. Willis (1621–75), English anatomist]

circulation (ser-kew-**lay**-shŏn) *n.* **1.** the movement of a fluid in a circular course, especially the passage of blood through the cardiovascular system. **2.** the system of vessels effecting this passage. *pulmonary c.* circulation of blood between the heart and lungs. Deoxygenated blood passes to the lungs from the right ventricle via the pulmonary artery; oxygenated blood returns to the left atrium via the pulmonary vein. *systemic c.* circulation of blood between the heart and all parts of the body except the lungs. Oxygenated blood leaves the aorta and deoxygenated blood returns into the vena cava. *See also* collateral circulation. —**circulatory** *adj.*

circum- *prefix denoting* around; surrounding.

circumcision (ser-kŭm-**sizh**-ŏn) *n.* surgical removal of the foreskin of the penis. This operation is usually performed for religious and ethnic reasons but is sometimes required for medical conditions, mainly phimosis and paraphimosis. *female c.* surgical removal of the clitoris, labia minora, and labia majora. *See* clitoridectomy, infibulation.

circumduction (ser-kŭm-**duk**-shŏn) *n.* a circular movement, such as that made by a limb.

circumflex nerve (ser-kŭm-fleks) *n.* a mixed sensory and motor nerve of the upper arm. It arises from the fifth and sixth cervical segments of the spinal cord and is distributed to the deltoid muscle of the shoulder and the overlying skin.

circumoral (ser-kŭm-or-ăl) *adj.* situated around the mouth.

cirrhosis (si-**roh**-sis) *n.* a condition in which the liver responds to injury or death of some of its cells by producing interlacing strands of fibrous tissue between which are nodules of regenerating cells. Causes include alcoholism (*alcoholic c.*), viral hepatitis (*postnecrotic c.*), chronic obstruction of the common bile duct (*secondary biliary c.*), autoimmune diseases (*primary biliary c., PBC*), and chronic heart failure (*cardiac c.*). Complications include portal hypertension, ascites, hepatic encephalopathy, and hepatoma. —**cirrhotic** *adj.*

cirs- (**cirso-**) *prefix denoting* a varicose vein.

cirsoid (ser-soid) *adj.* describing the distended knotted appearance of a varicose vein.

CIS *n. see* carcinoma in situ.

CISC *n. see* (clean) intermittent self-catheterization.

cisplatin (sis-**plat**-in) *n.* a heavy-metal compound; a cytotoxic drug that impedes cell division by damaging DNA. Administered intravenously, it is used in the treatment of testicular and ovarian tumours.

cisterna (sis-ter-nă) *n.* (*pl.* **cisternae**) **1.** one of the enlarged spaces beneath the arachnoid that act as reservoirs for cerebrospinal fluid. *c. magna* the largest of the cisternae, lying beneath the cerebellum and behind the medulla oblongata. **2.** a dilatation at the lower end of the thoracic duct, into which the great lymph ducts of the lower limbs drain.

citalopram (sit-**al**-ŏ-pram) *n.* an antidepressant drug that acts by prolonging the action of the neurotransmitter serotonin (5-hydroxytryptamine) in the brain (*see* SSRI). It is taken by mouth. Trade name: **Cipramil**.

citric acid (sit-rik) *n.* an organic acid found naturally in citrus fruits. Citric acid is formed in the first stage of the Krebs cycle. Formula: $CH_2(COOH)C(OH)(COOH)CH_2COOH$.

citric acid cycle *n. see* Krebs cycle.

Citrobacter (sit-roh-bak-ter) *n.* a genus of Gram-negative anaerobic rod-shaped bacteria widely distributed in nature. The organisms cause infections of the intestinal and urinary tracts, gall bladder, and the meninges that are usually secondary, occurring in the elderly, newborn, debilitated, and immunocompromised.

citrulline (sit-rŭ-lcen) *n.* an amino acid produced by the liver as a by-product during the conversion of ammonia to urea.

CJD *n. see* Creutzfeldt-Jakob disease.

clamp (klamp) *n.* a surgical instrument designed to compress a structure, such as a blood vessel or a cut end of the intestine. See illustration.

claudication (klaw-di-**kay**-shŏn) *n.* limping. *intermittent* c. a cramping pain in the calf and leg muscles, induced by exercise and relieved by rest, that is caused by an inadequate supply of blood to the affected muscles.

claustrophobia (klaw-strŏ-**foh**-biǎ) *n.* a morbid fear of enclosed places. *See also* phobia.

clavicle (klav-i-kǔl) *n.* the collar bone: a long slender curved bone, a pair of which form the front part of the shoulder girdle. Fracture of the clavicle is a common sports injury: the majority of cases require no treatment other than supporting the weight of the arm in a sling. —**clavicular** (klǎ-**vik**-yoo-ler) *adj.*

clavulanic acid (klav-yoo-lan-ik) *n.* a drug that interferes with the enzymes (penicillinases) that inactivate many penicillin-type antibiotics, such as amoxicillin. Combined with the antibiotic, clavulanic acid can overcome drug resistance.

clavus (klay-vŭs) *n.* a sharp pain in the head, as if a nail were being driven in.

claw-foot (klaw-fuut) *n.* an excessively arched foot, giving an unnaturally high instep. In most cases the cause is unknown, but the deformity may sometimes be due to an imbalance between the muscles flexing the toes and the shorter muscles that extend them. Medical name: **pes cavus**.

claw-hand (klaw-hand) *n.* flexion and contraction of the fingers with extension at the joints between the

noncrushing clamp

twin gastrointestinal clamp

Intestinal clamps

fingers and the hand, giving a claw-like appearance. The causes of claw-hand include injuries, syringomyelia, and leprosy. *See also* Dupuytren's contracture.

cleavage (kleev-ij) *n.* (in embryology) the process of repeated cell division of the fertilized egg to form a ball of cells that becomes the blastocyst.

cleft lip (harelip) (kleft) *n.* the congenital deformity of a cleft in the upper lip, on one or both sides of the midline. It is often associated with a cleft palate. Medical name: **cheiloschisis**.

cleft palate *n.* a fissure in the midline of the palate due to failure of the two sides to fuse in embryonic development. Only part of the palate may be affected, or the cleft may extend the full length with bilateral clefts at the front of the maxilla; it may be accompanied by a cleft lip and disturbance of tooth formation.

cleid- (cleido-, clid-, clido-) *prefix denoting* the clavicle (collar bone).

cleidocranial dysostosis (kly-doh-**kray**-niăl dis-os-**toh**-sis) *n.* a congenital defect of bone formation in which the skull bones ossify imperfectly and the collar bones (clavicles) are absent.

clemastine (klem-ă-steen) *n.* an antihistamine used to relieve the symptoms of hay fever and urticaria. It is administered by mouth. Trade names: **Aller-eze, Tavegil**.

Clifton Assessment Procedures for the Elderly (CAPE) (klif-tŏn) *n.* an assessment tool designed to assess quality of life and physical and cognitive dependency levels in the elderly.

climacteric (kly-**mak**-ter-ik) *n. see* menopause. *male c.* declining sexual drive and fertility in men, usually occurring around or after middle age.

clindamycin (klin-dă-**my**-sin) *n.* an antibiotic administered by mouth, injection, or topically to treat serious bacterial infections. Trade name: **Dalacin**.

clinic (klin-ik) *n.* **1.** an establishment or department of a hospital devoted to the treatment of particular diseases or the medical care of outpatients. **2.** a gathering of instructors, students, and patients, usually in a hospital ward, for the examination and treatment of the patients.

clinical audit (klin-i-kăl) *n.* a process by which doctors, nurses, and other health-care professionals systematically review the procedures used for diagnosis, care, and treatment, examining how associated resources are used and investigating the effects care has on the outcome and quality of life for the patient.

clinical governance (guv-er-năns) *n.* a system for making local health services responsive to patients and aiming to reduce variations in clinical practice, thus improving national standards. It consists of audit, continuing professional development, standard setting, workforce planning, complaints handling, user involvement, risk assessment, and research and development.

clinical medicine *n.* the branch of medicine dealing with the study of actual patients and the diagnosis and treatment of disease at the bedside, as opposed to the study of disease by pathology or other laboratory work.

clinodactyly (klin-oh-**dak**-tili) *n.* congenital deflection of one or more digits from the central axis of the hand or foot. Clinodactyly may affect both hands (or feet) and may be found in association with other congenital malformations.

clitoridectomy (klit-er-id-**ek**-tŏmi) *n.* surgical removal of the clitoris.

clitoris (**klit**-er-iss) *n.* the female counterpart of the penis, which contains erectile tissue (*see* corpus (cavernosum)) but is unconnected with the urethra. It becomes erect under conditions of sexual stimulation.

clitoromegaly (klit-er-oh-**meg**-ăli) *n.* abnormal development of the clitoris due to excessive exposure to androgens, either from abnormal endogenous production or exogenous administration.

cloaca (kloh-**ay**-kă) *n.* the most posterior part of the embryonic hindgut. It becomes divided into the rectum and the urinogenital sinus.

clomethiazole (chlormethiazole) (kloh-mi-**th'y**-ă-zohl) *n.* a sedative and hypnotic drug administered by mouth or injection to treat insomnia in the elderly (when associated with confusion, agitation, and restlessness) and drug withdrawal symptoms (especially in alcoholism). Trade name: **Heminevrin**.

clomifene (clomiphene) (**kloh**-mi-feen) *n.* a synthetic nonsteroidal compound (*see* anti-androgen) that induces ovulation and subsequent menstruation in women who fail to ovulate and stimulates increased ovulation (*see* superovulation) for in vitro fertilization. Trade name: **Clomid**.

clomipramine (kloh-**mip**-ră-meen) *n.* a drug administered by mouth or injection to treat various depressive states (*see* antidepressant). Trade name: **Anafranil**.

clonazepam (kloh-**naz**-ĕ-pam) *n.* a drug with anticonvulsant properties, administered by mouth or injection to treat epilepsy and other conditions involving seizures. Trade name: **Rivotril**.

clone (klohn) **1.** *n.* a group of cells (usually bacteria) descended from a single cell by asexual reproduction and therefore genetically identical to each other and to the parent cell. **2.** an organism derived from a single cell of its parent and therefore genetically identical to it. *gene c.* a group of identical genes produced by techniques of genetic engineering. **3.** *vb.* to form a clone.

clonic (**klon**-ik) *adj.* of, relating to, or resembling clonus. The term is most commonly used to describe the rhythmical limb movements seen as part of a convulsive epileptic seizure (*see* epilepsy).

clonidine (**kloh**-ni-deen) *n.* a drug administered by mouth or injection to treat high blood pressure (hypertension) and migraine. Trade names: **Catapres**, **Dixarit**.

clonus (**kloh**-nŭs) *n.* rhythmical contraction of a muscle in response to a suddenly applied and then sustained stretch stimulus. It is most readily obtained at the ankle and is usually a sign of disease in the brain or spinal cord.

clopidogrel (kloh-**pid**-oh-grel) *n.* a drug that reduces platelet aggregation. It is administered by mouth to prevent strokes or heart attacks in those at risk. Trade name: **Plavix**.

Clostridium (klo-strid-iŭm) *n.* a genus of mostly Gram-positive anaerobic spore-forming rodlike bacteria commonly found in soil and in the intestinal tract of humans and animals. *C. botulinum* a species that grows freely in badly preserved canned foods, producing a toxin causing serious food poisoning (*see* botulism). *C. tetani* a species that causes tetanus on contamination of wounds. *C. perfringens* (*Welch's bacillus*) a species that causes blood poisoning, food poisoning, and gas gangrene.

clotrimazole (kloh-trim-ă-zohl) *n.* an antifungal drug used to treat all types of fungal skin infections (including ringworm) and vaginal infections. It is applied to the infected part as a cream or solution or as vaginal pessaries. Trade name: **Canesten**.

clotting factors (klot-ing) *pl. n. see* coagulation factors.

clotting time *n. see* coagulation time.

clozapine (kloz-ă-peen) *n.* an atypical antipsychotic drug used in the treatment of schizophrenia and other disorders resistant to conventional antipsychotics. Administered by mouth, it is notable for the absence of tremors and repetitive movements that are associated with other antipsychotic drugs. In a few cases it may depress levels of white blood cells. Trade name: **Clozaril**.

clubbing (klub-ing) *n.* thickening of the tissues at the bases of the finger and toe nails so that the normal angle between the nail and the digit is filled in. In extreme cases the digit

end becomes bulbous like a club or drumstick. Clubbing is seen in some diseases of the heart and respiratory system and as a harmless congenital abnormality.

club-foot (klub-fuut) *n. see* talipes.

clumping (klump-ing) *n. see* agglutination.

cluster headache (klust-er) *n.* a variant of migraine more common in men than in women. The unilateral pain around one eye is very severe and lasts between 15 minutes and three hours. It is associated with drooping of the eyelid (ptosis), a bloodshot eye, and/or excessive production of tears in the eye.

cluttering (klut-er-ing) *n.* an erratic unrhythmical way of speaking in rapid jerky bursts. It can make speech hard to understand, and speech therapy is usually helpful. Unlike stammering, there are no repetitions or prolonged hesitations of speech.

Clutton's joint (klu-t'nz) *n.* a painless joint effusion in a child, usually in the knee, caused by inflammation of the synovial membranes due to congenital syphilis. [H. H. Clutton (1850–1909), British surgeon]

CMF *n.* cyclophosphamide, methotrexate, 5-fluorouracil: the combination of chemotherapy drugs used in standard treatment for breast cancer.

CML *n.* chronic myeloid leukaemia. *See* myeloid (leukaemia).

CMV *n. see* cytomegalovirus.

CNS *n. see* central nervous system.

COAD *n.* chronic obstructive airways disease (*see* chronic obstructive pulmonary disease).

coagulant (koh-ag-yoo-lănt) *n.* any substance capable of converting blood from a liquid to a solid state. *See* blood coagulation.

coagulase (koh-ag-yoo-layz) *n.* an enzyme, formed by disease-producing varieties of certain bacteria of the genus *Staphylococcus*, that causes blood plasma to coagulate. Staphylococci that are positive when tested for coagulase production are classified as belonging to the species *Staphylococcus aureus*.

coagulation (koh-ag-yoo-lay-shŏn) *n.* the process by which a colloidal liquid changes to a jelly-like mass. *See* blood coagulation.

coagulation factors (clotting factors) *pl. n.* a group of substances present in blood plasma that are responsible for the conversion of blood from a liquid to a solid state (*see* blood coagulation). Although they have specific names, most coagulation factors are referred to by an agreed set of Roman numerals (*see* Factor VIII, Factor IX, Factor XI).

coagulation time (clotting time) *n.* the time taken for blood or blood plasma to coagulate (*see* blood coagulation).

coagulum (koh-ag-yoo-lŭm) *n.* a mass of coagulated matter, such as that formed when blood clots.

coalesce (koh-ă-less) *vb.* to grow together or unite. —**coalescence** *n.*

coal-worker's pneumoconiosis (anthracosis) (kohl-wer-kerz) *n.* a lung disease caused by coal dust. It affects mainly coal miners but also other exposed workers, such as lightermen, if the lungs' capacity to accommodate and remove the particles is exceeded. *See* pneumoconiosis.

coarctation (koh-ark-tay-shŏn) *n.* (of the aorta) a congenital narrowing of a short segment of the aorta, resulting in high blood pressure in the upper part of the body and arms and low blood pressure in the legs. The defect is corrected surgically.

Coats' disease (kohts) *n.* a congenital anomaly of the blood vessels of the retina, which are abnormally dilated and leaking. This results in subretinal haemorrhage and massive exudation. [G. Coats (1876–1915), British ophthalmologist]

cobalt (koh-bawlt) *n.* a metallic element that forms part of the vitamin B_{12} molecule. Symbol: Co. *cobalt-60* (*radiocobalt*) a powerful emitter of gamma radiation, used in the radiation treatment of cancer (*see* radiotherapy, teletherapy).

cocaine (kŏ-kayn) *n.* an alkaloid, derived from the leaves of the coca plant (*Erythroxylon coca*) or prepared synthetically, sometimes used as a local anaesthetic in eye, ear, nose, and throat surgery. Since it may lead to psychological dependence, cocaine has largely been replaced by safer anaesthetics.

cocainism (koh-kayn-izm) *n.* **1.** the habitual use of, or addiction to, cocaine in order to experience its intoxicating effects. **2.** the mental and physical deterioration resulting from addiction to cocaine.

coccus (kok-ŭs) *n.* (*pl.* cocci) any spherical bacterium. *See* gonococcus, meningococcus, Micrococcus, pneumococcus, Staphylococcus, Streptococcus.

cocci- (coccyg-, coccygo-) *prefix denoting* the coccyx.

coccygodynia (coccydynia)

(kok-si-goh-**din**-iă) *n.* pain in the coccyx and the neighbouring area.

coccyx (**kok**-siks) *n.* (*pl.* **coccyges** or **coccyxes**) the lowermost element of the backbone: the vestigial human tail. It consists of four rudimentary *coccygeal vertebrae* fused to form a triangular bone that articulates with the sacrum. *See also* vertebra. —**coccygeal** (kok-**sij**-iăl) *adj.*

cochlea (**kok**-liă) *n.* the spiral organ of the labyrinth of the ear, which is concerned with the reception and analysis of sound. —**cochlear** (kok-li-er) *adj.*

cochlear duct (scala media) *n.* *see* scala.

cochlear implant *n.* a device to improve the hearing of profoundly deaf people who derive no benefit from conventional hearing aids. It consists of an electrode that is permanently implanted into the inner ear (cochlea). An external battery-powered device with a microphone and an electronic processing unit passes information to the electrode using radio-frequency waves.

cochlear nerve *n.* the nerve connecting the cochlea to the brain and therefore responsible for the nerve impulses relating to hearing. It forms part of the vestibulocochlear nerve.

Cockayne's syndrome (kok-**aynz**) *n.* a hereditary disorder (inherited as an autosomal recessive condition) associated with trisomy of chromosome no. 20. Clinical features include epidermolysis bullosa, dwarfism, mental retardation, and pigmentary degeneration of the retina. [E. A. Cockayne (1880–1956), British physician]

codeine (koh-deen) *n.* an analgesic derived from morphine but less potent as a pain killer and sedative and less toxic. It is administered by mouth or injection to relieve pain and also to suppress coughs.

cod liver oil (kod) *n.* a pale yellow oil, extracted from the livers of cod and related fish, that is rich in vitamins A and D and used in the treatment and prevention of deficiencies of these vitamins (e.g. rickets).

-coele *suffix denoting* **1.** a body cavity. **2.** *see* -cele.

coeli- (coelio-) *prefix denoting* the abdomen or belly.

coeliac (seel-i-ak) *adj.* of or relating to the abdominal region. *c. trunk* a branch of the abdominal aorta supplying the stomach, spleen, liver, and gall bladder.

coeliac disease *n.* a condition in which the small intestine fails to digest and absorb food. It is due to a permanent sensitivity of the intestinal lining to the protein gliadin, which is contained in gluten in the germ of wheat and rye and causes atrophy of the digestive and absorptive cells of the intestine. Symptoms include stunted growth, distended abdomen, and pale frothy foul-smelling stools. Medical name: **gluten enteropathy**.

coelioscopy (see-li-**os**-kŏpi) *n.* the technique of introducing an endoscope through an incision in the abdominal wall to examine the intestines and other organs within the abdominal cavity.

coenzyme (koh-en-zym) *n.* a nonprotein organic compound that, in the presence of an enzyme, plays an essential role in the reaction that is catalysed by the enzyme.

coffee-ground vomit (kof-ee-grownd) *n.* vomit containing gastric juices and small dark fragments of partly digested blood, indicating slow bleeding in the upper gastrointestinal tract.

Cogan's syndrome (koh-gănz) *n.* a disorder in which keratitis and iridocyclitis (*see* uveitis) are associated with tinnitus, vertigo, and bilateral sensorineural deafness. [D. G. Cogan (1908–93), US ophthalmologist]

cognition (kog-nish-ŏn) *n.* a group of mental activities (including perception, recognition, and judgment) that leads to awareness of an object or situation. *Compare* conation. —**cognitive** (kog-ni-tiv) *adj.*

cognitive psychology *n.* the school of psychology concerned with the ways in which knowledge is acquired, stored, correlated, and retrieved, by studying the mental processes underlying attention, concept formation, information processing, memory, and speech.

cognitive therapy *n.* a form of psychotherapy based on the belief that psychological problems are the products of faulty ways of thinking about the world. The therapist assists the patient to identify these false ways of thinking and to avoid them.

coitus (sexual intercourse, copulation) (koh-it-ŭs) *n.* sexual contact between a man and a woman during which the erect penis enters the vagina and is moved within it by pelvic thrusts until ejaculation occurs. **c. interruptus** an unreliable contraceptive method in which the penis is removed from the vagina before ejac-ulation of semen. *See also* orgasm. —**coital** *adj.*

col- (coli-, colo-) *prefix denoting* the colon.

colchicine (kol-chi-seen) *n.* a drug obtained from the meadow saffron (*Colchicum autumnale*), administered by mouth to relieve pain in attacks of gout and to prevent attacks of polyserositis.

cold (common cold) (kohld) *n.* a widespread infectious virus disease causing inflammation of the mucous membranes of the nose, throat, and bronchial tubes. Symptoms include a sore throat, stuffy or runny nose, headache, cough, and general malaise.

cold sore *n. see* herpes (simplex).

colectomy (kŏ-lek-tŏmi) *n.* surgical removal of the colon (*total c.*) or a segment of the colon (*partial c.*). *See also* hemicolectomy, proctocolectomy.

colestipol (kŏ-les-ti-pol) *n.* a drug that binds bile acids (*see* bile-acid sequestrant). It is administered by mouth to lower cholesterol levels in the blood in patients with hyperlipidaemia and primary hypercholesterolaemia. Trade name: **Colestid**.

colestyramine (cholestyramine) (koli-sty-ră-meen) *n.* a drug that binds bile acids (*see* bile-acid sequestrant). It is administered by mouth to relieve conditions due to irritant effects of bile acids (such as the itching that occurs in obstructive jaundice), to treat diarrhoea, and to lower blood levels of cholesterol and other fats. Trade names: **Questran, Questran Light**.

colic (kol-ik) *n.* severe abdominal pain, usually of fluctuating severity, with waves of pain seconds or a few minutes apart. *infantile c.* colic that is common among babies, due to wind in the intestine associated with feeding difficulties. *intestinal c.* colic due to partial or complete obstruction of the intestine or to constipation. Medical names: **enteralgia**, **tormina**. *See also* biliary (colic).

coliform bacteria (kol-i-form) *pl. n.* a group of Gram-negative rodlike bacteria that are normally found in the gastrointestinal tract and ferment the sugar lactose. It includes the genera *Enterobacter*, *Escherichia*, and *Klebsiella*.

colistin (kŏ-list-in) *n.* an antibiotic administered by mouth to sterilize the bowel before surgery. Trade name: **Colomycin**.

colitis (kŏ-ly-tis) *n.* inflammation of the colon. The usual symptoms are diarrhoea, sometimes with blood and mucus, and lower abdominal pain. *ischaemic c.* colitis caused by partial or temporary cessation of blood supply to the colon. *mucous c. see* irritable bowel syndrome. *pseudomembranous c.* colitis caused by overgrowth of the normal population of *Clostridium difficile*, which is a complication of therapy with some antibiotics. *ulcerative c.* (*UC*, *idiopathic proctocolitis*) colitis of varying severity in which the rectum (*see* proctitis) as well as a varying amount of the colon become inflamed and ulcerated; its cause is unknown.

collagen (kol-ă-jin) *n.* a protein that is the principal constituent of white fibrous connective tissue (as occurs in tendons). Collagen is also found in skin, bone, cartilage, and ligaments.

collagen disease *n.* an obsolete term for connective-tissue disease.

collar bone (kol-er) *n. see* clavicle.

collateral (kŏ-lat-er-ăl) **1.** *adj.* accessory or secondary. **2.** *n.* a branch (e.g. of a nerve fibre) that is at right angles to the main part.

collateral circulation *n.* **1.** an alternative route provided for the blood by secondary vessels when a primary vessel becomes blocked. **2.** the channels of communication between the blood vessels supplying the heart.

Colles' fracture (kol-iss) *n. see* fracture. [A. Colles (1773–1843), Irish surgeon]

collodion (kŏ-loh-diŏn) *n.* a syrupy solution of nitrocellulose in a mixture of alcohol and ether. When applied to minor wounds it evaporates to leave a thin clear transparent skin. Flexible collodion also contains camphor and castor oil, which allow the skin to stretch a little more.

colloid (kol-oid) *n.* a mixture in which particles of one component (diameter 10^{-6}–10^{-4} mm) are dispersed in a continuous phase of another component. —**colloidal** *adj.*

collyrium (ko-leer-iŭm) *n.* a medicated solution used to bathe the eyes.

coloboma (kolŏ-boh-mă) *n.* (*pl.* **colobomata**) a defect in the development of the eye causing abnormalities ranging in severity from a notch in the lower part of the iris, making the pupil pear-shaped, to defects behind the iris in the fundus. The enlarged pupil causes dazzle symptoms.

colon (koh-lŏn) *n.* the main part of the large intestine, which consists of four sections – the *ascending*, *transverse*, *descending*, and *sigmoid colons* (see illustration). The colon absorbs large amounts of water and electrolytes from the undigested food passed on from the small intestine. At intervals strong peristaltic movements move the dehydrated contents (faeces) towards the rectum. —**colonic** (koh-lon-ik) *adj*.

descending colon
transverse colon
ileum
hepatic flexure
splenic flexure
haustra
rectum
appendix
ascending colon
caecum
sigmoid colon

The colon

colonic irrigation *n*. washing out the contents of the large bowel by means of copious enemas, using either water, with or without soap, or other medication.

colonoscopy (koh-lŏn-os-kŏpi) *n*. a procedure for examining the interior of the entire colon and rectum using a flexible illuminated fibre-optic instrument (*colonoscope*) introduced through the anus.

colony (kol-ŏni) *n*. a discrete population or mass of microorganisms, usually bacteria, all of which are considered to have developed from a single parent cell. *See also* culture.

colorimeter (kul-ŏ-rim-it-er) *n*. an instrument for determining the concentration of a particular compound in a preparation by comparing the intensity of colour in it with that in a standard preparation of known concentration.

colostomy (kŏ-lost-ŏmi) *n*. a surgical operation in which a part of the colon is brought through the abdominal wall and opened in order to drain or decompress the intestine. The colostomy may be temporary, eventually being closed to restore continuity; or permanent, usually when the rectum or lower colon has been removed.

colostrum (kŏ-los-trŭm) *n*. the first secretion from the breast, occurring shortly after, or sometimes before, birth, prior to the secretion of true milk. It is a relatively clear fluid containing serum, white blood cells, and protective antibodies.

colour blindness (kul-er) *n*. any of various conditions in which certain colours are confused with one another. True lack of colour appreciation is extremely rare (*see* monochromat); the most common type of colour blindness is red-blindness (*see* Daltonism). *See also* deuteranopia, tritanopia.

colour flow ultrasound imaging *n*. *see* Doppler ultrasound.

colp- (colpo-) *prefix denoting* the vagina.

colpitis (kol-py-tis) *n.* inflammation of the vagina. *See* vaginitis.

colphysterectomy (kol-poh-hiss-ter-**ek**-tŏmi) *n.* surgical removal of the uterus through the vagina. *See* hysterectomy.

colpoperineorrhaphy (kol-poh-pe-ri-ni-o-**răf**i) *n.* an operation to repair tears in the vagina and the muscles surrounding its opening, particularly posteriorly.

colporrhaphy (kol-po-răfi) *n.* an operation designed to remove lax and redundant vaginal tissue and so reduce the diameter of the vagina in cases of prolapse of the anterior vaginal wall (*anterior c.*) or posterior vaginal wall (*posterior c.*).

colposcope (**vaginoscope**) (**kol**-poh-skohp) *n.* an instrument that is inserted into the vagina and permits visual examination of the cervix and the upper part of the vagina (vaginal vault). —**colposcopy** (kol-**pos**-kŏpi) *n.*

colposuspension (kol-poh-su-**spen**-shŏn) *n.* a surgical operation in which the upper part of the vaginal wall is fixed to the anterior abdominal wall by unabsorbable suture material. Performed through an abdominal incision, this sling operation is used in the surgical treatment of prolapse of the vaginal wall, particularly when stress incontinence exists. *See also* Stamey procedure.

colpotomy (kol-**pot**-ŏmi) *n.* an incision made into the wall of the vagina. This was formerly used to confirm the diagnosis of ectopic pregnancy, but has now been largely superseded by laparoscopy.

column (kol-ŭm) *n.* (in anatomy) any pillar-shaped structure, especially any of the tracts of grey matter found in the spinal cord.

coma (koh-mă) *n.* a state of unrousable unconsciousness.

comatose (koh-mă-tohs) *adj.* in a state of coma; unconscious.

combined therapy (kŏm-bynd) *n.* therapy that combines several types of treatment in order to improve results. It is usually a combination of surgery with radiotherapy and/or chemotherapy for the treatment of malignant tumours (*see* adjuvant therapy). *See also* sandwich therapy.

comedo (kom-i-doh) *n.* (*pl.* **comedones**) *see* blackhead.

commando operation (kŏ-mahn-doh) *n.* a major operation performed to remove a malignant tumour from the head and neck. Extensive dissection, often involving the face, is followed by reconstruction to restore function and cosmetic acceptability.

commensal (kŏ-men-săl) *n.* an organism that lives in close association with another of a different species without either harming or benefiting it. *Compare* symbiosis. —**commensalism** *n.*

comminuted fracture (kom-i-new-tid) *n. see* fracture.

Commission for Health Improvement (CHI) (kŏ-mish-ŏn) *n.* an independent inspectorate, covering England and Wales, that was set up in 1999 to ensure that government standards set through its health policies, national service frameworks, and the National Institute of Clinical Excellence (NICE) are being met.

commissure (kom-iss-yoor) *n.* **1.** a bundle of nerve fibres that crosses the midline of the central nervous system, often connecting similar structures on each side. **2.** any other tissue connecting two similar structures.

commotio retinae (kŏ-moh-shi-oh ret-i-nee) *n.* swelling of the retina associated with sudden reduction of vision, usually resulting from blunt trauma to the eye.

communicable disease (contagious disease, infectious disease) (kŏ-mew-nik-ăbŭl) *n.* any disease that can be transmitted from one person to another. This may occur by direct physical contact, by common handling of a contaminated object (*see* fomes), via a disease carrier, or by spread of infected droplets exhaled into the air.

community health (kŏ-mew-niti) *n.* preventive services, mainly outside the hospital, involving the surveillance of special groups of the population, such as preschool and school children, women, and the elderly, by means of routine clinical assessment and screening tests. *See also* child health clinic.

Community Health Council (CHC) *n.* (formerly, in Britain) a group of local residents appointed to voice the views of patients in relation to the National Health Service.

community hospital *n. see* hospital.

community medicine *n. see* public health medicine.

community midwife (domiciliary midwife) *n.* (in Britain) a registered nurse with special training in midwifery (both hospital and domiciliary practice). The midwife must be registered with the Nursing and Midwifery Council in order to practise; this requires regular refresher courses to supplement the basic qualification of *Registered Midwife (RM)*. Community midwives are attached to hospital obstetric units and their work includes home deliveries and antenatal and postnatal care in the community.

community nurses *pl. n.* (in Britain) a generic term for health visitors, community midwives, district nurses, and community psychiatric nurses. *See also* domiciliary services.

community paediatrician *n.* a consultant in paediatrics with special responsibility for the care of children outside the hospital. *See also* community health.

community physician *n. see* public health physician.

community services *pl. n. see* domiciliary services.

community trust *n.* an NHS trust that is concerned with the provision of community health services and, in some locations, mental health services.

compartment (kŏm-part-mĕnt) *n.* any one of the spaces in a limb that are bounded by bone and thick sheets of fascia and contain the muscles and other tissues of the limb. *c. syndrome* swelling of the muscles in a compartment, which raises the pressure within so that the blood supply to the muscle is cut off, causing ischaemia and further swelling. It is caused by trauma, damage to blood vessels, reperfusion after ischaemia, or tight casts or bandages. *See also* Volkmann's contracture.

compatibility (kŏm-pati-bil-iti) *n.*

the degree to which the body's defence systems will tolerate the presence of intruding foreign material, such as blood when transfused or a kidney when transplanted. *Compare* incompatibility. *See also* histocompatibility, immunity. —**compatible** *adj.*

compensation (kom-pen-**say**-shŏn) *n.* **1.** the act of making up for a functional or structural deficiency. For example, compensation for the loss of a diseased kidney is brought about by an increase in size of the remaining kidney, so restoring the urine-producing capacity. **2.** (in psychoanalysis) the act of exaggerating an approved character trait to make up for a weakness in an opposite trait.

complement (kom-pli-mĕnt) *n.* a system of proteins that interact with one another to aid the body's defences when antibodies combine with antigens. *See also* immunity.

complementary medicine (kom-pli-**ment**-ări) *n.* various forms of therapy that are viewed as complementary to conventional medicine. Previously, complementary therapies were regarded as an alternative to conventional therapies, and the two types were considered to be mutually exclusive (hence the former names *alternative medicine* and *fringe medicine*). However, many practitioners now have dual training in conventional and complementary therapies. There is very limited provision for complementary medicine within the confines of the National Health Service. *See* acupuncture, aromatherapy, chiropractic, homeopathy, naturopathy, osteopathy, reflexology, reiki.

complement fixation *n.* the binding of complement to the complex that is formed when an antibody reacts with a specific antigen. Because complement is taken up from the serum only when such a reaction has occurred, testing for the presence of complement after mixing a suspension of a known organism with a patient's serum can give confirmation of infection with a suspected organism.

complex (kom-pleks) *n.* (in psychoanalysis) an emotionally charged and repressed group of ideas and beliefs that is capable of influencing an individual's behaviour.

complication (kom-pli-**kay**-shŏn) *n.* a disease or condition arising during the course of or as a consequence of another disease.

compos mentis (kom-pŏs men-tis) *adj.* of sound mind; sane.

compress (kom-press) *n.* a pad of material soaked in hot or cold water and applied to an injured part of the body to relieve the pain of inflammation.

compressed air illness (caisson disease) (kŏm-prest) *n.* a syndrome occurring in people working under high pressure in diving bells or at great depths with breathing apparatus. On return to normal atmospheric pressure nitrogen dissolved in the bloodstream expands to form bubbles, causing pain (the *bends*) and blocking the circulation in small blood vessels in the brain and elsewhere (*decompression sickness*). Symptoms may be eliminated by returning the victim to a higher atmospheric pressure and reducing this gradually.

compression (kŏm-**presh**-ŏn) *n.* the state in which an organ, tissue, or part is subject to pressure. *cerebral c.* pressure on brain tissue from a cerebral tumour, intracranial haematoma, etc. *c. venography* see venography.

compulsion (kŏm-**pul**-shŏn) *n.* an obsession that takes the form of a motor act, such as repetitive washing based on a fear of contamination.

compulsory admission (kŏm-**pul**-ser-i) *n.* (in Britain) the entry and detention of a person within an institution without his consent, either because of mental illness (see Mental Health Acts) or severe social deprivation and self-neglect (see Section 47). *Compare* voluntary admission.

computerized tomography (CT) (kŏm-**pew**-tĕ-ryzd) *n.* a form of X-ray examination in which the X-ray source and detector (*CT scanner*) rotate around the object to be scanned and the information can be used to produce cross-sectional images by computer (a *CT scan*). A higher radiation dose is received by the patient than with some conventional X-ray techniques, but the diagnostic information obtained is far greater and should outweigh the risk. CT scanning is particularly useful in the head, chest, and abdomen.

conation (koh-**nay**-shŏn) *n.* the group of mental activities (including drives, will, and instincts) that leads to purposeful action. *Compare* cognition.

conception (kŏn-**sep**-shŏn) *n.* **1.** (in gynaecology) the start of pregnancy, when a male germ cell (sperm) fertilizes a female germ cell (ovum) in the Fallopian tube. **2.** (in psychology) an idea or mental impression.

conceptus (kŏn-**sep**-tŭs) *n.* the products of conception: the developing fetus and its enclosing membrane at all stages in the uterus.

concha (konk-ă) *n.* (*pl.* **conchae**) (in anatomy) any part resembling a shell. *c. auriculae* a depression on the outer surface of the pinna (auricle), which leads to the external auditory meatus of the outer ear. *See also* nasal (concha).

concordance (kŏn-**kor**-dănss) *n.* similarity of any physical characteristic that is found in both of a pair of twins.

concretion (kŏn-**kree**-shŏn) *n.* a stony mass formed within such an organ as the kidney, especially the coating of an internal organ or a foreign body with calcium salts. *See also* calculus.

concussion (kŏn-**kush**-ŏn) *n.* a condition caused by injury to the head, characterized by headache, confusion, and amnesia. These symptoms may be prolonged and constitute a *post-concussional syndrome. See also* (cerebral) contusion, punch-drunk syndrome.

condenser (kŏn-**den**-ser) *n.* (in microscopy) an arrangement of lenses beneath the stage of a microscope. It can be adjusted to provide correct focusing of light on the microscope slide.

conditioned reflex (kŏn-**dish**-ŏnd) *n.* a reflex in which the response occurs not to the sensory stimulus that normally causes it but to a separate stimulus, which has been learnt to be associated with it.

conditioning (kŏn-dish-ŏn-ing) *n.* the establishment of new behaviour by modifying the stimulus/response associations.

condom (kon-dŏm) *n.* a sheath made of latex rubber, plastic, or silk that is fitted over the penis during sexual intercourse. A condom is a reasonably reliable contraceptive; it also protects both partners against sexually transmitted diseases (including AIDS). *female c.* a similar device for women, designed to fit into the vagina.

conduct disorder (kon-dukt) *n.* a repetitive and persistent pattern of aggressive or otherwise antisocial behaviour. It is usually recognized in childhood or adolescence and can lead to antisocial personality disorder. Treatment is usually with behaviour therapy or family therapy.

conduction (kŏn-duk-shŏn) *n.* **1.** (in physics) the process in which heat is transferred through a substance from regions of higher to regions of lower temperature. **2.** (in physiology) the passage of a nerve impulse.

conductor (kŏn-duk-ter) *n.* **1.** (in physics) a substance capable of transmitting heat (e.g. copper, silver) or electricity. **2.** (in surgery) a grooved surgical director.

condyle (kon-dil) *n.* a rounded protuberance that occurs at the ends of some bones, e.g. the occipital bone, and forms an articulation with another bone.

condyloma (kon-di-loh-mǎ) *n.* (*pl.* **condylomata**) a raised wartlike growth. *c. acuminatum* (*pl. condylomata acuminata*) a wart, caused by human papillomavirus, found on the vulva, under the foreskin, or on the skin of the anal region. *c. latum* (*pl. condylomata lata*) a flat plaque occurring in the anogenital region in the secondary stage of syphilis.

cone (kohn) *n.* one of the two types of light-sensitive cells in the retina of the eye (*compare* rod). Cones are essential for acute vision and can also distinguish colours.

cone biopsy *n.* surgical removal, via a colposcope, of a cone-shaped segment of tissue from the cervix of the uterus. It may be performed if a cervical smear reveals evidence of cervical intraepithelial neoplasia (*see* CIN): the affected tissue is removed and examined microscopically for confirmation of the diagnosis.

confabulation (kŏn-fab-yoo-lay-shŏn) *n.* the invention of circumstantial but fictitious detail about events supposed to have occurred in the past. Usually this is to disguise a loss of memory; it typically occurs in Korsakoff's syndrome.

confection (kŏn-fek-shŏn) *n.* (in pharmacy) a sweet substance that is combined with a medicinal preparation to make it suitable for administration.

conflict (kon-flikt) *n.* (in psychology) the state produced when a stimulus produces two opposing reactions. Conflict has been used to explain the development of neurotic disorders, and the resolution of conflict remains an important part of psychoanalysis. *See also* conversion.

congenital (kŏn-jen-it'l) *adj.* describing a condition that is recognized at birth or that is believed to have been present since birth. Congenital malformations include all disorders present at birth whether they are inherited or caused by an environmental factor.

congenital adrenal hyperplasia (CAH) n. a family of autosomal recessive genetic disorders causing decreased activity of any of the enzymes involved in the synthesis of cortisol from cholesterol. Adrenal hyperplasia occurs due to excessive stimulation of the glands by ACTH (adrenocorticotrophic hormone) in response to the cortisol deficiency. The most serious consequence is adrenal crisis and/or severe salt wasting due to lack of cortisol and/or aldosterone. The condition is often easier to spot at birth in females, who may exhibit ambiguous genitalia due to high levels of testosterone in utero.

congenital dislocation of the hip (CDH) n. an abnormality of the hip joint, present at birth, in which the head of the femur is displaced or easily displaceable from the acetabulum, which is poorly developed. It frequently affects both hip joints. See also Barlow's manoeuvre, Ortolani manoeuvre.

congenital heart disease n. see blue baby.

congestion (kŏn-jes-chŏn) n. an accumulation of blood within an organ, which is the result of back pressure within its veins (for example congestion of the lungs and liver occurs in heart failure).

Congo red (kon-goh) n. a dark-red or reddish-brown pigment that becomes blue in acidic conditions. It is used as a histological stain.

coning (kohn-ing) n. prolapse of the brainstem through the foramen magnum of the skull as a result of

raised intracranial pressure: it is usually immediately fatal.

conization (ko-ny-zay-shŏn) n. surgical removal of a cone of tissue. The technique is commonly used in excising a portion of the cervix (neck) of the uterus (see cone biopsy) for the treatment of cervicitis or early cancer (carcinoma in situ).

conjoined twins (kŏn-joind) pl. n. see Siamese twins.

conjugate (conjugate diameter, true conjugate) (kon-jŭg-it) n. the distance between the front and rear of the pelvis measured from the most prominent part of the sacrum to the back of the pubic symphysis. It is estimated by subtracting 1.3–1.9 cm from the distance between the lower edge of the symphysis and the sacrum (the *diagonal c.*). If the true conjugate is less than about 10.2 cm, delivery of an infant through the natural passages may be difficult or impossible.

conjunctiva (kon-junk-ty-vă) n. the delicate mucous membrane that covers the front of the eye and lines the inside of the eyelids. **—conjunctival** adj.

conjunctivitis (pink eye) (kŏn-junk-ti-vy-tis) n. inflammation of the conjunctiva, which becomes red and swollen and produces a watery or pus-containing discharge. Conjunctivitis is caused by infection by bacteria or viruses, allergy, or physical or chemical irritation. *allergic* (or *vernal*) c. conjunctivitis of allergic origin, often associated with hay fever or other forms of atopy. *inclusion c.* a sexually transmitted form of conjunctivitis caused by *Chlamydia trachomatis*. It can be acquired by newborn infants as they pass through an infected birth canal. *See also* trachoma, ophthalmia (neonatorum).

connective tissue (kŏ-nek-tiv) *n.* the tissue that supports, binds, or separates more specialized tissues and organs or functions as a packing tissue of the body. It consists of an amorphous matrix of mucopolysaccharides (*ground substance*) in which may be embedded white (collagenous), yellow (elastic), and reticular fibres, fat cells, fibroblasts, mast cells, and macrophages. Forms of connective tissue include bone, cartilage, tendons, ligaments, and adipose, areolar, and elastic tissues.

connective-tissue disease *n.* any one of a group of diseases that are characterized by inflammatory changes in connective tissue. They include dermatomyositis, systemic and discoid lupus erythematosus, morphoea, polyarteritis nodosa, and rheumatoid arthritis.

Conn's syndrome (konz) *n.* a condition resulting from overproduction of the hormone aldosterone due to disease of the adrenal cortex. *See* aldosteronism. [W. J. Conn (1907–), US physician]

consanguinity (kon-sang-win-iti) *n.* relationship by blood; the sharing of a common ancestor within a few generations.

consensus management (kŏn-sen-sŭs) *n.* a style of management practised in the National Health Service, in which multidisciplinary management teams make decisions based on discussion and mutual agreement.

consequentialism (kon-si-kwen-shăl-izm) *n.* an ethical approach that stresses the importance of taking account of the objective effects or consequences of one's actions on other people and on the overall situation.

conservative treatment (kŏn-ser-vă-tiv) *n.* treatment aimed at preventing a condition from becoming worse, in the expectation that either natural healing will occur or progress of the disease will be so slow that no drastic treatment will be justified. *Compare* radical treatment.

consolidation (kŏn-soli-day-shŏn) *n.* **1.** the state of the lung in which the alveoli (air sacs) are filled with fluid produced by inflamed tissue, as in pneumonia. **2.** the stage of repair of a broken bone following callus formation, during which the callus is transformed by osteoblasts into mature bone.

constipation (kon-sti-pay-shŏn) *n.* a condition in which bowel evacuations occur infrequently, or in which the faeces are hard and small, or where passage of faeces causes difficulty or pain. Recurrent or long-standing constipation is treated by increasing dietary fibre (roughage), laxatives, or enemas.

constrictor (kŏn-strik-ter) *n.* any muscle that compresses an organ or causes a hollow organ or part to contract.

consultant (kŏn-sul-t'nt) *n.* a fully trained specialist in a branch of medicine who accepts total responsibility for patient care.

consumption (kŏn-sump-shŏn) *n.* any disease causing wasting of tissues, especially (formerly) pulmonary tuberculosis. **—consumptive** *adj.*

contact (kon-takt) *n.* transmission

of an infectious disease by touching or handling an infected person or animal (*direct c.*) or by inhaling airborne droplets, etc., containing the infective microorganism (*indirect c.*).

contact lenses *pl. n.* glass or plastic lenses worn directly against the eye, separated from it only by a film of tear fluid. Contact lenses are used mainly in place of glasses to correct errors of refraction, but they may be used for protection in some types of corneal disease.

contagious disease (kŏn-tay-jŭs) *n.* originally, a disease transmitted only by direct physical contact: now usually taken to mean any communicable disease.

continent diversion (kon-ti-nĕnt dy-ver-shŏn) *n.* the diversion and collection of urine, usually after cystectomy, by constructing a reservoir or pouch from a section of small or large intestine or a combination of both. This can be emptied by catheterization via a small stoma; a urinary drainage bag is not required.

continuing professional development (CPD) (kŏn-tin-yoo-ing) *n.* the concept that learning continues throughout one's life, both through educational courses and work experience and practice. Individuals are encouraged to identify their personal learning needs and to assess their progress in dynamic ways

continuous insulin infusion pump (kŏn-tin-yoo-ŭs) *n.* a device to deliver a continuous infusion of fast-acting insulin to the body instead of using repeated injections throughout the day. It is worn under

the clothing and connected to the skin by a tube and a fine needle.

continuous positive airways pressure (CPAP) *n.* an air pressure in the range 5–30 cm H_2O (1.2–7.5 mPa). It can be applied to the upper airways using a full face mask or a nasal mask only (nCPAP). It is used in high-dependency units to optimize oxygen delivery to patients who are being weaned from ventilators and on patients at home with sleep apnoea syndrome.

contra- *prefix denoting* against or opposite.

contraception (kon-tră-sep-shŏn) *n.* the prevention of unwanted pregnancy. *See* coitus (interruptus), condom, diaphragm, IUCD, IUS, oral contraceptive, postcoital (contraception), rhythm method, sterilization. —**contraceptive** *adj., n.*

contraction (kŏn-trak-shŏn) *n.* the shortening of a muscle in response to a motor nerve impulse. This generates tension in the muscle, usually causing movement.

contracture (kŏn-trak-cher) *n.* fibrosis of skeletal muscle or connective tissue producing shortening and resulting in deformity of a joint. *See also* Dupuytren's contracture, Volkmann's contracture.

contraindication (kon-tră-in-di-kay-shŏn) *n.* any factor in a patient's condition that makes it unwise to pursue a certain line of treatment.

contralateral (kon-tră-lat-er-ăl) *adj.* on or affecting the opposite side of the body.

contrast medium (contrast agent) (kon-trahst) *n.* a substance administered to enhance the visibility of structures (i.e. increase the contrast) during imaging. *positive c. m.* a contrast agent (e.g. barium sulphate) that increases the density of a structure in radiography. *negative c. m.* a contrast agent (e.g. gas) that decreases the density of a structure in radiography. *magnetic resonance c. m.* a contrast agent that contains either a positive contrast atom (usually gadolinium) to increase the signal or a negative contrast atom (such as iron) to decrease it. *ultrasound c. m.* a contrast medium consisting of tiny (1–10 µm diameter) bubbles of gas, which reflect back the sound waves strongly.

contrecoup (kon-trĕ-koo) *n.* injury of a part resulting from a blow on its opposite side. This may happen, for example, if a blow on the back of the head causes the front of the brain to be pushed against the inner surface of the skull.

controlled drug (CD) (kŏn-trohld) *n. see* Misuse of Drugs Act 1971.

contusion (kŏn-tew-zhŏn) *n. see* bruise. *cerebral c.* bruising of the brain, resulting from head injury or surgery. Clinical signs range from concussion to coma, reflecting the severity of the trauma.

convection (kŏn-vek-shŏn) *n.* the transfer of heat through a liquid or gas by movement of the heated portions of the liquid or gas.

convergence (kŏn-ver-jĕns) *n.* inward turning of the eyes to achieve fusion of separate images during near vision.

conversion (kŏn-ver-shŏn) *n.* (in psychiatry) the expression of conflict as physical symptoms.

conversion disorder *n.* a psychological disorder, known for-merly as *conversion hysteria*, in which a conflict or need manifests itself as an organic dysfunction or a physical symptom, such as blindness, deafness, loss of sensation, gait abnormalities, or paralysis of various parts of the body. None of these can be accounted for by organic disease.

convolution (kon-vŏ-loo-shŏn) *n.* a folding or twisting, such as one of the many that cause the fissures, sulci, and gyri of the surface of the cerebrum.

convulsion (kŏn-vul-shŏn) *n.* an involuntary contraction of the muscles producing contortion of the body and limbs. Rhythmic convulsions of the limbs are a feature of major epilepsy. *febrile c.* an epileptic-type seizure associated with a fever, which affects infants and young children and is usually caused by a viral infection.

Cooley's anaemia (koo-liz) *n. see* thalassaemia. [T. B. Cooley (1871–1945), US paediatrician]

Coombs' test (koomz) *n.* a means of detecting rhesus antibodies on the surface of red blood cells that precipitate proteins (globulins) in the blood serum. The test is used in the diagnosis of haemolytic anaemia. [R. R. A. Coombs (1921–), British immunologist]

COPD *n. see* chronic obstructive pulmonary disease.

co-phenotrope (koh-fen-ŏ-trohp) *n.* a drug administered by mouth in the treatment of diarrhoea. It consists of a mixture of diphenoxylate hydrochloride (an opioid that reduces peristalsis) and atropine (which relaxes the smooth muscle of the gut) in a ratio of 100 to 1. Trade names: **Lomotil**, **Tropergen**.

copper sulphate (kop-er) *n.* a salt of copper that, in solution, has been used as a fungicide and is a constituent of Fehling's and Benedict's solutions, used to test for the presence of glucose in the urine. Formula: $CuSO_4$.

copr- (copro-) *prefix denoting* faeces.

coprolalia (kop-rŏ-lay-liǎ) *n.* the repetitive speaking of obscene words. It can be involuntary, as part of the Gilles de la Tourette syndrome.

coprolith (kop-rŏ-lith) *n.* a mass of hard faeces within the colon or rectum, due to chronic constipation. It may become calcified.

coproporphyrin (kop-rŏ-por-fi-rin) *n.* a porphyrin compound that is formed during the synthesis of protoporphyrin IX. Coproporphyrin is excreted in the faeces in *hereditary coproporphyria*.

co-proxamol (koh-proks-ǎ-mol) *n.* an analgesic drug consisting of a combination of the drug paracetamol and the weakly narcotic drug dextropropoxyphene. It is administered by mouth. Trade names: **Distalgesic**, **Paxalgesic**.

copulation (kop-yoo-lay-shŏn) *n.* see coitus.

cor (kor) *n.* the heart. *c. pulmonale* enlargement of the right ventricle of the heart resulting from disease of the lungs or pulmonary arteries.

coracoid process (ko-rǎ-koid) *n.* a beaklike process that curves upwards and forwards from the top of the scapula, over the shoulder joint.

cord (kord) *n.* any long flexible structure, which may be solid or tubular. Examples include the spermatic cord, spinal cord, umbilical cord, and vocal cord.

cordectomy (kor-dek-tŏmi) *n.* surgical removal of a vocal cord or, more usually, a piece of the vocal cord (*partial c.*).

cordocentesis (kor-doh-sen-tee-sis) *n.* the removal of a sample of fetal blood by inserting a hollow needle through the abdominal wall of a pregnant woman, under ultrasound guidance, into the umbilical vein. The blood is subjected to chromosome analysis and biochemical and other tests to determine the presence of abnormalities. *See also* prenatal diagnosis.

cordotomy (chordotomy) (kor-dot-ŏmi) *n.* a surgical procedure for the relief of severe and persistent pain in the pelvis or lower limbs, in which the tracts of the spinal cord transmitting the sensation of pain to consciousness are severed in the cervical (neck) region.

corium (kor-iŭm) *n.* see dermis.

corn (korn) *n.* an area of hard thickened skin on or between the toes: a type of callosity produced by ill-fitting shoes.

cornea (korn-iǎ) *n.* the transparent circular part of the front of the eyeball. It refracts the light entering the eye onto the lens, which then focuses it onto the retina. —**corneal** (korn-iǎl) *adj.*

corneal graft *n.* see keratoplasty.

corneal topography *n.* see topography.

cornification (kor-ni-fi-kay-shŏn) *n.* see keratinization.

cornu (kor-new) *n.* (*pl.* **cornua**) (in anatomy) a horn-shaped structure. *See also* horn.

corona (kŏ-roh-nă) *n.* a crown or crownlike structure. **c. capitis** the crown of the head.

coronal (ko-rō-năl) *adj.* relating to the crown of the head or of a tooth. **c. plane** the plane that divides the body into dorsal and ventral parts. **c. suture** the immovable joint between the frontal and parietal bones (*see* skull).

coronary angiography (ko-rŏn-er-i) *n. see* angiography.

coronary arteries *pl. n.* the arteries supplying blood to the heart. They arise from the aorta, just above the aortic valve, and form branches that encircle the heart.

coronary artery bypass graft (CABG) *n.* an operation in which a segment of a coronary artery narrowed by atheroma is bypassed by an autologous section of healthy saphenous vein or internal mammary artery at thoracotomy. The improved blood flow resulting from one or more such grafts relieves angina pectoris and reduces the risk of myocardial infarction.

coronary care *n.* a type of intensive care developed in order to provide for the needs of critically ill and immediately postoperative patients with cardiac and coronary artery disease. **c. c. unit (CCU)** a designated ward in a hospital in which coronary care is given. *See* intensive care.

coronary heart disease (CHD) *n. see* ischaemic heart disease.

coronary thrombosis *n.* the formation of a blood clot (thrombus) in the coronary artery, which obstructs the flow of blood to the heart. *See* myocardial infarction.

coroner (ko-rŏn-er) *n.* the official who presides at an inquest, who must be either a medical practitioner or a lawyer of at least five years standing.

coronoid process (ko-rŏn-oid) *n.* **1.** a process on the upper end of the ulna. It forms part of the notch that articulates with the humerus. **2.** the process on the ramus of the mandible to which the temporalis muscle is attached.

corpus (kor-pŭs) *n.* (*pl.* **corpora**) any mass of tissue that can be distinguished from its surroundings. **c. callosum** the broad band of nervous tissue that connects the two cerebral hemispheres. **c. cavernosum** either of a pair of cylindrical blood sinuses that form the erectile tissue of the penis and clitoris. **c. luteum** the glandular tissue in the ovary that forms at the site of a ruptured Graafian follicle after ovulation. It secretes the hormone progesterone, which prepares the uterus for implantation. If implantation fails the corpus luteum degenerates. If an embryo becomes implanted the corpus luteum continues to secrete progesterone until the fourth month of pregnancy. **c. spongiosum** the blood sinus that surrounds the urethra of the male. Together with the corpora cavernosa, it forms the erectile tissue of the penis. **c. striatum** the part of the basal ganglia in the cerebral hemispheres of the brain consisting of the caudate nucleus and the lentiform nucleus.

corpuscle (kor-pŭs-ŭl) *n.* any small particle, cell, or mass of tissue.

corrective (kŏ-rek-tiv) *n.* any drug or agent that modifies the action of another substance.

Corrigan's pulse (water-ham-

mer pulse) (ko-ri-gănz) *n.* a pulse characterized by an initial surge followed by a sudden collapse, usually due to aortic regurgitation. [Sir D. J. Corrigan (1802–80), Irish physician]

cortex (kor-teks) *n.* (*pl.* **cortices**) the outer part of an organ, situated immediately beneath its capsule or outer membrane. —**cortical** (kor-ti-kăl) *adj.*

cortical Lewy body disease *n.* *see* Lewy bodies.

corticosteroid (corticoid) (kor-ti-koh-**steer**-oid) *n.* any steroid hormone synthesized by the adrenal cortex. *See* glucocorticoid, mineralocorticoid.

corticotrophin (kor-ti-koh-**troh**-fin) *n. see* ACTH.

corticotrophin-releasing hormone (CRH) *n.* a peptide hypothalamic hormone stimulating the release of ACTH (adrenocorticotrophic hormone) from the anterior pituitary. *CRH test* a test in which CRH is administered intravenously to analyse the ACTH response, which is excessive in cases of primary adrenal failure and suppressed in cases of anterior hypopituitarism.

cortisol (kor-ti-sol) *n.* a steroid hormone: the major glucocorticoid synthesized and released by the human adrenal cortex. It is important for normal carbohydrate metabolism and for the normal response to any stress. *See also* hydrocortisone.

cortisone (kor-tiz-ohn) *n.* a naturally occurring corticosteroid that is used mainly to treat deficiency of corticosteroid hormones in Addison's disease and following surgical removal of the adrenal glands. It is administered by mouth or injection and may cause serious side-effects such as stomach ulcers and muscle and bone damage.

Corynebacterium (kŏ-ry-ni-bak-teer-iŭm) *n.* a genus of Gram-positive, mostly aerobic, non-motile rodlike bacteria. *C. diphtheriae* (*Klebs-Loeffler bacillus*) the causative organism of diphtheria. It occurs in one of three forms: *gravis*, *intermedius*, and *mitis*.

coryza (cold in the head) (kŏ-ry-ză) *n.* a catarrhal inflammation of the mucous membrane in the nose caused by either a cold or hay fever. *See also* catarrh.

COSHH (control of substances hazardous to health) *n.* (in occupational health) legislation and resulting regulations concerning the duties and responsibilities of employers and employees to ensure that hazardous substances used in a workplace do not affect adversely the operatives themselves or their colleagues.

cost- (costo-) *prefix denoting* the rib(s).

costal (kos-t'l) *adj.* of or relating to the ribs. *c. cartilage* a cartilage that connects a rib to the breastbone (sternum).

costive (kost-iv) *adj.* constipated.

cot death (sudden infant death syndrome, SIDS) (kot) *n.* the sudden unexpected death of an infant less than two years old (peak occurrence between two and six months) from an unidentifiable cause. There appear to be many factors involved, the most important of which is the position in which the baby is laid to sleep: babies who sleep on their fronts (the prone position) have an increased risk.

co-trimoxazole (koh-tri-**moks**-ă-zohl) *n.* an antibacterial drug consisting of sulfamethoxazole (a sulphonamide) and trimethoprim. Co-trimoxazole is taken by mouth for treating urinary-tract, respiratory-tract, and gastrointestinal infections. Side-effects may be severe. Trade name: **Septrin**.

cotyledon (kot-i-lee-dŏn) *n.* any of the major convex subdivisions of the mature placenta. Each cotyledon contains a major branch of the umbilical blood vessels.

cotyloid cavity (kot-i-loid) *n. see* acetabulum.

coughing (kof-ing) *n.* a form of violent exhalation by which irritant particles in the airways can be expelled. Medical name: **tussis**.

coulomb (koo-lom) *n.* the SI unit of electric charge, equal to the quantity of electricity transferred by 1 ampere in 1 second. Symbol: C.

counselling (kown-sěl-ing) *n.* a method of approaching psychological difficulties in adjustment that aims to help the client work out his own problems.

counterextension (kownt-er-eks-ten-shŏn) *n.* traction on one part of a limb, while the remainder of the limb is held steady: used particularly in the treatment of a fractured femur.

counterirritant (kownt-er-i-ri-t'nt) *n.* an agent, such as methyl salicylate, that causes irritation when applied to the skin and is used in order to relieve more deep-seated pain or discomfort. —**counterirritation** *n.*

countertraction (kownt-er-trak-shŏn) *n.* the use of an opposing force to balance that being applied during traction, when a strong contin-

uous pull is applied, for example, to a limb so that broken bones can be kept in alignment during healing.

Cowper's glands (bulbourethral glands) (kow-perz) *pl. n.* a pair of small glands that open into the urethra at the base of the penis. Their secretion contributes to the seminal fluid. [W. Cowper (1666–1709), English surgeon]

cowpox (kow-poks) *n.* a virus infection of cows' udders, transmitted to humans by direct contact, causing very mild symptoms similar to smallpox. An attack confers immunity to smallpox. Medical name: **vaccinia**.

cox- (coxo-) *prefix denoting* the hip.

coxa (koks-ă) *n.* (*pl.* **coxae**) **1.** the hip bone. **2.** the hip joint. *c. valga* a deformity of the hip joint in which the angle between the neck and shaft of the femur is abnormally increased. *c. vara* a deformity of the hip joint in which the angle between the neck and shaft of the femur is abnormally decreased.

coxalgia (koks-al-jiă) *n.* **1.** pain in the hip joint. **2.** disease of the hip joint.

COX-2 inhibitor *n.* an anti-inflammatory drug (*see* NSAID) that blocks the action of the enzyme cyclo-oxygenase 2 (COX-2), which mediates the production of prostaglandin at sites of inflammation, especially in joints. COX-2 inhibitors are used in the treatment of arthritis (*see* celecoxib, rofecoxib).

Coxsackie virus (kok-sak-i) *n.* one of a group of RNA-containing viruses that are able to multiply in the gastrointestinal tract (*see* enterovirus). Type A viruses generally cause less severe diseases, although some cause meningitis and severe throat infections. Type B viruses cause inflammation or degeneration of brain or heart tissue and they can also attack the muscles of the chest wall, the bronchi, pancreas, thyroid, and conjunctiva. *See also* Bornholm disease, hand, foot, and mouth disease.

CPAP *n. see* continuous positive airways pressure.

CPD *n. see* continuing professional development.

C-peptide *n.* a peptide (so-called because of its C shape) formed when insulin is produced from its precursor molecule, proinsulin. As it remains detectable in the plasma much longer than insulin, it can be more easily assayed as a marker of the degree of insulin secretion.

CPK *n.* creatine phosphokinase: *see* creatine (kinase).

CPN *n.* community psychiatric nurse. *See* community nurses.

CPR *n. see* cardiopulmonary resuscitation.

crab louse (krab) *n. see* Phthirus.

cradle (kray-d'l) *n.* a framework of metal strips or other material that forms a cage over an injured part of the body of a patient lying in bed, to protect it from the pressure of the bedclothes.

cradle cap *n.* a common condition in young babies in which crusty white or yellow scales form a 'cap' on the scalp. It is treated by applying oil or using a special shampoo and usually resolves in the first year of life, although it may represent the start of seborrhoeic eczema.

cramp (kramp) *n.* prolonged painful contraction of a muscle. It is sometimes caused by an imbalance of the salts in the body, but is more often a result of fatigue, imperfect posture, or stress. *occupational c.* spasm in the muscles making it impossible to perform a specific task but allowing the use of these muscles for any other movement. *writer's c. see* dystonia.

crani- (cranio-) *prefix denoting* the skull.

cranial nerves (kray-niǎl) *pl. n.* the 12 pairs of nerves that arise directly from the brain and leave the skull through separate apertures. *Compare* spinal nerves.

craniometry (kray-ni-**om**-itri) *n.* the science or practice of measuring the differences in the size and shape of skulls.

craniopagus (dicephalus) (kray-ni-**op**-ǎgǔs) *n.* Siamese twins united by their heads.

craniopharyngioma (kray-ni-oh-fǎ-rinj-i-**oh**-mǎ) *n.* a brain tumour derived from remnants of *Rathke's pouch*, an embryologic structure from which the pituitary gland is partly formed.

craniostenosis (kray-ni-oh-sti-**noh**-sis) *n.* premature closing of the sutures and fontanelles between the cranial bones during development, resulting in the skull remaining abnormally small. *Compare* craniosynostosis.

craniosynostosis (kray-ni-oh-sin-os-**toh**-sis) *n.* premature fusion of some of the cranial sutures, usually before birth, so that the skull is unable to expand in certain directions to assume its normal shape under the influence of the growing brain. The skull may become elongated from front to back, broad and short,

craniotabes (kray-ni-oh-tay-beez) *n.* abnormal thinness and brittleness of the bones of the vault of the skull, occurring in children with rickets.

craniotomy (kray-ni-ot-ŏmi) *n.* **1.** surgical removal of a portion of the cranium, performed to expose the brain and meninges for inspection or biopsy or to relieve excessive intracranial pressure (as in a subdural haematoma). **2.** surgical perforation of the skull of a dead fetus during difficult labour, so that delivery may continue.

cranium (kray-niŭm) *n.* the part of the skeleton that encloses the brain. It consists of eight bones connected together by immovable joints (*see* skull). —**cranial** *adj.*

cream (kreem) *n.* a preparation for use on the skin consisting of an emulsion of oil in water, which may or may not contain medication. It rubs into the skin easily, tends to dry the skin, and also contains preservatives, which may be allergenic. *Compare* ointment.

creatine (kree-ă-teen) *n.* a product of protein metabolism found in muscle. *c. kinase* (CK, *c. phosphokinase, CPK*) an enzyme involved in the breakdown of creatine to creatinine, isomers of which originate in the brain and thyroid, skeletal muscle, and heart. Damage to these tissues results in increased levels of the isomer in the serum. *c. phosphate* (*phosphocreatine, phosphagen*) the phosphate of creatine, which acts as a store of high-energy phosphate in muscle and serves to maintain adequate amounts of ATP.

creatinine (kree-at-i-neen) *n.* a substance derived from creatine and creatine phosphate in muscle. Creatinine is excreted in the urine.

creatinuria (kree-at-in-yoor-iă) *n.* an excess of the nitrogenous compound creatine in the urine.

creatorrhoea (kree-at-ŏ-ree-ă) *n.* the passage of excessive nitrogen in the faeces due to failure of digestion or absorption in the small intestine. It is found particularly in pancreatic failure. *See* cystic fibrosis, pancreatitis.

Credé's method (kray-dayz) *n.* a technique for expelling the placenta from the uterus. With the uterus contracted, downward pressure is applied to the uterus through the abdominal wall in the direction of the birth canal. This method has now been largely replaced by the Brandt Andrews method. [K. S. F. Credé (1819–92), German gynaecologist]

Credit Accumulation Transfer System (kred-it) *n. see* CATS.

creeping eruption (larva migrans) (kreep-ing) *n.* a skin disease caused either by larvae of nematode worms (e.g. *Ancylostoma braziliense*) or by the maggots of certain flies. The larvae burrow within the skin tissues, their movements marked by long thin red lines that cause the patient intense irritation.

crepitation (rale) (krep-i-tay-shŏn) *n.* a soft fine crackling sound heard in the lungs through the stethoscope. Crepitations are not normally heard in healthy lungs.

crepitus (krep-itŭs) *n.* **1.** a crackling sound or grating feeling produced by bone rubbing on bone or roughened cartilage, detected on movement of an arthritic joint. **2.** a similar sound heard with a stethoscope over an inflamed lung when the patient breathes in.

cresol (kree-sol) *n.* a strong antiseptic effective against many microorganisms and used mostly in soap solutions as a general disinfectant. Cresol solutions irritate the skin and if taken by mouth are corrosive and cause pain, nausea, and vomiting.

crest (krest) *n.* a ridge or linear protuberance, particularly on a bone.

CREST syndrome (krest) *n.* a disease characterized by the association of calcinosis, Raynaud's phenomenon, (o)esophageal malfunction, sclerodactyly (tapering fingers), and telangiectasia. It represents a variant of systemic sclerosis and may be associated with severe pulmonary hypertension.

cretinism (kret-in-izm) *n.* a syndrome of dwarfism, mental retardation, and coarseness of the skin and facial features due to congenital hypothyroidism.

Creutzfeldt-Jakob disease (CJD) (kroits-felt yak-ob) *n.* a disease in which rapid progressive degeneration of brain tissue results in dementia and eventually death. It is thought to be caused by an abnormal prion protein (see spongiform encephalopathy). Most cases occur sporadically but some forms of CJD are inherited and a few are acquired. A variant form of acquired CJD (vCJD) has been linked with the consumption of beef from cattle infected with bovine spongiform encephalopathy (BSE). [H. G. Creutzfeldt (1885–1964) and A. M. Jakob (1884–1931), German psychiatrists]

CRF *n.* chronic renal failure.

CRH *n.* see corticotrophin-releasing hormone.

cribriform plate (krib-ri-form) *n.* see ethmoid bone.

cricoid cartilage (kry-koid) *n.* the cartilage, shaped like a signet ring, that forms part of the anterior and lateral walls and most of the posterior wall of the larynx.

cricoid pressure *n.* a technique in which a trained assistant presses downwards on the cricoid cartilage of a supine patient to aid endotracheal intubation.

cricothyroid membrane (kry-koh-**th'y**-roid) *n.* the fibrous tissue in the anterior aspect of the neck between the lower border of the thyroid cartilage (the 'Adam's apple') and the upper border of the cricoid cartilage, lying immediately below it. It is the site where certain emergency airway devices can be inserted.

cricothyroidotomy (kry-koh-**th'y**-roid-ot-ōmi) *n.* a technique for obtaining an emergency airway through the cricothyroid membrane when standard airway techniques have failed. *needle c.* cricothyroidotomy in which a large-bore intravenous cannula is inserted directly through the membrane. *surgical c.* cricothyroidotomy in which a surgical hole is made in the membrane and a cuffed tube, similar to a short endotracheal tube, is inserted directly.

cri-du-chat syndrome (kree-doo-sha) *n.* a congenital condition of severe mental retardation associated with an abnormal facial appearance, spasticity, and a characteristic catlike cry in infancy. It results from an abnormality in chromosome no. 5.

Crigler-Najjar syndrome (krygler **nah**-jar) *n.* a genetic disease in which the liver enzyme glucuronyl transferase, responsible for dealing with bilirubin, is absent. Large amounts of bilirubin accumulate in the blood, and the child becomes progressively more jaundiced. Life expectancy is usually less than two years. [J. F. Crigler (1919–) and V. A. Najjar (1914–), US paediatricians]

crisis (kry-sis) *n.* (*pl.* **crises**) **1.** the turning point of a disease, after which the patient either improves or deteriorates. Since the advent of antibiotics, infections seldom reach the point of crisis. **2.** the occurrence of sudden severe pain in certain diseases. *See also* Dietl's crisis. **3.** a state of psychological or physiological disequilibrium in which normal coping strategies and mechanisms have been suspended. Intervention may be required.

crista (krist-ă) *n.* (*pl.* **cristae**) **1.** the sensory structure within the ampulla of a semicircular canal within the inner ear. **2.** one of the infoldings of the inner membrane of a mitochondrion. **3.** any anatomical structure resembling a crest.

Crohn's disease (krohnz) *n.* a condition in which segments of the alimentary tract become inflamed, thickened, and ulcerated. It usually affects the terminal part of the ileum; its acute form (*acute ileitis*) sometimes mimics appendicitis. Chronic disease often causes partial obstruction of the intestine, leading to pain, diarrhoea, and malabsorption. Alternative names: **regional**

enteritis, regional ileitis. [B. B. Crohn (1884–1983), US physician]

cromoglicate (sodium cromoglicate, cromoglycate) (kroh-moh-**gly**-kayt) *n.* a drug used to prevent attacks of asthma and hay fever and to treat allergic conjunctivitis and other allergic conditions. It is administered as a nasal spray or eye drops. Trade names: **Cromogen, Intal, Rynacrom, Vividrin**.

cross-dressing (kros-dres-ing) *n. see* transvestism.

cross-infection (kros-in-fek-shŏn) *n.* the transfer of infection from one patient to another in hospital.

cross-sectional imaging (krossek-shŏn-ăl) *n.* any technique that produces an image in the form of a plane through the body with the structures cut across. *See* computerized tomography, magnetic resonance imaging, positron emission tomography, SPECT scanning, ultrasonography.

crotamiton (kroh-tă-my-tŏn) *n.* a drug that destroys mites and is used to treat scabies and similar skin infections and also to relieve itching. It is applied to the skin as a lotion or ointment. Trade name: **Eurax**.

croup (kroop) *n.* acute inflammation and obstruction of the respiratory tract, involving the larynx and main air passages, in young children (usually aged between six months and three years). The usual cause is a virus infection but bacterial secondary infection can occur. The symptoms are those of laryngitis, accompanied by harsh difficult breathing (*see* stridor), a characteristic barking cough, a rising pulse rate, restlessness, and cyanosis.

crown (krown) *n.* **1.** the part of a tooth normally visible in the mouth and usually covered by enamel. **2.** a dental restoration that covers most or all of the natural crown. **3.** *see* corona.

crowning (krown-ing) *n.* the stage of labour when only the upper part of the infant's head is visible, encircled by, and just passing through, the vaginal opening.

cruciate ligaments (krew-shi-ayt) *pl. n.* a pair (anterior and posterior) of ligaments inside each knee joint. Damage to the cruciate ligaments is a common sports injury, especially in football players.

crude rate (krood) *n.* the total number of events (e.g. cases of lung cancer) expressed as a percentage (or rate per 1000, etc.) of the whole population.

crural (kroor-ăl) *adj.* **1.** relating to the thigh or leg. **2.** relating to the crura cerebri (*see* crus).

crus (kruus) *n.* (*pl.* **crura**) an elongated process or part of a structure. *c. cerebri* one of two symmetrical nerve tracts situated between the medulla oblongata and the cerebral hemispheres.

crush syndrome (krush) *n.* the condition resulting from crushing accidents in which large areas of muscle are damaged, characterized by severe shock resulting from blood and fluid loss and oliguria leading to kidney failure.

cry- (cryo-) *prefix denoting* cold.

cryaesthesia (kry-iss-theez-iă) *n.* **1.** exceptional sensitivity to low temperature. **2.** a sensation of coldness.

cryoprecipitate (kry-oh-pri-sip-i-tăt) *n.* a precipitate produced by freezing and thawing under controlled conditions, such as the residue obtained from fresh frozen blood plasma that has been thawed at 4°C. This residue is used in the control of bleeding in haemophilia.

cryopreservation (kry-oh-prez-er-vay-shŏn) *n.* preservation of tissues by freezing.

cryoprobe (kry-oh-prohb) *n.* an instrument used in cryosurgery, which has a fine tip cooled by allowing carbon dioxide or nitrous oxide gas to expand within it.

cryoretinopexy (kry-oh-ret-i-noh-peks-i) *n.* the use of extreme cold to freeze areas of weak or torn retina in order to cause scarring and seal breaks. It is used in cryosurgery for retinal detachment.

cryosurgery (kry-oh-ser-jer-i) *n.* the use of extreme cold in a localized part of the body to freeze and destroy unwanted tissues. Cryosurgery is commonly used for the treatment of retinal detachment, the destruction of certain bone tumours, and the obliteration of skin blemishes. *See* cryoprobe.

cryotherapy (kry-oh-th'e-ră-pi) *n.* the use of cold in the treatment of disorders. *See* cryosurgery, hypothermia. *Compare* thermotherapy.

crypt (kript) *n.* a small sac, follicle, or cavity; for example, the crypts of Lieberkühn (*see* Lieberkühn's glands).

crypt- (crypto-) *prefix denoting* concealed.

cryptococcosis (torulosis) (krip-toh-kok-oh-sis) *n.* a disease caused by the fungus *Cryptococcus neoformans*, which attacks the lung, resulting in a solid tumour-like mass (*toruloma*). It may spread to the brain, leading to meningitis; this can occur as an opportunistic infection in those suffering from AIDS.

cryptogenic (krip-toh-jen-ik) *adj.* of obscure or unknown cause.

cryptomenorrhoea (krip-toh-men-ŏ-ree-ă) *n.* absence of blood flow when the internal symptoms of menstruation are present. The condition may arise because the hymen lacks an opening (*see* imperforate (hymen)) or because of some other obstruction.

cryptorchidism (cryptorchism) (krip-or-kid-izm) *n.* the condition in which the testes fail to descend into the scrotum and are retained within the abdomen or inguinal canal. —**cryptorchid** *adj., n.*

cryptosporidiosis (krip-toh-sper-id-i-oh-sis) *n.* an intestinal infection of mammals and birds caused by parasitic protozoa of the genus *Cryptosporidium*, which is usually transmitted to humans via farm animals. Ingestion of water or milk contaminated with infective oocysts results in severe diarrhoea and abdominal cramps, caused by release of a toxin. Most patients recover in 7–14 days, but the disease can persist in the immunocompromised (including AIDS patients), the elderly, and young children.

CSF *n. see* cerebrospinal fluid.

CSI *n. see* Caregiver Strain Index.

CSOM *n.* chronic suppurative otitis media. *See* otitis (media).

CSSD *n.* Central Sterile Supplies Department (in a hospital).

CT scanner *n. see* computerized tomography.

cubital (kew-bit'l) *adj.* relating to the elbow or forearm. *c. fossa* the depression at the front of the elbow.

cuboid bone (kew-boid) *n.* the outer bone of the tarsus, which articulates with the fourth and fifth metatarsal bones in front and with the calcaneus (heel bone) behind.

cuirass (kwi-ras) *n. see* respirator.

culdocentesis (kul-doh-sen-tee-sis) *n. see* colpotomy.

culdoscope (kul-doh-skohp) *n.* a tubular instrument with lenses and a light source, used for direct observation of the uterus, ovaries, and Fallopian tubes (*culdoscopy*). The instrument is passed through the wall of the vagina behind to the neck of the uterus. The culdoscope has now been largely replaced by the laparoscope.

Cullen sign (kul-ĕn) *n.* a bluish bruiselike appearance around the umbilicus, which is seen in acute pancreatitis. [T. S. Cullen (1868–1953), US gynaecologist]

culture (kul-cher) **1.** *n.* a population of microorganisms, usually bacteria, grown in a solid or liquid laboratory medium (*c. medium*), which is usually agar, broth, or gelatin. *stock c.* a permanent bacterial culture, from which subcultures are made. *See also* tissue (culture). **2.** *vb.* to grow bacteria or other microorganisms in cultures.

cumulative action (kew-mew-lă-tiv) *n.* the toxic effects of a drug produced by repeated administration of small doses at intervals that are not long enough for it to be either broken down or excreted by the body.

cuneiform bones (kew-ni-form) *pl. n.* three bones in the tarsus that articulate with the first, second, and third metatarsal bones in front. All three bones articulate with the navicular bone behind.

cupola (kew-pŏ-lă) *n.* **1.** the small dome at the end of the cochlea. **2.** any of several dome-shaped anatomical structures.

curare (kew-rar-i) *n.* an extract from the bark of South American trees (*Strychnos* and *Chondodendron* species) that relaxes and paralyses voluntary muscle. Curare was formerly employed to control the muscle spasms of tetanus and as a muscle relaxant in surgical operations.

curettage (kewr-i-tij) *n.* the scraping of the skin or the internal surface of an organ or body cavity by means of a spoon-shaped instrument (*curette*). Curettage is usually performed to remove diseased tissue or to obtain a specimen for diagnostic purposes. *See also* dilatation and curettage.

curette (kewr-et) *n. see* curettage.

curie (kewr-ee) *n.* a former unit for expressing the activity of a radioactive substance. It has been replaced by the becquerel. Symbol: Ci.

Curling's ulcers (ker-lingz) *pl. n.* gastric or duodenal ulcers associated with stress from severe injury or major burns. [T. B. Curling (1811–88), British surgeon]

Cushing's syndrome (kuush-ingz) *n.* the condition resulting from excess amounts of corticosteroid hormones in the body. Symptoms include weight gain, reddening of the face and neck, excess growth of body and facial hair, raised blood pressure, loss of mineral from the bones (osteoporosis), raised blood glucose levels, and sometimes mental disturbances. The syndrome may be due to overstimulation of the adrenal glands by excessive amounts of the hormone ACTH, secreted either by a tumour of the pituitary gland (*Cushing's disease*) or by a malignant tumour in the lung or elsewhere. [H. W. Cushing (1869–1939), US surgeon]

cusp (kusp) *n.* **1.** any of the cone-shaped prominences on the teeth, especially the premolars and molars. **2.** a pocket or fold of the membrane lining the heart or of the layer of the wall of a vein, several of which form a valve. When the blood flows backwards the cusps fill up and become distended, so closing the valve.

cutaneous (kew-tay-niŭs) *adj.* relating to the skin.

cuticle (kew-ti-kŭl) *n.* **1.** the epidermis of the skin. **2.** a layer of solid or semisolid material that is secreted by and covers an epithelium. **3.** a layer of cells, such as the outer layer of cells in a hair.

cutis (kew-tis) *n. see* skin.

CVA *n. see* cerebrovascular accident.

CVP *n. see* central venous pressure.

CVS *n. see* chorionic villus sampling.

CXR *n.* chest X-ray.

cyan- (cyano-) *prefix denoting* blue.

cyanide (sy-ă-nyd) *n.* any of the notoriously poisonous salts of hydrocyanic acid. Cyanides combine with and render inactive the enzymes of the tissues responsible for cellular respiration, and therefore they kill extremely quickly.

cyanocobalamin (vitamin B$_{12}$) (sy-ă-noh-koh-bal-ă-min) *n. see* vitamin B.

cyanosis (sy-ă-noh-sis) *n.* a bluish

discoloration of the skin and mucous membranes resulting from an inadequate amount of oxygen in the blood. Cyanosis is associated with heart failure, lung diseases, the breathing of oxygen-deficient atmospheres, and asphyxia. Cyanosis is also seen in blue babies, because of congenital heart defects. —**cyanotic** *adj.*

cybernetics (sy-ber-net-iks) *n.* the science of communication processes and automatic control systems in both machines and living things: a study linking the working of the brain and nervous system with the functioning of computers and automated feedback devices. *See also* bionics.

cycl- (cyclo-) *prefix denoting* **1.** cycle or cyclic. **2.** the ciliary body.

cyclical vomiting (sy-klik-ăl) *n.* recurrent attacks of vomiting, often associated with acidosis, occurring in children but with no apparent cause.

cyclitis (sy-kly-tis) *n.* inflammation of the ciliary body of the eye (*see* uveitis).

cyclizine (sy-kliz-een) *n.* a drug with antihistamine properties, administered by mouth to prevent and relieve nausea and vomiting in motion sickness, vertigo, disorders of the inner ear, and postoperative sickness. Trade name: **Valoid**.

cycloablation (sy-kloh-ă-blay-shŏn) *n.* the destruction of part of the ciliary body of the eye to reduce the production of aqueous humour and hence reduce intraocular pressure. It is used in the treatment of advanced glaucoma resistant to other forms of treatment.

cyclocryotherapy (sy-kloh-kry-

oh-th'e-ră-pi) *n.* the destruction of part of the ciliary body by freezing. It is used to reduce intraocular pressure in the control of glaucoma.

cyclodialysis (sy-kloh-dy-al-i-sis) *n.* separation of the ciliary body from its attachment to the sclera. This may result from trauma or it may be performed as part of an operation to treat glaucoma.

cyclopenthiazide (sy-kloh-pen-th'y-ă-zyd) *n.* a diuretic administered by mouth to treat oedema, high blood pressure, and heart failure. Trade name: **Navidrex**.

cyclopentolate (sy-kloh-pen-tŏ-layt) *n.* a drug, similar to atropine, that is used in eye drops to paralyse the ciliary muscles and dilate the pupil for eye examinations and to treat some types of eye inflammation. Trade names: **Minims Cyclopentolate**, **Mydrilate**.

cyclophosphamide (sy-kloh-fos-fă-myd) *n.* an alkylating agent administered by mouth or injection to treat a variety of cancers, often in combination with other cytotoxic drugs. It also has immunosuppressant properties and is used in treating rheumatoid arthritis and other conditions requiring reduced immune response. Trade name: **Endoxana**.

cyclophotoablation (sy-kloh-foh-toh-ă-blay-shŏn) *n.* the use of light or lasers to destroy the ciliary body of the eye in order to reduce production of aqueous humour and hence reduce intraocular pressure. It is used in the treatment of glaucoma.

cycloplegia (sy-kloh-plee-jiă) *n.* paralysis of the ciliary muscle of the eye (*see* ciliary body). This causes inability to alter the focus of the eye and is usually accompanied by paralysis of the muscles of the iris, resulting in fixed dilation of the pupil (mydriasis).

cycloserine (sy-kloh-**seer**-een) *n.* an antibiotic, active against a wide range of bacteria, that may be used as supporting treatment in tuberculosis. It is administered by mouth.

cyclosporin (sy-kloh-**spo**-rin) *n. see* ciclosporin.

cyclothymia (sy-kloh-**th'y**-miă) *n.* the occurrence of marked swings of mood from cheerfulness to misery. These fluctuations usually represent a personality disorder, and are not as great as those of manic-depressive psychosis.

cyclotomy (sy-**klot**-ŏmi) *n.* surgical incision of the ciliary body of the eye.

cyesis (sy-ee-sis) *n.* pregnancy. *See also* pseudocyesis.

cyn- (**cyno**-) *prefix denoting* a dog or dogs.

cyproheptadine (sy-proh-**hep**-tă-deen) *n.* a potent antihistamine administered by mouth to treat allergies and itching skin conditions and to prevent migraine attacks. Trade name: **Periactin**.

cyproterone (**cyproterone acetate**) (sy-proh-ter-ohn) *n.* a steroid drug that inhibits the effects of male sex hormones (*see* antiandrogen) and is used to treat various sexual disorders and advanced prostate cancer in men. It is administered by mouth. Trade names: **Androcur**, **Cyprostat**.

cyst (sist) *n.* **1.** an abnormal sac or closed cavity lined with epithelium and filled with liquid or semisolid matter. There are many varieties of cysts occurring in different parts of the body. *See* dermoid cyst, fimbrial cyst, hydatid, ovarian cyst, retention cyst, sebaceous cyst. **2.** a dormant stage produced during the life cycle of certain protozoan parasites of the alimentary canal, including *Giardia* and *Entamoeba*. **3.** a structure formed by and surrounding the larvae of certain parasitic worms.

cyst- (**cysto-**) *prefix denoting* **1.** a bladder, especially the urinary bladder. **2.** a cyst.

cystadenoma (sis-tad-i-**noh**-mă) *n.* an adenoma showing a cystic structure.

cystalgia (sis-**tal**-jiă) *n.* pain in the urinary bladder. This is common in cystitis and when there are stones in the bladder and is occasionally present in bladder cancer.

cystectomy (sis **tek**-tŏmi) *n.* surgical removal of the urinary bladder. Usually the ureters draining the urine from the kidneys are reimplanted into the ileum (*see* ileal conduit).

cysteine (sis-ti-een) *n.* a sulphur-containing amino acid that is an important constituent of many enzymes.

cystic (sis-tik) *adj.* **1.** of, relating to, or characterized by cysts. **2.** of or relating to the gall bladder or urinary bladder. *c. duct see* bile duct.

cysticercosis (sis-ti-ser-**koh**-sis) *n.* a disease caused by the presence of tapeworm larvae (*see* cysticercus) of the species *Taenia solium* in any of the body tissues. The presence of cysticerci in the muscles causes pain and weakness; in the brain the symptoms are more serious, including mental deterioration, paralysis, giddiness, epileptic attacks, and convulsions.

cysticercus (bladderworm) (sis-ti-ser-kŭs) *n.* a larval stage of some tapeworms in which the scolex and neck are invaginated into a large fluid-filled cyst. *See* cysticercosis.

cystic fibrosis (CF, fibrocystic disease of the pancreas, mucoviscidosis) *n.* a hereditary disease affecting cells of the exocrine glands; the faulty gene responsible has been identified as lying on chromosome no. 7 and is recessive, i.e. both parents of the patient can be carriers without being affected by the disease. The abnormality results in the production of thick mucus, which obstructs the intestinal glands (causing meconium ileus in newborn babies), pancreas (causing deficiency of pancreatic enzymes resulting in malabsorption and failure to thrive), and bronchi (causing bronchiectasis). Respiratory infections, which may be severe, are a common complication.

cystine (sis-teen) *n. see* amino acid.

cystinosis (sis-ti-noh-sis) *n.* an inborn defect in the metabolism of amino acids, leading to abnormal accumulation of the amino acid cystine in the blood, kidneys, and lymphatic system. *See also* Fanconi syndrome.

cystinuria (sis-tin-yoor-iă) *n.* an inborn error of metabolism resulting in excessive excretion of the amino acid cystine in the urine due to a defect of reabsorption by the kidney tubules. It may lead to the formation of cystine stones in the kidney.

cystitis (sis-ty-tis) *n.* inflammation of the urinary bladder, often caused by infection. It is usually accompanied by the desire to pass urine frequently, with a degree of burning.

cystitome (sis-ti-tohm) *n.* a small knife with a tiny curved or hooked blade, used to cut the lens capsule in some operations for cataract.

cystocele (sis-tŏ-seel) *n.* prolapse of the base of the bladder in women. It is usually due to weakness of the pelvic floor after childbirth and causes bulging of the anterior wall of the vagina on straining.

cystography (sis-tog-răfi) *n.* X-ray examination of the urinary bladder after the injection of a contrast medium. The X-ray photographs or films thus obtained are known as *cystograms*.

cystolithiasis (sis-toh-lith-I-ă-sis) *n.* the presence of stones (calculi) in the urinary bladder. The stones cause pain, the passage of bloody urine, and interruption of the urinary stream and should be removed surgically. *See* calculus.

cystometer (sis-tom-it-er) *n.* an apparatus for measuring pressure within the bladder. —**cystometry** *n.*

cystopexy (vesicofixation) (sis-toh-peksi) *n.* a surgical operation to fix the urinary bladder (or a portion of it) in a different position. It may be performed as part of the repair or correction of a prolapsed bladder.

cystoplasty (sis-toh-plasti) *n.* the operation of enlarging the capacity of the bladder by incorporating a segment of bowel. **clam** *c.* an operation in which the bladder is cut across longitudinally from one side of the neck to the other side through the dome (fundus) of the bladder and a length of ileum or colon is inserted as a patch. *See also* ileocaecocystoplasty, ileocystoplasty.

cystoscopy (sis-tos-kŏpi) *n.* examination of the bladder by means of an instrument (*cystoscope*) inserted via the urethra.

cystostomy (sis-tost-ŏmi) *n.* the operation of creating an artificial opening between the bladder and the anterior abdominal wall. This provides a temporary or permanent drainage route for urine.

cystotomy (sis-tot-ŏmi) *n.* surgical incision into the urinary bladder, usually by cutting through the abdominal wall above the pubic symphysis (*suprapubic c.*).

cyt- (**cyto-**) *prefix denoting* **1.** cell(s). **2.** cytoplasm.

cytarabine (sy-ta-ră-been) *n.* a cytotoxic drug that is used to suppress the symptoms of some types of leukaemia. It is administered by injection and can damage the normal bone marrow, leading to various blood cell disorders. Trade name: **Cytosar**

-cyte *suffix denoting* a cell.

cytochemistry (sy-toh-**kem**-istri) *n.* the study of chemical compounds and their activities in living cells.

cytogenetics (sy-toh-ji-**net**-iks) *n.* a science that links the study of inheritance (genetics) with that of cells (cytology); it is concerned mainly with the study of the chromosomes, especially their origin, structure, and functions.

cytokinesis (sy-toh-ki-**nee**-sis) *n.* see karyokinesis.

cytology (sy-tol-ŏji) *n.* the study of the structure and function of cells. *aspiration c.* the aspiration of specimens of cells from tumours or cysts through a hollow needle, using a sy-

ringe, and their subsequent examination under the microscope after suitable preparation (by staining, etc.). *cervical c.* the microscopic examination of cells obtained by scraping the cervix. *See* cervical (smear). *exfoliative c.* the microscopic examination of cells that have already been shed, used in the diagnosis of various diseases. *See also* liquid-based cytology. —**cytological** *adj.*

cytolysis (sy-tol-i-sis) *n.* the breakdown of cells, particularly by destruction of their outer membranes.

cytomegalovirus (CMV) (sy-toh-meg-ă-loh-vy-rŭs) *n.* a virus belonging to the herpesvirus group. It normally causes only mild symptoms, but in immunocompromised individuals its effects can be more severe; if contracted by a pregnant woman it may give rise to congenital mental handicap in her child.

cytometer (sy-tom-it-er) *n.* an instrument for determining the number of cells in a given quantity of fluid, such as blood, cerebrospinal fluid, or urine. *See* haemocytometer.

cytopenia (sy-toh-pee-niă) *n.* a deficiency of one or more of the various types of blood cells. *See* eosinopenia, erythropenia, lymphopenia, neutropenia, pancytopenia, thrombocytopenia.

cytoplasm (sy-toh-plazm) *n.* the jelly-like substance that surrounds the nucleus of a cell. *See also* protoplasm. —**cytoplasmic** *adj.*

cytosine (sy-toh-seen) *n.* one of the nitrogen-containing bases (*see* pyrimidine) that occurs in the nucleic acids DNA and RNA.

cytosome (sy-toh-sohm) *n.* the part of a cell that is outside the nucleus.

cytotoxic drug (sy-toh-**toks**-ik) *n.*
a drug that damages or destroys
cells and is used to treat various
types of cancer. There are various
classes of cytotoxic drugs, including
alkylating agents, antimetabolites,
anthracycline antibiotics, vinca alkaloids, and platinum compounds
(e.g. carboplatin). They destroy cancer cells by inhibiting cell division
but also affect normal cells, causing
side-effects, particularly in bone
marrow, skin, stomach lining, and
fetal tissue; dosage must therefore
be carefully controlled.

cytotoxin (sy-toh-**toks**-in) *n.* any
substance that has a toxic action on
specific cells.

Dd

dacarbazine (da-kah-bă-zeen) *n.* a drug administered by injection in the treatment of certain cancers, including Hodgkin's disease and malignant melanoma. Trade name: **DTIC-Dome**.

dacry- (dacryo-) *prefix denoting* **1.** tears. **2.** the lacrimal apparatus.

dacryoadenitis (dak-ri-oh-ad-i-ny-tis) *n.* inflammation of the tear-producing gland. *See* lacrimal (apparatus).

dacryocystitis (dak-ri-oh-sis-ty-tis) *n.* inflammation of the lacrimal sac, usually occurring when the duct draining the tears into the nose is blocked. *See* lacrimal (apparatus).

dacryocystorhinostomy (DCR) (dak-ri-oh-sis-toh-ry-nost-ōmi) *n.* an operation to relieve blockage of the nasolacrimal duct (which drains tears into the nose), in which a communication is made between the lacrimal sac and the nose by removing the intervening bone. *See* dacryocystitis, lacrimal (apparatus).

dacryolith (dak-ri-oh-lith) *n.* a stone in the lacrimal canaliculus or lacrimal sac. *See* lacrimal (apparatus).

dacryoma (dak-ri-oh-mă) *n.* a harmless tumour-like swelling obstructing any of the ducts associated with the lacrimal apparatus.

dactinomycin (actinomycin D) (dak-ti-noh-my-sin) *n.* a cytotoxic drug (an antibiotic) used mainly to treat cancers in children. It is administered by injection. Trade name: **Comegen Lyovac**.

dactyl- *prefix denoting* the digits (fingers or toes).

dactylion (dak-til-iŏn) *n. see* dactyly.

dactylitis (dak-ti-ly-tis) *n.* inflammation of a finger or toe caused by bone infection (as in tuberculous osteomyelitis) or rheumatic disease or seen in infants with sickle-cell disease.

dactylology (dak-ti-lol-ŏji) *n.* the representation of speech by finger movements: sign language.

Daltonism (protanopia) (dawl-tŏn-izm) *n.* red-blindness: a defect in colour vision in which a person cannot distinguish between reds and greens. The term has been used to refer to colour blindness in general. [J. Dalton (1766–1844), British chemist]

danazol (dan-ă-zol) *n.* a synthetic progestogen that inhibits the secretion by the pituitary gland of gonadotrophins. Administered by mouth, it is used to treat precocious puberty, breast enlargement in males (gynaecomastia), excessively heavy menstrual periods, and endometriosis. Trade name: **Danol**.

D and C *n. see* dilatation and curettage.

dandruff (dan-druf) *n.* visible scaling from the surface of the scalp, associated with the presence of the yeast *Pityrosporum ovale*. It is the precursor of seborrhoeic eczema of the scalp, in which there is a degree of inflammation in addition to the greasy scaling. Dandruff can be controlled by shampoos containing tar, selenium sulphide, zinc pyrithione, or imidazole antifungals. Medical name: **pityriasis capitis**.

Dandy-Walker syndrome (dandi **wawk**-er) *n*. a form of cerebral palsy in which the cerebellum is usually the part of the brain affected. It leads to unsteadiness of balance and an abnormal gait and may be associated with hydrocephalus. [W. E. Dandy (1886–1946) and A. E. Walker (1907–), US surgeons]

dangerous drugs (dayn-jer-ŭs) *pl. n. see* Misuse of Drugs Act 1971.

dantrolene (dan-troh-leen) *n*. a muscle relaxant drug used to relieve muscle spasm in such conditions as cerebral palsy, multiple sclerosis, or spinal cord injury. It is administered by mouth or by injection. Trade name: **Dantrium**.

dapsone (dap-sohn) *n*. a drug (*see* sulphone) administered by mouth or injection to treat leprosy and dermatitis herpetiformis.

dark adaptation (dark) *n*. the changes that take place in the retina and pupil of the eye enabling vision in very dim light. *See* rod. *Compare* light adaptation.

daunorubicin (daw-noh-**roo**-bi-sin) *n*. an anthracycline antibiotic that interferes with DNA synthesis and is used in the treatment of acute leukaemia. It is administered by injection.

dawn phenomenon (Somogyi effect) (dawn) *n*. the phenomenon of high fasting blood-sugar levels in the morning due to an unrecognized hypoglycaemic episode during the night in a person with diabetes. The episode has resulted in an outpouring of regulatory hormones (e.g. adrenaline, glucagon), which have increased the blood sugar to supernormal levels.

day blindness (day) *n*. comparatively good vision in poor light but poor vision in good illumination. The condition is usually congenital and associated with poor visual acuity and defective colour vision. Medical name: **hemeralopia**. *Compare* night blindness.

day-case surgery *n*. surgical procedures that can be performed in a single day, without the need to admit the patient for an overnight stay in hospital. Examples include removal of many breast lesions, dilatation and curettage, and operations for hernia and varicose veins. Special units are established in many hospitals.

day hospital *n. see* hospital.

DCIS *n. see* (ductal) carcinoma in situ.

DDT (chlorophenothane, dicophane) *n*. a powerful insecticide that was formerly widely used. The quantities now present in the environment – in the form of stores accumulated in animal tissues – have led to its use being restricted.

de- *prefix denoting* **1.** removal or loss. **2.** reversal.

dead space (ded) *n*. **1.** any part of the respiratory tract containing air that does not participate in the exchange of oxygen and carbon dioxide. **2.** a cavity that remains in an incompletely closed wound, in which blood may accumulate and delay healing.

deafness (def-nis) *n.* partial or total loss of hearing in one or both ears. *conductive d.* deafness that is due to a defect in the conduction of sound from the external ear to the inner ear. This may be due to perforations of the eardrum, fluid or infection in the middle ear (*see* glue ear, otitis (media)), or disorders of the small bones in the middle ear (ossicles). *sensorineural. d. (perceptive d.)* deafness that may be due to a lesion of the cochlea in the inner ear, the auditory nerve, or the auditory centres in the brain. *See also* cochlear implant, hearing aid, hearing therapy, Rinne's test, Weber's test.

deamination (dee-ami-nay-shŏn) *n.* a process that occurs in the liver during the metabolism of amino acids. The amino group (–NH$_2$) is removed from an amino acid and converted to ammonia, which is ultimately converted to urea and excreted.

death (deth) *n.* absence of vital functions. *brain d.* permanent functional death of the centres in the brainstem that control breathing, heart rate, and other vital reflexes (including pupillary responses). Usually two independent medical opinions are required before brain death is agreed, but organs such as kidneys may then legally be removed for transplantation surgery before the heart has stopped.

death certificate *n.* a medical certificate stating the cause of a person's death, usually also stating the deceased's marital status, occupation, and age.

debility (di-bil-iti) *n.* physical weakness; loss of strength and power.

debridement (di-breed-měnt) *n.* the process of cleaning an open wound by removal of foreign material and dead tissue, so that healing may occur without hindrance.

debrisoquine (deb-ris-oh-kween) *n.* a potent drug administered by mouth to treat high blood pressure (hypertension). Trade name: **Declinax**.

dec- (deca-) *prefix denoting* ten.

decalcification (dee-kal-sifi-kay-shŏn) *n.* loss or removal of calcium salts from a bone or tooth.

decapitation (di-kapi-tay-shŏn) *n.* removal of the head, usually the head of a dead fetus to enable delivery to take place. This procedure is now very rare.

decapsulation (decortication) (dee-kaps-yoo-lay-shŏn) *n.* the surgical removal of a capsule from an organ; for example, the stripping of the membrane that envelops the kidney or of the inflammatory capsule that encloses a chronic abscess, as in the treatment of empyema.

decay (di-kay) *n.* (in bacteriology) the decomposition of organic matter due to microbial action.

deci- *prefix denoting* a tenth.

decidua (di-sid-yoo-ă) *n.* the modified mucous membrane that lines the wall of the uterus during pregnancy and is shed with the afterbirth at parturition (*see* endometrium). *d. basalis* the region of the decidua where the embryo is attached. *d. capsularis* the thin layer of the decidua that covers the embryo. *d. parietalis* the region of the decidua that is not in contact with the embryo. —**decidual** *adj.*

decompensation (dee-kom-pen-say-shŏn) *n.* inability of the heart to maintain an adequate circulation in the face of an increased workload or some structural defect.

decomposition (dee-kom-pŏ-zish-ŏn) *n.* the gradual disintegration of dead organic matter, usually foodstuffs or tissues, by the chemical action of bacteria and/or fungi.

decompression (dee-kŏm-presh-ŏn) *n.* **1.** the reduction of pressure on an organ or part of the body by surgical intervention. Raised pressure in the fluid of the brain can be lowered by cutting into the dura mater; cardiac compression – the abnormal presence of blood or fluid round the heart – can be cured by cutting the pericardium. **2.** the gradual reduction of atmospheric pressure for deep-sea divers. *See* compressed air illness.

decompression sickness *n. see* compressed air illness.

decongestant (dee-kŏn-jest-ănt) *n.* an agent that reduces or relieves nasal congestion. Most nasal decongestants are sympathomimetic drugs, which are applied either locally, in the form of nasal sprays or drops, or taken by mouth.

decortication (dee-kor-ti-kay-shŏn) *n.* **1.** the removal of the outside layer (cortex) from an organ or structure, such as the kidney. **2.** an operation for removing the blood clot and scar tissue that forms after bleeding into the chest cavity. **3.** *see* decapsulation.

decubitus (di-kew-bit-ŭs) *n.* the recumbent position. *d. ulcer see* bedsore.

decussation (dee-kus-ay-shŏn) *n.* a point at which two or more structures of the body cross to the opposite side. The term is used particularly for the point at which nerve fibres cross over in the central nervous system.

deep vein thrombosis (DVT) *n. see* phlebothrombosis.

defecation (def-i-kay-shŏn) *n.* the expulsion of faeces through the anus.

defence mechanism (di-fenss) *n.* the means whereby an undesirable impulse can be avoided or controlled. Defence mechanisms include repression, projection, reaction formation, sublimation, and splitting.

deferent (def-er-ĕnt) *adj.* **1.** carrying away from or down from. **2.** relating to the vas deferens.

defervescence (def-er-ves-ĕns) *n.* the disappearance of a fever, a process that may occur rapidly or take several days.

defibrillation (dee-fib-ri-lay-shŏn) *n.* administration of a controlled electric shock to restore normal heart rhythm in cases of cardiac arrest due to ventricular fibrillation. *See* defibrillator.

defibrillator (dee-fib-ri-lay-ter) *n.* the apparatus used for issuing a measured electrical current to a patient's heart in defibrillation. Defibrillators may be semi- or fully automated to recognize abnormal rhythms and to deliver the appropriate shock, fully operator-dependent, or implanted into the patient's body like a pacemaker.

defibrination (dee-fib-ri-nay-shŏn) *n.* the removal of fibrin, one of the plasma proteins that causes coagulation, from a sample of blood.

deficiency disease (di-fish-ĕn-si) *n.* any disease caused by the lack of an essential nutrient in the diet. Such nutrients include vitamins, essential amino acids, and essential fatty acids.

degeneration (di-jen-er-ay-shŏn) *n.* the deterioration and loss of specialized function of the cells of a tissue or organ. The changes may be caused by a defective blood supply or by disease. Degeneration may involve the deposition of calcium salts, of fat (*see* fatty degeneration), or of fibrous tissue in the affected organ or tissue. *See also* infiltration.

deglutition (dee-gloo-tish-ŏn) *n. see* swallowing.

dehiscence (di-hiss-ĕns) *n.* a splitting open, as of a surgical wound.

dehydration (dee-hy-dray-shŏn) *n.* loss or deficiency of water in body tissues. The condition may result from inadequate water intake and/or from excessive removal of water from the body; for example, by sweating, vomiting, or diarrhoea.

dehydroepiandrosterone (DHEA) (dee-hy-droh-epi-an-dros-ter-ohn) *n.* a weak androgen produced and secreted by the adrenal glands after adrenal maturation (*see* adrenarche). It is largely converted to dehydroepiandrosterone sulphate and androstenedione. All three of these molecules can cause a degree of mild androgenation but can also be converted in the circulation to the more potent androgens testosterone and dihydrotestosterone.

dehydrogenase (dee-hy-droj-ĕ-nayz) *n. see* oxidoreductase.

déjà vu (day-zha-vew) *n.* a vivid psychic experience in which immediately contemporary events seem to be a repetition of previous happenings. It is a symptom of some forms of epilepsy. *See also* jamais vu.

delayed suture (delayed primary closure) (di-layd) *n.* a technique used in the closure of contaminated wounds and wounds associated with tissue necrosis, such as are produced by missile injuries. The superficial layers of the wound are left open, to be closed later when the tissues have been cleaned.

Delhi boil (del-i) *n. see* oriental sore.

delirium (di-li-ri-ŭm) *n.* an acute disorder of the mental processes accompanying organic brain disease. It may be manifested by delusions, disorientation, hallucinations, or extreme excitement and occurs in metabolic disorders, intoxication, deficiency diseases, and infections. *d. tremens* a psychosis caused by alcoholism, usually seen as a withdrawal syndrome in chronic alcoholics. Features include anxiety, tremor, sweating, and vivid hallucinations.

delivery (di-liv-ĕri) *n. see* labour.

delta cells (del-tă) *pl. n.* the cells in the islets of Langerhans that produce somatostatin and pancreatic polypeptide. *Compare* alpha cells, beta cells.

deltoid (del-toid) *n.* a thick triangular muscle that covers the shoulder joint. It is responsible for raising the arm from the side of the body. See illustration.

delusion (di-loo-zhŏn) *n.* an irrationally held belief that cannot be altered by rational argument. It may be a symptom of manic-depressive

clavicle

scapula

teres major

deltoid

humerus

The deltoid muscle

psychosis, schizophrenia, or an organic psychosis. *See also* paranoia.

Delusions Rating Scale (DRS) *n.* a tool to estimate the extent and effect of delusions in patients by means of a structured interview.

demarcation (dee-mar-**kay**-shŏn) *n.* the marking of a limit or boundary. *line of d.* a red or black line marking the boundary between necrotic and healthy tissue in gangrene.

demeclocycline (dee-mek-loh-sy-kleen) *n.* an antibiotic that is active against a wide range of bacteria and is administered by mouth to treat various infections. Trade name: **Ledermycin**.

dementia (di-**men**-shă) *n.* a chronic or persistent disorder of behaviour and higher intellectual function due to organic brain disease. It is marked by memory disorders, changes in personality, deterioration in personal care, impaired reasoning ability, and disorientation.

d. with Lewy bodies the second most common cause of dementia after Alzheimer's disease. *See* Lewy bodies. *multi-infarct d.* dementia resulting from the destruction of brain tissue by a series of small strokes. *presenile d.* dementia that occurs in young or middle-aged people. *See* Alzheimer's disease, Pick's disease.

demi- *prefix denoting* half.

demography (di-**mog**-răfi) *n.* the study of the populations of the world, their racial make-up, movements, birth rates, death rates, and other factors affecting the quality of life within them.

demulcent (di-**mul**-sĕnt) *n.* a soothing agent that protects the mucous membranes and relieves irritation.

demyelination (dee-my-ĕ-li-**nay**-shŏn) *n.* damage to the myelin sheaths surrounding the nerve fibres in the central or peripheral nervous system. Demyelination may be a primary disorder, as in multiple sclerosis.

dendrite (**den**-dryt) *n.* one of the shorter branching processes of the cell body of a neurone, which makes contact with other neurones at synapses and carries nerve impulses from them into the cell body.

dendritic ulcer (den-**drit**-ik) *n.* a branching ulcer of the surface of the cornea caused by herpes simplex virus.

denervation (de-ner-**vay**-shŏn) *n.* interruption of the nerve supply to the muscles and skin. A denervated area of skin loses all forms of sensation and its subsequent ability to heal and renew its tissues may be impaired.

dengue (breakbone fever)

deodorant

(deng-i) *n.* a viral disease that occurs throughout the tropics and subtropics; it is transmitted to humans principally by the mosquito *Aëdes aegypti*. Symptoms include severe pains in the joints and muscles, headache, fever, and an irritating rash.

denial (di-ny-ăl) *n.* a psychological process in which an individual refuses to accept an aspect of reality. It is seen particularly in dying patients who refuse to accept their impending death.

Denis Browne splint (den-iss brown) *n.* a splint used for the correction of club-foot in early infancy. [Sir Denis J. W. Browne (1892–1967), British orthopaedic surgeon]

dens (denz) *n.* a tooth or tooth-shaped structure.

dent- (denti-, dento-) *prefix denoting* the teeth.

dental auxiliary (den-t'l) *n.* any of various assistants to a dentist, now referred to as *professionals complementary to dentistry*. A *dental hygienist* performs scaling and instruction in oral hygiene under the prescription of the dentist. A *dental nurse* helps the dentist at the chairside by preparing materials, passing instruments, and aspirating fluids from the patient's mouth. A *dental technician* constructs dentures, crowns, and orthodontic appliances in the laboratory for the dentist. A *dental therapist* performs treatment on children under the direction of a dentist in the community dental services and in hospitals.

dental caries *n. see* caries.

dental nurse *n. see* dental auxiliary.

dentate (den-tayt) *adj.* **1.** having teeth. **2.** serrated; having toothlike projections.

dentifrice (dent-i-fris) *n.* a powder or paste for cleaning the teeth. Toothpastes contain a fine abrasive, flavouring materials, and (usually) fluoride. Some contain antimicrobials.

dentine (den-teen) *n.* a hard tissue that forms the bulk of a tooth. The dentine of the crown is covered by enamel and that of the root by cementum.

dentistry (den-tist-ri) *n.* the profession concerned with care and treatment of diseases of the teeth, gums, and jaws.

dentition (den-tish-ŏn) *n.* the number, type, and arrangement of the teeth as a whole in the mouth. *permanent d.* the 32 teeth usually present by the age of 21, made up of incisors, canines, premolars, and molars. *primary d.* the teeth of young children, which are progressively lost in preparation for the eruption of the permanent teeth. It consists of 20 teeth, made up of incisors, canines, and molars only. See illustration.

denture (den-cher) *n.* a removable plate or frame bearing one or more false teeth. *complete d.* a denture replacing all the teeth in one jaw. *partial d.* a denture replacing some teeth, designed to restore function to the remaining teeth.

deodorant (dee-oh-der-ănt) *n.* an agent that reduces or removes unpleasant body odours by destroying bacteria that live on the skin and break down sweat. Deodorant preparations often contain an antiseptic.

molars | incisors | molars
canines | canines

Primary dentition

R — L

premolars | incisors | premolars
molars | canines | canines | molars

Permanent dentition

deontology (dee-on-**tol**-ŏji) *n.* an ethical approach stating that certain things must be done or principles followed, without consideration of whether or not this will lead to the best consequences in the particular circumstances.

deoxycholic acid (dee-oks-i-koh-lik) *n. see* bile acids.

deoxycorticosterone (dee-oks-i-kor-ti-koh-**steer**-ohn) *n.* a hormone, synthesized and released by the adrenal cortex, that regulates salt and water balance. *See also* corticosteroid.

deoxyribonucleic acid (dee-oks-i-ry-boh-new-**klee**-ik) *n. see* DNA.

Department of Health (DOH) (di-**part**-mĕnt) *n.* a department of central government that supports the Secretary of State for Health in meeting his or her obligations, which include the National Health Service and the promotion and protection of the health of the nation.

dependence (drug dependence) (di-**pen**-dăns) *n.* **1.** the physical and/or the psychological effects produced by the habitual taking of certain drugs, characterized by a compulsion to continue taking the drug. *physical d.* dependence in which withdrawal of the drug causes specific symptoms (*withdrawal symptoms*), such as sweating, vomiting, or tremors, that are reversed by further doses. It may be induced by alcohol, morphine, heroin, and cocaine. *psychological d.* dependence in which repeated use of a drug induces reliance on it for a state of well-being and contentment, but there are no physical withdrawal symptoms if use of the drug is stopped. It may be induced by nicotine in tobacco, cannabis, and such drugs as barbiturates and amphetamines. **2.** a state of reliance on others for aspects of self-care, sometimes used as a measure of nursing workload.

depersonalization (dee-per-sŏ-nă-ly-**zay**-shŏn) *n.* a state in which a person feels himself becoming unreal or strangely altered, or feels that his mind is becoming separated from his body. Severe feelings of depersonalization occur in conditions such as anxiety neurosis, schizophrenia, and epilepsy. *See also* derealization, out-of-the-body experience.

depilatory (di-**pil**-ă ter-i) *n.* an agent applied to the skin to remove hair.

depolarization (dee-poh-lă-ry-**zay**-shŏn) *n.* the sudden surge of charged particles across the membrane of a nerve cell or of a muscle cell that accompanies a physicochemical change in the membrane and cancels out, or reverses, its resting potential to produce an action potential.

depot injection (dep-oh) *n.* the administration of a sustained-action drug formulation that allows slow release and gradual absorption, so that the active agent can act for much longer periods than is possible with standard injections.

Depot injections are usually given deep into a muscle.

depressant (di-pres-ănt) *n.* an agent that reduces the normal activity of any body system or function. Drugs such as general anaesthetics, barbiturates, and opiates are depressants of the central nervous system and respiration.

depression (di-presh-ŏn) *n.* a mental state characterized by excessive sadness. Activity can be agitated or retarded and sleep, appetite, and concentration can be disturbed. Loss or frustration cause depression, which may be prolonged and disproportionate (*dysthymic disorder*; formerly called *depressive neurosis*). Manic-depressive psychosis causes very severe depression, a major affective disorder. Treatment for depression is with antidepressant drugs, cognitive therapy, and/or psychotherapy. *See also* postnatal (depression).

depressor (di-pres-er) *n.* **1.** a muscle that causes lowering of part of the body. **2.** a nerve that lowers blood pressure.

dequalinium (dek-wă-lin-iŭm) *n.* an antiseptic, active against some bacteria and fungi, used as lozenges to treat mouth and throat infections. Trade names: **Dequadin**, **Labosept**.

Derbyshire neck (dar-bi-sher) *n.* endemic goitre that was once common in Derbyshire due to lack of iodine in the soil and water.

derealization (dee-riă-ly-zay-shŏn) *n.* a feeling of unreality in which the environment is experienced as unreal and strange. It occurs in association with depersonalization or with the conditions that cause depersonalization.

dereism (dee-ri-izm) *n.* undirected fantasy thinking that fails to respect the realities of life. It may be a feature of schizophrenia.

derm- (**derma-, dermo-, dermat(o)-**) *prefix denoting* the skin.

-derm *suffix denoting* **1.** the skin. **2.** a germ layer.

dermal (der-măl) *adj.* relating to or affecting the skin, especially the dermis.

dermatitis (der-mă-ty-tis) *n.* an inflammatory condition of the skin, especially one in which outside agents play a primary role (*compare* eczema). *allergic contact d.* dermatitis in which skin changes resembling those of eczema develop as a delayed reaction to contact with a particular allergen. The commonest example in women is *nickel d.* from jewellery, jean studs, etc.; in men *chromium d.* is relatively common (cement is the usual source). *d. herpetiformis* an uncommon very itchy rash with symmetrical blistering, especially on the knees, elbows, buttocks, and shoulders. It is associated with gluten sensitivity. *primary irritant d.* a condition that may occur in anyone who has sufficient contact with such irritants as acids, alkalis, solvents, and (especially) detergents. It is the commonest cause of *occupational d.* in hairdressers, nurses, cooks, etc. *See also* napkin rash. *seborrhoeic d. see* (seborrhoeic) eczema.

dermatochalasis (der-mă-toh-kă-lay-sis) *n.* redundant eyelid skin, which may cause drooping of the upper lid. It occurs as a result of ageing and is therefore seen only in

middle-aged and elderly people. *Compare* blepharochalasis.

dermatoglyphics (der-mă-toh-glif-iks) *n.* **1.** the patterns of finger, palm, toe, and sole prints, which are unique to each individual. Abnormalities are found in those with chromosomal aberrations, e.g. Down's syndrome. **2.** the study of these patterns, which is of use in medicine, criminology, and anthropology.

dermatology (der-mă-tol-ŏji) *n.* the medical specialty concerned with the diagnosis and treatment of skin disorders. —**dermatological** *adj.* —**dermatologist** *n.*

dermatome (der-mă-tohm) *n.* a surgical instrument used for cutting thin slices of skin in some skin grafting operations.

dermatomycosis (der-mă-toh-my-koh-sis) *n.* any infection of the skin caused by fungi.

dermatomyositis (der-mă-toh-my-oh-**sy**-tis) *n.* an inflammatory disorder of the skin and underlying tissues, including the muscles. A bluish-red skin eruption occurs on the face, scalp, neck, shoulders, and knuckles and is later accompanied by severe swelling. The condition is one of the connective-tissue diseases; it is often associated with internal cancer in adults, though not in children.

dermatophyte (der-mă-toh-fyt) *n.* any fungus belonging to the genera *Microsporum*, *Epidermophyton*, or *Trichophyton*, which cause ringworm. *See also* tinea.

dermatosis (der-mă-toh-sis) *n.* any disease of skin, particularly one without inflammation. *juvenile plantar d.* a condition in which the skin on the front of the sole becomes red, glazed, and symmetrically cracked. It affects children up to the age of 14 and is believed to be related to the wearing of trainers.

dermis (corium) (der-mis) *n.* the true skin: the thick layer of living tissue that lies beneath the epidermis. —**dermal** *adj.*

dermographism (der-moh-graf-izm) *n.* a local reaction caused by pressure on the skin. People with such highly sensitive skin can 'write' on it with a finger or blunt instrument, the pressure producing weals.

dermoid cyst (dermoid) (dermoid) *n.* a cyst containing hair, hair follicles, and sebaceous glands, usually found at sites marking the fusion of developing sections of the body in the embryo.

Descemet's membrane (dess-ē-mayz) *n.* the membrane that forms the deepest layer of the stroma of the cornea of the eye. The endothelium lies between it and the aqueous humour. [J. Descemet (1732– 1810), French anatomist]

desensitization (dee-sen-si-ty-zay-shŏn) *n.* **1.** (**hyposensitization**) a method for reducing the effects of a known allergen by injecting, over a period, gradually increasing doses of the allergen, until resistance is built up. *See* allergy. **2.** a technique used in the behaviour therapy of phobic states. The thing that is feared is very gradually introduced to the patient, in conjunction with relaxation therapy, so that he or she is able to cope with progressively closer approximations to it.

desferrioxamine (dess-ferri-oks-ă-meen) *n.* a drug that combines with iron in body tissues and fluids and is administered by injection to treat iron poisoning or diseases that involve iron storage in parts of the body (*see* haemochromatosis). Trade name: **Desferal**.

desmoid tumour (dez-moid) *n.* a dense connective-tissue tumour with a dangerous propensity for repeated local recurrence after treatment. Intra-abdominal desmoids have an association with familial adenomatous polyposis.

desmopressin (dess-moh-press-in) *n.* a synthetic derivative of vasopressin that causes a decrease in urine output. It is taken orally, intranasally, or intravenously to treat diabetes insipidus, nocturnal enuresis, mild haemophilia, and von Willebrand's disease. Trade names: **DDAVP, Desmotabs, Desmospray**.

desogestrel (dess-oh-jee-strĕl) *n.* a progestogen used in various oral contraceptives, usually in combination with an oestrogen. Trade names: **Marvelon, Mercilon**.

desoximetasone (dess-oxi-met-ă-zohn) *n.* a corticosteroid applied to the skin as a cream or ointment to reduce inflammation and pruritus. Trade name: **Stiedex**.

desquamation (dess-kwă-may-shŏn) *n.* the process in which the outer layer of the epidermis of the skin is removed by scaling.

detached retina (di-tacht) *n.* *see* retinal detachment.

detergent (di-ter-jĕnt) *n.* a synthetic cleansing agent that removes all impurities from a surface by reacting with grease and suspended particles, including bacteria and other microorganisms.

detoxication (detoxification) (dee-toksi-kay-shŏn) *n.* **1.** the process by which toxic substances are removed or toxic effects neutralized. It is one of the functions of the liver. **2.** the 'drying-out' of a patient suffering from alcoholism.

detrition (di-trish-ŏn) *n.* the process of wearing away solid bodies (e.g. bones) by friction or use.

detritus (di-try-tŭs) *n.* particles of matter produced by disintegration, tissue death, etc.

detrusor muscle (di-troo-ser) *n.* the muscle of the urinary bladder wall. Its function is assessed by urodynamic investigation (*see* urodynamics).

detumescence (dee-tew-mes-ĕns) *n.* **1.** the reverse of erection, whereby the erect penis or clitoris becomes flaccid after orgasm. **2.** subsidence of a swelling.

deut- (deuto-, deuter(o)-) *prefix* denoting two, second, or secondary.

deuteranopia (dew-ter-ă-noh-piă) *n.* a defect in colour vision in which reds, yellows, and greens are confused. *Compare* tritanopia.

developmental delay (di-vel-ŏp-men-t'l) *n.* considerable delay in the physical or mental development of children when compared with their peers. There are many causes. *Global delay* describes the state of a child whose overall development is slow in all areas.

developmental disorder *n.* any one of a group of conditions that arise in infancy or childhood and are characterized by delays in biologically determined psychological functions, such as language. In *pervasive* conditions (e.g. autism) many types of development are involved; in *specific* disorders, (such as dyslexia) the handicap is an isolated problem.

developmental milestones *pl. n.* skills gained by a developing child, which should be achieved by a given age. Examples include smiling by six weeks and sitting unsupported by eight months. Failure to achieve a particular milestone by a given age is indicative of developmental delay.

deviation (dee-vi-ay-shŏn) *n.* **1.** (in ophthalmology) any abnormal position of one or both eyes. Deviations of both eyes may occur in brain disease. Deviations of one eye come into the category of squint (*see* strabismus). *dissociated vertical d.* an acquired condition, chiefly associated with infantile esotropia (convergent strabismus), in which one eye looks upwards when it is covered. **2.** *see* sexual deviation.

Devic's disease (dev-iks) *n. see* neuromyelitis optica. [E. Devic (1869–1930), French physician]

DEXA *n.* dual-energy X-ray absorptiometry: a method of measuring bone density based on the proportion of a beam of photons that passes through the bone.

dexamethasone (deks-ă-meth-ă-zohn) *n.* a corticosteroid drug administered by mouth or injection or as eye or ear drops principally to treat severe allergies, skin and eye diseases, rheumatic and other inflammatory conditions, and hormone and blood disorders. Trade names: **Decadron**, **Maxidex**.

dexamfetamine (dexamfetamine) (deks-am-fet-ămin) *n. see* amphetamines.

dextr- (dextro-) *prefix denoting* **1.**

the right side. **2.** (in chemistry) dextrorotation.

dextran (deks-tran) *n.* a carbohydrate, consisting of branched chains of glucose units, that is a storage product of bacteria and yeasts. Preparations of dextran solution are used in transfusions, in order to increase the volume of plasma.

dextrin (deks-trin) *n.* a carbohydrate formed as an intermediate product in the digestion of starch by the enzyme amylase. Dextrin is used in the preparation of pharmaceutical products and surgical dressings.

dextrocardia (deks-troh-**kar**-diă) *n.* a congenital defect in which the position of the heart is a mirror image of its normal position, with the apex of the ventricles pointing to the right.

dextromoramide (deks-troh-**mor**-ă-myd) *n.* an analgesic administered by mouth, injection, or as suppositories to relieve moderate or severe pain. Dextromoramide is similar to morphine and can cause morphine-type dependence. Trade name: **Palfium**.

dextropropoxyphene (deks-troh-prŏ-**poks**-i-feen) *n.* an analgesic administered by mouth to relieve mild or moderate pain. Trade name: **Doloxene**.

dextrose (deks-trohz) *n. see* glucose.

DHEA *n. see* dehydroepiandrosterone.

dhobie itch (doh-bi) *n.* a fungal infection of the skin that chiefly affects the groin but may spread to the thighs and buttocks. It is caused by certain species of *Trichophyton* and *Epidermophyton*. Medical name: **tinea cruris**. *See also* tinea.

DI *n.* donor insemination (*see* artificial insemination).

di- *prefix denoting* two or double.

dia- *prefix denoting* **1.** through. **2.** completely or throughout. **3.** apart.

diabetes (dy-ă-bee-teez) *n.* any disorder of metabolism causing excessive thirst and the production of large volumes of urine. *d. insipidus* a rare form of diabetes that is due to deficiency of the pituitary hormone vasopressin (antidiuretic hormone). *d. mellitus* (**DM**) a disorder of carbohydrate metabolism in which sugars in the body are not oxidized to produce energy due to lack of the pancreatic hormone insulin. The accumulation of sugar leads to its appearance in the blood (hyperglycaemia), then in the urine; symptoms include thirst, loss of weight, and the excessive production of urine. The use of fats as an alternative source of energy leads to disturbances of the acid-base balance, ketosis, and eventually to *diabetic coma*. The diet must be controlled, with adequate carbohydrate for the body's needs; lack of balance in the diet leads to hypoglycaemia. In *type 1* (or *insulin-dependent*) *d. mellitus*, which usually starts in childhood or adolescence, patients are entirely dependent on injections of insulin for survival. In *type 2* (*noninsulin-dependent* or *maturity-onset*) *d. mellitus*, either the pancreas retains some ability to produce insulin, but this is inadequate for the body's needs, or the body becomes resistant to the effects of insulin; oral hypoglycaemic drugs or insulin may be required. Type 2 diabetes usually occurs after the age of 40, but a rare form, *maturity-onset d.*

of the young (MODY), develops in people under 25. *Type 3* (or *gestational*) *d. mellitus* develops during pregnancy. —**diabetic** (dy-ă-bet-ik) *adj., n.*

diabetic amyotrophy *n. see* amyotrophy.

diabetic hand syndrome *n.* the combination of features, often found in the hands of long-standing diabetic subjects, consisting of Dupuytren's contractures, knuckle pads, carpal tunnel syndrome, cheiroarthropathy, and sclerosing tenosynovitis.

diabetic honeymoon period *n.* a well-recognized period just after the diagnosis of type 1 diabetes mellitus when only very low insulin doses are required to control the condition. It will last for months to a few years.

diabetic nephropathy *n. see* nephropathy.

diabetic neuropathy *n. see* neuropathy.

diabetic retinopathy *n. see* retinopathy.

diagnosis (dy-ăg-noh-sis) *n.* the process of determining the nature of a disorder by considering the patient's signs and symptoms, medical background, and – where necessary – results of laboratory tests and X-ray examinations. *differential d.* diagnosis of a condition whose signs and/or symptoms are shared by various other conditions. *See also* prenatal diagnosis. *Compare* prognosis. —**diagnostic** (dy-ăg-noss-tik) *adj.*

diagnostic peritoneal lavage *n.* the instillation of saline directly into the abdominal cavity and its subsequent aspiration a few minutes later. If the fluid is bloodstained

on recovery an intra-abdominal haemorrhage is indicated. This is a useful diagnostic tool in trauma patients.

dialyser (dy-ă-ly-zer) *n.* a piece of apparatus for separating components of a liquid mixture by dialysis, used especially in haemodialysis.

dialysis (dy-al-i-sis) *n.* a method of separating particles of different dimensions in a liquid mixture, using a thin semipermeable membrane. A solution of the mixture is separated from distilled water by the membrane; the solutes pass through the membrane into the water while the proteins, etc., are retained. The principle of dialysis is used in treating kidney failure (*see* haemodialysis). *peritoneal d.* the use of the peritoneum as a semipermeable membrane by patients with kidney failure, either continuously or intermittently, employed when haemodialysis is not appropriate.

diamorphine (dy-ă-mor-feen) *n.* a pharmaceutical preparation of heroin: a powerful narcotic analgesic used for the relief of severe pain.

diapedesis (dy-ă-pĕ-dee-sis) *n.* migration of cells through the walls of blood capillaries into the tissue spaces. Diapedesis is an important part of the reaction of tissues to injury (*see* inflammation).

diaphoresis (dy-ă-fer-ee-sis) *n.* the process of sweating, especially excessive sweating. *See* sweat.

diaphoretic (sudorific) (dy-ă-fer-et-ik) *n.* a drug, such as pilocarpine, that causes an increase in sweating. Antipyretic drugs also have diaphoretic activity.

diaphragm (dy-ă-fram) *n.* **1.** (in anatomy) a thin musculomembranous dome-shaped muscle that separates the thoracic and abdominal cavities. It plays an important role in breathing. There are openings in the diaphragm through which the oesophagus, blood vessels, and nerves pass. **2.** a hemispherical rubber cap fitted inside the vagina over the neck (cervix) of the uterus as a contraceptive. When combined with the use of a chemical spermicide the diaphragm provides reasonably reliable contraception.

diaphysis (dy-af-i-sis) *n.* the body, or shaft, of a long bone, consisting of a thick cylinder of compact bone surrounding a large medullary cavity. *Compare* epiphysis. —**diaphysial** (dy-ă-fiz-iăl) *adj.*

diarrhoea (dy-ă-ree-ă) *n.* frequent bowel evacuation or the passage of abnormally soft or liquid faeces. Its causes include intestinal infections, other forms of intestinal inflammation, anxiety, and the irritable bowel syndrome. Severe or prolonged diarrhoea may lead to excess losses of fluid, salts, and nutrients in the faeces.

diarthrosis (synovial joint) (dy-arth-**roh**-sis) *n.* a freely movable joint. The ends of the adjoining bones are covered with a thin cartilaginous sheet, and the bones are linked by a ligament lined with synovial membrane, which secretes synovial fluid. See illustration.

diastase (dy-ă-stayz) *n.* an enzyme that hydrolyses starch in barley grain to produce maltose during the malting process. It has been used to aid the digestion of starch in some digestive disorders.

diastasis (dy-ast-ă-sis) *n.* dislocation of bones at an immovable or slightly movable joint, as at the pubic symphysis.

diastema (dy-ă-stee-mă) *n.* a space between two teeth.

diastole (dy-ast-ŏ-li) *n.* the period between two contractions of the heart, when the muscle of the heart relaxes and allows the chambers to fill with blood. *See also* blood pressure, systole. —**diastolic** (dy-ă-stol-ik) *adj.*

diastolic pressure *n.* see blood pressure.

diathermy (dy-ă-therm-i) *n.* the production of heat in a part of the body by means of a high-frequency electric current passed between two electrodes placed on the patient's skin. The heat generated can be used in the treatment of deep-seated pain in rheumatic and arthritic conditions. *d. knife* a knife generating heat that coagulates blood and is used to make bloodless surgical incisions. *d. snare* (or *needle*) an electrically heated snare (or needle)

synovial
membrane

cartilage

synovial
cavity

ligament
forming
capsule

A synovial joint

used to destroy unwanted tissue and to remove small superficial neoplasms. *See also* electrosurgery.

diathesis (dy-ath-i-sis) *n*. a higher than average tendency to acquire certain diseases, such as allergies, rheumatic diseases, or gout. Such diseases may run in families, but they are not inherited.

diazepam (dy-az-ē-pam) *n*. a long-acting benzodiazepine, administered by mouth or injection, used to treat acute anxiety, delirium tremens, epilepsy, and muscle spasms. It is also used as a premedication. Trade names: **Diazemuls, Valium.**

diazoxide (dy-ă-zok-syd) *n*. a drug used to lower blood pressure in patients with hypertension and also used to treat conditions in which the levels of blood sugar are low. It is administered by mouth or (for hypertension) injection. Trade name: **Eudemine.**

DIC *n*. *see* disseminated intravascular coagulation.

dicephalus (dy-sef-ă-lŭs) *n*. *see* craniopagus.

dichromatic (dy-kroh-mat-ik) *adj*. describing the state of colour vision of those who can appreciate only two of the three primary colours. *Compare* trichromatic.

Dick test (dik) *n*. a test for susceptibility to scarlet fever. [G. F. Dick (1881–1967) and G. R. H. Dick (1881–1963), US physicians]

diclofenac (dy-kloh-fen-ak) *n*. an anti-inflammatory drug (*see* NSAID) used to relieve joint pain in osteoarthritis, rheumatoid arthritis, and ankylosing spondylitis. It is administered by mouth or injection or

topically. Trade names: **Volraman, Voltarol.**

Diconal (dy-kŏ-năl) *n*. *see* dipipanone.

dicophane (dy-koh-fayn) *n*. *see* DDT.

dicrotism (dy-krŏ-tizm) *n*. a condition in which the pulse is felt as a double beat for each contraction of the heart. It may be seen in typhoid fever. —**dicrotic** (dy-krot-ik) *adj*.

dicycloverine (dicyclomine) (dy-sy-klŏ-vě-reen) *n*. an anticholinergic drug that reduces spasms of smooth muscle and is administered by mouth to relieve peptic ulcer, infantile colic, colitis, and related conditions. Trade name: **Merbentyl.**

didanosine (ddI) (dy-dan-ŏ-seen) *n*. an antiviral drug that is administered by mouth to prolong the lives of patients with AIDS and HIV infection. Possible side-effects include damage to nerves, severe pancreatitis, nausea, vomiting, and headache. Trade name: **Videx.**

didym- (didymo-) *prefix denoting* the testis.

diet (dy-ĕt) *n*. the mixture of foods that a person eats. *balanced d*. a diet that contains the correct proportions of all the nutrients.

dietary fibre (roughage) (dy-it-er-i) *n*. the part of food that cannot be digested and absorbed to produce energy. Foods with a high fibre content include wholemeal cereals and flour, root vegetables, nuts, and fruit. Dietary fibre is considered by some to be helpful in the prevention of such diseases as diverticulosis, constipation, appendicitis, obesity, and diabetes mellitus.

dietetics (dy-i-tet-iks) *n*. the application of the principles of nutrition to the selection of food and the feeding of individuals and groups.

diethylcarbamazine (dy-eth-il-kar-**bam**-ă-zeen) *n.* an anthelmintic drug that is administered by mouth in the treatment of filariasis and loiasis.

diethylstilbestrol (dy-eth-il-stil-**bes**-tröl) *n.* a synthetic female sex hormone (*see* oestrogen) administered by mouth or as pessaries to relieve menstrual disorders and symptoms of the menopause, to treat prostate and breast cancer, and to suppress lactation. Trade names: **Apstil, Tampovagan**.

Dietl's crisis (dee-t'lz) *n.* acute obstruction of a kidney causing severe pain in the loins. The obstruction usually occurs at the junction of the renal pelvis and the ureter, causing the kidney to become distended with accumulated urine (*see* hydronephrosis). [J. Dietl (1804–78), Polish physician]

differential diagnosis (dif-er-en-shăl) *n. see* diagnosis.

differential leucocyte count (differential blood count) *n.* a determination of the proportions of the different kinds of white cells (leucocytes) present in a sample of blood. The information often aids diagnosis of disease.

differentiation (dif-er-en-shi-ay-shŏn) *n.* **1.** (in embryology) the process in which embryonic development during which unspecialized cells or tissues become specialized for particular functions. **2.** (in oncology) the degree of similarity of tumour cells to the structure of the organ from which the tumour arose. Tumours are classified as well, moderately, or poorly differentiated.

diffusion (di-**few**-zhŏn) *n.* the mixing of one liquid or gas with another by the random movement of their particles.

diflunisal (dy-**floo**-ni-săl) *n.* an anti-inflammatory drug (*see* NSAID) derived from salicylic acid and used to control symptoms in osteoarthritis and other painful conditions. It is administered by mouth. Trade name: **Dolobid**.

di George syndrome (dee-**jorj**) *n.* a hereditary condition resulting in an inability to fight infections (immunodeficiency) associated with absence of the parathyroid and thymus glands, abnormalities of the heart, and low levels of calcium. *See also* CATCH-22. [A. M. di George (1921–), US paediatrician]

digestion (dy-**jes**-chŏn) *n.* the process in which ingested food is broken down in the alimentary canal into a form that can be absorbed and assimilated by the tissues of the body.

digit (**dij**-it) *n.* a finger or toe.

digital (**dij**-it-ăl) *adj.* **1.** relating to a finger or toe. **2.** relating to or designating information that can be represented by a series of numbers. **d. hearing aid** *see* hearing aid. **d. image** an electronically produced image, such as an image produced by digital radiography, made up of pixels, each of which has numbers to represent its position and shade. *See* digitization. **d. radiography** *see* radiography. **d. subtraction** a technique used in X-ray examination, most commonly of blood vessels, in which a digitized image taken before addition of the contrast medium is subtracted by computer from the images taken after contrast injection. Only the outline of the blood vessel remains on the image, enabling blood-vessel anatomy and blood supply to an organ to be demonstrated more clearly.

digitalis (dij-i-tay-lis) *n.* an extract from the dried leaves of foxgloves (*Digitalis* species), which contains various substances, including digitoxin and digoxin, that stimulate heart muscle.

digitalization (dij-it-ă-ly-zay-shŏn) *n.* the administration of a derivative of digitalis to a patient with heart failure until the optimum level has been reached in the heart tissues.

digitization (dij-it-I-zay-shŏn) *n.* (in radiology) the representation of analogue images (i.e. images produced by X-ray machines, CT scanners, MRI scanners, or ultrasound probes) as a set of numerical values, which enables their electronic manipulation, storage, and transfer via computer links in the form of digital images.

digitoxin (dij-i-toks-in) *n.* a drug that increases heart muscle contraction and is administered by mouth or injection in heart failure. It is slow-acting but the effects are prolonged.

digoxin (dy-goks-in) *n.* a drug that increases heart muscle contraction and is administered by mouth or injection in heart failure. It is rapidly effective and the effects are short-lived. Trade name: **Lanoxin**.

dihydrocodeine (dy-hy-drŏ-koh-deen) *n.* a drug administered by mouth or injection to relieve pain and suppress coughs (*see* analgesic, antitussive). Trade name: **DHC Continus**.

dilatation (dy-lă-tay-shŏn) *n.* the enlargement or expansion of a hollow organ (such as a blood vessel) or cavity.

dilatation and curettage (D and C) *n.* an operation in which the cervix (neck) of the uterus is dilated, using a dilator, and the lining (endometrium) of the uterus is lightly scraped off with a curette (*see* curettage). It is performed for a variety of reasons, including removal of cysts or tumours and examination of the endometrium in the diagnosis of gynaecological disorders.

dilator (dy-lay-ter) *n.* **1.** an instrument used to enlarge a body opening or cavity. **2.** a drug, applied either locally or systemically, that causes expansion of a structure. *See also* vasodilator. **3.** a muscle that, by its action, opens an aperture or orifice in the body.

dill water (dil) *n.* a preparation containing a volatile oil extracted from the dill plant (*Anethum graveolens*), used to treat flatulence in infants.

diltiazem (dil-ti-ă-zem) *n.* a calcium antagonist that is used in the treatment of effort-associated angina and high blood pressure (hypertension). It acts as a vasodilator and is administered by mouth. Trade names: **Adizem, Dilzem, Tildiem,** etc.

dimercaprol (BAL, British Anti-Lewisite) (dy-mer-kap-rol) *n.* a drug that combines with metals in the body and is administered by injection to treat poisoning by antimony, arsenic, bismuth, gold, mercury, and thallium.

dimeticone (dimethicone) (dy-met-i-kohn) *n.* a silicone preparation used externally to prevent undue drying of the skin and to protect it against irritating external agents. It is commonly used to prevent napkin rash in babies. Trade names: **Conotrane, Siopel**. *See also* simethicone.

dinoprostone (dy-noh-**prost**-ohn) *n.* a prostaglandin drug used mainly to induce labour. It is administered as a vaginal tablet or gel. Trade names: **Propess, Prostin E2**.

dioctyl sodium sulphosuccinate (docusate sodium) (dy-**ok**-tyl soh-di-ŭm sul-foh-**suk**-si-nayt) *n.* a softening agent that is given by mouth or in suppositories, often together with a laxative, to relieve constipation. It is also used in solution to soften ear wax.

diode laser (dy-ohd) *n. see* laser.

dioptre (dy-**op**-ter) *n.* the unit of measurement of the power of refraction of a lens. One dioptre is the power of a lens that brings parallel light rays to a focus at a point one metre from the lens, after passing through it.

diphenhydramine (dy-fen-hy-**dră**-meen) *n.* an antihistamine with sedative properties administered by mouth to induce sleep. It may be combined with other drugs in cough mixtures.

diphtheria (dif-**theer**-iă) *n.* an acute highly contagious infection, caused by the bacterium *Corynebacterium diphtheriae*, that generally affects the throat but occasionally affects other mucous membranes and the skin. Early symptoms are a sore throat, weakness, and mild fever; later, a soft grey membrane forms across the throat, constricting the air passages and causing difficulty in breathing and swallowing. Bacteria multiply at the site of infection and release a toxin into the bloodstream, which damages heart and nerves. An effective immunization programme has now made diphtheria rare in most Western countries (*see also* Schick test).

diphtheroid (dif-ther-oid) *adj.* resembling diphtheria (especially the membrane formed in diphtheria) or the bacteria that cause it.

diphyllobothriasis (dy-fil-oh-bo-thry-ă-sis) *n.* an infestation of the intestine with the broad tapeworm, *Diphyllobothrium latum*, which sometimes causes nausea, malnutrition, diarrhoea, and anaemia resulting from impaired absorption of vitamin B_{12} through the gut.

dipipanone (dy-**pip**-ă-nohn) *n.* a potent opioid analgesic administered by mouth in combination with cyclizine (as *Diconal*) to relieve severe pain.

dipl- (diplo-) *prefix denoting* double.

diplacusis (dip-lă-**kew**-sis) *n.* perception of a single sound as double owing to a defect of the cochlea in the inner ear.

diplegia (dy-**plee**-jă) *n.* paralysis involving both sides of the body and affecting the legs more severely than the arms. *cerebral d.* a form of cerebral palsy in which there is widespread damage, in both cerebral hemispheres, of the brain cells that control the movements of the limbs. —**diplegic** *adj.*

diplococcus (dip-loh-**kok**-ŭs) *n.* any of a group of nonmotile parasitic spherical bacteria that occur in pairs. The group includes the pneumococcus.

diploë (**dip**-loh-ee) *n.* the lattice-like

tissue that lies between the inner and outer layers of the skull.

diploid (dip-loid) *adj.* describing cells, nuclei, or organisms in which each chromosome except the Y sex chromosome is represented twice. *Compare* haploid. —**diploid** *n.*

diplopia (di-ploh-piǎ) *n.* double vision: the simultaneous awareness of two images of the one object. It is usually due to limitation of movement of one eye, which may be caused by a defect of the nerves or muscles controlling eye movement or a mechanical restriction of eyeball movement in the orbit. Double vision that does not disappear on covering one eye can be caused by early cataract (*see also* polyopia).

dipsomania (dip-sŏ-may-niǎ) *n.* morbid and insatiable craving for alcohol, occurring in paroxysms. Only a small proportion of alcoholics show this symptom. *See* alcoholism.

dipyridamole (dy-py-rid-ǎ-mohl) *n.* a drug that dilates the blood vessels of the heart and reduces platelet aggregation. It is given by mouth to prevent thrombosis around prosthetic heart valves. Trade name: **Persantin**.

direct observed therapy (DOT) (di-rekt) *n.* antituberculosis therapy in which the drugs are administered by a nurse practitioner.

director (di-rek-ter) *n.* an instrument used to guide the extent and direction of a surgical incision.

dis- *prefix denoting* separation.

disability (dis-ǎ-bil-iti) *n.* a loss or restriction of functional ability or activity as a result of impairment of the body or mind. *See also* handicap.
—**disabled** (dis-ay-bŭld) *adj.*

disaccharide (dy-sak-ǎ-ryd) *n.* a carbohydrate consisting of two linked monosaccharide units. The most common disaccharides are maltose, lactose, and sucrose.

disarticulation (dis-ar-tik-yoo-lay-shŏn) *n.* separation of two bones at a joint. This may be the result of an injury or it may be done by the surgeon at operation in the course of amputation.

disc (disk) *n.* (in anatomy) a rounded flattened structure, such as an intervertebral disc or the optic disc.

discission (dis-sizh-ŏn) *n.* an obsolete operation for cataract in which the lens capsule was ruptured by a fine knife or needle to allow the substance of the lens to be absorbed naturally into the surrounding fluid of the eye.

discoid lupus erythematosus (DLE) (dis-koid) *n.* *see* lupus (erythematosus).

discrete (dis-kreet) *adj.* composed of several parts: describing lesions that are separate and do not run into each other.

disease (di-zeez) *n.* a disorder with a specific cause and recognizable signs and symptoms; any bodily abnormality or failure to function properly, except that resulting directly from physical injury (the latter, however, may open the way for disease).

disimpaction (dis-im-pak-shŏn) *n.* the process of separating the broken ends of a bone when they have been forcibly driven together during a fracture.

disinfectant (dis-in-fek-tǎnt) *n.* an agent that destroys or removes bacteria and other microorganisms and

dissociative disorder

is used to cleanse surgical instruments and other objects. Examples are cresol, hexachlorophene, and phenol.

disinfection (dis-in-fek-shŏn) *n.* the process of eliminating infective microorganisms from contaminated instruments, clothing, or surroundings by the use of physical means or chemicals (disinfectants).

disinfestation (dis-in-fes-tay-shŏn) *n.* the destruction of insect pests and other animal parasites. This generally involves the use of insecticides.

dislocation (luxation) (dis-lŏ-kay-shŏn) *n.* displacement from their normal position of bones meeting at a joint such that there is complete loss of contact of the joint surfaces. The bones are restored to their normal positions by manipulation under local or general anaesthesia (*see* reduction). *Compare* subluxation.

disopyramide (dy-soh-py-rǎ-myd) *n.* a drug administered by mouth or injection to treat various heart conditions involving abnormal heart rates. Trade names: **Dirythmin SA, Rythmodan**.

disorientation (dis-or-i-ĕn-tay-shŏn) *n.* the state produced by loss of awareness of space, time, or personality. It can occur as the result of drugs, anxiety, or organic disease (such as dementia or Korsakoff's syndrome).

dispensary (dis-pen-ser-i) *n.* a place where medicines are made up by a pharmacist according to the doctor's prescription and dispensed to patients.

dispensing practice (dis-pen-sing **prak**-tis) *n.* (in Britain) a general practice in which doctors re-

ceive special allowances under the terms of the National Health Service for dispensing the medications they prescribe for their patients.

dissection (dis-sek-shŏn) *n.* the cutting apart and separation of the body tissues along the natural divisions of the organs and different tissues in the course of an operation. Dissection of corpses is carried out for the study of anatomy.

disseminated (dis-sem-in-ayt-id) *adj.* widely distributed in an organ (or organs) or in the whole body. The term may refer to disease organisms or to pathological changes.

disseminated intravascular coagulation (DIC) *n.* a condition resulting from overstimulation of the blood-clotting mechanisms in response to disease or injury, such as severe infection, malignancy, acute leukaemia, burns, severe trauma, abruptio placentae, or intrauterine fetal death. The overstimulation results in generalized blood coagulation and excessive consumption of coagulation factors. The resulting deficiency of these may lead to spontaneous bleeding.

disseminated sclerosis *n. see* multiple sclerosis.

dissociation (dis-soh-si-ay-shŏn) *n.* (in psychiatry) the process whereby thoughts and ideas can be split off from consciousness and may function independently, allowing conflicting opinions to be held at the same time about the same object. Dissociation may be the main factor in cases of dissociative fugue and multiple personalities (*see* dissociative disorder). —**dissociative** (dis-soh-shǎ-tiv) *adj.*

dissociative disorder *n.* any one

of a group of extreme defence mechanisms that include amnesia, fugue, multiple personality disorder, and trancelike states with severely reduced response to external stimuli. *See also* dissociation.

distal (dis-t'l) *adj.* (in anatomy) situated away from the origin or point of attachment or from the median line of the body. *Compare* proximal.

Distalgesic (dis-t'l-jee-sik) *n. see* co-proxamol.

distichiasis (dis-ti-ky-ă-sis) *n.* a very rare condition in which there is an extra row of eyelashes behind the normal row. They may rub on the cornea.

distigmine (dy-stig-meen) *n.* an anticholinesterase drug used to treat myasthenia gravis. It is administered by mouth. Trade name: **Ubretid**.

distraction (dis-trak-shŏn) *n.* **1.** (in orthopaedics) increasing the distance between two joint surfaces or the two ends of a divided bone. **2.** (in psychiatry) a diversional therapy that can enable procedures to be carried out with the patient in a state of relaxation.

distraction test *n.* a hearing test used for screening infants between the ages of six and ten months. One examiner sits in front of the infant and gains its attention, while a second examiner, situated just behind the infant, makes a sound at the level of the infant's ear to one side or the other. If the infant can hear it turns in the direction of the sound.

district nurse (home nurse) (**dis**-trikt) *n.* (in Britain) a nurse with special training in domiciliary services. District nurses are usually employed by a community trust but

may also be allocated to a designated general practice (*see* attachment).

disulfiram (dy-**sul**-fi-ram) *n.* a drug administered by mouth in the treatment of chronic alcoholism. It acts as a deterrent by producing unpleasant effects, such as headache, nausea, and vomiting, when taken with alcohol. Trade name: **Antabuse**.

dithranol (**dith**-ră-nol) *n.* a drug applied to the skin as an ointment or paste to treat psoriasis. It may irritate the skin on application. Trade names: **Alphodith**, **Dithrolan**.

diuresis (dy-yoor-ee-sis) *n.* increased secretion of urine by the kidneys. This normally follows the drinking of more fluid than the body requires, but it can be stimulated by the administration of a diuretic.

diuretic (dy-yoor-et-ik) *n.* a drug that increases the volume of urine produced by promoting the excretion of salts and water from the kidney. Diuretics are used in the treatment of oedema and high blood pressure. **loop** *d.* a diuretic, such as furosemide, that acts by inhibiting reabsorption of sodium and potassium in Henle's loop. **potassium-sparing** *d.* a diuretic, such as amiloride, that prevents excessive loss of potassium at the distal convoluted tubules. **thiazide** *d.* a diuretic, such as bendroflumethiazide, that acts by preventing the reabsorption of sodium and potassium in the distal kidney tubules.

diurnal (dy-ern-ăl) *adj.* occurring during the day.

divarication (dy-va-ri-kay-shŏn) *n.* the separation or stretching of bodily structures. **rectus** *d.* stretching of the rectus abdominis muscle, a common condition associated with pregnancy or obesity.

divaricator (dy-va-ri-kay-ter) *n.* **1.** a scissor-like surgical instrument used to divide portions of tissue into two separate parts during an operation. **2.** a form of retractor used to open out the sides of an abdominal incision and facilitate access.

divergence (dy-**ver**-jĕns) *n.* (in ophthalmology) movement of the eyes away from the midline. **d. excess** a type of divergent strabismus in which the eyes are deviated outwards more when looking in the distance than for near vision. **d. insufficiency** a type of convergent strabismus in which the eyes are deviated slightly inwards only when looking in the distance.

diverticular disease (dy-ver-tik-yoo-ler) *n.* a condition in which there are diverticula (*see* diverticulum) in the colon associated with lower abdominal pain and disturbed bowel habit. The pain is due to spasm of the muscle of the intestine and not to inflammation of the diverticula (*compare* diverticulitis).

diverticulitis (dy-ver-tik-yoo-**ly**-tis) *n.* inflammation of a diverticulum, most commonly of one or more colonic diverticula. This type of diverticulitis is caused by infection and causes lower abdominal pain with diarrhoea or constipation. A Meckel's diverticulum may sometimes become inflamed due to infection, causing symptoms similar to appendicitis. *Compare* diverticular disease.

diverticulosis (dy-ver-tik-yoo-**loh**-sis) *n.* a condition in which diverticula exist in a segment of the in-

testine without evidence of inflammation (*compare* diverticulitis).

diverticulum (dy-ver-**tik**-yoo-lŭm) *n.* (*pl.* **diverticula**) a sac or pouch formed at weak points in the walls of the alimentary tract. **colonic d.** a diverticulum that affects the colon. They are sometimes associated with abdominal pain or altered bowel habit (*see* diverticular disease, diverticulitis). **jejunal d.** a diverticulum that affects the small intestine. They are often multiple and may give rise to abdominal discomfort and malabsorption. **Meckel's d.** a diverticulum that occurs in the ileum as a congenital abnormality. It may become inflamed, mimicking appendicitis, or it may form a peptic ulcer, causing pain, bleeding, or perforation.

division (di-**vizh**-ŏn) *n.* the separation of an organ or tissue into parts by surgery.

dizygotic twins (dy-zy got-ik) *pl. n. see* twins.

DKA *n. see* (diabetic) ketoacidosis.

DLE *n. see* (discoid) lupus erythematosus.

DM *n. see* diabetes (mellitus).

DMD *n.* Duchenne muscular dystrophy: *see* muscular dystrophy.

DMSA *n.* dimercaptosuccinic acid, which when labelled with technetium-99m is used as a tracer to obtain scintigrams of the kidney, by means of a gamma camera, particularly to show scarring resulting from infection and to assess the relative quantity of functioning tissue in each kidney.

DNA (deoxyribonucleic acid) *n.* the genetic material of nearly all living organisms, which controls heredity and is located in the cell nucleus (*see* chromosome, gene). DNA is a nucleic acid composed of two strands made up of units called nucleotides, wound around each other into a double helix. The DNA molecule can make exact copies of itself by the process of replication, thereby passing on the genetic information to the daughter cells when the cell divides.

DNAse *n.* an enzyme that catalyses the cleavage of DNA. A genetically engineered form, recombinant human DNAse (*dornase alfa*), is administered by inhalation in the treatment of cystic fibrosis to reduce the viscosity of the sticky secretions in the lungs. Trade name: **Pulmozyme.**

dobutamine (doh-bew-tă-meen) *n.* a sympathomimetic drug used to assist in the management of heart failure. It increases the force of contraction of the ventricles and improves the heart output and it may be given by continuous intravenous drip. Trade names: **Dobutrex, Posiject.**

docetaxel (dos-i-taks-ĕl) *n.* a cytotoxic anticancer drug (*see* taxane) administered by intravenous infusion for the treatment of advanced breast cancer and non-small-cell lung cancer. Trade name: **Taxotere.**

Doctor (dok-ter) *n.* **1.** the title given to a recipient of a higher university degree than a Master's degree, usually a Doctor of Philosophy (PhD or DPhil) degree. The degree Medicinae Doctor (MD) is awarded by some British universities as a research degree to those with a first degree in medicine. **2.** a courtesy title given to a qualified medical

practitioner, i.e. one who has been registered by the General Medical Council.

docusate sodium (dok-yoo-sayt) *n. see* dioctyl sodium sulphosuccinate.

Döderlein's bacillus (ded-er-lynz) *n.* the bacterium *Lactobacillus acidophilus*, occurring normally in the vagina and its secretions. *See* Lactobacillus. [A. S. G. Döderlein (1860–1941), German obstetrician and gynaecologist]

DOH *n. see* Department of Health.

dolich- (dolicho-) *prefix denoting* long.

dolichocephaly (doli-koh-sef-ăli) *n.* the condition of having a relatively long skull, with a cephalic index of 75 or less. —**dolichocephalic** *adj.*

dolor (dol-er) *n.* pain: one of the four classical signs of inflammation in a tissue. *See also* calor, rubor, tumor.

dolorimetry (dol-er-im-itri) *n.* the measurement of pain. *See* algesimeter.

domiciliary midwife (dom-i-sil-yeri) *n. see* community midwife.

domiciliary services *pl. n.* (in Britain) health and social services that are available in the home and are distinguished from hospital-based services.

dominant (dom-i-nănt) *adj.* (in genetics) describing a gene (or its corresponding characteristic) whose effect is shown in the individual whether its allele is the same or different. *autosomal d. see* autosomal (dominant). *Compare* recessive. —**dominant** *n.*

domperidone (dom-pe-ri-dohn) *n.* an antiemetic drug used especially to reduce the nausea and vomiting caused by other drugs (e.g. anti-cancer drugs). It is administered by mouth or suppository. Trade name: **Motilium**.

Donald-Fothergill operation (Fothergill's operation, Manchester operation) (don-ăld *foth*-er-gil) *n*. a surgical operation consisting of anterior colporrhaphy, amputation of the cervix, and colpoperineorrhaphy. It is performed for genital prolapse. [A. Donald (1860–1933) and W. E. Fothergill (1865–1926), British gynaecologists]

donepezil (don-ep-i-zil) *n*. *see* acetylcholinesterase inhibitor.

donor (doh-ner) *n*. a person who makes his own tissues or organs available for use by someone else. For example, a donor may provide blood for transfusion or a kidney for transplantation. *d. insemination see* artificial insemination.

dopa (doh-pă) *n*. dihydroxyphenylalanine: a physiologically important compound that forms an intermediate stage in the synthesis of catecholamines from the essential amino acid tyrosine. The laevorotatory form, levodopa, is administered for the treatment of parkinsonism.

dopamine (doh-pă-meen) *n*. a catecholamine derived from dopa that functions as a neurotransmitter, acting on specific dopamine receptors and also on adrenergic receptors throughout the body; it also stimulates the release of noradrenaline from nerve endings. Dopamine is used as a drug to increase the strength of contraction of the heart in heart failure, shock, severe trauma, and septicaemia. It is administered by injection in carefully controlled dosage.

Doppler ultrasound (dop-ler) *n*. a diagnostic technique utilizing the fact that the frequency of ultrasound waves changes when they are reflected from a moving surface. It is used to study the flow in blood vessels and the movement of such structures as heart valves. The frequency detector may be part of the ultrasound imaging probe, which displays an image of the anatomy on a TV screen. Simultaneously, the Doppler signal from a particular point on the image can be displayed next to the anatomical position using a split screen (*duplex imaging*). Direction and velocity of blood flow can each be allocated to different colours and displayed on a colour monitor over the anatomical image (*colour flow ultrasound imaging*). [C. J. Doppler (1803–53), Austrian physicist]

dornase alfa (dor-nayz) *n*. *see* DNAse.

dors- (dorsi-, dorso-) *prefix denoting* **1**. the back. **2**. dorsal.

dorsal (dor-săl) *adj*. relating to or situated at or close to the back of the body or to the posterior part of an organ.

dorsiflexion (dor-si-flek-shŏn) *n*. backward flexion of the foot or hand or their digits; i.e. bending towards the upper surface.

dorsoventral (dor-soh-ven-trăl) *adj*. (in anatomy) extending from the back (dorsal) surface to the front (ventral) surface.

dorsum (dor-sŭm) *n*. **1**. the back. **2**. the upper or posterior surface of a part of the body.

dorzolamide (dor-zol-ă-myd) *n*. a carbonic anhydrase inhibitor used to reduce intraocular pressure in the treatment of glaucoma. It is administered as eye drops, sometimes in combination with timolol. Trade names: **Cosopt**, **Trusopt**.

dose (dohs) *n.* a carefully measured quantity of a drug that is prescribed by a doctor to be given to a patient at any one time.

dosimeter (doh sim-it-er) *n.* **1.** a device to measure the intensity of a radiation source. **2.** a device to record the amount of radiation received by workers exposed to X-rays or other radiation.

dosimetry (doh-sim-itri) *n.* **1.** the calculation of appropriate radiation doses for treating given conditions, usually cancer in different parts of the body. **2.** the measurement of the dose received by a patient having a diagnostic technique involving ionizing radiation or by a radiation worker in his or her employment.

DOT *n. see* direct observed therapy.

double contrast (dub-ŭl) *n.* a technique usually used in X-ray examinations of the bowel, to enhance the quality of the image. Barium sulphate contrast medium is used to coat the bowel wall; the bowel is then distended with gas.

double vision *n. see* diplopia.

douche (doosh) *n.* a forceful jet of water used for cleaning any part of the body, most commonly the vagina.

Down's syndrome (downz) *n.* a condition resulting from a genetic abnormality in which an extra chromosome is present (there are three no. 21 chromosomes instead of the usual two), giving a total of 47 chromosomes rather than the normal 46. The chances of having a Down's child are higher with increasing maternal age. Affected individuals share certain clinical features, including a characteristic flat facial appearance with slanting eyes (as in the Mongolian races, which gave the former name, *mongolism*, to the condition), broad hands with short fingers and a single crease across the palm, malformed ears, eyes with a speckled iris (*Brushfield spots*), and short stature. Many individuals also have a degree of mental handicap, although the range of ability is wide and some individuals are of normal intelligence. Medical name: **trisomy 21**. [J. L. H. Down (1828–96), British physician]

doxapram (doks-ă-pram) *n.* a drug that stimulates breathing. Administered by mouth or injection, it is used to raise the level of consciousness in comatose patients so that they can be encouraged to cough up bronchial secretions. Trade name: **Dopram**.

doxazosin (doks-az-oh-sin) *n.* an alpha-blocker drug used to treat high blood pressure. It is administered by mouth. Trade name: **Cardura**.

doxepin (doks-ĕ-pin) *n.* a drug administered by mouth to relieve depression, especially when this is associated with anxiety (*see* antidepressant), and applied topically to relieve itching associated with eczema. Trade names: **Sinequan**, **Xepin**.

doxorubicin (doks-oh-roo-bi-sin) *n.* an anthracycline antibiotic isolated from *Streptomyces peucetius caesius* and used mainly in the treatment of leukaemia and various other forms of cancer. It is administered by injection or infusion and can be given as a lipid formulation to transport the drug to its target; side-effects include bone marrow depression, baldness, gastrointestinal disturbances, and heart damage.

doxycycline (doks-i-sy-kleen) *n*. an antibiotic administered by mouth to treat infections caused by a wide range of bacteria and other microorganisms. Trade name: **Vibramycin**.

DPT vaccine *n*. a combined vaccine against diphtheria, whooping cough (pertussis), and tetanus organisms, prepared from their toxoids and other antigens. See Appendix 8.

DR *n*. see (digital) radiography.

dracontiasis (drak-on-ty-ă-sis) *n*. a tropical disease caused by the parasitic nematode *Dracunculus medinensis* (*see* guinea worm). The disease is transmitted to humans via contaminated drinking water. The worm migrates to the skin surface and eventually forms a large blister, usually on the legs or arms, which bursts and may ulcerate and become infected.

Dracunculus (dra-kunk-yoo-lŭs) *n*. see guinea worm.

dragee (dra-zhay) *n*. a pill that has been coated with sugar.

drain (drayn) **1.** *n*. a device, usually a tube or wick, used to draw fluid from an internal body cavity to the surface. Suction can be applied through a tube drain to increase its effectiveness. **2.** *vb*. see drainage.

drainage (drayn-ij) *n*. the drawing off of fluid from a cavity in the body, usually fluid that has accumulated abnormally. *See also* drain.

drastic (dras-tik) *n*. any agent causing a major change in a body function.

draw-sheet (draw-sheet) *n*. a sheet placed beneath a patient in bed that may be pulled under the patient when one portion has been soiled or becomes uncomfortably wrinkled.

drepanocyte (sickle cell) (drep-ă-noh-syt) *n*. see sickle-cell disease.

drepanocytosis (drep-ă-noh-sy-toh-sis) *n*. see sickle-cell disease.

dressing (dres-ing) *n*. material applied to a wound or diseased part of the body, with or without medication, to give protection and assist healing.

drill (dril) *n*. (in dentistry) a rotary instrument used to remove tooth substance, particularly in the treatment of caries.

drip (intravenous drip) (drip) *n*. apparatus for the continuous injection (transfusion) of blood, plasma, saline, glucose solution, or other fluid into a vein. The fluid flows under gravity from a suspended bottle through a tube ending in a hollow needle inserted into the patient's vein. Many infusions are now controlled by electronically regulated infusion pumps.

dropsy (drop-si) *n*. see oedema.

DRS *n*. see Delusions Rating Scale.

drug (drug) *n*. any substance that affects the structure or functioning of a living organism. Drugs are widely used for the prevention, diagnosis, and treatment of disease and for the relief of symptoms.

drug dependence *n*. see dependence.

drusen (macular drusen) (droo-sĕn) *pl. n*. white or yellow deposits of hyalin in Bruch's membrane of the choroid. They are often associated with macular degeneration.

dry mouth (dry) *n.* a condition that occurs as a result of reduced salivary flow from a variety of causes, including Sjögren's syndrome, connective-tissue disease, diabetes, excision or absence of a major salivary gland, or radiotherapy to the head that destroys the salivary glands. Medical name: **xerostomia**.

DSH *n.* deliberate self-harm. *See* (attempted) suicide, parasuicide.

DTPA *n.* diethylenetriaminepentaacetic acid, which when labelled with technetium-99m is used as a tracer to obtain scintigrams of the kidney over a period of time, by means of a gamma camera, to show function and reflux.

DU *n. see* duodenal ulcer.

Duchenne muscular dystrophy (DMD) (dew-shen) *n. see* muscular dystrophy. [G. B. A. Duchenne (1806–75), French neurologist]

Ducrey's bacillus (doo-krayz) *n.* the bacterium *Haemophilus ducreyi*. *See* Haemophilus. [A. Ducrey (1860–1940), Italian dermatologist]

duct (dukt) *n.* a tubelike structure or channel, especially one for carrying glandular secretions.

ductal carcinoma in situ (DCIS) (duk-t'l) *n. see* carcinoma in situ.

ductless gland (dukt-lis) *n. see* endocrine gland.

ductule (duk-tewl) *n.* a small duct or channel.

ductus arteriosus (duk-tŭs arteer-i-oh-sŭs) *n.* a blood vessel in the fetus connecting the pulmonary artery directly to the ascending aorta, so bypassing the pulmonary circulation. It normally closes after birth. *patent d. a.* (*PDA*) failure of the ductus to close, producing a continuous murmur and consequences similar to those of a septal defect.

dumbness (dum-nis) *n. see* mutism.

Dumdum fever (dum-dum) *n. see* kala-azar.

dumping syndrome (dump-ing) *n.* a group of symptoms that sometimes occur after stomach operations, particularly gastrectomy (*postgastrectomy syndrome*). After a meal, especially one rich in carbohydrate, the patient feels faint, weak, and nauseous, has a rapid pulse, and may sweat and become pale.

Duncan disease (dun-kǎn) *n. see* X-linked lymphoproliferative syndrome. [Duncan family, in whom the disease was first studied]

duo- *prefix denoting* two.

duoden- (duodeno-) *prefix denoting* the duo

duodenal ulcer (DU) (dew-ŏ-deen-ǎl) *n.* an ulcer in the duodenum, caused by the action of acid and pepsin on the duodenal lining (mucosa) of a susceptible individual. Symptoms include pain in the upper abdomen and vomiting; complications include bleeding (*see* haematemesis), perforation, and obstruction due to scarring (*see* pyloric stenosis). *See also* Helicobacter.

duodenoscope (dew-ŏ-deen-ŏ-skohp) *n.* a fibreoptic or video instrument for examining the interior of the duodenum. An end-viewing instrument is used for most examinations, but a side-viewing instrument is used for ERCP. The end-viewing instrument is also used for examination of the stomach (*gas-

troduodenoscope) and it is usual to combine the two examinations (*gastroduodenoscopy*).

duodenostomy (dew-ŏ-di-nost-ŏmi) *n.* an operation in which the duodenum is brought through the abdominal wall and opened, usually in order to introduce food. *See also* gastroduodenostomy.

duodenum (dew-ŏ-deen-ŭm) *n.* the first of the three parts of the small intestine. It extends from the pylorus of the stomach to the jejunum. The duodenum receives bile from the gall bladder and pancreatic juice from the pancreas. —**duodenal** *adj.*

duplex imaging (dew-pleks) *n. see* Doppler ultrasound.

Dupuytren's contracture (dew-pwee-trahnz) *n.* a flexion deformity of the fingers (usually the ring and little fingers) caused by contracture of the fascia in the palm and fingers. [Baron G. Dupuytren (1777–1835), French surgeon]

dura (**dura mater, pachymeninx**) (dewr-ă) *n.* the thickest and outermost of the three meninges surrounding the brain and spinal cord. —**dural** *adj.*

DVT *n.* deep vein thrombosis. *See* phlebothrombosis.

dwarfism (dworf-izm) *n.* abnormally short stature. The most common cause is achondroplasia. Dwarfism may also be caused by a deficiency of growth hormone due to a defect in the pituitary gland; a genetic defect in the response to growth hormone; thyroid deficiency (*see* cretinism); such chronic diseases as rickets; renal failure; and intestinal malabsorption.

dydrogesterone (dy-droh-jest-er-ohn) *n.* a synthetic female sex hor-

mone (*see* progestogen) administered by mouth to treat menstrual abnormalities (such as dysmenorrhoea) and infertility and to prevent miscarriage. Trade name: **Duphaston**.

dynamic splintage (dy-nam-ik splint-ij) *n.* a technique that retains the essentials of splinting but allows some controlled movement of the restrained body part.

dynamometer (dy-nă-mom-it-er) *n.* a device for recording the force of a muscular contraction. A small hand-held dynamometer may be used to record the strength of a patient's grip.

-dynia *suffix denoting* pain.

dys- *prefix denoting* difficult, abnormal, or impaired.

dysaesthesiae (dis-iss-theez-i-ee) *pl. n.* the abnormal and sometimes unpleasant sensations felt by a patient with partial damage to sensory nerve fibres when his skin is stimulated. *Compare* paraesthesiae.

dysarthria (dis-arth-riă) *n.* a speech disorder in which the pronunciation is unclear although the language content and meaning are normal.

dysbarism (dis-bar-izm) *n.* any clinical syndrome due to a difference between the atmospheric pressure outside the body and the pressure of air or gas within a body cavity. *See* compressed air illness.

dyschezia (dis-kee-ziă) *n.* a form of constipation resulting from a long period of voluntary suppression of the urge to defecate. The rectum becomes distended with faeces and bowel movements are difficult or painful.

dyschondroplasia (**Ollier's dis-**

ease) (dis-kon-droh-**play**-ziă) *n.* a condition due to faulty ossification of cartilage, resulting in development of many benign cartilaginous tumours (*see* chondroma). The bones involved may become stunted and deformed and there is a risk of developing malignant tumours (*see* chondrosarcoma).

dyschromatopsia (dis-kroh-mă-**top**-siă) *n.* any defect of colour vision.

dyscoria (dis-**kor**-iă) *n.* any abnormality in the shape of the pupil of the eye.

dyscrasia (dis-**kray**-ziă) *n.* an abnormal state of the body or part of the body, especially one due to abnormal development or metabolism.

dysdiadochokinesis (adiadochokinesis) (dis-dy-ad-ŏ-koh-ki-**nee**-sis) *n.* clumsiness in performing rapidly alternating movements. It is a sign of disease of the cerebellum or its intracerebral connections.

dysentery (dis-ĕn-tri) *n.* an infection of the intestinal tract causing severe diarrhoea with blood and mucus. *amoebic d.* (*amoebiasis*) dysentery caused by the protozoan *Entamoeba histolytica*. It is mainly confined to tropical and subtropical countries. *bacillary d.* dysentery caused by bacteria of the genus *Shigella*. Epidemics are common in overcrowded insanitary conditions. *Compare* cholera.

dysfunction (dis-**funk**-shŏn) *n.* impairment or abnormality in the functioning of an organ. —**dysfunctional** (dis-**funk**-shŏn-ăl) *adj.*

dysfunctional uterine bleeding *n. see* menorrhagia.

dysgenesis (dis-**jen**-i-sis) *n.* faulty development.

dysgerminoma (germinoma, gonocytoma) (dis-jer-mi-noh-mă) *n.* a malignant tumour of the ovary, thought to arise from primitive germ cells; it is homologous to the seminoma of the testis. The tumours are very sensitive to radiotherapy.

dysgraphia (dis-**graf**-iă) *n. see* agraphia.

dyshormonogenesis (dis-hor-moh-noh-jen-i-sis) *n.* a group of inherited disorders of thyroid hormone synthesis resulting in low levels of thyroxine and triiodothyronine and high levels of thyroid-stimulating hormone, with consequent goitre formation, resulting in cretinism or milder forms of hypothyroidism.

dyskariosis (dis-ka-ri-**oh**-sis) *n.* the abnormal condition of a cell that has a nucleus showing the features characteristic of the earliest stage of malignancy. It may be seen, for example, in the squamous and columnar epithelial cells of a cervical smear.

dyskinesia (dis-ki-nee-ziă) *n.* a group of involuntary movements, including chorea and dystonia, that appear to be a fragmentation of the normal smoothly controlled limb and facial movements. *tardive d.* dyskinesia of the facial muscles, tongue, and limb muscles, associated with long-term medication with phenothiazines or certain other antipsychotic drugs.

dyslalia (dis-**lay**-liă) *n.* a speech disorder in which the patient uses a vocabulary or range of sounds that is peculiar to him or her.

dyslexia (dis-**leks**-ia) *n.* a developmental disorder selectively affecting a child's ability to learn to read and write. The condition can create serious educational problems. It is sometimes called *specific d.*, *developmental reading disorder*, or *developmental word blindness* to distinguish it from acquired difficulties with reading and writing. *Compare* alexia. —**dyslexic** *adj.*

dyslogia (dis-**loh**-jiă) *n.* disturbed and incoherent speech. This may be due to dementia, aphasia, mental retardation, or mental illness.

dysmenorrhoea (dis-men-ŏ-**ree**-ă) *n.* painful menstruation. *primary* (*spasmodic*) *d.* dysmenorrhoea that begins with the first period and is heralded by cramping lower abdominal pains starting just before or with the menstrual flow and continuing during menstruation. It is often associated with nausea, vomiting, headache, faintness, and symptoms of peripheral vasodilatation. *secondary* (*congestive*) *d.* dysmenorrhoea that usually affects older women who complain of a congested ache with lower abdominal cramps, which usually start from a few days to two weeks before menstruation. Causes include pelvic inflammatory disease, endometriosis, fibroids, and the presence of an IUCD.

dysostosis (dis-oss-**toh**-sis) *n.* the abnormal formation of bone or the formation of bone in abnormal places, such as a replacement of cartilage by bone.

dyspareunia (dis-pă-**roo**-niă) *n.* painful or difficult sexual intercourse experienced by a woman. Psychological or physical factors may be responsible (*see* vaginismus).

dyspepsia (indigestion) (dis-**pep**-siă) *n.* disordered digestion: usually applied to pain or discomfort in the lower chest or abdomen after eating and sometimes accompanied by nausea or vomiting. —**dyspeptic** *adj.*

dysphagia (dis-**fay**-jiă) *n.* a condition in which the action of swallowing is either difficult to perform, painful (*see* odynophagia), or in which swallowed material seems to be held up in its passage to the stomach.

dysphasia (dis-**fay**-ziă) *n. see* aphasia.

dysphemia (dis-**fee**-miă) *n. see* stammering.

dysphonia (dis-**foh**-niă) *n.* difficulty in voice production. This may be due to a disorder of the larynx, pharynx, tongue, or mouth, or it may be psychogenic. *Compare* dysarthria, aphasia.

dysplasia (alloplasia, heteroplasia) (dis-**play**-ziă) *n.* abnormal development of skin, bone, or other tissues. *fibrous d.* dysplasia in which bony tissue is replaced by fibrous tissue, resulting in a tendency to pathological fracture. *See also* bronchopulmonary (dysplasia). —**dysplastic** (dis-**plas**-tik) *adj.*

dyspnoea (disp-**nee**-ă) *n.* laboured or difficult breathing. Dyspnoea can be due to obstruction to the flow of air into and out of the lungs (as in bronchitis and asthma), various diseases affecting the tissue of the lung, or heart disease.

dyspraxia (dis-**praks**-iă) *n. see* apraxia.

dysrhythmia (dis-**rith**-miă) *n.* abnormality in a rhythm, such as the rhythm of speech or of brain waves as recorded on an EEG.

dyssocial personality (dis-soh-shăl) *n. see* antisocial personality disorder.

dyssynergia (asynergia) (dis-sin-**er**-jiă) *n.* lack of coordination, especially clumsily uncoordinated movements found in patients with disease of the cerebellum. **bladder sphincter** *d.* incoordination of micturition due to spinal cord damage in multiple sclerosis.

dysthymic disorder (dis-**th**'y-mik dis-or-der) *n. see* depression.

dystocia (dis-**toh**-siă) *n.* difficult birth. It may be caused by abnormalities in the fetus (*fetal d.*), such as excessive size or malpresentation, or by abnormalities in the mother (*maternal d.*), such as an abnormally small pelvis or failure of the uterine muscles to contract.

dystonia (dis-**toh**-niă) *n.* muscle dysfunction characterized by spasms or abnormal muscle contraction. Forms of dystonia include torticollis, blepharospasm, and writer's cramp. Another form is a postural disorder often associated with disease of the basal ganglia in the brain. —**dystonic** *adj.*

dystrophia adiposogenitalis (dis-**troh**-fiă adi-poh-soh-jen-i-**tahl**-iss) *n. see* Fröhlich's syndrome.

dystrophia myotonica (myotonic dystrophy) (my-ŏ-**ton**-ikă) *n.* a type of muscular dystrophy in which the muscle weakness and wasting is accompanied by an unnatural prolongation of the muscular contraction after any voluntary effort (*see* myotonia). The disease can affect both sexes (as it is inherited as an autosomal dominant character).

dystrophy (dystrophia) (dis-trŏ-fi) *n.* a disorder of an organ or tissue, usually muscle, due to impaired nourishment of the affected part. *See also* Becker muscular dystrophy, Fuchs' endothelial dystrophy, muscular dystrophy.

dysuria (dis-yoor-iă) *n.* difficult or painful urination. This is usually associated with urgency and frequency of urination if it is due to cystitis or urethritis.

Ee

Eagle-Barrett syndrome (ee-gĕl ba-rĕt) *n. see* prune belly syndrome.

ear (eer) *n.* the sense organ concerned with hearing and balance. Sound waves, transmitted from the outside into the external auditory meatus, cause the eardrum (tympanic membrane) to vibrate. The small bones (ossicles) of the middle ear – the malleus, incus, and stapes – transmit the sound vibrations to the fenestra ovalis, which leads to the inner ear (*see* labyrinth). Inside the cochlea the sound vibrations are converted into nerve impulses. Pressure within the ear is released through the Eustachian tube. The semicircular canals, saccule, and utricle – also in the inner ear – are all concerned with balance.

earache (eer-ayk) *n. see* otitis, otalgia.

eardrum (eer-drum) *n. see* tympanic membrane.

earwax (eer-waks) *n. see* cerumen.

EB *n. see* epidermolysis bullosa.

EBM *n.* expressed breast milk.

Ebola virus (i-boh-lă) *n.* a virus re-

Structure of the ear

sponsible for an acute infection in humans with features similar to those of Marburg disease. Transmission is by contact with infected blood and other body fluids. The mortality rate is 53–88%, but intensive treatment (including rehydration) in the early stages of the disease can halt its rapid and usually irreversible progression to haemorrhaging of internal organs.

EBP n. see evidence-based practice.

Ebstein's anomaly (eb-stynz) n. a form of congenital heart disease affecting the right side of the heart: the muscle is unusually thin and the heart valves are abnormal. It can cause breathlessness, failure to thrive, cyanosis, and abnormal heart rhythms. If mild, it may be asymptomatic and life expectancy is normal. If severe, corrective surgery may be necessary. [W. Ebstein (1836–1912), German physician]

eburnation (ee-ber-**nay**-shŏn) n. the wearing down of the cartilage at the articulating surface of a bone, exposing the underlying bone and leading to bone sclerosis. This is an end result of osteoarthritis.

EB virus (EBV) n. see Epstein-Barr virus.

ec- prefix denoting out of or outside.

ecbolic (ek-**bol**-ik) n. an agent, such as oxytocin, that induces childbirth by stimulating contractions of the uterus.

ecchondroma (ek-kon-**droh**-mă) n. (pl. **ecchondromata**) a benign cartilaginous tumour (see chondroma) that protrudes beyond the margins of a bone. Compare enchondroma.

ecchymosis (eki-**moh**-sis) n. a bruise: an initially bluish-black mark on the skin, resulting from the release of blood into the tissues either through injury or through the spontaneous leaking of blood from the vessels.

eccrine (ek-ryn) adj. describing sweat glands that are distributed all over the body. They are densest on the soles of the feet and the palms of the hands. Compare apocrine.

ecdysis (ek-**dy**-sis) n. the act of shedding skin; desquamation.

ECF n. see extracellular (fluid).

ECG n. see electrocardiogram.

echinococciasis (echinococcosis) (i-ky-noh-kŏ-ky-ă-sis) n. see hydatid disease.

Echinococcus (i-ky-nŏ-**kok**-ŭs) n. a genus of small parasitic tapeworms. Adults are found in the intestines of dogs, wolves, or jackals. If the eggs are swallowed by humans, the resulting larvae may cause hydatid disease. Two species causing this condition are E. granulosus and E. multilocularis.

echocardiography (ek-oh-kar-di-**og**-răfi) n. the use of ultrasound waves to investigate and display the action of the heart as it beats. Used in the diagnosis and assessment of congenital and acquired heart diseases, it is safe, painless, and reliable. Doppler e. a technique for calculating blood flow and pressure within the heart and great vessels by observing the reflection of ultrasound from moving red blood cells. M-mode e. a technique using a single beam of ultrasound to produce a nonanatomical image that permits precise measurement of cardiac dimensions. real-time e. a technique using a pulsed array of ultrasound beams to build up a moving image on a TV monitor of the chambers and valves of the heart. *transoesophageal e.* echocardiography in which the ultrasound probe is mounted on an oesophageal endoscope, allowing the probe to be placed directly against the back of the heart, enabling improved visualization of posterior structures.

echoencephalography (ek-oh-en-sef-ă-log-răfi) *n.* investigation of structures within the skull by detecting the echoes of ultrasonic pulses.

echokinesis (ek-oh-ki-nee-sis) *n.* see echopraxia.

echolalia (ek-oh-lay-liă) *n.* pathological repetition of the words spoken by another person. It may be a symptom of language disorders, autism, catatonia, or Gilles de la Tourette syndrome.

echopraxia (echokinesis) (ek-oh-praks-iă) *n.* pathological imitation of the actions of another person. It may be a symptom of catatonia.

echovirus (ek-oh-vy-rŭs) *n.* one of a group of about 30 RNA-containing viruses originally isolated from the human intestinal tract. These viruses were termed *enteric cytopathic human orphan* viruses and are the cause of some neurological disorders. *Compare* reovirus.

ECI *n. see* Experience of Caregiving Inventory.

eclabium (ek-lay-biŭm) *n.* the turning outward of a lip.

eclampsia (i-klamp-siă) *n.* the occurrence, in a woman with preeclampsia, of one or more convulsions not caused by other conditions, such as epilepsy or cerebral haemorrhage. The onset of convulsions may be preceded by a sudden rise in blood pressure and/or a sudden increase in oedema and development of oliguria. The convulsions are usually followed by coma. Eclampsia is a threat to both mother and baby and must be treated immediately.

ecmnesia (ek-nee-ziă) *n.* loss of memory for recent events that does not extend to more remote ones: a common symptom of old age.

ECMO *n. see* extracorporeal (membrane oxygenation).

ECoG *n. see* electrocochleography.

ecology (bionomics) (ee-kol-ŏji) *n.* the study of the relationships between humans, plants and animals, and the environment. —**ecological** *adj.* —**ecologist** *n.*

econazole (ee-kon-ă-zohl) *n.* an antifungal drug used to treat ringworm and candidosis. It is administered as a cream, lotion, spray powder, or vaginal pessary. Trade names: **Ecostatin, Pevaryl.**

écraseur (ay-kra-zer) *n.* a surgical device, resembling a snare, that is used to sever the base of a tumour during its surgical removal.

ecstasy (ek-stă-si) *n.* a sense of extreme well-being and bliss. While not necessarily pathological, it can be caused by epilepsy (especially of the temporal lobe) or by schizophrenia.

Ecstasy *n.* the street name for methylenedioxymethamphetamine (MDMA), a mildly hallucinogenic drug that generates feelings of euphoria in those who take it. Its most common side-effect is hyperthermia; drinking large quantities of water to combat the intense thirst produced by taking the drug may result in fatal damage to the body's fluid balance. Its manufacture, sale, use, and possession are illegal.

ECT *n. see* electroconvulsive therapy.

ect- (ecto-) *prefix denoting* outer or external.

ectasia (ectasis) (ek-tay-ziă) *n.* the dilatation of a tube, duct, or hollow organ.

ecthyma (ek-th'y-mă) *n.* an infection of the skin, usually caused by both *Streptococcus pyogenes* and *Staphylococcus aureus*, in which the full thickness of the epidermis is involved (*compare* impetigo). Ecthyma heals slowly and causes scarring.

ectoderm (ek-toh-derm) *n.* the outer of the three germ layers of the early embryo. It gives rise to the nervous system and sense organs, the teeth and lining of the mouth, and the epidermis and its associated structures (hair, nails, etc.). —**ectodermal** *adj.*

ectomorphic (ek-toh-**mor**-fik) *adj.* describing a body type that is relatively thin, with a large skin surface in comparison to weight. —**ectomorph** *n.* —**ectomorphy** *n.*

-ectomy *suffix denoting* surgical removal of a segment or all of an organ or part.

ectoparasite (ek-toh-**pa**-ră-syt) *n.* a parasite that lives on the outer surface of its host. *Compare* endoparasite.

ectopia (ek-toh-piă) *n.* **1.** the misplacement, due either to a congenital defect or injury, of a bodily part. **2.** the occurrence of something in an unnatural location (*see* ectopic

beat, ectopic pregnancy). —**ectopic** (ek-top-ik) *adj.*

ectopic beat (extrasystole) *n.* a heartbeat due to an impulse generated somewhere in the heart outside the sinoatrial node. They may be produced by any heart disease, by nicotine from smoking, or by caffeine from excessive tea or coffee consumption; they are common in normal individuals. *See* arrhythmia.

ectopic pregnancy (extrauterine pregnancy) *n.* the development of a fetus at a site other than in the uterus. The most common type of ectopic pregnancy occurs in Fallopian tubes that become blocked or inflamed (*tubal* or *oviducal pregnancy*). The growth of the fetus may cause the tube to rupture and bleed. In many cases the fetus dies within three months of conception. Medical name: **eccyesis**.

ectro- *prefix denoting* congenital absence.

ectrodactyly (ek-troh-**dak**-ti-li) *n.* congenital absence of all or part of one or more fingers.

ectromelia (ek-troh-**mee**-liă) *n.* congenital absence or gross shortening (aplasia) of the long bones of one or more limbs. *See also* amelia, hemimelia, phocomelia.

ectropion (ek-**troh**-pi-ŏn) *n.* turning out of the eyelid, away from the eyeball.

eczema (eks-imă) *n.* a common itchy skin disease characterized by reddening (erythema) and vesicle formation, which may lead to weeping and crusting. Outside agents do not play a primary role (*compare* dermatitis), but in some contexts the terms 'dermatitis' and 'eczema' are used interchangeably. *atopic e.* eczema that affects up to 20% of the population and is associated with asthma and hay fever. *discoid* (or *nummular*) *e.* a type of eczema that is characterized by coin-shaped lesions and occurs only in adults. *gravitational* (or *stasis*) *e.* eczema associated with poor venous circulation. *seborrhoeic e.* (*seborrhoeic dermatitis*) eczema that involves the scalp, eyelids, nose, and lips and is associated with the presence of *Pityrosporum* yeasts and is especially common in patients with AIDS. *See also* pompholyx. —**eczematous** (eks-em-ă-tŭs) *adj.*

EDD *n.* expected date of delivery.

edentulous (ee-den-choo-lŭs) *adj.* lacking teeth: usually applied to people who have lost some or all of their teeth.

edetate (ee-di-tayt) *n.* a salt of the compound *ethylenediaminetetra-acetic acid* (*EDTA*), used as a chelating agent in the treatment of poisoning. *dicobalt e.* an antidote to cyanide, administered by intravenous injection as soon as possible after poisoning. *sodium calcium e.* a drug used to treat poisoning by heavy metals, such as lead and strontium.

edrophonium (ed-roh-foh-niŭm) *n.* an anticholinesterase drug that is administered by injection in a test for diagnosis of myasthenia gravis.

EDTA (ethylenediaminetetra-acetic acid) *n. see* edetate.

EDV *n. see* end-diastolic volume.

Edwards' syndrome (ed-wădz) *n.* the condition of a baby born with multiple congenital abnormalities, including mental retardation, due to trisomy of chromosome no. 18.

[J. H. Edwards (1928–), British geneticist]

EEG (electroencephalogram) *n. see* electroencephalography.

effector (i-fek-ter) *n.* any structure or agent that brings about activity in a muscle or gland. The term is also used for the muscle or gland itself.

efferent (ef-er-ĕnt) *adj.* **1.** designating nerves or neurones that convey impulses from the brain or spinal cord to muscles, glands, and other effectors. **2.** designating vessels or ducts that drain fluid from an organ or part. *Compare* afferent.

effleurage (ef-ler-*ahzh*) *n.* a form of massage in which the hands are passed continuously and rhythmically over a patient's skin in one direction only, with the aim of increasing blood flow in that direction and aiding the dispersal of any swelling due to oedema.

effort syndrome (ef-ert) *n.* a condition of marked anxiety about the condition of one's heart and circulatory system. This is accompanied by a heightened consciousness of heartbeat and respiration, which in turn is worsened by the anxiety it induces.

effusion (i-few-zhŏn) *n.* **1.** the escape of pus, serum, blood, lymph, or other fluid into a body cavity. **2.** fluid that has escaped into a body cavity.

eformoterol (ef-or-moh-ter-ol) *n. see* formoterol.

egg cell (eg) *n. see* ovum.

ego (eg-oh) *n.* (in psychoanalysis) the part of the mind that develops from a person's experience of the outside world and is most in touch with external realities.

Ehlers-Danlos syndrome (ay-lerz **dan**-los) *n.* any one of a rare group of inherited (autosomal dominant or autosomal recessive) disorders of the connective tissue involving abnormal or deficient collagen. The skin is very elastic but also very fragile: it bruises easily and scars poorly, the scars often being paper-thin. The joints tend to be very mobile (double-jointed) and dislocate easily. In some types the uterus or bowel can rupture or the valves in the heart can be weaker than normal. [E. L. Ehlers (1863–1937), Danish dermatologist; H. A. Danlos (1844–1912), French dermatologist]

Ehrlich's theory (**air**-liks) *n.* an early theory of antibody production, postulating that receptor groups with side chains were carried on cells and combined with antigens. The receptors were then thrown off the cell and became antibodies in the circulation. [P. Ehrlich (1854–1915), German bacteriologist]

EIA *n.* exercise-induced asthma. *See* asthma.

eidetic (I-**det**-ik) *adj. see* imagery.

Eisenmenger reaction (I-zĕn-meng-er) *n.* a condition in which pulmonary hypertension is associated with a septal defect, so that blood flows from the right to the left side of the heart or from the pulmonary artery to the aorta. Oxygen-depleted blood enters the general circulation, which results in cyanosis and polycythaemia. [V. Eisenmenger (1864–1932), German physician]

ejaculation (i-jak-yoo-**lay**-shŏn) *n.* the discharge of semen from the erect penis at the moment of sexual climax (orgasm) in the male.

Ekbom's syndrome (ek-bomz) *n. see* restless legs syndrome. [K. A. Ekbom (1907–77), Swedish neurologist]

elastic cartilage (i-**lasst**-ik) *n. see* cartilage.

elastic tissue *n.* strong extensible flexible connective tissue rich in yellow *elastic fibres*. Elastic tissue is found in the dermis of the skin, in arterial walls, and in the walls of the alveoli of the lungs.

elastin (i-**lasst**-in) *n.* protein forming the major constituent of elastic tissue fibres.

elastography (i-lasst-**og**-răfi) *n.* an ultrasonic imaging technique that displays the elasticity of soft tissues. It has been found useful in demonstrating abnormalities of both muscle and breast tissue.

elation (exaltation) (i-**lay**-shŏn) *n.* a state of cheerful excitement and enthusiasm. Marked elation of mood is a characteristic of mania or hypomania.

elbow (el-boh) *n.* the joint in the arm formed between the ulna and part of the radius and the humerus.

Electra complex (i-**lek**-trǎ) *n.* the unconscious sexual feelings of a girl for her father, accompanied by aggressive feelings for her mother. *Compare* Oedipus complex.

electrocardiogram (ECG) (i-lek-troh-**kar**-di-oh-gram) *n.* a recording of the electrical activity of the heart on a moving paper strip. The ECG tracing is recorded by means of an electrocardiograph (*see* electrocardiography). It aids in the diagnosis of heart disease, which may produce characteristic changes in the ECG.

electrocardiography (i-lek-troh-kar-di-og-răfi) *n.* a technique for recording the electrical activity of the heart. Electrodes connected to the recording apparatus (*electrocardiograph*) are placed on the skin of the four limbs and chest wall; the record itself is called an electrocardiogram (ECG).

electrocardiophonography (i-lek-troh-kar-di-oh-fō-nog-răfi) *n.* a technique for recording heart sounds and murmurs simultaneously with the ECG. The sound is picked up by a microphone placed over the heart. The tracing is a *phonocardiogram*.

electrocautery (i-lek-troh-kaw-ter-i) *n.* the destruction of diseased or unwanted tissue by means of a needle or snare that is electrically heated.

electrocoagulation (i-lek-troh-koh-ag-yoo-lay-shŏn) *n.* the coagulation of tissues by means of a high-frequency electric current concentrated at one point as it passes through them.

electrocochleography (ECoG) (i-lek-troh-kok-li-og-răfi) *n.* a test to measure electrical activity produced within the cochlea in response to a sound stimulus. It is used in the diagnosis of Ménière's disease and other forms of sensorineural deafness.

electroconvulsive therapy (ECT, electroplexy) (i-lek-troh-kŏn-vul-siv) *n.* a treatment for severe depression and occasionally

P wave due to atrial contraction
Q, R, S, and T waves due to ventricular activity

Typical electrocardiograms

for schizophrenia and mania. A convulsion is produced by passing an electric current through the brain; it is modified by giving a muscle relaxant drug and an anaesthetic.

electrode (i-lek-trohd) *n.* any part of an electrical conductor or recording device that is used to apply electric current to a part of the body or collect electrical activity (e.g. from the heart or brain).

electrodesiccation (i-lek-troh-dess-i-**kay**-shŏn) *n. see* fulguration.

electroencephalogram (EEG) (i-lek-troh-en-**sef**-ă-lŏ-gram) *n. see* electroencephalography.

electroencephalography (i-lek-troh-en-sef-ă-**log**-răfi) *n.* the technique for recording the electrical activity from different parts of the brain and converting it into a tracing called an *electroencephalogram* (*EEG*). The machine that records this activity is known as an *encephalograph*. Electroencephalography is mostly used in the diagnosis and management of epilepsy and sleep disorders.

electroglottography (i-lek-troh-glot-og-răfi) *n.* a method of assessing laryngeal function using external recording electrodes.

electrolarynx (i-lek-troh-**la**-rinks) *n.* a battery-powered electrical vibrator that helps people to speak after laryngectomy.

electrolysis (i-lek-**trol**-i-sis) *n.* **1.** the chemical decomposition of a substance (*see* electrolyte) into positively and negatively charged ions (*see* anion, cation) when an electric current is passed through it. **2.** destruction of tissue, especially hair follicles (*see* epilation), by the passage of an electric current.

electrolyte (i-lek-trŏ-lyt) *n.* a solution that produces ions; for example, sodium chloride solution consists of free sodium and free chloride ions. In medical usage electrolyte usually means the ion itself; thus the *serum electrolyte level* is the concentration of separate ions (sodium, potassium, chloride, bicarbonate, etc.) in the circulating blood. *See also* anion, cation.

electromyography (EMG) (i-lek-troh-my-og-răfi) *n.* continuous recording of the electrical activity of a muscle by means of electrodes inserted into the muscle fibres. The tracing is displayed on an oscilloscope.

electron (i-lek-tron) *n.* a negatively charged particle in an atom, one or more of which orbit around the positively charged nucleus of the atom.

electron microscope *n.* a microscope that uses a beam of electrons as a radiation source for viewing the specimen. The resolving power (ability to register fine detail) is a thousand times greater than that of an ordinary light microscope.

electron volt *n.* a unit of energy equal to the increase in the energy of an electron when it passes through a rise in potential of one volt. Symbol: eV.

electrooculography (i-lek-troh-ok-yoo-**log**-răfi) *n.* an electrical method of recording eye movements by means of tiny electrodes attached to the skin at the inner and outer corners of the eye. The recording is an *electrooculogram* (*EOG*).

electroplexy (i-lek-troh-pleks-i) *n. see* electroconvulsive therapy.

electroretinography (i-lek-troh-ret-in-og-răfi) *n.* a method of recording changes in the electrical potential of the retina when it is stimulated by light; the recording is an *electroretinogram* (ERG). One electrode is placed on the eye in a contact lens and the other is usually attached to the back of the head.

electrosurgery (i-lek-troh-**serj**-er-i) *n.* the use of a high-frequency electric current from a fine wire electrode (a diathermy knife) to cut tissue. The ground electrode is a large metal plate. When used correctly, little heat spreads to the surrounding tissues, in contrast to electrocautery.

electrotherapy (i-lek-troh-**th'e**-ră-pi) *n.* the passage of electric currents through the body's tissues to stimulate the functioning of nerves and the muscles that they supply. *See also* faradism, galvanism.

electuary (i-**lek**-tew-er-i) *n.* a pharmaceutical preparation in which the drug is made up into a paste with syrup or honey.

element (**el**-i-měnt) *n.* a substance, such as carbon, nitrogen, or oxygen, that cannot be decomposed into simpler substances. All the atoms of an element have the same number of protons. *See also* isotope, trace element.

elephantiasis (el-i-făn-**ty**-ă-sis) *n.* gross enlargement of the skin and underlying connective tissues caused by obstruction of the lymph vessels. Obstruction is commonly caused by the parasitic filarial worms *Wuchereria bancrofti* and *Brugia malayi*. The parts most commonly affected are the legs but the scrotum, breasts, and vulva may also be involved. *See also* filariasis.

elevator (**el**-i-vay-ter) *n.* **1.** an instrument that is used to raise a depressed broken bone. *periosteal e.* an instrument used in orthopaedics to strip the fibrous tissue (periosteum) covering bone. **2.** a lever-like instrument used to ease a tooth or root out of its socket during extraction.

elimination (i-lim-i-**nay**-shŏn) *n.* (in physiology) the process of excretion of metabolic waste products from the blood by the kidneys and urinary tract.

ELISA *n. see* enzyme-linked immunosorbent assay.

elixir (i-**liks**-er) *n.* a preparation containing alcohol (ethanol) or glycerine, which is used as the vehicle for bitter or nauseous drugs.

elliptocytosis (i-lip-toh-sy-**toh**-sis) *n.* the presence of significant numbers of abnormal elliptical red cells (*elliptocytes*) in the blood.

em- *prefix. see* en-.

emaciation (i-may-si-ay-shŏn) *n.* wasting of the body, caused by such conditions as malnutrition or cancer.

emasculation (i-mas-kew-**lay**-shŏn) *n.* strictly, surgical removal of the penis. The term is often used to mean loss of male characteristics, as a result of castration or emotional stress.

embalming (im-**bahm**-ing) *n.* the preservation of a dead body by the introduction of chemical compounds that delay putrefaction.

embolectomy (em-bŏ-**lek**-tŏmi) *n.* surgical removal of an embolus in order to relieve arterial obstruction.

embolism (em-bŏl-izm) *n.* the condition in which an embolus becomes lodged in an artery and obstructs its blood flow. Treatment is by anticoagulant therapy; major embolism is treated by embolectomy or strep-tokinase. *pulmonary e.* obstruction of the pulmonary artery by an embolus, usually a blood clot derived from phlebothrombosis of the leg veins. Large emboli result in acute heart failure. *systemic e.* embolism affecting any artery except the pulmonary artery. The embolus is often a blood clot formed in the heart in mitral valve disease or following myocardial infarction. *See also* air embolism.

embolization (therapeutic embolization) (em-bol-I-**zay**-shŏn) *n.* the introduction of occluding material, such as microspheres, into an artery in order to reduce or obstruct blood flow in such conditions as congenital arteriovenous malformations, angiodysplasia, malignant tumours, or arterial rupture. *bilateral uterine arterial e.* embolization

of the uterine artery for the treatment of postpartum haemorrhage and fibroids and to terminate abdominal and cervical pregnancies.

embolus (em-bŏ-lŭs) *n.* (*pl.* **emboli**) material, such as a blood clot, fat, air, amniotic fluid, or a foreign body, that is carried by the blood from one point in the circulation to lodge at another point (*see* embolism).

embrocation (em-broh-**kay**-shŏn) *n.* a lotion that is rubbed onto the body for the treatment of sprains and strains.

embryo (em-bri-oh) *n.* an animal at an early stage of development, before birth (see illustration). In humans the term refers to the products of conception within the uterus up to the eighth week of development, during which time all the main or-

A developing embryo

gans are formed. *Compare* fetus.
—**embryonic** (em-bri-on-ik) *adj.*

embryology (em-bri-ol-ŏji) *n.* the study of growth and development of the embryo and fetus from fertilization of the ovum until birth. —**embryological** *adj.*

embryoscopy (em-bri-os-kŏpi) *n.* examination of an embryo or fetus during the first 12 weeks of pregnancy by means of a fibreoptic endoscope inserted through the cervix. Direct visualization of the embryo or fetus permits the diagnosis of malformations.

emesis (em-i-sis) *n. see* vomiting.

emetic (i-met-ik) *n.* an agent that causes vomiting, such as ipecacuanha or common salt.

EMG *n. see* electromyography.

eminence (emin-ĕns) *n.* a projection, often rounded, on an organ or tissue, particularly on a bone.

emissary veins (em-iss-er-i) *pl. n.* a group of veins within the skull that drain blood from the venous sinuses of the dura mater to veins outside the skull.

emission (i-mish-ŏn) *n.* the flow of semen from the erect penis, usually occurring while the subject is asleep (*nocturnal e.*).

EMLA cream (em-lă) *n.* a cream containing a *eutectic* mixture of local anaesthetics. Applied to the skin as a thick coating and left for 90 minutes, it gives a helpful degree of local anaesthesia, allowing blood samples to be taken and facilitating biopsy procedures in young children.

emmetropia (em-i-troh-piă) *n.* the state of refraction of the normal eye, in which parallel light rays are brought to a focus on the retina with the accommodation relaxed. *Compare* ametropia, hypermetropia, myopia.

emollient (i-mol-iĕnt) *n.* an agent that soothes and softens the skin, such as lanolin or liquid paraffin. Emollients are used alone as moisturizers to lessen the need for active drug therapy (such as corticosteroids for eczema) and in skin preparations as a base for more active drugs, such as antibiotics.

emotion (i-moh-shŏn) *n.* a state of arousal that can be experienced as pleasant or unpleasant. Emotions can have three components: for example, fear can involve an unpleasant subjective experience, an increase in physiological measures such as heart rate, and a tendency to flee from the situation provoking the fear.

empathy (em-pă-thi) *n.* the ability to understand the thoughts and emotions of another person.

emphysema (em-fi-see-mă) *n.* air in the tissues. *pulmonary e.* emphysema in which the alveoli of the lungs are enlarged and damaged, which reduces the surface area for the exchange of oxygen and carbon dioxide. Severe emphysema causes breathlessness, which is made worse by infections. *surgical e.* emphysema in which air escapes into surrounding tissues through wounds or surgical incisions, usually into the tissues of the chest and neck from leaks in the lungs or oesophagus. Bacteria may form gas in soft tissues.

empirical (im-pi-ri-kăl) *adj.* describing a system of treatment based on experience or observation, rather than of logic or reason.

empyema (pyothorax) (em-py-ee-mă) *n.* pus in the pleural cavity, usually secondary to infection in the lung or in the space below the diaphragm.

emulsion (i-mul-shŏn) *n.* a preparation in which fine droplets of one liquid (such as oil) are dispersed in another liquid (such as water). In pharmacy medicines are prepared in the form of emulsions to disguise the taste of an oil, which is dispersed in a flavoured liquid.

EN *n.* see enrolled nurse.

en- (em-) *prefix denoting* in; inside.

enalapril (en-al-ă-pril) *n.* a drug administered by mouth for the treatment of high blood pressure (hypertension). It inhibits the action of angiotensin, which results in decreased vasopressor (blood-vessel constricting) activity and decreased aldosterone secretion. Trade name: *Innovace*.

enamel (i-nam-ĕl) *n.* the extremely hard outer covering of the crown of a tooth, which consists of crystalline hydroxyapatite.

enarthrosis (en-arth-roh-sis) *n.* a ball-and-socket joint, e.g. the shoulder joint. Such a joint always involves a long bone, which is thus allowed to move in all planes.

encapsulated (in-kaps-yoo-layt-id) *adj.* (of an organ, tumour, bacterium, etc.) enclosed in a capsule.

encephal- (encephalo-) *prefix denoting* the brain.

encephalin (enkephalin) (en-sef-ă-lin) *n.* a peptide occurring naturally in the brain and having effects resembling those of morphine or other opiates. See also endorphin.

encephalitis (en-sef-ă-ly-tis) *n.* inflammation of the brain. It may be caused by a viral or bacterial infection or it may be part of an allergic response to a systemic viral illness or vaccination (*see* encephalomyelitis). **e. lethargica** a form of viral encephalitis that is marked by headache and drowsiness, progressing to coma (hence its popular name – *sleepy sickness*). It can cause postencephalitic parkinsonism. *See also* Rasmussen's encephalitis.

encephalocele (en-sef-ă-loh-seel) *n.* protrusion of the brain through a defect in the bones of the skull. *See* neural tube defects.

encephalography (en-sef-ă-log-răfi) *n.* any of various techniques for recording the structure of the brain or the activity of the brain cells. *See* echoencephalography, electroencephalography, pneumoencephalography.

encephaloid (en-sef-ă-loid) *adj.* having the appearance of brain tissue.

encephaloma (en-sef-ă-loh-mă) *n.* a brain tumour.

encephalomalacia (en-sef-ă-loh-mă-lay-shiă) *n.* softening of the brain.

encephalomyelitis (en-sef-ă-loh-my-ĕ-ly-tis) *n.* an acute inflammatory disease affecting the brain and spinal cord. **acute disseminated e.** a form of delayed tissue hypersensitivity provoked by a mild infection or vaccination 7–10 days earlier.

encephalomyelopathy (en-sef-ă-loh-my-ĕ-lop-ă-thi) *n.* any condition in which there is widespread disease of the brain and spinal cord.

encephalon (en-sef-ă-lon) *n.* see brain.

encephalopathy (en-sef-ă-lop-ă-thi) *n.* any of various diseases that affect the functioning of the brain. *See also* hepatic (encephalopathy), spongiform encephalopathy, Wernicke's encephalopathy.

enchondroma (en-kon-**droh**-mă) *n.* (*pl.* **enchondromata**) a benign cartilaginous tumour (*see* chondroma) occurring in the growing zone of a bone and not protruding beyond its margins. *Compare* ecchondroma.

encopresis (en-koh-**pree**-sis) *n.* incontinence of faeces. The term is used for faecal soiling in a child who has gained bowel control but passes formed stools in unacceptable places.

encounter group (in-**kown**-ter) *n.* a form of group psychotherapy. The emphasis is on encouraging close relationships between group members and on the expression of feelings.

encysted (en-**sist**-id) *adj.* enclosed in a cyst.

end- (endo-) *prefix denoting* within or inner.

endarterectomy (end-ar-ter-**ek**-tŏmi) *n.* a surgical 're-bore' of an artery that has become obstructed by atheroma with or without a blood clot (thrombus); the former operation is known as *thromboendarterectomy*. The inner part of the wall is removed together with any clot that is present. *carotid e.* endarterectomy of one or more of the carotid arteries.

endarteritis (end-ar-ter-**I**-tis) *n.* chronic inflammation of the inner portion of the wall of an artery, which most often results from late syphilis. Thickening of the wall produces progressive arterial obstruc-

tion and symptoms from reduced blood supply to the affected part.

end artery (end) *n.* the terminal branch of an artery, which does not communicate with other branches.

endaural (end-or-ăl) *adj.* within the ear, especially relating to the external auditory meatus of the outer ear.

end-diastolic volume (EDV) (end-dy-ă-**stol**-ik) *n.* the volume of blood contained by the ventricles at the end of diastole when the chambers are full.

endemic (en-**dem**-ik) *adj.* occurring frequently in a particular region or population: applied to diseases that are generally or constantly found among people in a particular area. *Compare* epidemic, pandemic.

endemic syphilis *n. see* bejel.

endemiology (en-dee-mi-**ol**-ŏji) *n.* the study of endemic disease.

endocarditis (en-doh-kar-**dy**-tis) *n.* inflammation of the endocardium and heart valves. It is most often due to rheumatic fever or bacterial infection (*bacterial e.*). The main features are fever, changing heart murmurs, heart failure, and embolism. *See also* subacute bacterial endocarditis.

endocardium (en-doh-**kar**-diŭm) *n.* a delicate membrane that lines the heart and is continuous with the lining of arteries and veins. —**endocardial** *adj.*

endocervicitis (en-doh-ser-vi-**sy**-tis) *n.* inflammation of the membrane lining the cervix (neck) of the uterus, usually caused by infection. The condition is accompanied by a thick mucoid discharge.

endocervix (en-doh-**ser**-viks) *n.* the

mucous membrane lining the cervix of the uterus.

endochondral (en-doh-**kon**-drǎl) *adj.* within the material of a cartilage.

endocrine gland (ductless gland) (**end**-oh-kryn) *n.* a gland that manufactures one or more hormones and secretes them directly into the bloodstream (and not through a duct to the exterior). Endocrine glands include the pituitary, thyroid, parathyroid, and adrenal glands, the ovary and testis, the placenta, and part of the pancreas.

endocrinology (en-doh-kri-**nol**-ŏji) *n.* the study of the endocrine glands and the hormones they secrete. —**endocrinologist** *n.*

endoderm (**end**-oh-derm) *n.* the inner of the three germ layers of the early embryo, which gives rise to the lining of most of the alimentary canal and its associated glands, the lining of the bronchi and alveoli of the lung, and most of the urinary tract. —**endodermal** (en-doh-**der**-mǎl) *adj.*

endodermal sinus tumour *n.* a rare tumour of fetal remnants of the ovaries or testes.

endogenous (en-**doj**-in-ŭs) *adj.* arising within or derived from the body. *Compare* exogenous.

endolymph (**end**-oh-limf) *n.* the fluid that fills the membranous labyrinth of the ear.

endolysin (en-**dol**-i-sin) *n.* a substance within a cell that has a specific destructive action against bacteria.

endometrial (en-doh-**mee**-tri-ǎl) *adj.* relating to or affecting the lining of the uterus (endometrium). *e.*

ablation an operation to remove the entire endometrium, usually to treat menorrhagia. It is performed under local anaesthetic by means of laser ablation, electrocoagulation, balloon heating methods, microwaves, or cryotherapy. *e. aspiration* the removal, by means of suction, of a sample of endometrial tissue for diagnostic purposes. *e. hyperplasia* an increase in the thickness of the cells of the endometrium, usually due to prolonged exposure to unopposed oestrogen (e.g. from HRT or an oestrogen-secreting tumour). Atypical cells may be present.

endometriosis (en-doh-mee-tri-oh-sis) *n.* the presence of tissue similar to the kind lining the uterus (endometrium) at other sites in the pelvis or, rarely, throughout the body. The condition causes pelvic pain and severe dysmenorrhoea.

endometritis (en-doh-mi-**try**-tis) *n.* inflammation of the endometrium due to acute or chronic infection. It may be caused by foreign bodies, bacteria, viruses, or parasites. Chronic endometritis may be responsible for the contraceptive action of IUCDs.

endometrium (en-doh-**mee**-tri-ŭm) *n.* the mucous membrane lining the uterus. It becomes thicker and more vascular during the latter part of the menstrual cycle and much of it breaks down and is lost in menstruation. If pregnancy becomes established the endometrium becomes the decidua.

endomorphic (en-doh-**mor**-fik) *adj.* describing a body type that is relatively fat, with highly developed viscera and weak muscular and skeletal development. **—endomorph** n. **—endomorphy** n.

endomyocarditis (en-doh-my-oh-kar-**dy**-tis) n. an acute or chronic inflammatory disorder of the muscle and lining membrane of the heart. The principal causes are rheumatic fever and virus infections. There is enlargement of the heart, murmurs, embolism, and frequently arrhythmias.

endomysium (en-doh-**miz**-iŭm) n. the fine connective tissue sheath that surrounds a single muscle fibre.

endoneurium (en-doh-**newr**-iŭm) n. the layer of fibrous tissue that separates individual fibres within a nerve.

endoparasite (en-doh-pa-ră-syt) n. a parasite that lives inside its host, for example in the liver, lungs, gut, or other tissues of the body. Compare ectoparasite.

endophthalmitis (end-off-thal-**my**-tis) n. inflammation, usually due to infection, within the eye.

endoplasmic reticulum (ER) (en-doh-**plaz**-mik) n. a system of membranes present in the cytoplasm of cells. It is the site of manufacture of proteins and lipids and is concerned with the transport of these products within the cell (see also Golgi apparatus).

end organ n. a specialized structure at the end of a peripheral nerve, such as the taste buds in the tongue, acting as a receptor for a particular sensation.

endorphin (en-dor-fin) n. one of a group of peptides that occur naturally in the brain and have pain-relieving properties similar to those of the opiates. See also encephalin.

endoscope (end-oh-skohp) n. any instrument, such as an auriscope or a gastroscope, used to obtain a view of the interior of the body. Most endoscopes consist of a tube with a light at the end and an optical system or a miniature video camera for transmitting an image to the examiner's eye. See also fibrescope. **—endoscopic** (en-doh-**skop**-ik) adj. **—endoscopy** (en-dos-kŏ-pi) n.

endoscopic retrograde cholangiopancreatography n. see ERCP.

endospore (end-oh-spor) n. the resting stage of certain bacteria, particularly species of the genera Bacillus and Clostridium.

endostapler (end-oh-stay-pler) n. a stapling instrument (see staple) used endoscopically for purposes of fixing tissues or joining them together.

endosteum (en-dos-tiŭm) n. the membrane that lines the marrow cavity of a bone.

endothelioma (en-doh-th'ee-ll-ohmă) n. any tumour arising from or resembling endothelium.

endothelium (en-doh-**th'ee**-li-um) n. the single layer of cells that lines the heart, blood vessels, and lymphatic vessels. It is derived from embryonic mesoderm. Compare epithelium. **—endothelial** adj.

endotoxin (en-doh-**toks**-in) n. a poison generally harmful to all body tissues, contained within certain Gram-negative bacteria and released only when the bacterial cell is broken down or dies and disintegrates. Compare exotoxin.

endotracheal (ET) (en-doh-tray-ki-ăl) adj. within or through the trachea. e. tube a tube inserted into the trachea to maintain a patent airway. *See also* intubation.

end-plate (end-playt) *n.* the area of muscle cell membrane immediately beneath the motor nerve ending at a neuromuscular junction.

end-stage renal failure (ESRF) (end-stayj) *n.* the most advanced stage of kidney failure, which is reached when the glomerular filtration rate (GFR) falls to 5 ml/min (normal GFR = 120 ml/min).

end-systolic volume (ESV) (end-sis-tol-ik) *n.* the volume of blood that remains in the ventricles after systole when the heart is fully contracted.

enema (en-im-ă) *n.* (*pl.* **enemata** or **enemas**) a quantity of fluid infused into the rectum through a tube passed into the anus. *barium e.* an enema using barium sulphate, given to demonstrate the large bowel by X-ray. For double contrast, gas is pumped through the tube to distend the large bowel before the radiographs are taken. *evacuant e.* an enema using soap or olive oil to remove faeces. *small-bowel e. see* small bowel. *therapeutic e.* an enema used to insert drugs into the rectum.

enervation (en-er-vay-shŏn) *n.* **1.** weakness; loss of strength. **2.** the surgical removal of a nerve.

engagement (in-gayj-mĕnt) *n.* (in obstetrics) the stage of pregnancy that occurs when the presenting part of the fetus has descended into the mother's pelvis. Engagement of the fetal head occurs when the widest part has passed through the pelvic inlet.

enhanced role (en-hahnst) *n.* (of the nurse) *see* extended role.

enkephalin (en-kef-ă-lin) *n. see* encephalin.

enophthalmos (en-off-thal-mŏs) *n.* a condition in which the eye is abnormally sunken into the socket.

enostosis (en-os-toh-sis) *n.* a benign growth within a bone.

enoximone (en-oks-i-mohn) *n.* an inotropic drug used in heart failure to increase the force and output of the heart. It is administered by injection. Trade name: **Perfan**.

enrolled nurse (EN) (en-rohld) *n.* (in the UK) a nurse who has undergone a two-year programme of nursing education (*see* second-level nurse). Entry to the second-level part of the Register may be in general, mental, or mental handicap nursing in England and Wales. In Scotland and Northern Ireland there is generic training for second-level qualification.

ensiform cartilage (en-si-form) *n. see* xiphoid process.

ENT *n.* ear, nose, and throat. *See* otorhinolaryngology.

Entamoeba (ent-ă-mee-bă) *n.* a genus of widely distributed amoebae. *E. coli* a harmless intestinal parasite. *E. gingivalis* a species found between the teeth; it is associated with periodontal disease and gingivitis. *E. histolytica* a species that invades the intestinal wall, causing amoebic dysentery and ulceration; infection of the liver with this species (amoebic hepatitis) is common in tropical countries.

enter- (entero-) *prefix denoting* the intestine.

enteral (en-ter-ăl) *adj.* of or relating to the intestinal tract. *e. feeding see* nutrition.

enteralgia (en-ter-**al**-jiă) *n. see* colic.

enterectomy (en-ter-**ek**-tŏmi) *n.* surgical removal of part of the intestine.

enteric (en-te-rik) *adj.* relating to or affecting the intestine. *e. fever see* paratyphoid fever, typhoid fever.

enteric-coated *adj.* describing tablets that are coated with a substance that enables them to pass through the stomach to the intestine unchanged.

enteritis (en-ter-**I**-tis) *n.* inflammation of the small intestine, usually causing diarrhoea. *infective e.* enteritis caused by viruses or bacteria. *radiation e.* enteritis caused by X-rays or radioactive isotopes. *See also* Crohn's disease (regional enteritis), gastroenteritis.

enterobiasis (oxyuriasis) (en-ter-oh-by-ă-sis) *n.* a disease, common in children throughout the world, caused by the parasitic nematode *Enterobius vermicularis* (*see* threadworm) in the large intestine. The worms do not cause any serious lesions of the gut wall although, rarely, they may provoke appendicitis. Enterobiasis responds well to treatment with piperazine compounds.

Enterobius (Oxyuris) (en-ter-oh-biŭs) *n. see* threadworm.

enterocele (en-ter-oh-seel) *n.* a hernia of the pouch of Douglas (between the rectum and uterus) into the upper part of the posterior vaginal wall.

enteroclysis (en-ter-oh-**kly**-sis) *n.* small-bowel enema (*see* small bowel).

enterococcus (en-ter-oh-**kok**-ŭs) *n.* any bacterium of the genus *Strep-*

tococcus that inhabits the human intestine.

enterocolitis (en-ter-oh-kŏ-**ly**-tis) *n.* inflammation of the colon and small intestine. *See also* colitis, enteritis, necrotizing enterocolitis.

enterogenous (en-ter-**oj**-i-nŭs) *adj.* borne by or carried in the intestine.

enterokinase (en-ter-oh-**ky**-nayz) *n.* the former name for enteropeptidase.

enterolith (en-ter-oh-lith) *n.* a stone within the intestine. It usually builds up around a gallstone or a swallowed fruit stone.

enteron (en-ter-on) *n.* the intestinal tract.

enteropathy (en-ter-**op**-ă-thi) *n.* disease of the small intestine. *See also* coeliac disease (gluten enteropathy).

enteropeptidase (en-ter-oh pep-ti-dayz) *n.* an enzyme secreted by the glands of the small intestine that acts on trypsinogen to produce trypsin.

enteroptosis (en-ter-op toh-sis) *n.* a condition in which loops of intestine (especially transverse colon) are in a low anatomical position.

enterorrhaphy (en-ter-o-ră-fi) *n.* the surgical procedure of stitching an intestine that has either perforated or been divided during an operation.

enteroscope (en-ter-oh-skohp) *n.* an illuminated optical instrument used to inspect the interior of the small intestine. The image is transmitted through a fibreoptic bundle or by a tiny video-camera. The *push* type is introduced by guidance under direct vision. The *sonde* type has an inflatable balloon that pulls the instrument through the length of the intestine by peristalsis. The enteroscope is useful in diagnosing the cause of haemorrhage of the small intestine or of strictures. —**enteroscopy** (en-ter-os-kŏpi) n.

enterostomy (en-ter-ost-ŏmi) n. an operation in which the small intestine is brought through the abdominal wall and opened (see duodenostomy, jejunostomy, ileostomy) or is joined to the stomach (gastroenterostomy) or to another loop of small intestine (enteroenterostomy).

enterotomy (en-ter-ot-ŏmi) n. surgical incision into the intestine.

enterotoxin (en-ter-oh-toks-in) n. a poisonous substance that has a particularly marked effect upon the gastrointestinal tract, causing vomiting, diarrhoea, and abdominal pain.

enterovirus (en-ter-oh-vy-rŭs) n. any virus that enters the body through the gastrointestinal tract, multiplies there, and then (generally) invades the central nervous system. Enteroviruses include Coxsackie viruses and polioviruses.

enterozoon (en-ter-oh-zoh-on) n. any animal species inhabiting or infecting the gut of another. See also endoparasite.

enthesis (en-th'ee-sis) n. **1.** the site of insertion of tendons and ligaments into bones. **2.** insertion of synthetic inorganic material to replace lost tissue.

enthesopathy (en-theez-op-ă-thi) n. any rheumatic disease resulting in inflammation of entheses. Ankylosing spondylitis, psoriatic arthritis, and Reiter's disease are examples.

entrapment neuropathy (en-trap-mĕnt) n. pain, muscle wasting, and paralysis resulting from pressure on a nerve in conditions in which it is subjected to compression by surrounding structures. See carpal tunnel syndrome.

entropion (en-troh-pi-on) n. inturning of the eyelid towards the eyeball. The lashes may rub against the eye and cause irritation (see trichiasis).

enucleation (i-new-kli-ay-shŏn) n. a surgical operation in which an organ, tumour, or cyst is completely removed. In ophthalmology it is an operation in which the eyeball is removed but the other structures in the socket are left in place prior to fitting an artificial eye.

enuresis (en-yoor-ee-sis) n. the involuntary passing of urine, especially bedwetting by children at night (nocturnal e.). See also incontinence. —**enuretic** (en-yoor-et-ik) adj.

environment (in-vyr-ŏn-mĕnt) n. any or all aspects of the surroundings of an organism, both internal and external, which influence its growth, development, and behaviour.

Environmental Health Officer (EHO) (in-vyr-ŏn-men-tăl) n. a person, employed by a local authority, who has special training in such aspects of environmental health and pollution as housing, sanitation, food, clean air, and water supplies (formerly known as a Public Health Inspector).

environmental hearing aid n. see hearing aid.

enzyme (en-zym) n. a protein that, in small amounts, speeds up the rate of a biological reaction without itself being used up in the reaction (i.e. it acts as a catalyst). Enzymes are essential for the normal functioning and development of the body. Failure in the production or activity of a single enzyme may result in metabolic disorders; such disorders are often inherited and some have serious effects. —**enzymatic** *adj.*

enzyme-linked immunosorbent assay (ELISA) *n.* a sensitive technique for measuring the amount of a substance. An antibody that will bind to the substance is produced; the amount of an easily measured enzyme that then binds to the antibody complex enables accurate measurement.

EOG *n. see* electrooculography.

eonism (ee-ŏ-nizm) *n.* the adoption of female manners and dress by a man. *See* transsexualism, transvestism.

eosin (ee-oh-sin) *n.* a red acidic dye, produced by the reaction of bromine and fluorescein, used to stain biological specimens for microscopical examination.

eosinopenia (ee-oh-sin-oh-**pee**-niă) *n.* a decrease in the number of eosinophils in the blood.

eosinophil (ee-oh-**sin**-ŏ-fil) *n.* a variety of white blood cell distinguished by the presence in its cytoplasm of coarse granules that stain orange-red with Romanowsky stains. Eosinophils are capable of ingesting foreign particles and are involved in allergic responses and host defence against parasites.

eosinophilia (ee-oh-sin-ŏ-**fil**-iă) *n.* an increase in the number of eosinophils in the blood. Eosinophilia occurs in response to certain drugs and in a variety of dis-

eases, including allergies, parasitic infestations, and certain forms of leukaemia.

eparterial (ep-ar-**teer**-iăl) *adj.* situated on or above an artery.

ependyma (ep-**en**-dim-ă) *n.* the extremely thin membrane, composed of cells of the glia (*ependymal cells*), that lines the ventricles of the brain and the choroid plexuses. It is responsible for helping to form cerebrospinal fluid. —**ependymal** *adj.*

ependymoma (ep-en-di-**moh**-mă) *n.* a cerebral tumour derived from the glial ependymal cells. It may obstruct the flow of cerebrospinal fluid, causing a hydrocephalus.

ephebiatrics (i-fee-bi-**at**-riks) *n.* the branch of medicine concerned with the common disorders of children and adolescents. *Compare* paediatrics.

ephedrine (ef-i-drin) *n.* a drug that causes constriction of blood vessels and widening of the bronchial passages (*see* sympathomimetic). It is used mainly as a nasal decongestant, being administered (alone or in combination with other drugs) as nose drops or by mouth.

epi- *prefix denoting* above or upon.

epiblepharon (epi-**blef**-er-on) *n.* an abnormal fold of skin, present from birth, stretching across the eye just above the lashes of the upper eyelid or in front of them in the lower lid. It usually disappears within the first year of life.

epicanthus (epicanthic fold) (epi-**kanth**-ŭs) *n.* a vertical fold of skin from the upper eyelid that covers the inner corner of the eye. It occurs abnormally in certain congenital conditions, e.g. Down's syndrome. —**epicanthal, epicanthic** *adj.*

epicardium (epi-kar-diŭm) *n.* the outermost layer of the heart wall, enveloping the myocardium. It is a serous membrane that forms the inner layer of the serous pericardium. —**epicardial** *adj.*

epicondyle (epi-kon-dyl) *n.* the protuberance above a condyle at the end of an articulating bone.

epicranium (epi-kray-niŭm) *n.* the structures that cover the cranium, i.e. all layers of the scalp.

epicranius (epi-kray-ni-ŭs) *n.* the muscle of the scalp.

epicritic (epi-krit-ik) *adj.* describing or relating to sensory nerve fibres responsible for the fine degrees of sensation, as of temperature and touch. *Compare* protopathic.

epidemic (epi-dem-ik) *n.* a sudden outbreak of infectious disease that spreads rapidly through the population, affecting a large proportion of people. *Compare* endemic, pandemic. —**epidemic** *adj.*

epidemiology (epi-dee-mi-ol-ŏji) *n.* the study of the occurrence, distrib-

ution, and control of infectious and noninfectious diseases in populations, including all forms of disease that relate to the environment and ways of life.

epidermis (epi-der-mis) *n.* the outer layer of the skin, which is divided into four layers (see illustration). The top three layers are continually renewed as cells from the continuously dividing Malpighian layer are gradually pushed outwards and become progressively impregnated with keratin (*see* keratinization). —**epidermal** *adj.*

epidermoid cyst (epi-der-moid) *n. see* sebaceous cyst.

epidermolysis bullosa (EB) (epi-der-mol-i-sis buul-oh-să) *n.* any one of a group of genetically determined disorders characterized by blistering of skin and mucous membranes. In the simple forms the blistering is induced by injury. In the more serious (dystrophic) forms the blistering may occur spontaneously; some of the dystrophic forms of the disease are fatal.

Epidermophyton (epi-der-mof-i-

A section of epidermis

tŏn) *n.* a genus of fungi that grow on the skin, causing tinea (ringworm). *See also* dermatophyte.

epidiascope (epi-dy-ă-skohp) *n.* an apparatus for projecting a greatly magnified image of an object, such as a specimen on a microscope slide, on to a screen.

epididymectomy (epi-did-i-mek-tŏmi) *n.* the surgical removal or excision of the epididymis.

epididymis (epi-did-i-mis) *n.* (*pl.* **epididymides**) a highly convoluted tube, about seven metres long, that connects the testis to the vas deferens. The spermatozoa are moved along the tube and are stored in the lower part until ejaculation. —**epididymal** *adj.*

epididymitis (epi-did-i-my-tis) *n.* inflammation of the epididymis. The usual cause is infection spreading down the vas deferens from the bladder or urethra. The inflammation may spread to the testicle (*epididymo-orchitis*).

epididymovasostomy (epi-did-i-moh-vayz-os-tŏmi) *n.* the operation of connecting the vas deferens to the epididymis to bypass obstruction of the latter. It is performed in an attempt to cure azoospermia caused by this blockage.

epidural (extradural) (epi-dewr-ăl) *adj.* on or over the dura mater. *e. anaesthesia* suppression of sensation in the lower part of the body by injecting a local anaesthetic into the epidural space, which anaesthetizes spinal nerve roots. It is used especially to provide pain relief during childbirth or to reduce the need for deep general anaesthesia. *e. space* the space between the dura mater and

the spinal cord and the vertebral canal.

epigastrium (epi-gas-tri-ŭm) *n.* the upper central region of the abdomen. —**epigastric** *adj.*

epigastrocele (epi-gas-troh-seel) *n.* a hernia through the upper central abdominal wall.

epiglottis (epi-glot-iss) *n.* a thin leaf-shaped flap of cartilage, covered with mucous membrane, that is situated immediately behind the root of the tongue. It covers the entrance to the larynx during swallowing.

epiglottitis (epi-glot-I-tis) *n.* an infection of the epiglottis, which swells and causes obstruction of the upper airways. It usually occurs in children under seven years old, but is much less common since the Hib vaccine was introduced.

epikeratophakia (epi-ke-ră-toh-fay-kiă) *n.* eye surgery to correct errors of refraction in which the curvature of the cornea is altered using donor corneal tissue, which has been frozen and shaped using a lathe to produce a tissue lens that is then sutured onto the cornea.

epilation (epi-lay-shŏn) *n.* the removal of a hair by its roots. This can be done mechanically or by electrolysis; lasers for epilation are now available.

epilepsy (ep-i-lep-si) *n.* any one of a group of disorders of brain function characterized by recurrent attacks that have a sudden onset. Seizures may be generalized or partial. Generalized seizures may take the form of major (*tonic-clonic* or *grand mal*) seizures. The tonic phase begins when the patient falls to the ground unconscious with his muscles in a state of spasm. This is replaced by the convulsive movements of the clonic phase, when the tongue may be bitten and urinary incontinence may occur. Minor or *petit mal* seizures (*absences*) are brief spells of unconsciousness, lasting for a few seconds, during which posture and balance are maintained and the eyes stare blankly. A form of partial idiopathic epilepsy, they seldom appear before the age of three or after adolescence and often subside spontaneously in adult life, although they may be followed by the onset of major epilepsy. *focal e.* epilepsy caused by structural disease of the brain. *idiopathic e.* epilepsy that is not associated with structural damage to the brain. *Jacksonian e.* focal motor epilepsy in which the convulsive movements may spread from the thumb to the hand, arm, and face. *temporal lobe* (or *psychomotor*) *e.* focal epilepsy caused by disease in the cortex of the temporal lobe or the adjacent parietal lobe of the brain. Its symptoms include hallucinations of smell, taste, sight, and hearing, paroxysmal disorders of memory, and automatism. —**epileptic** (epi-**lep**-tik) *adj.*, *n.*

epileptiform (epi-**lep**-ti-form) *adj.* resembling an epileptic attack.

epileptogenic (epi-lep-toh-**jen**-ik) *adj.* having the capacity to provoke epileptic seizures.

epiloia (epi-**loi**-ă) *n. see* tuberous (sclerosis).

epimenorrhagia (epi-men-ŏ-**ray**-jiă) *n. see* menorrhagia.

epimenorrhoea (epi-men-ŏ-**ree**-ă) *n.* menstruation at shorter intervals than is normal.

epinephrine (epi-**nef**-rin) *n. see* adrenaline.

epineurium (epi-**newr**-iŭm) *n.* the outer sheath of connective tissue that encloses the bundles (fascicles) of fibres that make up a nerve.

epiphenomenon (epi-fin-**om**-inŏn) *n.* an unusual symptom or event that may occur simultaneously with a disease but is not necessarily directly related to it. *Compare* complication.

epiphora (i-**pif**-er-ă) *n.* watering of the eye, in which tears flow onto the cheek. It is due to some abnormality of the tear drainage system: *see* lacrimal (apparatus).

epiphysis (i-**pif**-i-sis) *n.* **1.** the end of a long bone, which is initially separated by cartilage from the shaft (diaphysis) of the bone and develops separately. It eventually fuses with the diaphysis to form a complete bone. **2.** *see* pineal gland. —**epiphyseal** (epi-**fiz**-iăl) *adj.*

epiphysitis (ep-ifi-**sy**-tis) *n.* inflammation of the epiphysis of a long bone.

epiplo- *prefix denoting* the omentum.

epiplocele (i-**pip**-loh-seel) *n.* a hernia that contains omentum.

epiploon (i-**pip**-loh-on) *n. see* omentum.

episclera (epi-**skleer**-ă) *n.* the outermost covering of the sclera of the eye, which provides nutritional support to the sclera.

episcleritis (epi-skleer-**I**-tis) *n.* inflammation of the outermost layer of the sclera of the eyeball, resulting in a red painful eye that is sensitive to light.

episio- *prefix denoting* the vulva.

episiorrhaphy (ep-izi-o-**răfi**) *n.* stitching together the margins of a tear in the tissues around the vaginal opening.

episiotomy (ep-izi-ot-ŏmi) *n.* an incision into the perineum during a difficult birth. The aim is to make delivery easier and to avoid extensive tearing of adjacent tissues.

epispadias (epi-**spay**-di-ăs) *n.* a congenital abnormality in which the opening of the urethra is on the dorsal (upper) surface of the penis. Surgical correction is carried out in infancy.

epistaxis (epi-**staks**-iss) *n.* bleeding from the nose, which may be caused by low-grade bacterial infection of the front of the nose, hypertension, clotting disorders, or tumours of the nose or sinuses.

epithalaxia (epi-thal-**aks**-iă) *n.* loss of layers of epithelial cells from the lining of the intestine.

epithelialization (epi-th'ee-li-ă-ly-zay-shŏn) *n.* the growth of epithelium over the surface of a wound, which marks the final stage of healing.

epithelioma (epi-th'ee-li-**oh**-mă) *n.* a tumour of epithelium: a former name for carcinoma.

epithelium (epi-**theel**-iŭm) *n.* the tissue that covers the external surface of the body and lines hollow structures (except blood and lymphatic vessels). Epithelium may be either *simple*, consisting of a single layer of cells; *stratified*, consisting of several cell layers; or *pseudostratified*, in which the cells appear to be arranged in layers but in fact share a common basement membrane. See illustration. *See also* endothelium, mesothelium. —**epithelial** *adj.*

eponym (ep-ŏ-nim) *n.* a disease,

Stratified squamous epithelium, surface view above and sectional view below

basement membrane
Simple cuboidal epithelium

goblet cell

Ciliated columnar epithelium

basement membrane
Pseudostratified ciliated epithelium

Types of epithelium

structure, or species named after a particular person, usually the person who first discovered or described it. —**eponymous** (i-pon-i-mŭs) *adj*.

epoprostenol (ee-poh-pros-ti-nol) *n*. a prostaglandin drug used immediately before and during renal dialysis to prevent clotting of blood in the shunt. It is administered by intravenous injection.

Epstein-Barr virus (EB virus, EBV) (ep-styn bar) *n*. the virus, belonging to the herpesvirus group, that is the causative agent of glandular fever. It is also implicated in Burkitt's lymphoma, Hodgkin's disease, and hepatitis. [Sir M. A. Epstein (1921–) and Y. M. Barr (1932–), British pathologists]

epulis (ep-yoo-lis) *n*. a swelling on the gum.

equi- *prefix denoting* equality.

equinia (i-kwin-iă) *n*. *see* glanders.

Erb's palsy (erbz) *n*. weakness or paralysis of the shoulder and arm caused by injury to the upper roots of a baby's brachial plexus during birth. The muscles of the shoulder and the flexors of the elbow are paralysed and the arm hangs at the side internally rotated at the shoulder. [W. H. Erb (1840–1921), German neurologist]

ERCP *n*. endoscopic retrograde cholangiopancreatography; a technique in which a catheter is passed through a duodenoscope into the ampulla of Vater of the common bile duct and injected with a radiopaque medium to outline the pancreatic duct and bile ducts radiologically.

erectile (i-rek-tyl) *adj*. capable of causing erection or becoming erect.

The penis is composed largely of erectile tissue.

erection (i-rek-shŏn) *n*. the sexually active state of the penis, which becomes enlarged and rigid (due to the erectile tissue being swollen with blood). The term is also applied to the clitoris.

erepsin (i-rep-sin) *n*. a mixture of protein-digesting enzymes (*see* peptidase) secreted by the intestinal glands. It is part of the succus entericus.

ERG *n*. *see* electroretinography.

erg- (ergo-) *prefix denoting* work or activity.

ergocalciferol (er-goh-kal-sif-er-ol) *n*. *see* vitamin D.

ergograph (er-gŏ-grahf) *n*. an apparatus for recording the work performed by the muscles of the body when undergoing activity.

ergometrine (er-goh-met-reen) *n*. a drug that stimulates contractions of the uterus. It is administered by injection to assist labour and (combined with oxytocin) to control bleeding following incomplete abortion.

ergonomics (er-gŏ-nom-iks) *n*. the study of humans in relation to their work and working surroundings.

ergosterol (er-gos-ter-ol) *n*. a plant sterol that, when irradiated with ultraviolet light, is converted to ergocalciferol (vitamin D$_2$). *See* vitamin D.

ergot (er-got) *n*. a fungus (*Claviceps purpurea*) that grows on rye. It produces several important alkaloids, including ergotamine and ergometrine. *See also* ergotism.

ergotamine (er-got-ă-meen) *n*. a drug that causes constriction of blood vessels and is used to relieve migraine. It is administered by mouth or in suppositories. Trade names: **Cafergot, Migril**.

ergotism (er-gŏ-tizm) *n.* poisoning caused by eating rye infected with the fungus ergot. The chief symptom is gangrene of the fingers and toes, with diarrhoea and vomiting, nausea, and headache.

erogenous (i-roj-in-ŭs) *adj.* describing certain parts of the body, the physical stimulation of which leads to sexual arousal.

erosion (i-roh-zhŏn) *n.* an eating away of surface tissue by physical or chemical processes, including those associated with inflammation. *cervical e.* an abnormal area of epithelium that may develop at the cervix of the uterus due to tissue damage caused at childbirth or by attempts at abortion. *dental e.* loss of surface tooth substance, usually caused by repeated application of acid. It may result from excessive intake of citrus or carbonated drinks or citrus fruits or from regurgitation of acid from the stomach.

erot- (eroto-) *prefix denoting* sexual desire or love.

ERPC *pl. n.* evacuated retained products of conception.

eructation (i-ruk-tay-shŏn) *n.* belching: the sudden raising of gas from the stomach.

eruption (i-rup-shŏn) *n.* **1.** the outbreak of a rash. **2.** (in dentistry) the emergence of a growing tooth from the gum into the mouth.

ERV *n.* see (expiratory) reserve volume.

erysipelas (e-ri-sip-ilăs) *n.* a streptococcal infection of the skin, especially the face, characterized by redness and swelling. The affected areas usually have sharply defined margins, which can differentiate erysipelas from the otherwise similar cellulitis.

erysipeloid (e-ri-sip-i-loid) *n.* an infection of the skin and underlying tissues with the bacterium *Erysipelothrix insidiosa*, developing usually in people handling fish, poultry, or meat. It is normally confined to a finger or hand, which becomes reddened; sometimes systemic illness develops.

erythema (e-ri-theem-ă) *n.* flushing of the skin due to dilatation of the blood capillaries in the dermis. *e. ab igne* a reticular pigmented rash on the lower legs or elsewhere caused by persistent exposure to radiant heat. *e. multiforme* a condition characterized by so-called target lesions that may be recurrent and follow herpes simplex infection. *e. nodosum* a condition characterized by tender bruiselike swellings on the shins. It is often associated with streptococcal infection.

erythr- (erythro-) *prefix denoting* **1.** redness. **2.** erythrocytes.

erythraemia (e-ri-three-miă) *n.* see polycythaemia (vera).

erythrasma (e-ri-thraz-mă) *n.* a chronic skin infection due to the bacterium *Corynebacterium minutissimum*, occurring in such areas as the armpits, where skin surfaces are in contact.

erythroblast (i-rith-roh-blast) *n.* any of a series of nucleated cells (*see* normoblast) that pass through a succession of stages of maturation to form red blood cells (erythrocytes). *See also* erythropoiesis.

erythroblastosis (i-rith-roh-blas-

toh-sis) *n.* the presence in the blood of erythroblasts. *e. foetalis* a severe but rare haemolytic anaemia affecting newborn infants due to destruction of the infant's red blood cells by factors present in the mother's serum. It is usually caused by incompatibility of the rhesus blood groups between mother and infant (*see* rhesus factor).

erythrocyanosis (i-rith-roh-sy-ă-noh-sis) *n.* mottled purplish discoloration on the legs and thighs. The condition is worse in cold weather. Weight loss is the best treatment as it reduces the insulating effect of a thick layer of fat.

erythrocyte (red blood cell, RBC) (i-rith-roh-syt) *n.* a blood cell containing the pigment haemoglobin, the principal function of which is to transport oxygen. There are normally about 5×10^{12} erythrocytes per litre of blood.

erythrocyte sedimentation rate *n. see* ESR.

erythrocytosis (i-rith-roh-sy-toh-sis) *n.* an increase in the number of red blood cells (erythrocytes) in the blood. *See* polycythaemia.

erythroderma (exfoliative dermatitis) (i-rith-roh-der-mă) *n.* abnormal reddening, flaking, and thickening of the skin affecting a wide area of the body.

erythroedema (i-rith-ri-dee-mă) *n. see* pink disease.

erythromycin (i-rith-roh-my-sin) *n.* an antibiotic used to treat infections caused by a wide range of bacteria and other microorganisms. It is administered by mouth or injection or topically. Trade names: **Erymax**, **Erythrocin**.

erythropenia (i-rith-roh-pee-niă)

n. a reduction in the number of red blood cells (erythrocytes) in the blood.

erythroplasia (i-rith-roh-play-ziă) *n.* an abnormal red patch of skin that occurs particularly in the mouth or on the genitalia and is precancerous.

erythropoiesis (i-rith-roh-poi-ee-sis) *n.* the process of red blood cell (erythrocyte) production, which normally occurs in the blood-forming tissue of the bone marrow. *See also* haemopoiesis.

erythropoietin (haemopoietin) (i-rith-roh-**poi**-ĕ-tin) *n.* a hormone secreted by certain cells in the kidney in response to a reduction in the amount of oxygen reaching the tissues. Erythropoietin increases and controls the rate of red cell production (erythropoiesis).

erythropsia (e-ri-throp-siă) *n.* red vision: a symptom sometimes experienced after removal of a cataract and also in snow blindness.

Esbach's albuminometer (ess-bahks) *n.* a graduated glass tube used for measuring the amount of albumin in a specimen of urine. [G. H. Esbach (1843–90), French physician]

eschar (ess-kar) *n.* a scab or slough, as produced by the action of heat or a corrosive substance on living tissue.

Escherichia (esh-er-ik-iă) *n.* a genus of Gram-negative, generally motile, rodlike bacteria that are found in the intestines of humans and many animals. *E. coli* a species that is usually not harmful but some strains of which cause gastrointestinal infections. *E. coli O157* a pathogenic serotype causing colitis, which may give rise to the complications of haemolytic uraemic syndrome or thrombocytopenic purpura.

Esmarch's bandage (ess-marks) *n.* a rubber or elastic bandage that is wound tightly around a limb in order to force blood out from an area in which an operation is to be performed in a blood-free field. [J. F. A. von Esmarch (1823–1908), German surgeon]

esotropia (ess-oh-troh-piǎ) *n.* convergent strabismus: a type of squint.

espundia (mucocutaneous leishmaniasis) (ess-puun-diǎ) *n.* a disease of the skin and mucous membranes caused by the parasitic protozoan *Leishmania braziliensis* (*see* leishmaniasis), occurring in South and Central America.

ESR (erythrocyte sedimentation rate) *n.* the rate at which red blood cells (erythrocytes) settle out of suspension in blood plasma, measured under standardized conditions. The ESR increases in rheumatic diseases, chronic infections, and malignant disease, and thus provides a valuable screening test for these conditions.

ESRF *n. see* end-stage renal failure.

essence (ess-ěns) *n.* a solution consisting of an essential oil dissolved in alcohol.

essential (i-sen-shǎl) *adj.* describing a disorder that is not apparently attributable to an outside cause.

essential amino acid *n.* an amino acid that is essential for normal growth and development but cannot be synthesized by the body and must therefore be obtained from protein in the diet. *See* amino acid.

essential fatty acid *n.* one of a group of unsaturated fatty acids that are essential for growth but cannot be synthesized by the body. The essential fatty acids are *linoleic*, *linolenic*, and *arachidonic acids*.

essential oil *n.* a volatile oil derived from an aromatic plant. Essential oils are used in various pharmaceutical preparations. *See also* aromatherapy.

ESV *n. see* end-systolic volume.

ESWL *n.* extracorporeal shock-wave lithotripsy. *See* lithotripsy.

ET *adj. see* endotracheal.

etacrynic acid (ethacrynic acid) (et-ǎ-krin-ik) *n.* a loop diuretic administered by injection to treat fluid retention (oedema), such as that associated with heart failure and kidney and liver disorders. Trade name: **Edecrin**.

ethambutol (eth-am-bew-tol) *n.* a drug administered by mouth in the treatment of tuberculosis, in conjunction with other drugs.

ethanol (ethyl alcohol) (eth ǎ nol) *n. see* alcohol.

ether (ee-ther) *n.* a volatile liquid formerly used as an anaesthetic administered by inhalation. It also has laxative action when administered by mouth.

ethics (eth-iks) *n.* a code of principles governing correct behaviour, which in the nursing profession includes behaviour towards patients and their families, visitors, and colleagues.

ethinylestradiol (eth-i-nyl-ee-strǎ-dy-ol) *n.* a synthetic female sex hormone (*see* oestrogen) mainly used (in combination with a progestogen) in oral contraceptives.

ethmoid bone (eth-moid) *n.* a bone

in the floor of the cranium that contributes to the nasal cavity and orbits. The part of the ethmoid forming the roof of the nasal cavity (the *cribriform plate*) is pierced with the many small holes through which the olfactory nerves pass. *See also* nasal (concha). skull.

ethnology (eth-nol-ŏji) *n.* the study of the different races of mankind, concerned mainly with cultural and social differences between groups and the problems that arise from their particular ways of life. —**ethnic** (eth-nik) *adj.*

ethosuximide (eth-oh-suks-i-myd) *n.* an anticonvulsant drug administered by mouth to control epileptic seizures. Trade names: **Emeside, Zarontin.**

ethyl chloride (chloroethane) *n.* a volatile liquid used chiefly as a local anaesthetic applied topically to the skin before minor surgery. Formula: C_2H_5Cl.

etidronate (et-i-droh-nayt) *n. see* bisphosphonates.

etiology (ee-ti-ol-ŏji) *n. see* aetiology.

etoposide (e-top-oh-syd) *n.* a cytotoxic drug derived from an extract of the mandrake plant. It is administered intravenously or by mouth, primarily in the treatment of bronchial carcinoma, lymphomas, and testicular tumours. Trade name: **Vepesid.**

etynodiol (ethynodiol) (et-I-nohdy-ol) *n.* a synthetic female sex hormone (*see* progestogen) that is used in progestogen-only oral contraceptives. Trade name: **Femulen.**

eu- *prefix denoting* **1.** good, well, or easy. **2.** normal.

EUA *n.* examination under anaesthetic.

eucalyptol (yoo-kă-lip-tol) *n.* a volatile oil that has a mild irritant effect on the mucous membranes of the mouth and digestive system. It is taken as pastilles or inhaled as vapour to relieve catarrh.

eugenics (yoo-jen-iks) *n.* the science that is concerned with the improvement of the human race by means of the principles of genetics.

eumenorrhoea (yoo-men-ŏ-ree-ă) *n.* regular menstruation. This does not necessarily indicate regular ovulation.

eunuch (yoo-nŭk) *n.* a male who has undergone castration.

eupepsia (yoo-pep-siă) *n.* the state of normal or good digestion.

euphoria (yoo-for-iă) *n.* a state of cheerfulness and well-being. A morbid degree of euphoria is characteristic of mania and hypomania. *See also* ecstasy, elation.

euplastic (yoo-plast-ik) *adj.* describing a tissue that heals quickly after injury.

Eustachian tube (pharyngotympanic tube) (yoo-stay-shŏn) *n.* the tube that connects the middle ear to the pharynx. It allows the pressure on the inner side of the eardrum to remain equal to the external pressure. [B. Eustachio (1520–74), Italian anatomist]

euthanasia (yooth-ăn-ay-ziă) *n.* the act of taking life to relieve suffering. *active e.* euthanasia achieved by active steps, usually the administration of a drug. *passive e.* euthanasia achieved by the deliberate withholding of treatment that might prevent death. *voluntary e.* euthanasia produced at the request of the patient.

euthyroid (yoo-th'y-roid) *adj.* having a normally functioning thyroid gland. *Compare* hyperthyroidism, hypothyroidism. —**euthyroidism** *n.*

euthyroid sick syndrome (sick euthyroid syndrome) *n.* a syndrome in which the level of triiodothyronine is markedly reduced, thyroxine is slightly reduced, and thyroid-stimulating hormone is reduced or normal. It is commonly seen in nonthyroidal illness, due to altered metabolism and transport of the thyroid hormones.

evacuation (i-vak-yoo-ay-shŏn) *n.* removal of the contents of a cavity, especially the emptying of the bowels (defecation).

evacuator (i-vak-yoo-ay-ter) *n.* a device for sucking fluid out of a cavity. Evacuators may be used to empty the bladder of unwanted material during such operations as the removal of a calculus or transurethral prostatectomy.

evaluation (i-val-yoo-ay-shŏn) *n.* the final stage of the nursing process, in which the effects of nursing interventions are compared with the goals or objectives set in the care plan. *See* expected outcome.

eventration (ee-ven-tray-shŏn) *n.* **1.** protrusion of the intestines through the abdominal wall. **2.** abnormal elevation of part of the diaphragm due to a congenital weakness.

eversion (i-ver-shŏn) *n.* a turning outward. *e. of the cervix* a condition in which the edges of the neck (cervix) of the uterus turn outward after having been torn during childbirth.

evidence-based practice (EBP) (ev-i-dĕns-bayst) *n.* health care provided on the basis of the effectiveness of interventions in relation to the cost-effectiveness of health outcomes.

evisceration (i-vis-er-ay-shŏn) *n.* **1.** (in surgery) *a.* the removal of part of the viscera. *b.* the protrusion of an organ through a surgical incision. **2.** (in ophthalmology) an operation in which the contents of the eyeball are removed, the empty outer envelope (sclera) being left behind. *Compare* enucleation.

Ewing's tumour (Ewing's sarcoma) (yoo-ingz) *n.* a malignant bone tumour arising in the bone marrow. It usually affects the femur but is liable to spread to other bones and to the lung. It is most common in children and adolescents. [J. Ewing (1866–1943), US pathologist]

ex- (exo-) *prefix denoting* outside or outer.

exacerbation (eks-ass-er-bay-shŏn) *n.* an increase in the severity of a disorder, marked by an increase in the intensity of its symptoms and signs.

exaltation (eg-zawl-tay-shŏn) *n. see* elation.

exanthem (eks-anth-ĕm) *n.* a rash or eruption, such as that occurring in measles. *e. subitum see* roseola (infantum). —**exanthematous** (eks-an-th'em-ătŭs) *adj.*

exchange transfusion (iks-chaynj) *n.* a technique for treating haemolytic disease in newborn infants. Blood is withdrawn from the baby (via the umbilical vein) and replaced by an equal amount of donor blood compatible with the mother's blood.

excimer laser (ek-sy-mer) *n. see* laser.

excise (ek-syz) *vb.* to cut out tissue, an organ, or a tumour from the body. —**excision** (ek-si-zhŏn) *n.*

excitation (eks-i-tay-shŏn) *n.* (in neurophysiology) the triggering of a conducted impulse in the membrane of a muscle cell or nerve fibre.

excoriation (iks-kor-i-ay-shŏn) *n.* the destruction and removal of the surface of the skin or the covering of an organ by scraping, the application of a chemical, or other means.

excrescence (iks-kress-ĕns) *n.* an abnormal outgrowth on the surface of the body, such as a wart.

excreta (iks-kree-tă) *n.* any waste material discharged from the body, especially faeces.

excretion (iks-kree-shŏn) *n.* the removal of the waste products of metabolism from the body, mainly through the action of the kidneys. Excretion also includes the loss of water, salts, etc. through the sweat glands, the loss of carbon dioxide and water vapour from the lungs, and the egestion of faeces.

exemestane (eks-i-mess-tayn) *n. see* aromatase inhibitor.

exenteration (eks-en-ter-ay-shŏn) *n.* (in ophthalmology) an operation in which all the contents of the eye socket (orbit) are removed, leaving only the bony walls intact.

exercise (eks-er-syz) *n.* any activity resulting in physical exertion that is intended to maintain physical fitness, to condition the body, or to correct a physical deformity. Exercises may be done actively by the person or passively by a therapist.

aerobic e. an exercise intended to increase oxygen consumption (as in running) and to benefit the lungs and cardiovascular system. *isometric e.* an exercise in which the muscles contract but there is no movement; this is induced when a limb is made to push against something rigid and is designed to improve muscle tone. *isotonic e.* an exercise in which the muscles contract and there is movement, but the force remains the same; this improves joint mobility and muscle strength.

exfoliation (eks-foh-li-ay-shŏn) *n.* **1.** flaking off of the upper layers of the skin. **2.** separation of a surface epithelium from the underlying tissue. **3.** the natural shedding of primary teeth. —**exfoliative** *adj.*

exhalation (expiration) (eks-hă-lay-shŏn) *n.* the act of breathing air from the lungs out through the mouth and nose.

exhibitionism (eksi-bish-ŏn-izm) *n.* exposure of the genitals to another person, as a sexually deviant act. The word is often broadened to mean public flaunting of any quality of the individual.

exo- *prefix. see* ex-.

exocrine gland (eks-oh-kryn) *n.* a gland that discharges its secretion by means of a duct, which opens onto an epithelial surface. Examples of exocrine glands are the sebaceous and sweat glands. *See also* secretion.

exogenous (eks-soj-in-ŭs) *adj.* originating outside the body or part of the body: applied particularly to substances in the body that are derived from the diet rather than built up by the body's own processes of metabolism. *Compare* endogenous.

exomphalos (ek-som-fă-lŭs) *n.* an umbilical hernia.

exophthalmic goitre (Graves's disease) (eks-off-thal-mik) *n. see* thyrotoxicosis.

exophthalmos (eks-off-thal-mos) *n.* protrusion of the eyeballs in their sockets. This can result from injury or disease of the eyeball or socket but is most commonly associated with overactivity of the thyroid gland (*see* thyrotoxicosis). —**exophthalmic** *adj.*

exostosis (eks-os-toh-sis) *n.* a benign outgrowth of bone with a cap of cartilage, arising from the surface of a bone. *See* osteoma.

exotic (ig-zot-ik) *adj.* describing a disease occurring in a region of the world far from where it might be expected.

exotoxin (eks-oh-toks-in) *n.* a highly potent poison, often harmful to only a limited range of tissues, that is produced by a bacterial cell and secreted into its surrounding medium. Exotoxins are produced by the bacteria causing botulism, diphtheria, and tetanus. *Compare* endotoxin.

exotropia (eks-oh-troh-piă) *n.* divergent strabismus: a type of squint.

expected outcome (iks-pekt-id) *n.* a statement in the care plan of what the nursing intervention is intended to achieve, usually described in terms of the patient's expected behaviour. *See* behavioural objective.

expectorant (iks-pek-ter-ănt) *n.* a drug that enhances the secretion of sputum by the air passages so that it is easier to cough up. Expectorants are used in cough mixtures; they act by increasing the bronchial secre-

tion or make it less viscous (*see* mucolytic).

expectoration (iks-pek-ter-ay-shŏn) *n.* the act of spitting out material brought into the mouth by coughing.

Experience of Caregiving Inventory (ECI) (iks-peer-i-ĕns) *n.* a tool used by mental health nurses and others to assess the burden of caring and the coping among members of a patient's family.

experiential learning (iks-peer-i-en-shăl) *n.* learning by experiencing a situation or a simulated situation, as in role playing, and then reflecting on that experience.

expiration (eks-per-ay-shŏn) *n.* **1.** the act of breathing out air from the lungs: exhalation. **2.** dying.

explant (eks-plahnt) **1.** *n.* live tissue transferred from the body (or any organism) to a suitable artificial medium for culture. **2.** *vb.* to transfer live tissue for culture outside the body. —**explantation** *n.*

exploration (eks-plŏ-ray-shŏn) *n.* (in surgery) an investigative operation on a wound, tissue, or cavity to determine the cause of symptoms. —**exploratory** (iks-plo-ră-ter-i) *adj.*

exposure (iks-poh-zher) *n.* (in behaviour therapy) a method of treating fears and phobias that involves confronting the individual with the feared object or situation, either gradually (*see* desensitization, graded self-exposure) or suddenly (*see* flooding).

expression (iks-presh-ŏn) *n.* **1.** the appearance of the face, reflecting the individual's physical or emotional state. **2.** expulsion by pressing or squeezing, as of milk from the breast after pregnancy or the fetus or placenta from the uterus at childbirth.

expulsive haemorrhage (eks-**pul**-siv) *n.* sudden bleeding from the choroid and retina of the eye, usually during a surgical procedure or trauma. This may force the ocular tissue out of the wound and is potentially one of the most devastating intraoperative complications of ocular surgery.

exsanguination (iks-sang-win-ay-shŏn) *n.* **1.** depriving the body of blood; for example, as a result of an accident causing severe bleeding. **2.** a technique for providing a bloodless field to facilitate certain operative procedures. **3.** the removal of blood from a part (usually a limb) before stopping the inflow of blood (by tourniquet). —**exsanguinate** *vb.*

exsufflation (eks-suf-**lay**-shŏn) *n.* the forcible removal of secretions from the air passages by some form of suction apparatus.

extended role (enhanced role) (iks-**ten**-did) *n.* (of the nurse) activities concerned with patients, either in hospital or the community, that are appropriate for delegation by doctors to nurses. Agreement on the delegated responsibilities is reached locally by consultation between medical and nursing professions.

extension (iks-**ten**-shŏn) *n.* **1.** the act of extending or stretching, especially the muscular movement by which a limb is straightened. **2.** the application of traction to a fractured or dislocated limb in order to restore it to its normal position.

extensor (iks-**ten**-ser) *n.* any muscle that causes the straightening of a limb or other part.

exteriorization (iks-teer-i-er-I-**zay**-shŏn) *n.* a surgical procedure in which an organ is brought from its normal site to the surface of the body, as in colostomy.

exteroceptor (eks-ter-oh-sep-ter) *n.* a sensory nerve, ending in the skin or a mucous membrane, that is responsive to stimuli from outside the body. *See also* chemoreceptor, receptor.

extinction (iks-**tink**-shŏn) *n.* (in psychology) the weakening of a conditioned reflex that takes place if it is not maintained by reinforcement.

extirpation (eks-ter-**pay**-shŏn) *n.* the complete surgical removal of tissue, an organ, or a growth.

extra- *prefix denoting* outside or beyond.

extracapsular (eks-tră-**kaps**-yoo-ler) *adj.* outside or not involving a capsule. *e. extraction* surgical removal of a cataract in which the capsule of the lens is left behind. *e. fracture* a fracture, especially of the hip, that does not involve the joint capsule.

extracellular (eks-tră-**sel**-yoo-ler) *adj.* situated or occurring outside cells. *e. fluid* (*ECF*) the fluid surrounding cells.

extracorporeal (eks-tră-kor-**por**-iăl) *adj.* situated or occurring outside the body. *e. circulation* the circulation of the blood outside the body, as through a heart-lung machine or an artificial kidney (*see* haemodialysis). *e. membrane oxygenation* (*ECMO*) a rescue treatment for otherwise fatal respiratory failure in newborn babies or infants due to prematurity or overwhelming septicaemia. It involves prolonged cariopulmonary bypass to support gas exchange.

extract (eks-trakt) *n.* a preparation containing the pharmacologically active principles of a drug, made by evaporating a solution of the drug in water, alcohol, or ether.

extraction (iks-trak-shŏn) *n.* **1.** the surgical removal of a part of the body. Extraction of teeth is usually achieved by applying extraction forceps to the crown or root of the tooth to dislocate it from its socket. **2.** the act of pulling out a baby from the body of its mother during childbirth.

extradural (eks-tră-dewr-ăl) *adj. see* epidural.

extraembryonic membranes (eks-tră-em-bree-on-ik) *pl. n.* the membranous structures that surround the embryo and contribute to the placenta and umbilical cord. They include the amnion, chorion, allantois, and yolk sac.

extrapleural (eks-tră-ploor-ăl) *adj.* relating to the tissues of the chest wall outside the parietal pleura.

extrapyramidal system (eks-tră-pi-ram-i-d'l) *n.* the system of nerve tracts and pathways connecting the cerebral cortex, basal ganglia, thalamus, cerebellum, reticular formation, and spinal neurones in complex circuits not included in the pyramidal system. The extrapyramidal system is mainly concerned with the regulation of stereotyped reflex muscular movements.

extrasystole (eks-tră-sis-tŏ-li) *n. see* ectopic beat.

extrauterine (eks-tră-yoo-teryn) *adj.* outside the uterus.

extravasation (iks-trav-ă-say-shŏn) *n.* the leakage and spread of blood or fluid from vessels into the surrounding tissues, which follows injury, burns, inflammation, and allergy.

extraversion (eks-tră-ver-shŏn) *n. see* extroversion.

extrinsic factor (eks-trin-sik) *n.* an old name for vitamin B$_{12}$.

extrinsic muscle *n.* a muscle, such as any of those controlling movements of the eyeball, that has its origin some distance from the part it acts on.

extroversion (eks-trŏ-ver-shŏn) *n.* **1. (extraversion)** an enduring personality trait characterized by interest in the outside world rather than the self. People high in extroversion (*extroverts*) are gregarious and outgoing, prefer to change activities frequently, and are not susceptible to permanent conditioning. *Compare* introversion. **2.** a turning inside out of a hollow organ, such as the uterus (which sometimes occurs after childbirth).

extrovert (eks-trŏ-vert) *n. see* extroversion.

exudation (eks-yoo-day-shŏn) *n.* the slow escape of liquid (the *exudate*) containing proteins and white cells through the walls of intact blood vessels, usually as a result of inflammation. Exudation is a normal part of the body's defence mechanisms.

eye (I) *n.* the organ of sight: a three-layered roughly spherical structure specialized for receiving and responding to light (see illustration). Light enters the eye through the cornea, which refracts it through the aqueous humour onto the lens. By accommodation light is focused through the vitreous humour onto

conjunctiva

eyelash
iris
lens

aqueous
humour

cornea

suspensory
ligament

ciliary body

sclera

choroid

vitreous humour

blind spot
optic nerve

retina

extrinsic
muscle

The eye (sagittal section)

the retina. Here light-sensitive cells (*see* cone, rod) send nerve impulses to the brain via the optic nerve.

eyeball (I-bawl) *n.* the body of the eye, which is roughly spherical, is bounded by the sclera, and lies in the orbit. Its movements are controlled by three pairs of extrinsic eye muscles.

eyelid (I-lid) *n.* the protective covering of the eye. Each eye has two eyelids consisting of skin, muscle, connective tissue (*tarsus*), and sebaceous glands (*meibomian* or *tarsal glands*). Each eyelid is lined with membrane (*see* conjunctiva) and fringed with eyelashes. Anatomical names: **blepharon**, **palpebra**.

eyestrain (I-strayn) *n.* a sense of fatigue brought on by use of the eyes for prolonged close work or in persons who have an uncorrected error of refraction. Symptoms are usually aching or burning of the eyes, accompanied by headache. Medical name: **asthenopia**.

eye tooth *n. see* canine.

Ff

F 1. *symbol for* Fahrenheit. **2.** *symbol for* farad.

face-lift (fays-lift) *n.* plastic surgery designed to correct sagging facial tissues. Eyelid drooping can be corrected at the same procedure.

facet (fas-it) *n.* a small flat surface on a bone, especially a surface of articulation.

facet syndrome *n.* a syndrome caused by dislocation of the articulating surface of the vertebrae, resulting in pain and muscle spasm.

facial nerve (fay-shǎl) *n.* the seventh cranial nerve (VII): a mixed sensory and motor nerve that supplies the muscles of facial expression, the taste buds of the front part of the tongue, the sublingual salivary glands, and the lacrimal glands.

-facient *suffix denoting* causing or making.

facies (fay-shi-eez) *n.* facial expression, often a guide to a patient's state of health as well as his emotions. **adenoid f.** the vacant look, with the mouth drooping open, seen in adenoids. **Hippocratic f.** the sallow face, sagging and with listless staring eyes, that some read as the expression of approaching death.

Factor V Leiden (ly-děn) *n.* an inherited mutation in the gene coding for coagulation Factor V, which results in an increased susceptibility to develop venous thrombosis.

Factor VIII (antihaemophilic factor, AHF) (fak-ter) *n.* a coagulation factor normally present in blood. Deficiency of the factor, which is inherited by males from their mothers, results in haemophilia A.

Factor IX (Christmas factor) *n.* a coagulation factor normally present in the blood. Deficiency of the factor results in haemophilia B.

Factor XI *n.* a coagulation factor normally present in blood. Deficiency of the factor is inherited, but rarely causes spontaneous bleeding. However, bleeding does occur after surgery or trauma to the blood vessels.

facultative (fak-ŭl-tă-tiv) *adj.* describing an organism, such as a parasite, that is not restricted to one way of life. *Compare* obligate.

faecalith (fee-kă-lith) *n.* a small hard mass of faeces, found particularly in the vermiform appendix: a cause of inflammation.

faeces (fee-seez) *n.* the waste material that is eliminated through the anus. It is formed in the colon and consists of a solid or semisolid mass of undigested food remains (chiefly cellulose) mixed with bile pigments (which are responsible for the colour), bacteria, various secretions (e.g. mucus), and some water. —**faecal** (fee-kǎl) *adj.*

Fahrenheit temperature (fa-rěn-hyt) *n.* temperature expressed on a scale in which the melting point of ice is assigned a temperature of 32° and the boiling point of water a temperature of 212°. The formula for converting from Fahrenheit (F) to Celsius (C) is: C = 5/9(F − 32). *See also* Celsius temperature. [G. D. Fahrenheit (1686–1736), German physicist]

failure to thrive (FTT) (fayl-yer tŏ thryv) *n.* failure of an infant to grow satisfactorily compared with the average for that community. It is detected by regular measurements and plotting on centile charts. It can be the first indication of a serious underlying condition, such as kidney or heart disease or malabsorption, or it may result from problems at home, particularly nonaccidental injury.

fainting (faynt-ing) *n. see* syncope.

Fairbank's splint (fair-banks) *n.* a splint used for the correction of Erb's palsy in infants. It immobilizes the affected arm with the shoulder abducted and externally rotated, the elbow bent at 90°, and the forearm and wrist held in a supine position. [T. J. Fairbank, British orthopaedic surgeon]

falciform ligament (fal-si-form) *n.* a fold of peritoneum separating the right and left lobes of the liver and attaching it to the diaphragm and the anterior abdominal wall as far as the umbilicus.

Fallopian tube (oviduct, uterine tube) (fă-loh-piăn) *n.* either of a pair of tubes that conduct ova from the ovary to the uterus (*see* reproductive system). The ovarian end opens into the abdominal cavity via a funnel-shaped structure with fimbriae surrounding the opening. The ovum is fertilized near the ovar-

ian end of the tube. [G. Fallopius (1523–63), Italian anatomist]

falloposcope (fă-loh-poh-skohp) *n.* a narrow flexible fibreoptic endoscope used to view the inner lining of the Fallopian tubes. —**falloposcopy** *n.*

Fallot's tetralogy (fal-ohz) *n. see* tetralogy of Fallot.

falx (falx cerebri) (falks) *n.* a sickle-shaped fold of the dura mater that dips inwards from the skull in the midline, between the cerebral hemispheres.

familial (fă-mil-iăl) *adj.* describing a condition or character that is found in some families but not in others. It is often inherited. *f. adenomatous polyposis see* polyposis.

family planning (fam-ili) *n.* **1.** the use of contraception to limit or space out the numbers of children born to a couple. **2.** provision of contraceptive methods within a community or nation.

family therapy *n.* a form of psychotherapy in which all family members are seen together in order to clarify and modify the ways they relate together.

famotidine (fam-oh-ti-deen) *n.* an H_2-receptor antagonist (*see* antihistamine) used for the treatment of duodenal ulcers and conditions of excessive gastric acid secretion, such as the Zollinger-Ellison syndrome. It is administered by mouth or intravenously. Trade name: **Pepcid**.

Fanconi's anaemia (fan-koh-niz) *n.* an autosomal recessive disorder characterized by severe aplastic anaemia and an increased predisposition to malignancy. It also causes mental retardation, poor growth, skeletal abnormalities, and kidneys of an unusual shape or in an unusual position. [G. Fanconi (1892–1979), Swiss paediatrician]

Fanconi syndrome *n.* a disorder of the proximal kidney tubules, which may be inherited or acquired and is most common in children. It is characterized by the urinary excretion of large amounts of amino acids, glucose, and phosphates. Symptoms may include osteomalacia, rickets, muscle weakness, and cystinosis. [G. Fanconi]

fantasy (fan-tă-si) *n.* a complex sequence of imagination in which several imaginary elements are woven together into a story. An excessive preoccupation with one's own imaginings may be symptomatic of a difficulty in coping with reality.

farad (fa-răd) *n.* the SI unit of capacitance, equal to the capacitance of a capacitor between the plates of which a potential difference of 1 volt appears when it is charged with 1 coulomb of electricity. Symbol: F.

faradism (fa-ră-dizm) *n.* the use of induced rapidly alternating electric currents to stimulate nerve and muscle activity. *See also* electrotherapy.

farcy (far-si) *n. see* glanders.

farinaceous (fa-ri-nay-shŭs) *adj.* starchy; describing foods rich in starch (e.g. flour, bread, cereals) or diets based on these foods.

farmer's lung (far-merz) *n.* an occupational lung disease caused by allergy to fungal spores that grow in inadequately dried stored hay, straw, or grain, which then becomes mouldy. An acute reversible form can develop a few hours after exposure; a chronic form, with the grad-

ual development of irreversible breathlessness, occurs with or without preceding acute attacks.

FAS *n. see* fetal alcohol syndrome.

fascia (fash-iă) *n.* (*pl.* **fasciae**) connective tissue that envelops organs and tissues, forms sheaths for muscles, and is found immediately beneath the skin.

fasciculation (fă-sik-yoo-lay-shŏn) *n.* brief spontaneous contraction of a few muscle fibres, which is seen as a flicker of movement under the skin. It is most often associated with disease of the lower motor neurones (e.g. motor neurone disease).

fasciculus (fascicle) (fă-sik-yoo-lŭs) *n.* a bundle, e.g. of nerve or muscle fibres.

fasciitis (fash-i-I-tis) *n.* inflammation of fascia. It may result from bacterial infection or from a rheumatic disease, such as Reiter's syndrome or ankylosing spondylitis. *See* necrotizing fasciitis, plantar (fasciitis).

Fasciola (fas-i-oh-lă) *n.* a genus of flukes. *F. hepatica* the liver fluke, which normally lives as a parasite of sheep and other herbivorous animals but sometimes infects humans (*see* fascioliasis).

fascioliasis (fas-i-oh-ly-ă-sis) *n.* an infestation of the bile ducts and liver with the liver fluke, *Fasciola hepatica*. Symptoms include fever, dyspepsia, vomiting, loss of appetite, abdominal pain, and coughing; the liver may also be extensively damaged.

fastigium (fas-tij-iŭm) *n.* the highest point of a fever.

fat (neutral fat) (fat) *n.* a substance that consists chiefly of triglycerides and is the principal form in which energy is stored by the body (see adipose tissue). It also serves as an insulating material beneath the skin and around certain organs. See also brown fat, fatty acid, lipid.

fatal familial insomnia (fay-t'l) *n.* an autosomal dominant disorder due to a mutation in the gene for the prion protein (PrP): it is an example of a spongiform encephalopathy. Patients present with intractable progressive insomnia, disturbances of the autonomic nervous system, and eventually dementia.

fatigue (fă-teeg) *n.* **1.** mental or physical tiredness, following prolonged or intense activity. Muscle fatigue may be due to the waste products of metabolism accumulating in the muscles faster than they can be removed by the venous blood. **2.** the inability of an organism, an organ, or a tissue to give a normal response to a stimulus until a certain recovery period has elapsed.

fatty acid (fat-i) *n.* an organic acid such as oleic acid or stearic acid. Fatty acids are the fundamental constituents of many important lipids, including triglycerides. Some fatty acids can be synthesized by the body; others (see essential fatty acid) must be obtained from the diet. See also fat.

fatty degeneration *n.* deterioration in the health of a tissue due to the deposition of abnormally large amounts of fat in its cells. It may be caused by incorrect diet, excessive alcohol consumption, or a shortage of oxygen in the tissues.

fauces (faw-seez) *n.* the opening leading from the mouth into the pharynx. It is surrounded by the *glossopalatine arch* (which forms the anterior pillars of the fauces) and the *pharyngopalatine arch* (the posterior pillars).

favism (fay-vizm) *n.* an inherited defect in the enzyme glucose-6-phosphate dehydrogenase causing the red blood cells to become sensitive to a chemical in broad beans. It results in destruction of red blood cells (haemolysis), which may lead to severe anaemia, requiring blood transfusion. Favism occurs in parts of the Mediterranean and Iran. See also glucose-6-phosphate dehydrogenase deficiency.

favus (fay-vŭs) *n.* a type of ringworm of the scalp, caused by the fungus *Trichophyton schoenleinii*. Favus, which is rare in Europe, is typified by yellow crusts forming honeycomb-like masses.

FBC *n. see* (full) blood count.

FBS *n. see* (fasting) blood sugar.

fear (feer) *n.* an emotional state evoked by threat of danger. It is usually characterized by unpleasant subjective experiences; physiological changes, such as increased heart rate and sweating; and behavioural changes, such as avoidance of fear-producing objects or situations. See also phobia.

Fear Questionnaire (FQ) *n.* a 16-item questionnaire used to assess anxiety utilizing a Likert scale. It can be self-administered.

febricula (fi-brik-yoo-lă) *n.* a fever of low intensity or short duration.

febrifuge (feb-ri-fewj) *n.* a treatment or drug that reduces or prevents fever. See antipyretic.

febrile (fee-bryl) *adj.* relating to or affected with fever.

feedback (feed-bak) *n.* the coupling of the output of a process to the input. Feedback mechanisms are important in regulating many physiological processes; for example, hormone output and enzyme-mediated reactions. *negative f.* a mechanism in which high levels of a substance (e.g. a circulating hormone) inhibit a further increase in its production (e.g. by reducing production of its releasing factors). *positive f.* a mechanism in which a rise in the output of a substance is associated with an increase in the output of another substance.

Fehling's test (fay-lingz) *n.* a test used for detecting the presence of sugar in urine; it has now been replaced by better and easier methods. [H. von Fehling (1812–85), German chemist]

Felty's syndrome (fel-tiz) *n.* enlargement of the spleen (*see* hypersplenism) associated with rheumatoid arthritis, characterized by a decrease in the numbers of white blood cells and frequent infections. [A. R. Felty (1895–1964), US physician]

feminization (fem-i-ny-zay-shŏn) *n.* the development of female secondary sexual characteristics (enlargement of the breasts, loss of facial hair, and fat beneath the skin) in the male, either as a result of an endocrine disorder or of hormone therapy.

femoral (fem-er-ăl) *adj.* of or relating to the thigh or to the femur. *f. artery* an artery arising from the external iliac artery. It runs down the front medial aspect of the thigh, passing into the back of the thigh two-thirds of the way down. *f. epi-*

physis the growth area of the upper end of the femur; partial dislocation leads to deformity of the head of the bone and premature degeneration of the hip joint. *f. neck* the narrowed end of the femur, which carries the head: the commonest site of fracture of the leg in elderly women. *f. nerve* the nerve that supplies the quadriceps muscle at the front of the thigh and receives sensation from the front and inner sides of the thigh. *f. triangle* (*Scarpa's triangle*) a triangular depression on the inner side of the thigh bounded by the sartorius and adductor longus muscles and the inguinal ligament. The pulse can be felt here as the femoral artery lies over the depression.

femur (thigh bone) (fee-mer) *n.* a long bone between the hip and the knee. The head of the femur articulates with the acetabulum of the hip bone; the lower end articulates with the tibia.

fenbufen (fen-bew-fĕn) *n.* an anti-inflammatory drug (*see* NSAID) used to relieve inflammation and the resulting pain and stiffness. It is administered by mouth. Trade name: **Lederfen**.

fenestra (fi-nes-trä) *n.* (in anatomy) an opening resembling a window. *f. ovalis* (*f. vestibuli*) the opening between the middle ear and the vestibule of the inner ear. *f. rotunda* (*f. cochleae*) the opening between the scala tympani of the cochlea and the middle ear.

fenestration (fen-i-stray-shŏn) *n.* a surgical operation in which a new opening is formed in the bony labyrinth of the inner ear as part of the treatment of deafness due to otosclerosis. It is now rarely performed, having been superseded by stapedectomy.

fenofibrate (fen-oh-**fy**-brayt) *n.* a drug used for treating hyperlipidaemia (*see* fibrate). It is administered by mouth. Trade names: **Lipantril, Supralip**.

fenoprofen (fen-oh-**proh**-fēn) *n.* an analgesic drug that also reduces inflammation (*see* NSAID) and is administered by mouth to treat arthritic conditions. Trade name: **Fenopron**.

fermentation (fer-men-tay-shŏn) *n.* the biochemical process by which organic substances, particularly carbohydrates, are decomposed by the action of enzymes to provide chemical energy, as in the production of alcohol.

ferning (fern-ing) *n.* a test to determine if the amniotic membrane surrounding the fetus has ruptured in late pregnancy. A typical pattern of amniotic fluid crystallization occurs when the amniotic fluid dries.

ferri- (ferro-) *prefix denoting* iron.

ferrous sulphate (fe-rŭs) *n.* an iron salt administered by mouth to treat or prevent iron-deficiency anaemia. Similar preparations used to treat anaemia include *ferrous fumarate* and *ferrous succinate*.

fertility rate (fer-til-iti) *n.* the number of live births occurring in a year per 1000 women of child-bearing age (usually 15 to 44 years of age).

fertilization (fer-ti-ly-**zay**-shŏn) *n.* the fusion of a spermatozoon and an ovum to form a zygote.

FESS *n. see* functional endoscopic sinus surgery.

fester (fes-ter) *vb.* (of superficial wounds) to become inflamed, with the formation of pus.

festination (fes-ti-**nay**-shŏn) *n.* the short tottering steps that characterize the gait of a patient with parkinsonism.

fetal alcohol syndrome (FAS) (fee-t'l) *n.* head and facial abnormalities and possibly mental retardation in a fetus due to intrauterine growth retardation caused by maternal over-consumption of alcohol during pregnancy.

feticide (fee-ti-syd) *n.* the destruction of a fetus in the uterus; for example by injection of a lethal substance into the fetal heart to achieve a late-stage termination of pregnancy.

fetishism (fet-i-shizm) *n.* sexual attraction to an inappropriate object (known as a *fetish*). This may be a part of the body, clothing, or other objects (e.g. leather handbags or rubber sheets). Treatment can involve psychotherapy or behaviour therapy. *See also* sexual deviation.

feto- *prefix denoting* a fetus.

fetor (foetor) (fee-ter) *n.* an unpleasant smell. *f. oris* bad breath (*see* halitosis).

fetoscopy (fi-tos-kŏpi) *n.* inspection of the fetus before birth by passing a special fibreoptic instrument (a *fetoscope*) through the abdomen of a pregnant woman into her uterus. Usually performed in the 18th–20th week of gestation, it allows the inspection of the fetus for visible abnormalities and blood sampling by inserting a hollow needle under direct vision into a placental blood vessel. *See* prenatal diagnosis.

fetus (foetus) (fee-tŭs) *n.* a mammalian embryo during the later stages of development within the uterus; in humans it is an unborn child from its eighth week of development. *f. papyraceous* a twin fetus that has died in the uterus and become flattened and mummified. —**fetal** *adj.*

FEV *n.* see forced expiratory volume.

fever (pyrexia) (fee-ver) *n.* a rise in body temperature above the normal, i.e. above an oral temperature of 98.6°F (37°C) or a rectal temperature of 99°F (37.2°C), usually caused by bacterial or viral infection. Fever is generally accompanied by shivering, headache, nausea, constipation, or diarrhoea. *intermittent f.* a periodic rise and fall in body temperature, as in malaria. *remittent f.* a fever in which body temperature fluctuates but does not return to normal. *See also* relapsing fever.

FFP *n.* fresh frozen plasma.

fibr- (fibro-) *prefix denoting* fibres or fibrous tissue.

fibrate (fy-brayt) *n.* any of a class of drugs that are capable of reducing concentrations of triglycerides and low-density lipoproteins in the blood; they also tend to raise the levels of the beneficial high-density lipoproteins. Fibrates are used for treating hyperlipidaemia. *See* bezafibrate, ciprofibrate, fenofibrate, gemfibrozil.

fibre (fy-ber) *n.* **1.** (in anatomy) a threadlike structure, such as a muscle cell, a nerve fibre, or a collagen fibre. **2.** (in dietetics) *see* dietary fibre. —**fibrous** (fy-brŭs) *adj.*

fibre optics *n.* the use of fibres for the transmission of light images. Synthetic fibres with special optical properties can be used in instruments to relay pictures of the inside of the body for direct observation or photography. *See* fibrescope. —**fibreoptic** *adj.*

fibrescope (fy-ber-skohp) *n.* an endoscope that uses fibre optics for the transmission of images from the interior of the body. Being flexible, fibrescopes can be introduced into relatively inaccessible cavities of the body.

fibril (fy-bril) *n.* a very small fibre or a constituent thread of a fibre. —**fibrillar, fibrillary** *adj.*

fibrillation (fy-bril-ay-shŏn) *n.* a rapid and chaotic beating of the many individual muscle fibres of the heart, which is consequently unable to maintain effective synchronous contraction. The affected part of the heart then ceases to pump blood. *atrial f.* (AF) a common type of arrhythmia that results in rapid and irregular heart and pulse rates. The main causes are atherosclerosis, chronic rheumatic heart disease, and hypertensive heart disease. *ventricular f.* (VF) fibrillation that causes the heart to stop beating (*see* cardiac arrest). It is most commonly the result of myocardial infarction.

fibrin (fib-rin) *n.* the final product of the process of blood coagulation, produced by the action of the enzyme thrombin on a soluble precursor fibrinogen. Fibrin molecules link together to give a fibrous meshwork that forms the basis of a blood clot.

fibrinogen (fi-brin-ŏ-jĕn) *n.* a substance (*see* coagulation factors), present in blood plasma, that is acted upon by the enzyme thrombin to produce the insoluble protein fibrin in the final stage of blood coagulation.

fibrinolysin (fib-ri-**nol**-i-sin) n. see plasmin.

fibrinolysis (fib-ri-**nol**-i-sis) n. the process by which blood clots are removed from the circulation, involving digestion of the insoluble protein fibrin by the enzyme plasmin.

fibrinolytic (fib-rin-ŏ-**lit**-ik) adj. describing a group of drugs that are capable of breaking down the protein fibrin, which is the main constituent of blood clots, and are therefore used to disperse blood clots (thrombi) that have formed within the circulation. They include streptokinase, alteplase, and *reteplase* (Rapilysin).

fibroadenoma (fy-broh-ad-in-oh-ma) n. see adenoma.

fibroblast (fy-broh-blast) n. a widely distributed cell in connective tissue that is responsible for the production of both the ground substance and the precursors of collagen, elastic fibres, and reticular fibres.

fibrocartilage (fy-broh-**kar**-ti-lij) n. a tough kind of cartilage in which there are dense bundles of fibres in the matrix.

fibrochondritis (fy-broh-kon-**dry**-tis) n. an inflammation of fibrocartilage.

fibrocyst (fy-broh-sist) n. a benign tumour of fibrous connective tissue containing cystic spaces. —**fibrocystic** (fy-broh-**sis**-tik) adj.

fibrocystic disease of the pancreas n. see cystic fibrosis.

fibrocyte (fy-broh-syt) n. an inactive cell present in fully differentiated connective tissue. It is derived from a fibroblast.

fibroelastosis (fy-broh-ee-las-**toh**-sis) n. overgrowth or disturbed growth of the yellow (elastic) fibres in connective tissue. *endocardial f.* overgrowth and thickening of the wall of the heart's left ventricle.

fibroid (fy-broid) **1. (fibromyoma, uterine fibroid)** n. a benign tumour of fibrous and muscular tissue, one or more of which may develop in the muscular wall of the uterus. Fibroids often cause pain and excessive menstrual bleeding; in some cases they can be removed surgically. **2.** adj. resembling or containing fibres.

fibroma (fy-broh-mă) n. (pl. **fibromas** or **fibromata**) a nonmalignant tumour of connective tissue.

fibromyalgia (fy-broh-my-**al**-jiă) n. a disorder characterized by pain in the fibrous tissue components of muscles without any inflammation (*compare* fibromyositis). Widespread aching and stiffness are accompanied by extreme fatigue and often associated with headache and various other symptoms. Fibromyalgia is frequently triggered by anxiety, stress, sleep deprivation, and straining or overuse of muscles; it appears to be closely related to CFS/ME.

fibromyoma (fy-broh-my-**oh**-mă) n. see fibroid.

fibromyositis (fy-broh-my-oh-**sy**-tis) n. general inflammation of fibromuscular tissue.

fibroplasia (fy-broh-**play**-ziă) n. the production of fibrous tissue, occurring normally during the healing of wounds. See also retrolental fibroplasia.

fibrosarcoma (fy-broh-sar-**koh**-mă) n. a malignant tumour of connective tissue, derived from fibroblasts. Fibrosarcomas may arise in

finasteride

soft tissue or bone; they can affect any organ but are most common in the limbs, particularly the leg.

fibrosis (fy-broh-sis) n. thickening and scarring of connective tissue, most often a consequence of inflammation or injury. *pulmonary interstitial f.* thickening and stiffening of the lining of the alveoli causing progressive breathlessness. *See also* cystic fibrosis, retroperitoneal fibrosis.

fibrositis (fy-brŏ-sy-tis) n. inflammation of fibrous connective tissue, especially an acute inflammation of back muscles and their sheaths, causing pain and stiffness.

fibula (fib-yoo-lă) n. the long thin outer bone of the lower leg. The head of the fibula articulates with the tibia just below the knee; the lower end projects laterally and articulates with one side of the talus.

field of vision (feeld) n. *see* visual field.

FIGO staging n. a classification drawn up by the International Fed eration of Gynaecology and Obstetrics to define the extent of spread of cancers of the ovary, uterus, and cervix.

filament (fil-ă-mĕnt) n. a very fine threadlike structure, such as a chain of bacterial cells. —**filamentous** (fil-ă-ment-ŭs) adj.

filaria (fil-air-iă) n. (pl. **filariae**) any of the long threadlike nematode worms that, as adults, are parasites of the connective and lymphatic tissues of humans and capable of causing disease. They include the genera *Brugia*, *Loa*, *Onchocerca*, and *Wuchereria*. *See also* microfilaria. —**filarial** adj.

filariasis (fil-er-I-ă-sis) n. a disease, common in the tropics and subtropics, caused by the presence in the lymph vessels of the filariae *Wuchereria bancrofti* and *Brugia malayi*. The lymph vessels eventually become blocked, causing the surrounding tissues to swell (*see* elephantiasis).

filiform (fil-i-form) adj. shaped like a thread. *f. papillae* threadlike papillae on the tongue.

filipuncture (fil-I-punk-cher) n. the insertion of a fine wire thread into an aneurysm in order to cause clotting of the blood within it.

filling (fil-ing) n. (in dentistry) the operation of inserting a specially prepared substance into a cavity drilled in a tooth, often in the treatment of dental caries.

filtration (fil-tray-shŏn) n. the passage of a liquid through a porous filter in order to separate the solids or suspended particles within it.

filum (fy-lŭm) n. a threadlike structure. *f. terminale* the slender tapering terminal section of the spinal cord.

fimbria (fim-briă) n. (pl. **fimbriae**) a fringe or fringelike process, such as any of the finger-like projections that surround the opening of the ovarian end of the Fallopian tube. —**fimbrial** (fim-bri-ăl) adj.

fimbrial cyst n. a simple cyst of the fimbria of the Fallopian tube.

finasteride (fin-ass-tĕ-ryd) n. a drug that causes shrinkage of the prostate gland. It is administered by mouth both to relieve the symptoms of urinary retention caused by an enlarged gland obstructing the outflow of urine from the bladder and to reduce the risk of urinary retention. Trade name: **Proscar**.

fingerprint (fing-er-print) *n.* the distinctive pattern of minute ridges in the outer horny layer of the skin. Every individual has a unique pattern of loops, whorls, or arches. *See also* dermatoglyphics.

first aid (ferst) *n.* procedures used in an emergency to help a wounded or ill patient before the arrival of a doctor or admission to hospital.

first intention *n. see* intention.

first-level nurse *n.* a person who has completed a programme of nursing education that includes the study of life and nursing sciences, clinical experience for effective practice and direction of nursing care, and preparation for a leadership role. A first-level nurse is responsible for planning, providing, and evaluating nursing care in all settings for the promotion of health, prevention of illness, and care and rehabilitation of the sick, and also for supervising students during their practice experiences. *See* nurse.

fission (fish-ŏn) *n.* a method of asexual reproduction in which the body of a protozoan or bacterium splits into two equal parts (*binary f.*), as in the amoebae, or more than two equal parts (*multiple f.*).

fissure (fish-er) *n.* **1.** (in anatomy) a groove or cleft. **2.** (in pathology) a cleftlike defect in the skin or mucous membrane caused by some disease process. *anal f.* a break in the skin lining the anal canal, usually as a consequence of constipation, causing pain during bowel movements and sometimes bleeding. **3.** (in dentistry) a naturally occurring groove in the enamel on the surface of a tooth, especially a molar. It is a common site of dental caries.

fistula (fiss-tew-lă) *n.* (*pl.* **fistulae**) an abnormal communication between two hollow organs or between a hollow organ and the exterior. Many fistulae are caused by infection or injury, but there are a number of other causes. *anal f.* an opening between the anal canal and the surface of the skin that may develop after an abscess in the rectum has burst (*see* ischiorectal abscess). *arteriovenous f.* a surgical connection between an artery and a vein, usually in a limb, to create arterial and venous access for haemodialysis. *biliary f.* a fistula that may develop as a complication of gall bladder surgery. *gastrocolic f.* a fistula between the colon and the stomach that may result from malignant growth or ulceration. *rectovaginal f.* an opening between the rectum and vagina that occurs as a congenital abnormality. *vesicovaginal f.* an opening between the bladder and the vagina causing urinary incontinence. It may result from damage during surgery, radiation damage following radiotherapy for pelvic malignancy, or prolonged obstructed labour.

fit (fit) *n.* a sudden attack. The term is commonly used specifically for the seizures of epilepsy but it is also used more generally, e.g. a fit of coughing.

fixation (fiks-ay-shŏn) *n.* **1.** (in psychoanalysis) a failure of psychological development, in which traumatic events prevent a child from progressing to the next developmental stage. *See also* psychosexual development. **2.** a procedure for the hardening and preservation of tissues or microorganisms to be examined under a microscope.

fixator (fiks-ay-ter) *n.* an apparatus used to immobilize a fracture. *external f.* a rigid frame that connects pins passed through the skin into the bone above and below a fracture. It is used particularly to treat some open fractures and also for limb lengthening.

flaccid (flak-sid) *adj.* **1.** flabby and lacking in firmness. **2.** characterized by a decrease in muscle tone (e.g. *f. paralysis*). —**flaccidity** (flak-sid-iti) *n.*

flagellate (flaj-ĕl-ayt) *n.* a type of protozoan with one or more flagella projecting from its body surface, by means of which it is able to swim. Some flagellates are parasites of humans. *See* trypanosomiasis, Leishmania, giardiasis, Trichomonas.

flagellum (flă-jel-ŭm) *n.* (pl. **flagella**) a fine long whiplike thread attached to certain types of cell (e.g. spermatozoa and flagellates) Flagella are responsible for the movement of the organisms to which they are attached.

flail chest (flayl) *n.* instability of a segment of the ribcage due to fracture of two or more ribs in two or more places, resulting from trauma. It is often associated with underlying lung trauma or pneumothorax.

flap (flap) *n.* (in surgery) a strip of tissue dissected away from the underlying structures but left attached at one end so that it retains its blood and nerve supply in a pedicle. The flap is then used to repair a defect in another part of the body or to cover the end of a bone in an amputated limb. It is detached from its original site when it has healed into the new one.

flare (flair) *n.* **1.** reddening of the skin that spreads outwards from a focus of infection or irritation in the skin. **2.** the red area surrounding an urticarial weal.

flashback (flash-bak) *n.* vivid involuntary reliving of the perceptual abnormalities experienced during a previous episode of drug intoxication, including hallucinations and derealization.

flat-foot (flat-fuut) *n.* absence of the arching of the foot, so that the sole lies flat upon the ground. It may be present in infancy or be acquired in adult life. Medical name: **pes planus.**

flatulence (flat-yoo-lĕns) *n.* **1.** the expulsion of gas or air from the stomach through the mouth; belching. **2.** a sensation of abdominal distension. —**flatulent** *adj.*

flatus (flay-tŭs) *n.* intestinal gas, composed partly of swallowed air and partly of gas produced by bacterial fermentation of intestinal contents.

flatworm (platyhelminth) (flat-werm) *n.* any of the flat-bodied worms, including the flukes and tapeworms. Both these groups contain many parasites of medical importance.

flav- (flavo-) *prefix denoting* yellow.

flea (flee) *n.* a small wingless bloodsucking insect with a laterally compressed body and long legs adapted for jumping. Adult fleas are temporary parasites on birds and mammals and those species that attack humans (*Pulex, Xenopsylla,* and *Nosopsyllus*) may be important in the transmission of various diseases. Their bites may become a focus of infection.

flecainide (flek-ay-nyd) *n.* a drug used to control irregular heart rhythms. It is administered by mouth or injection. Trade name: **Tambocor**.

flexibilitas cerea (fleks-i-**bil**-i-tas **seer**-iă) *n.* a feature of catatonic patients in which the limbs may be moved passively by another person into positions that are then retained for hours on end. *See* catatonia.

flexion (flek-shŏn) *n.* the bending of a joint so that the bones forming it are brought towards each other. *plantar f.* the bending of the toes (or fingers) downwards, towards the sole (or palm). *See also* dorsiflexion.

Flexner's bacillus (fleks-nerz) *n.* the bacterium *Shigella flexneri*, which causes a form of bacillary dysentery. [S. Flexner (1863–1946), US pathologist]

flexor (fleks-er) *n.* any muscle that causes bending of a limb or other part.

flexure (flek-sher) *n.* a bend in an organ or part, such as the *hepatic* and *splenic flexures* of the colon.

floaters (floh-terz) *pl. n.* opacities in the vitreous humour of the eye, which cast a shadow on the retina and are therefore seen as dark shapes against a bright background in good illumination.

floccillation (flok-si-lay-shŏn) *n.* see carphology.

flocculation (flok-yoo-lay-shŏn) *n.* a reaction in which normally invisible material leaves solution to form a coarse suspension or precipitate. *See also* agglutination.

flooding (flud-ing) *n.* **1.** excessive bleeding from the uterus, as in menorrhagia or miscarriage. **2.** (implosion) (in psychology) a method of treating phobias in which the patient is exposed intensively and at length to the feared object, either in reality or fantasy.

floppy baby syndrome (flop-i) *n. see* amyotonia congenita.

flowmeter (floh-mee-ter) *n.* an instrument for measuring the flow of a liquid or gas. *laser Doppler f.* an instrument for measuring blood flow through tissue (e.g. skin) utilizing a laser beam.

flucloxacillin (floo-kloks-ă-**sil**-in) *n.* a semisynthetic penicillin, readily absorbed when taken by mouth, which is effective against bacteria that produce penicillinase. Trade name: **Floxapen**.

fluconazole (floo-**kon**-ă-zohl) *n.* an antifungal drug used to treat candidosis in any part of the body, externally or internally. It is administered by mouth. Trade name: **Diflucan**.

fluctuation (fluk-tew-**ay**-shŏn) *n.* the characteristic feeling of a wave motion produced in a fluid-filled part of the body by an examiner's fingers. If fluctuation is present when a swelling is examined, this is an indication that there is fluid within.

flucytosine (floo-sy-toh-seen) *n.* an antifungal drug that is effective against systemic infections, including cryptococcosis and candidosis. It is administered by mouth or infusion.

fludrocortisone (floo-droh-**kor**-tiz-ohn) *n.* a synthetic mineralocorticoid (*see* corticosteroid) administered by mouth to treat disorders of the adrenal glands. Trade name: **Florinef**.

fluke (flook) *n.* any of the parasitic flatworms that belong to the group Trematoda. Adult flukes are parasites of humans, occurring in the liver (*Fasciola*), lungs (*see* paragonimiasis), gut (*see* heterophyiasis), and blood vessels (*Schistosoma*) and often cause serious disease.

flumazenil (floo-maz-i-nil) *n.* a benzodiazepine antagonist drug, used in anaesthesia to reverse the effects of benzodiazepines on the nervous system. It is administered by injection. Trade name: **Anexate**.

flunisolide (floo-nis-oh-lyd) *n.* an anti-inflammatory corticosteroid drug used in the prevention and treatment of hay fever. It is administered as a nasal spray. Trade name: **Syntaris**.

flunitrazepam (floo-ni-traz-ĕ-pam) *n.* a benzodiazepine drug used for the short-term treatment of insomnia. It is administered by mouth. Trade name: **Rohypnol**.

fluocinonide (floo-ŏ-sin-oh-nyd) *n.* a synthetic corticosteroid used topically to reduce inflammation. It is applied to the skin as a cream, gel, ointment, or solution. Trade name: **Metosyn**.

fluorescein sodium (floo-er-ess-i-in) *n.* a water-soluble orange dye that glows with a brilliant green colour when blue light is shone on it. A dilute solution is used to detect defects in the surface of the cornea, since it stains areas where the epithelium is not intact. *See* angiography.

fluorescence (floo-er-ess-ĕns) *n.* the emission of light by a material as it absorbs radiation from outside.

The radiation absorbed may be visible or invisible (e.g. ultraviolet rays or X-rays). *See* fluoroscope. —**fluorescent** *adj.*

fluoridation (floo-er-id-ay-shŏn) *n.* the addition of fluoride to drinking water in order to reduce dental caries. Drinking water with a fluoride ion content of one part per million is effective in reducing caries throughout life when given during the years of tooth development. *See also* fluorosis.

fluoride (floo-eryd) *n.* a compound of fluorine. The incorporation of fluoride ions in the enamel of teeth makes them more resistant to dental caries. Fluoride may be applied through fluoridation or topically in toothpaste or by a dentist.

fluoroscope (floo-er-ŏ-skohp) *n.* historically, an instrument by which X-rays were projected through a patient onto a fluorescent screen enabling the resultant image to be viewed directly by the radiologist. However, as this resulted in high radiation doses for the radiologist, for diagnostic purposes the screen has been replaced by an image intensifier and TV monitor. —**fluoroscopy** (floo-er-os-kŏ-pi) *n.*

fluorosis (floo-er-oh-sis) *n.* the effects of high fluoride intake. When the level of fluoride in the water supply is above 2 parts per million the enamel of teeth becomes mottled. At above 8 parts per million, calcification of ligaments occurs. *See also* fluoridation.

fluorouracil (floo-er-oh-yoor-ă-sil) *n.* a drug that prevents cell growth (*see* antimetabolite) and is used in the treatment of cancers of the digestive system and breast; it is usually administered by injection. Fluorouracil is also applied as a cream to treat certain skin conditions, including skin cancer.

fluoxetine (floo-oks-i-teen) *n.* an antidepressant drug that acts by prolonging the action of the neurotransmitter serotonin (5-hydroxytryptamine) in the brain (*see* SSRI). It is administered by mouth. Trade name: **Prozac**.

flupentixol (flupenthixol) (floopen-tiks-ol) *n.* an antipsychotic drug used to treat schizophrenia and other psychoses. It is administered by mouth and by injection. Trade names: **Depixol, Fluanxol**.

fluphenazine (floo-fen-ă-zeen) *n.* a phenothiazine antipsychotic drug used for the treatment of schizophrenia and other psychotic disorders. It is administered by mouth or injection. Trade names: **Modecate, Moditen**.

flurazepam (floor-az-ĕ-pam) *n.* a benzodiazepine drug administered by mouth to treat insomnia and sleep disturbances (*see* hypnotic). Trade name: **Dalmane**.

flurbiprofen (fler-bip-roh-fen) *n.* an analgesic that relieves inflammation (*see* NSAID), used in the treatment of rheumatoid arthritis and osteoarthritis and to prevent contraction of the pupil during eye surgery. Trade names: **Froben, Ocufen**.

flutamide (floo-tă-myd) *n.* an antiandrogen commonly used in the treatment of prostate cancer, sometimes alone or in combination with LHRH analogues. It is taken by mouth.

flutter (flut-er) *n.* a disturbance of

normal heart rhythm, less rapid and less chaotic than fibrillation.

fluvastatin (floo-vas-tă-tin) *n.* a drug used to reduce abnormally high levels of cholesterol and other lipids in the blood (*see* statin). It is taken by mouth. Trade name: **Lescol**.

fluvoxamine (floo-voks-ă-meen) *n.* an antidepressant drug that acts by prolonging the action of the neurotransmitter serotonin (5-hydroxytryptamine) in the brain (*see* SSRI). It is taken by mouth. Trade name: **Faverin**.

flux (fluks) *n.* an abnormally copious flow from an organ or cavity.

fly (fly) *n.* a two-winged insect belonging to the order Diptera. The mouthparts of flies are adapted for sucking and sometimes also for piercing and biting. Fly larvae (maggots) may infest human tissues and cause disease (*see* myiasis).

focal distance (foh-kăl) *n.* (of the eye) the distance between the lens and the point behind the lens at which light from a distant object is focused.

focus (foh-kŭs) **1.** *n.* the point at which rays of light converge after passing through a lens. **2.** *n.* the principal site of an infection or other disease. **3.** *vb.* (in ophthalmology) to accommodate (*see* accommodation).

foetus (fee-tŭs) *n. see* fetus.

folic acid (pteroylglutamic acid) (foh-lik) *n.* a B vitamin that is important in the synthesis of nucleic acids. The metabolic role of folic acid is interdependent with that of vitamin B_{12} (both are required by rapidly dividing cells) and a deficiency of one may lead to deficiency of the other. A deficiency of folic acid results in the condition of megaloblastic anaemia. Good sources of folic acid are liver, yeast extract, and green leafy vegetables; increased intake shortly before conception and during the first three months of pregnancy helps prevent spina bifida and other congenital malformations in the fetus.

folie à deux (communicated insanity) (fol-i a der) *n.* a condition in which two people who are closely involved with each other share a system of delusions.

folinic acid (foh-**lin**-ik) *n.* a derivative of folic acid involved in purine synthesis. Administered by mouth or by injection, it is used to reverse the biological effects of methotrexate, and so prevent excessive toxicity (*f. a.* rescue), and to potentiate the action of fluorouracil. Trade names: **Lederfolin, Refolinon**.

follicle (fol-ikŭl) *n.* a small secretory cavity, sac, or gland. *See also* Graafian follicle, hair (follicle). —**follicular** (fŏ-lik-yoo-ler) *adj.*

follicle-stimulating hormone (FSH) *n.* a hormone (*see* gonadotrophin) synthesized and released by the anterior pituitary gland. FSH stimulates ripening of the follicles in the ovary and formation of sperm in the testes. It is administered by injection to treat sterility.

folliculitis (fŏ-lik-yoo-**ly**-tis) *n.* inflammation of hair follicles in the skin, commonly caused by infection. *See also* sycosis.

fomentation (foh-men-tay-shŏn) *n. see* poultice.

fomes (foh-meez) *n.* (*pl.* **fomites**) any object that is used or handled by a person with a communicable

disease and may therefore become contaminated with the infective organisms and transmit the disease to a subsequent user. Common fomites are towels, bed-clothes, cups, and money.

fontanelle (fon-tă-nel) *n.* an opening in the skull of a fetus or young infant due to incomplete ossification of the cranial bones and the resulting incomplete closure of the sutures. *anterior f.* the opening at the junction of the coronal, frontal, and sagittal sutures. *posterior f.* the opening at the junction of the sagittal and lambdoidal sutures.

Fontanelles in the skull of a newborn infant (from above)

food poisoning (food) *n.* an illness affecting the digestive system that results from eating food contaminated either by bacteria or bacterial toxins or, less commonly, by poisonous chemicals such as lead or mercury. It can also be caused by eating poisonous fungi, berries, etc. Symptoms include vomiting, diarrhoea, abdominal pain, and nausea.

Food-borne infections are caused by bacteria of the genus *Salmonella*, *Campylobacter*, and *Listeria* in foods of animal origin. Toxin-producing bacteria causing food poisoning include those of the genus *Staphylococcus*, which rapidly multiply in warm foods; pathogenic *Escherichia coli*; and the species *Clostridium perfringens*, which multiplies in reheated cooked meals. *See also* botulism, gastroenteritis.

foot (fuut) *n.* the terminal organ of the lower limb. It comprises the seven bones of the tarsus, the five metatarsal bones, and the phalangeal bones plus the surrounding tissues.

foot drop (fuut-drop) *n.* inability to keep the foot at right angles to the leg, caused by paralysis of the anterior leg muscles, pressure of bedclothes, or insufficient support for the sole of the foot when the leg is splinted.

foramen (fo-ray-men) *n.* (*pl.* **foramina**) an opening or hole, particularly in a bone. **apical f.** the small opening at the apex of a tooth. **f. magnum** a large hole in the occipital bone through which the spinal cord passes. **f. ovale** the opening between the two atria of the fetal heart, which allows blood to flow from the right to the left side of the heart by displacing a membranous valve.

forced expiratory volume (FEV) (forst iks-pir-ă-ter-i vol-yoom) *n.* the volume of air exhaled in a given period (usually limited to 1 second in tests of vital capacity). FEV is reduced in patients with obstructive airways disease and diminished lung volume.

forced vital capacity (FVC) *n. see* vital capacity.

forceps (for-seps) *n.* a pincer-like instrument designed to grasp an ob-

bone holding forceps

volsella

sinus forceps

dissecting forceps

dressing forceps

obstetrical forceps

dental extraction forceps

Types of forceps

ject so that it can be held firm or pulled. Specially designed forceps are used by surgeons and dentists in operations (see illustration).

forebrain (for-brayn) *n.* the furthest forward division of the brain, consisting of the diencephalon and the two cerebral hemispheres.

foregut (for-gut) *n.* the front part of the embryonic gut, which gives rise to the oesophagus, stomach, and part of the small intestine.

forensic medicine (fer-en-sik) *n.* the branch of medicine concerned with the scientific investigation of the causes of injury and death in unexplained circumstances, particularly when criminal activity is suspected.

forequarter amputation (for-kwor-ter) *n.* an operation involving removal of an entire arm, including the scapula and clavicle. It is usually performed for soft tissue or bone sarcomas arising from the upper arm or shoulder. *Compare* hindquarter amputation.

foreskin (for-skin) *n. see* prepuce.

forewaters (for-waw-terz) *n.* the amniotic fluid that escapes from the uterus through the vagina when that part of the amnion lying in front of the presenting part of the fetus ruptures, either spontaneously or by amniotomy. Spontaneous rupture is usual in labour but rupture may occur before labour starts (premature rupture of membranes).

formaldehyde (for-mal-di-hyd) *n.* the aldehyde derivative of formic acid, formerly used as a vapour to sterilize and disinfect rooms and such items as mattresses and blankets. The toxic vapour is produced by boiling formalin in an open container or using it in a sealed autoclave.

formalin (for-mă-lin) *n.* a solution containing 40% formaldehyde in water, used as a sterilizing agent and, in pathology, as a fixative.

formestan (for-mi-stan) *n. see* aromatase inhibitor.

formication (for-mi-kay-shŏn) *n.* a prickling sensation said to resemble the feeling of ants crawling over the skin. It is sometimes a symptom of drug intoxication and can also be reported by patients with Parkinson's disease or multiple sclerosis.

formoterol (eformoterol) (for-moh-ter-ol) *n.* a sympathomimetic drug used as a long-acting bronchodilator to treat asthma. Formoterol is formulated in powder form for administration by inhaler. Trade names: **Foradil, Oxis Turbohaler.**

formula (form-yoo-lă) *n.* **1.** a representation of the structure of a chemical compound using symbols and subscript numbers for the atoms it contains (e.g. H_2O for water; CO_2 for carbon dioxide). **2.** a prescription for a drug.

formulary (form-yoo-ler-i) *n.* a compendium of formulae used in the preparation of medicinal drugs.

fornix (for-niks) *n.* (*pl.* **fornices**) an arched or vaultlike structure. *f. cerebri* a triangular structure of white matter in the brain, situated between the hippocampus and hypothalamus. *f. of the vagina* any of three vaulted spaces at the top of the vagina, around the cervix of the uterus.

Forrest screening (fo-rist) *n.* the UK national breast screening programme, in which regular mammography is available for all women between the ages of 50 and 64. It enables the early diagnosis of breast cancer in order to improve treatment and reduce mortality. [Sir P. Forrest (1923–), Scottish surgeon]

forward parachute reflex (forwuud) *n.* a reflex action of the body that develops by five to six months and never disappears. If the body is held by the waist face down and lowered, the arms and legs extend automatically.

foscarnet (fos-kar-net) *n.* an antiviral drug used to treat infections caused by herpesviruses, including cytomegaloviruses, that are resistant to aciclovir, especially in patients with AIDS. It is administered by intravenous injection.

fossa (fos-ă) *n.* (*pl.* **fossae**) a depression or hollow. *cubital f.* the triangular hollow at the front of the elbow joint. *iliac f.* the depression in the inner surface of the ilium. *pituitary f.* the hollow in the sphenoid bone in which the pituitary gland is situated. *tooth f.* a pit in the enamel on the surface of a tooth.

Fothergill's operation *n. see* Donald-Fothergill operation.

fourchette (foor-shet) *n.* a thin fold of skin at the back of the vulva.

fovea (foh-viă) *n.* (in anatomy) a small depression, especially the shallow pit in the retina at the back of the eye. It contains a large number of cones and is therefore the area of greatest acuity of vision. *See also* macula (lutea).

FQ *n. see* Fear Questionnaire.

fracture (frak-cher) *n.* breakage of a bone, either complete or incomplete. Treatment includes realignment of the bone ends and immobi-

lization by external splints or internal fixation. *cervical f.* a fracture of a vertebra in the neck, with effects ranging from minor, requiring no treatment, to paralysis and instant death. *Colles' f.* a fracture of the distal (far) end of the radius, which is displaced backwards and upwards to produce a 'dinner fork' deformity. Avulsion of the ulnar styloid process usually takes place as well. *comminuted f.* a fracture in which the bone is broken into more than two pieces. *greenstick f.* an incomplete break in a bone occurring in children. *impacted f.* a fracture in which the bone ends are driven into each other. *march f.* a fracture through the neck of the second or third metatarsal bone, associated with excess walking. *open f.* a fracture in which the overlying skin is perforated and there is a wound extending to the fracture site. *pathological f.* fracture of a diseased or abnormal bone, usually resulting from a force insufficient to fracture a normal bone. *Pott's f.* a fracture of the lower end of the fibula accompanied by a fracture of the malleolus of the tibia. *simple f.* a clean break with little damage to surrounding tissues. *Smith's f.* a fracture just above the wrist, across the distal (far) end of the radius. The hand and wrist below the fracture are displaced forwards. See illustration.

fraenectomy (free-nek-tŏmi) *n. see* frenectomy.

fraenum (free-nŭm) *n. see* frenum.

fragile-X syndrome (fraj-yl-eks) *n.* a major genetic disorder caused by an abnormality in an X chromosome. The fragile-X syndrome is second only to Down's syndrome as a

Colles'

comminuted

greenstick

impacted

open

Pott's

Types of fracture

cause of mental retardation. It predominantly affects males, but about one-third of the females with this mutation on one of their two X chromosomes are also mentally retarded.

fragilitas (frä-jil-i-tas) *n.* abnormal brittleness or fragility. *f. crinium* brittleness of the hair. *f. ossium* brittleness of the bones (*see* osteogenesis (imperfecta)).

framboesia (fram-bee-ziä) *n. see* yaws.

framycetin (fra-my-see-tin) *n.* an antibiotic used mainly in the form of an ointment, cream, or eye or ear drops to treat skin, eye, and ear infections. Trade names: **Sofradex**, **Soframycin**.

fraternal twins (frä-ter-nål) *pl. n. see* twins.

FRC *n. see* functional residual capacity.

freckle (frek-ĕl) *n.* a small harmless brown spot on the skin, commonly seen on exposed areas of fair-skinned people, due to excessive production of melanin without an increase in melanocytes after exposure to sunlight. *Compare* lentigo.

free association (free) *n.* (in psychoanalysis) a technique in which the patient is encouraged to pursue a particular train of ideas as they enter his or her consciousness. *See also* association of ideas.

Freiburg's disease (fry-bergz) *n.* osteochondritis affecting the head of the second metatarsal bone. [A. H. Freiburg (1868–1940), US orthopaedic surgeon]

Frei test (fry) *n.* a rarely used diagnostic test for the sexually transmitted disease lymphogranuloma venereum. [W. S. Frei (1885–1943), German dermatologist]

fremitus (frem-i-tŭs) *n.* vibrations or tremors in a part of the body, detected by palpation or auscultation. The term is most commonly applied to vibrations perceived through the chest when a patient breathes, speaks (*vocal f.*), or coughs.

frenectomy (fraenectomy) (free-nek-tomi) *n.* an operation to remove the frenum, including the underlying fibrous tissue.

frenulum (fren-yoo-lŭm) *n. see* frenum.

frenum (fraenum, frenulum) (free-nŭm) *n.* **1.** any of the folds of mucous membrane under the tongue or between the gums and the upper or lower lips. **2.** any of several other structures of similar appearance.

frequency (free-kwĕn-si) *n.* (of urine) the passage of urine more than seven times a day. *See* lower urinary tract symptoms.

Freudian (froi-di-ăn) *adj.* relating to or describing the work and ideas of Sigmund Freud (1856–1939): applied particularly to the school of psychiatry based on his teachings (*see* psychoanalysis).

friar's balsam (fry-erz) *n.* a tincture of benzoin, balsam of Tolu, storax, aloes, and various other plant extracts, the vapour of which is inhaled to relieve bronchitis.

friction murmur (friction rub) (frik-shŏn) *n.* a scratching sound, heard over the heart with the aid of the stethoscope, in patients who have pericarditis. It results from the two inflamed layers of the pericardium rubbing together during activity of the heart.

Friedländer's bacillus (freed-len-derz) *n.* a Gram-negative rodlike bacterium, *Klebsiella pneumoniae*, that causes a form of pneumonia. [K. Friedländer (1847–87), German pathologist]

Friedreich's ataxia (freed-ryks) *n. see* ataxia. [N. Friedreich (1825–82), German neurologist]

frigidity (fri-jid-iti) *n.* lack of sexual desire or inability to achieve orgasm, especially in a woman.

fringe medicine (frinj) *n. see* complementary medicine.

frog plaster (frog) *n.* a plaster of Paris splint used to maintain the legs in their correct position after a congenital dislocation of the hip has been corrected by manipulation.

Fröhlich's syndrome (frer-liks) *n.* a disorder of the hypothalamus affecting males: the boy is overweight with sexual development absent and disturbances of sleep and appetite. Medical name: **dystrophia adiposogenitalis**. [A. Fröhlich (1871–1953), Austrian neurologist]

Froin's syndrome (frwahnz) *n.* a condition in which the cerebrospinal fluid (CSF) displays a combination of yellow colour and high protein content. It is characteristic of a block to the spinal circulation of CSF caused by a tumour. [G. Froin (1874–1932), French physician]

frontal (frun-t'l) *adj.* **1.** of or relating to the forehead. *f. bone* the bone forming the forehead and the upper parts of the orbits. *f. sinuses see* paranasal sinuses. **2.** denoting the anterior part of a body or organ. *f. lobe* the anterior part of each cerebral hemisphere, extending as far back as the deep central sulcus of its upper and outer surface.

frostbite (frost-byt) *n.* damage to the tissues caused by freezing. The affected parts, usually the nose, fingers, or toes, become pale and numb. Ice forms in the tissues, which may thus be destroyed, and amputation may become necessary. Frostbitten skin is highly susceptible to bacterial infection.

frozen shoulder (adhesive capsulitis) (froh-zĕn) *n.* chronic painful stiffness of the shoulder joint. This may follow injury, a stroke, or myocardial infarction or may gradually develop for no apparent reason. *See also* capsulitis.

frozen watchfulness *n.* the state of a child who is unresponsive to its surroundings but is clearly aware of them. Frozen watchfulness is usually a marker of child abuse.

fructose (fruk-tohz) *n.* a simple sugar found in honey and in such fruit as figs. Fructose is one of the two sugars in sucrose.

fructosuria (levulosuria) (fruk-tohz-yoor-iă) *n.* the presence of fructose (levulose) in the urine.

frusemide (frus-ĕ-myd) *n. see* furosemide.

FSH *n. see* follicle-stimulating hormone.

FTT *n. see* failure to thrive.

Fuchs' endothelial dystrophy (fooks) *n.* a hereditary condition in which the endothelium of the cornea fails to function with age; it results in thickening and swelling of the cornea and hence reduced vision. [E. Fuchs (1851–1913), German ophthalmologist]

fuchsin (magenta) (fook-sin) *n.* any one of a group of reddish to purplish dyes used in staining bacteria for microscopic observation and capable of killing various disease-causing microorganisms.

-fuge *suffix denoting* an agent that drives away, repels, or eliminates.

fugue (fewg) *n.* a period of memory loss during which the patient leaves his usual surroundings and wanders aimlessly or starts a new life elsewhere. It is often preceded by psychological conflict and depression (*see* dissociative disorder) or it may be associated with organic mental disease.

fulguration (electrodesiccation) (ful-gewr-ay-shŏn) *n.* the destruction with a diathermy instrument of warts, growths, or unwanted areas of tissue, particularly inside the bladder.

fulminating (fulminant, fulgurant) (ful-min-ayt-ing) *adj.* describing a condition or symptom that is of very sudden onset, severe, and of short duration.

fumigation (few-mig-ay-shŏn) *n.* the use of gases or vapours, such as formaldehyde or chlorine, to bring about disinfestation of clothing, buildings, etc.

functional disorder (funk-shŏn-ăl) *n.* a condition in which a patient complains of symptoms for which no physical cause can be found. Such a condition is frequently an indication of a psychiatric disorder. *Compare* organic (disorder).

functional endoscopic sinus surgery (FESS) *n.* surgery of the paranasal sinuses using endoscopes. Routes of sinus drainage and aeration that are blocked by disease are cleared and enlarged, allowing the rest of the sinuses to return to normal.

functional independence

measure *n.* a table recommended by the WHO for assessing the degree of whole-person disability, being particularly useful for judging the extent of recovery from serious injury. It has five grades, ranging from 0 (fully independent) to 4 (completely dependent).

Functional Recovery Index *n.* an international index, published by the World Health Organization, that grades the degree of recovery after serious injury.

functional residual capacity (FRC) *n.* the volume of air that remains in the lungs after normal expiration.

fundoplication (fun-doh-pli-kay-shŏn) *n.* a surgical operation for gastro-oesophageal reflux disease in which the upper part of the stomach is wrapped around the lower oesophagus.

fundoscopy (ophthalmoscopy) (fund-os-kŏpi) *n.* examination of the interior of the eye by means of an ophthalmoscope.

fundus (fun-dŭs) *n.* **1.** the base of a hollow organ: the part farthest from the opening. **2.** the interior concavity forming the back of the eyeball, opposite the pupil.

fungicide (fun-ji-syd) *n.* an agent that kills fungi. *See also* antifungal.

fungoid (fung-oid) **1.** *adj.* resembling a fungus. **2.** *n.* a fungus-like growth.

fungus (fung-ŭs) *n.* (*pl.* fungi) a simple organism (formerly regarded as a plant) that lacks the green pigment chlorophyll. Fungi include the yeasts, rusts, moulds, and mushrooms. Some species infect and cause disease in humans. Some yeasts are a good source of vitamin

B and many antibiotics are obtained from the moulds (*see* penicillin). *See also* yeast. **—fungal** *adj.*

funiculitis (few-nik-yoo-ly-tis) *n.* inflammation of the spermatic cord.

funiculus (few-nik-yoo-lùs) *n.* **1.** any of the three main columns of white matter found in each lateral half of the spinal cord. **2.** a bundle of nerve fibres enclosed in a sheath. **3.** (formerly) the spermatic cord or umbilical cord.

funis (few-nis) *n.* (in anatomy) any cordlike structure, especially the umbilical cord.

funnel chest (fun-èl) *n.* a developmental abnormality in which the sternum is depressed and the ribs and costal cartilages curve inwards. Medical name: **pectus excavatum.**

furor (fewr-or) *n.* indiscriminate violence and destructiveness, occurring especially during a period of mental confusion due to epilepsy.

furosemide (frusemide) (fewr-os-ĕ-myd) *n.* a loop diuretic administered by mouth or injection to treat fluid retention (oedema) associated with heart, liver, or kidney disease and also high blood pressure. Trade name: **Lasix.**

furuncle (fewr-ung-kŭl) *n. see* boil.

furunculosis (fewr-unk-yoo-loh-sis) *n.* the occurrence of several boils (furuncles) at the same time, usually caused by *Staphylococcus aureus* infection.

fusidic acid (few-sid-ik) *n.* a steroid antibiotic used to treat staphylococcal skin and eye infections. It is administered topically. Trade names: **Fucidin, Fucithalmic.**

fusiform (few-zi-form) *adj.* spindle-shaped; tapering at both ends.

fusion (few-zhŏn) *n.* **1.** the joining together of two structures by surgery. For example, fusion of two or more vertebrae is performed to stabilize an unstable spine. **2.** the joining together of two structures by growth. Fusion of the epiphyses during development is the cause of arrested growth of stature.

FVC *n. see* (forced) vital capacity.

Gg

GABA *n.* see gamma-aminobutyric acid.

GAD *n.* see glutamic acid decarboxylase.

gag (gag) *n.* (in medicine) an instrument that is placed between a patient's teeth to keep his mouth open.

gag reflex (pharyngeal reflex) *n.* a normal reflex action caused by contraction of pharynx muscles when the soft palate or posterior pharynx is touched. The reflex is used to test the integrity of the vagus and glossopharyngeal nerves.

gait (gayt) *n.* a manner of walking. *ataxic g.* an unsteady uncoordinated walk due to disease of the sensory nerves or cerebellum. *See* ataxia. *cerebellar g.* a staggering walk due to disease of the cerebellum. *spastic g.* a stiff shuffling walk in which the legs are held together.

galact- (galacto-) *prefix denoting* **1.** milk. **2.** galactose.

galactagogue (gă-lak-tă-gog) *n.* an agent that stimulates the secretion of milk or increases milk flow.

galactocele (gă-lak-toh-seel) *n.* **1.** a breast cyst containing milk, caused by closure of a milk duct. **2.** an accumulation of milky liquid in the sac surrounding the testis (*see* hydrocele).

galactorrhoea (gă-lak-toh-ree-ă) *n.* **1.** abnormally copious milk secretion. **2.** secretion of milk after breast feeding has been stopped.

galactosaemia (gă-lak-toh-see-miă) *n.* an inborn inability to utilize the sugar galactose, which in consequence accumulates in the blood. Untreated, affected infants fail to thrive and become mentally retarded, but if galactose is eliminated from the diet growth and development may be normal.

galactose (gă-lak-tohz) *n.* a simple sugar and a constituent of the milk sugar lactose. Galactose is converted to glucose in the liver.

galantamine (gă-lant-ă-meen) *n.* see acetylcholinesterase inhibitor.

galea (gay-liă) *n.* **1.** a helmet-shaped anatomical part. **2.** a type of head bandage.

galenical (gă-len-ikăl) *n.* a pharmaceutical preparation of a drug of animal or plant origin.

gallamine (gal-ă-meen) *n.* a drug administered by injection to produce muscle relaxation during anaesthesia (*see* muscle relaxant). Trade name: **Flaxedil.**

gall bladder (gawl) *n.* a pear-shaped sac (7–10 cm long), lying underneath the right lobe of the liver, in which bile is stored (*see* illustration). The gall bladder is a common site of stone formation (*see* gallstone).

Gallie's operation (gal-iz) *n.* an operation in which strips of fascia taken from the thigh are used as suturing material to repair a hernia. [W. E. Gallie (1882–1959), Canadian surgeon]

gallipot (gal-i-pot) *n.* a small pot for holding lotions or ointments.

gallium (gal-iŭm) *n.* a silvery metallic element. A radioisotope of gallium can be used for the detection of lymphomas and areas of infection (such as an abscess) following intravenous injection. Symbol: Ga.

gallstone (gawl-stohn) *n.* a hard mass composed of bile pigments, cholesterol, and calcium salts, in varying proportions, that can form in the gall bladder. They may cause severe pain (*see* biliary (colic)) or they may pass into the common bile duct and cause obstructive jaundice or cholangitis. Treatment is usually by surgical removal of the gall bladder (*see* cholecystectomy) or by removing the stones themselves, which can be either dissolved using bile salts given by mouth, or shattered by ultrasound waves.

galvanism (gal-vă-nizm) *n.* (formerly) any form of medical treatment using electricity. *interrupted*

hepatic duct — pancreatic duct

gall bladder —

cystic duct —

common bile duct —

duodenum —

orifice of common bile duct and pancreatic duct —

— pancreas

The gall bladder and pancreas

g. a form of electrotherapy in which direct current is used to stimulate the activity of nerves or the muscles they supply. *See also* faradism.

galvanometer (gal-vă-**nom**-it-er) *n.* an instrument for measuring the strength of an electric current.

gamete (gam-eet) *n.* a mature sex cell: the ovum of the female or the spermatozoon of the male. Gametes are haploid, containing half the normal number of chromosomes.

gamete intrafallopian transfer (GIFT) (intră-fă-**loh**-piăn) *n.* a procedure for assisting conception, suitable for women whose Fallopian tubes are normal but in whom some other factor, such as endometriosis, prevents conception. Using needle aspiration, under laparoscopic or ultrasonic guidance, ova are removed from the ovary. After being mixed with the partner's spermatozoa, they are introduced into a Fallopian tube, where fertilization takes place. The fertilized ovum is subsequently implanted in the uterus. A similar procedure is used in *zygote intrafallopian transfer* (*ZIFT*), except that fertilization occurs in vitro and the zygote is introduced into a Fallopian tube.

gametocide (gam-i-toh-syd) *n.* a drug that kills gametocytes.

gametocyte (gă-**meet**-oh-syt) *n.* any of the cells that are in the process of developing into gametes by undergoing gametogenesis.

gametogenesis (gam-i-toh-**jen**-i-sis) *n.* the process by which spermatozoa and ova are formed. In both sexes the precursor cells undergo meiosis, which halves the number of chromosomes. *See* oogenesis, spermatogenesis.

gamgee tissue (gam-jee) *n.* a thick layer of absorbent cotton between two layers of gauze, used as a surgical dressing.

gamma-aminobutyric acid (GABA) (gam-ă-ă-meen-oh-bew-ti-rik) *n.* an amino acid found in the central nervous system, predominantly in the brain, where it acts as an inhibitory neurotransmitter.

gamma camera *n.* a piece of apparatus that detects radioactivity in the form of gamma rays emitted by radioactive isotopes that have been introduced into the body as tracers. The position of the source of the radioactivity can be plotted and displayed on a TV monitor or photographic film. *See* scintillator.

gammaglobulin (gam-ă-glob-yoo-lin) *n.* any of a class of proteins (*see* globulin) present in the blood plasma. Almost all gammaglobulins are immunoglobulins.

gamma rays *pl. n.* electromagnetic radiation of wavelengths shorter than X-rays, given off by certain radioactive substances. Gamma rays used in nuclear medicine have higher energy than diagnostic X-rays and greater penetration; higher doses are used in radiotherapy. Gamma rays are harmful to living tissues and can be used to sterilize certain materials and to kill bacteria as a means of food preservation.

gamo- *prefix denoting* marriage.

ganciclovir (gan-sy-kloh-veer) *n.* an antiviral drug used to treat severe cytomegalovirus infections, mainly in patients with AIDS. It is administered by mouth, injection, or as eye drops. Trade names: **Cymevene, Virgan**.

gangli- (ganglio-) *prefix denoting* a ganglion.

ganglion (gang-li-ŏn) *n.* (*pl.* **ganglia**) **1.** (in neurology) any structure containing a collection of nerve cell bodies and often also numbers of synapses. Ganglia are found in the sympathetic and parasympathetic nervous systems. Within the central nervous system certain well-defined masses of nerve cells are called ganglia (*see* basal ganglia). **2.** an abnormal but harmless swelling (cyst) that sometimes forms in tendon sheaths, especially at the wrist.

ganglionectomy (gang-li-ŏn-ek-tŏmi) *n.* surgical removal of a ganglion cyst.

gangrene (gang-reen) *n.* death and decay of part of the body due to deficiency or cessation of blood supply. The causes include disease, injury, or atheroma in major blood vessels, frostbite or severe burns, and diseases such as diabetes mellitus and Raynaud's disease. *dry g.* death and withering of tissues caused simply by a cessation of local blood circulation. *moist g.* death and putrefactive decay of tissue caused by bacterial infection. *See also* gas gangrene.

Ganser state (pseudodementia) (gan-ser) *n.* a syndrome characterized by approximate answers, i.e. the patient gives absurdly false replies to questions, but the reply shows that the question has been understood. The condition is due to conversion disorder or to conscious malingering. [S. J. M. Ganser (1853–1931), German psychiatrist]

Gardnerella (gard-ner-el-ă) *n.* a genus of anaerobic bacteria. *G. vaginalis* a cause of vaginitis and, in pregnant women, of late miscarriage.

Gardner's syndrome (gard-nerz) *n.* a variant form of familial adenomatous polyposis in which polyps in the colon are associated with fibromas and osteomas (benign tumours), especially of the skull and jaw, and multiple sebaceous cysts. [E. J. Gardner (1909–), US physician]

gargle (gar-gŭl) **1.** *n.* a medicated solution used for washing the mouth and throat. **2.** *vb.* to apply a gargle by holding it in the throat and exhaling through it.

gargoylism (gar-goil-izm) *n.* see Hunter's syndrome, Hurler's syndrome.

gas (gas) *n.* a fluid whose physical state is such that the forces of attraction between its constituent atoms and molecules are very weak. It therefore has no definite shape or volume. *laughing g. see* nitrous oxide.

gas gangrene *n.* death and decay of wound tissue infected by the soil bacterium *Clostridium perfringens.* Toxins produced by the bacterium cause putrefactive decay of connective tissue with the generation of gas.

Gasserian ganglion (gas-eer-iăn) *n.* a ganglion on the sensory root of the trigeminal nerve, deep within the skull. [J. L. Gasser (1723–65), Austrian anatomist]

gastr- (**gastro-**) *prefix denoting* the stomach.

gastralgia (gas-tral-jiă) *n.* pain in the stomach.

gastrectomy (gas-trek-tŏmi) *n.* a surgical operation in which the whole or a part of the stomach is removed. *partial* (or *subtotal*) *g.* an operation in which the upper third or half of the stomach is joined to the duodenum or small intestine. *See also* Billroth's operation. *total g.* an operation usually performed for stomach cancer, in which the oesophagus is joined to the duodenum.

gastric (gas-trik) *adj.* relating to or affecting the stomach. *g. glands* tubular glands in the mucous membrane of the stomach wall that secrete gastric juice. *g. juice* the liquid secreted by the gastric glands, containing hydrochloric acid, mucin, rennin, and pepsinogen. The acid acts on pepsinogen to produce the digestive enzyme pepsin. The acidity of the stomach contents also kills unwanted bacteria and other organisms that have been ingested with the food. *g. ulcer* an ulcer in the stomach, caused by the action of acid, pepsin, and bile on the stomach lining. Symptoms include vomiting and pain in the upper abdomen soon after eating, and such complications as bleeding (*see* haematemesis), perforation, and obstruction due to scarring may occur. *See also* Helicobacter.

gastrin (gas-trin) *n.* a hormone produced in the mucous membrane of the pyloric region of the stomach. Its secretion is stimulated by the presence of food. It is circulated in the blood to the rest of the stomach, where it stimulates the production of gastric juice.

gastrinoma (gas-tri-noh-mă) *n.* a rare tumour that secretes excess amounts of the hormone gastrin, causing the Zollinger-Ellison syndrome. Such tumours most frequently occur in the pancreas; about half of them are malignant.

gastritis (gas-**try**-tis) *n.* inflammation of the lining (mucosa) of the stomach. *acute g.* gastritis in which vomiting occurs, caused by ingesting excess alcohol or other irritating or corrosive substances. *atrophic g.* gastritis in which the stomach lining is atrophied. *chronic g.* gastritis that is usually caused by the bacterium *Helicobacter pylori* but may be associated with smoking and chronic alcoholism or be caused by bile entering the stomach from the duodenum. It has no definite symptoms, but the patient is liable to develop gastric ulcers or stomach cancer.

gastrocele (gas-troh-seel) *n.* a hernia of the stomach.

gastrocnemius (gas-trok-**nee**-miŭs) *n.* a muscle that forms the greater part of the calf of the leg. It

- femur
- fibula
- tibia
- gastrocnemius
- soleus
- Achilles tendon

Gastrocnemius and soleus muscles

flexes the knee and foot (so that the toes point downwards).

gastrocolic reflex (gas-troh-**kol**-ik) *n.* a wave of peristalsis produced in the colon by introducing food into a fasting stomach.

gastroduodenoscopy (gas-troh-dew-ŏ-di-**nos**-kŏ-pi) *n.* the technique of viewing the inside of the stomach and duodenum with a fibreoptic or video endoscope.

gastroduodenostomy (gas-troh-dew-ŏ-di-**nost**-ŏmi) *n.* a surgical operation in which the duodenum is joined to an opening made in the stomach in order to bypass an obstruction or to facilitate the exit of food from the stomach after vagotomy. *See also* duodenostomy.

gastroenteritis (gas-troh-enter-**I**-tis) *n.* inflammation of the stomach and intestine. It is usually due to acute infection by viruses or bacteria or to food-poisoning toxins and causes vomiting and diarrhoea. Fluid loss is sometimes severe, especially in infants, and intravenous fluid replacement may be necessary.

gastroenterology (gas-troh-enter-**ol**-ŏji) *n.* the study of gastrointestinal disease, which includes disease of any part of the digestive tract and also of the liver, biliary tract, and pancreas.

gastroenterostomy (gas-troh-enter-**ost**-ŏmi) *n.* a surgical operation in which the small intestine is joined to an opening made in the stomach. The usual technique is gastroduodenostomy.

gastroileac reflex (gas-troh-**il**-i-ak) *n.* the relaxation of the ileocaecal valve caused by the presence of food in the stomach.

gastrointestinal (GI) (gas-troh-in-**test**-i-năl) *adj.* denoting, relating to, or affecting the stomach and intestines.

gastrojejunostomy (gas-troh-ji-joo-**nost**-ŏmi) *n.* a surgical operation in which the jejunum is joined to an opening made in the stomach.

gastrolith (**gas**-trŏ-lith) *n.* a stone in the stomach, which usually builds up around a bezoar.

gastro-oesophageal reflux (GOR) (gas-troh-ee-sof-ă-jee-ăl) *n.* a condition in which the stomach contents reflux into the oesophagus because of impairment of the usual mechanisms preventing this. *g.-o.r. disease* the syndrome caused by abnormal gastro-oesophageal reflux, including symptoms of heartburn, regurgitation, and odynophagia, in which oesophagitis may be present.

gastropexy (gas-troh-**peks**-i) *n.* surgical attachment of the stomach to the abdominal wall.

gastroplasty (**gas**-troh-plasti) *n.* surgical alteration of the shape of the stomach without removal of any part, especially in order to reduce the size of the stomach in the treatment of morbid obesity.

gastroptosis (gas-trop-**toh**-sis) *n.* a condition in which the stomach hangs low in the abdomen.

gastroschisis (gas-tros-**ki**-sis) *n.* a congenital defect in the abdominal wall, which fails to close to the right of a normal umbilical cord. Gut prolapses through the defect and has no covering.

gastroscope (**gas**-trŏ-skohp) *n.* an illuminated optical instrument used to inspect the interior of the stomach. Modern instruments transmit the image through a fibreoptic bundle or by a tiny video camera, allowing all areas of the stomach to be seen and photographed and specimens to be taken for microscopic examination. Therapeutic procedures may be performed. —**gastroscopy** (gas-**tros**-kŏ-pi) *n.*

gastrostomy (gas-**trost**-ŏmi) *n.* a surgical procedure in which an opening is made into the stomach from the outside. It is usually performed to allow food and fluid to be poured directly into the stomach when swallowing is impossible because of disease or obstruction of the oesophagus. *percutaneous endoscopic g. (PEG)* gastrostomy performed using an endoscope to guide insertion of the feeding tube.

gastrotomy (gas-**trot**-ŏmi) *n.* a procedure during abdominal surgery in which the stomach is opened, usually to allow inspection of the interior, to remove a foreign body, or to allow the oesophagus to be approached from below.

gastrula (**gas**-troo-lă) *n.* an early stage in the development of many animal embryos. The gastrula consists of a double-layered ball of cells formed by invagination and movement of cells in the preceding single-layered stage (blastula) in the process of *gastrulation.*

Gaucher's disease (goh-**shayz**) *n.* a genetically determined disease, inherited as a recessive condition, resulting from the deposition of fatty compounds in the brain and other tissues (especially bone). It causes mental retardation, abnormal limb posture and spasticity, and difficulty with swallowing. [P. C. E. Gaucher (1854–1918), French physician]

gauze (gawz) *n*. thin open-woven material used in several layers for the preparation of dressings and swabs.

gavage (gav-ah*zh*) *n*. forced feeding: any means used to get an unwilling or incapacitated patient to take in food by mouth, especially via a stomach tube.

GCS *n*. Glasgow coma scale (*see* Glasgow scoring system).

Geiger counter (gy-ger kownt-er) *n*. a device for detecting and measuring the level of radioactivity of a substance. [H. Geiger (1882–1945), German physicist]

gel (jel) *n*. a colloidal suspension that has set to form a jelly. Some insoluble drugs are administered in the form of gels.

gelatin (jel-ă-tin) *n*. a jelly-like substance formed when tendons, ligaments, etc. containing collagen are boiled in water. Gelatin has been used in medicine as a source of dietary protein, in pharmacy for the manufacture of capsules and suppositories, and in bacteriology for preparing culture media.

gemeprost (jem-ĕ-prost) *n*. a prostaglandin drug, administered as a vaginal pessary to terminate pregnancy. It causes powerful contractions of the uterus at any stage of pregnancy.

gemfibrozil (jem-fy-broh-zil) *n*. a drug used to treat hyperlipidaemia that has not responded to diet, weight reduction, or exercise (*see* fibrate). It is administered by mouth. Trade name: **Lopid**.

gene (jeen) *n*. the basic unit of genetic material, which is carried at a particular place on a chromosome. Originally it was regarded as the unit of inheritance and mutation but is now usually defined as a sequence of DNA or RNA that acts as the unit controlling the formation of a single polypeptide chain. In diploid organisms, including humans, genes occur as pairs of alleles (*see* dominant, recessive). *See also* (gene) clone, gene therapy.

General Health Questionnaire (GHQ) (jen-er-ăl) *n*. a tool used to assess symptoms of neurosis.

generalized anxiety disorder (jen-ĕr-ă-lyzd) *n*. a state of inappropriate and sometimes severe anxiety, without adequate cause, that lasts for at least six months. Symptoms include breathlessness, palpitations, sweating, clammy hands, dry mouth, and globus hystericus. Treatment is with beta blockers, antihistamines, and antidepressants.

general paralysis of the insane (GPI) *n*. a late consequence of syphilitic infection. The symptoms are those of a dementia and spastic weakness of the limbs. Deafness, epilepsy, and dysarthria may occur.

general practitioner (GP) (prak-tish-ŏn-er) *n*. a doctor who is the main agent of primary care, through whom patients make first contact with health services for a new episode of illness or fresh developments of chronic diseases. Advice and treatment are provided for those who do not require the expertise of a consultant or other specialist services of hospitals (*see* secondary care). *See also* group practice.

generic (jin-e-rik) *adj*. **1.** denoting a drug name that is not protected by a trademark. **2.** of or relating to a genus.

-genesis *suffix denoting* origin or development.

gene therapy *n.* treatment directed to curing genetic disease by introducing normal genes into patients to overcome the effects of defective genes, using techniques of genetic engineering. At present, gene therapy is most feasible for treating disorders caused by a defect in a single recessive gene, such as adenosine deaminase (ADA) deficiency, severe combined immune deficiency, and cystic fibrosis. Gene therapy for certain types of cancer is also undergoing clinical trials.

genetic code (ji-net-ik) *n.* the code in which genetic information is carried by DNA and messenger RNA. This information determines the sequence of amino acids in every protein and thereby controls the nature of all proteins made by the cell.

genetic counselling *n.* the procedure by which patients and their families are given advice about the nature and consequences of inherited disorders, the possibility of becoming affected or having affected children, and the various options that are available to them for the prevention, diagnosis, and management of such conditions.

genetic engineering (recombinant DNA technology) *n.* the techniques involved in altering the characteristics of an organism by inserting genes from another organism into its DNA. This altered DNA is known as *recombinant DNA*. For example, the human genes for insulin, interferon, and growth hormone production have been incorporated into bacterial DNA to enable the commercial production of these substances.

genetics (ji-net-iks) *n.* the science of inheritance. It attempts to explain the differences and similarities between related organisms and the ways in which characters are passed from parents to their offspring. *See also* cytogenetics, Mendel's laws.

genetic screening *n.* screening tests to discover individuals whose genotypes are associated with specific diseases. Such individuals may later develop the disease itself or pass it on to their children (*see* carrier).

geni- (genio-) *prefix denoting* the chin.

-genic *suffix denoting* **1.** producing. **2.** produced by.

genicular (ji-nik-yoo-ler) *adj.* relating to the knee joint: applied to arteries that supply the knee.

genital (jen-i-t'l) *adj.* relating to the reproductive organs or to reproduction.

genitalia (jen-i-tay-liǎ) *pl. n.* the reproductive organs of either the male or the female, particularly the external parts of the reproductive system. *See also* vulva.

genito- *prefix denoting* the reproductive organs.

genitourinary (jen-i-toh-yoor-in-er-i) *adj.* of or relating to the organs of reproduction and excretion. **g. medicine** (*GUM*) the branch of medicine concerned with the study and treatment of sexually transmitted diseases.

genodermatosis (jen-oh-der-mǎ-toh-sis) *n.* any genetically determined skin disorder, such as ichthyosis, neurofibromatosis, or xeroderma pigmentosum.

genome (jen-ohm) *n.* the total genetic material of an organism, comprising the genes contained in its chromosomes; sometimes the term is used for the basic haploid set of chromosomes of an organism. The human genome comprises 23 pairs of chromosomes. *See also* Human Genome Project.

genotype (jen-oh-typ) *n.* **1.** the genetic constitution of an individual or group, as determined by the particular set of genes it possesses. **2.** the genetic information carried by a pair of alleles, which determines a particular characteristic. *Compare* phenotype.

gentamicin (jen-tă-my-sin) *n.* an aminoglycoside antibiotic used to treat infections caused by a wide range of bacteria. It can be administered by injection or applied in a cream to the skin or in drops to the ears and eyes. Trade names: **Cidomycin, Garamycin, Genticin**.

gentian violet (jen-shăn vy-ŏ-lit) *n.* a dye used to stain tissues and microorganisms for microscopical study and also as a topically applied antiseptic.

genu (jen-yoo) *n.* **1.** the knee. *g. valgum see* knock-knee. *g. varum see* bow-legs. **2.** any bent anatomical structure resembling the knee. —**genual** *adj.*

genucubital position (knee-elbow position) (jen-yoo-kew-bit'l) *n.* the buttocks-up position commonly assumed by patients undergoing anorectal examinations.

genupectoral position (knee-chest position) (jen-yoo-pek-ter-ăl) *n.* the position of a patient in which the weight of the body is supported on the knees and chest. *See* position.

genus (jen-ŭs) *n.* (*pl.* **genera**) a category used in the classification of animals and plants. A genus consists of several closely related and similar species; for example the genus *Canis* includes the dog, wolf, and jackal.

geographical tongue (jee-oh-graf-i-kăl) *n.* glossitis in which areas of erythema change from day to day.

ger- (gero-, geront(o)-) *prefix denoting* old age.

geriatrics (je-ri-at-riks) *n.* the branch of medicine concerned with the diagnosis and treatment of disorders that occur in old age and with the care of the aged. *See also* gerontology. —**geriatrician** (je-ri-ă-trish-ăn) *n.*

germ (jerm) *n.* any microorganism, especially one that causes disease. *See also* infection.

German measles (jer-măn) *n.* a mild highly contagious virus infection, mainly of childhood. Symptoms include headache, sore throat, and slight fever, followed by swelling and soreness of the neck and the eruption of a rash of minute pink spots, spreading from the face and neck to the rest of the body. German measles can cause fetal malformations during early pregnancy. Medical name: **rubella**. *Compare* scarlet fever.

germ cell (gonocyte) *n.* **1.** any of the embryonic cells that have the potential to develop into spermatozoa or ova. **2.** a gamete.

germicide (jerm-i-syd) *n.* an agent that destroys microorganisms, particularly those causing disease. *See* antibiotic, antifungal, antiseptic, disinfectant.

germinal (jer-min-ǎl) *adj.* **1.** relating to the early developmental stages of an embryo or tissue. **2.** relating to a germ.

germ layer *n.* any of the three distinct types of tissue found in the very early stages of embryonic development (*see* ectoderm, endoderm, mesoderm).

gerontology (je-ron-tol-ǒji) *n.* the study of the changes in the mind and body that accompany ageing and the problems associated with them.

Gerstmann-Straussler-Scheinker syndrome (gerst-măn strowsler shyn-ker) *n.* an autosomal dominant condition that resembles Creutzfeldt-Jakob disease (CJD). Patients present with ataxia and dysarthria and later develop dementia. They continue to deteriorate over several years, in contrast with patients with CJD, who deteriorate rapidly over periods of less than 12 months. [J. G. Gerstmann (1887–1969), Austrian neurologist]

gestaltism (gěsh-talt-izm) *n.* a school of psychology that regards mental processes as wholes (*gestalts*) that cannot be broken down into constituent parts. From this was developed *gestalt therapy*, which aims at achieving a suitable gestalt within the patient that includes all facets of functioning.

gestation (jes-tay-shǒn) *n.* the period during which a fertilized egg cell develops into a baby that is ready to be delivered. *See also* pregnancy.

gestational diabetes mellitus

(type 3 diabetes) (jes-tay-shǒn-ǎl) *n. see* diabetes.

gestodene (jes-toh-deen) *n.* a progestogen used in oral contraceptives in combination with an oestrogen. Trade names: **Femodene, Minulet.**

GFR *n. see* glomerular filtration rate.

GH *n. see* growth hormone.

GHIH *n.* growth-hormone inhibiting hormone (*see* somatostatin).

Ghon's focus (gonz) *n.* the lesion produced in the lung of a previously uninfected person by tubercle bacilli. It is a small focus of granulomatous inflammation, which may become visible on a chest X-ray if it grows large enough or if it calcifies. [A. Ghon (1866–1936), Czech pathologist]

GHQ *n. see* General Health Questionnaire.

GI *adj. see* gastrointestinal.

giant cell (jy-ǎnt) *n.* any large cell, such as a megakaryocyte. Giant cells may have one or many nuclei.

giant-cell arteritis *n. see* arteritis.

giardiasis (lambliasis) (jy-ar-dy-ǎ-sis) *n.* a disease caused by the parasitic protozoan *Giardia lamblia* in the small intestine. Symptoms include diarrhoea, nausea, bellyache, flatulence, and the passage of pale fatty stools (steatorrhoea). The disease is particularly common in children; it responds well to oral doses of metronidazole.

gibbus (gibbosity) (gib-ǔs) *n.* a sharply angled curvature of the backbone, resulting from collapse of a vertebra. Infection with tuberculosis was a common cause.

GIFT *n. see* gamete intrafallopian transfer.

gigantism (jy-gan-tizm) *n.* abnormal growth causing excessive height, most commonly due to over-secretion during childhood of growth hormone (somatotrophin) by the pituitary gland. *See also* acromegaly.

GIK regime *n. see* Alberti regime.

Gilbert's syndrome (*zh*eel-bairz) *n.* familial unconjugated hyper-bilirubinaemia: a condition caused by an inherited congenital defi-ciency of the enzyme UDP glu-curonyl transferase in the liver cells. Patients become mildly jaun-diced, especially if they fast or have some minor infection. [N. A. Gilbert (1858–1927), French physician]

Gilles de la Tourette syn-drome (Tourette syndrome) (*zh*eel dĕ la toor-et) *n.* a condition of severe and multiple tics, including vocal tics, grunts, and involuntary obscene speech (coprolalia). The pa-tient may also involuntarily repeat the words or imitate the actions of others (*see* palilalia). The condition usually starts in childhood and be-comes chronic; the causes are un-known. [G. Gilles de la Tourette (1857–1904), French neurologist]

Gilliam's operation (gil-i-ămz) *n.* an operation to correct retroversion of the uterus in which the round lig-aments are shortened. [D. T. Gilliam (1844–1923), US gynaecologist]

gingiv- (gingivo-) *prefix denoting* the gums.

gingiva (jin-jiv-ă) *n.* (*pl.* **gingivae**) the gum: the layer of dense connec-tive tissue and overlying mucous membrane that covers the alveolar bone and necks of the teeth. —**gin-gival** *adj.*

gingivectomy (jin-ji-vek-tŏmi) *n.* the surgical removal of excess gum tissue. It is a specific procedure of periodontal surgery.

gingivitis (jin-ji-vy-tis) *n.* inflam-mation of the gums, which become swollen and bleed easily, caused by plaque at the necks of the teeth.

ginglymus (hinge joint) (jing-li-mŭs) *n.* a form of diarthrosis that al-lows angular movement in one plane only. Examples are the knee joint and the elbow joint.

girdle (ger-d'l) *n.* (in anatomy) an encircling or arching arrangement of bones. *See also* pelvic girdle, shoulder girdle.

Girdlestone's operation (ger-d'l-stohnz) *n.* an operation in which the head of the femur and part of the ace-tabulum are removed and a mass of muscle is sutured between the bone ends. It is performed for osteoarthritis. [G. R. Girdlestone (1881–1950), British surgeon]

glabella (glă-bel-ă) *n.* the smooth rounded surface of the frontal bone in the middle of the forehead, be-tween the two eyebrows.

gladiolus (glad-i-oh-lŭs) *n.* the mid-dle and largest segment of the ster-num.

gland (gland) *n.* an organ or group of cells that is specialized for synthe-sizing and secreting certain fluids, either for use in the body or for ex-cretion. *See* endocrine gland, exo-crine gland, secretion.

glanders (equinia) (glan-derz) *n.* an infectious disease of horses, don-keys, and mules that is caused by the bacterium *Pseudomonas mallei* and can be transmitted to humans. Symptoms include fever and in-flammation of the lymph nodes (a form of the disease known as *farcy*), skin, and nasal mucous membranes.

Administration of antibiotics is usually effective.

glandular fever (glan-dew-ler) *n.* an infectious disease, caused by the Epstein-Barr virus, that affects the lymph nodes in the neck, armpits, and groin; it mainly affects adolescents and young adults. Symptoms include swelling and tenderness of the lymph nodes, fever, headache, a sore throat, lethargy, and loss of appetite. Glandular fever is diagnosed by the presence of large numbers of monocytes in the blood. Medical name: **infectious mononucleosis**.

glans (glans penis) (glanz) *n.* the acorn-shaped end part of the penis, formed by the expanded end of the corpus spongiosum. The term glans is also applied to the end of the clitoris.

glare (glair) *n.* the undesirable effects of scattered stray light on the retina, causing reduced contrast and visual performance as well as annoyance and discomfort.

Glasgow scoring system (Glasgow coma scale, GCS) (glahz-goh skor-ing) *n.* a numerical system used to estimate a patient's level of consciousness after head injury. Each of the following are numerically graded: eye opening (1–4), motor response (1–6), and verbal response (1–5). The higher the score, the greater the level of consciousness: a score of 7 indicates a coma.

glatiramer (glǎ-ti-rǎ-mer) *n.* a drug that modifies the body's immune response and is used to reduce the frequency of relapses in people with relapsing/remitting multiple sclerosis. It is administered by subcutaneous injection. Trade name: **Copaxone**.

glaucoma (glaw-koh-mǎ) *n.* a condition in which loss of vision occurs because of an abnormally high pressure in the eye. *angle-closure* (or *acute*) *g.* primary glaucoma in which there is a sudden rise in pressure due to blockage of the angle between the junction of the cornea and sclera and the margin of the iris, where aqueous humour usually drains from the eye. It is accompanied by pain and marked blurring of vision. *open-angle* (or *chronic simple*) *g.* a more common form of primary glaucoma in which the pressure increases gradually, usually without producing pain, and the visual loss is insidious. *primary g.* glaucoma that occurs without any other ocular disease. It is an important cause of blindness. *secondary g.* glaucoma that may occur when other ocular disease impairs the normal circulation of the aqueous humour and causes the intraocular pressure to rise.

Gleason grade (glee-sŏn) *n.* the grade (from one to five) given to an area of prostate cancer, reflecting the level of differentiation of the tumour. Higher grades indicate poorer differentiation. [D. F. Gleason (1920–   ), US pathologist]

Gleason score *n.* a numerical score from two to ten, which is the sum of the two Gleason grades given to the most common and second most common pattern of prostate cancer seen in the tumour. [D. F. Gleason]

gleet (gleet) *n.* a discharge of purulent mucus from the penis or vagina resulting from chronic gonorrhoea.

glenohumeral (glee-noh-hew-mer-ǎl) *adj.* relating to the glenoid cavity and the humerus: the region of the shoulder joint.

glenoid cavity (glenoid fossa) (glee-noid) *n.* the socket of the shoulder joint: the pear-shaped cavity at the top of the scapula into which the head of the humerus fits.

gli- (glio-) *prefix denoting* **1.** glia. **2.** a glutinous substance.

glia (neuroglia) (glee-ă) *n.* the special connective tissue of the central nervous system. Glial cells outnumber the neurones by between five and ten to one, and make up some 40% of the total volume of the brain and spinal cord. —**glial** *adj.*

glibenclamide (gly-ben-klă-myd) *n.* a drug that reduces the level of sugar in the blood and is administered by mouth to treat noninsulin-dependent (type 2) diabetes (*see* sulphonylurea). Trade names: **Daonil, Euglucon.**

gliclazide (gly-klă-zyd) *n.* a sulphonylurea oral hypoglycaemic drug used in the treatment of noninsulin-dependent (type 2) diabetes. Trade name: **Diamicron.**

glioblastoma (gly-oh-blast-oh-mă) *n.* the most aggressive type of brain tumour derived from glial tissue. Its rapid enlargement destroys normal brain cells, with a progressive loss of function, and raises intracranial pressure, causing headache, vomiting, and drowsiness.

glioma (gly-oh-mă) *n.* any tumour of glial cells in the nervous system. The term is sometimes used for all tumours that arise in the central nervous system.

gliomyoma (gly-oh-my-oh-mă) *n.* a tumour composed of nervous and muscular tissue.

glipizide (glip-i-zyd) *n.* a drug used

to control high blood-glucose levels (hyperglycaemia) in patients with noninsulin-dependent diabetes after dietary control has failed (*see* sulphonylurea). It is administered by mouth. Trade names: **Glibenese, Minodiab.**

Glivec (glee-vek) *n. see* imatinib.

globin (gloh-bin) *n.* a polypeptide, found in the body, that can combine with iron-containing haem groups to form haemoglobin and myohaemoglobin.

globulin (glob-yoo-lin) *n.* one of a group of simple proteins that are soluble in dilute salt solutions and can be coagulated by heat. *serum g.* any of the different globulins present in the blood, including gammaglobulins. Some have important functions as antibodies (*see* immunoglobulin). *See also* hormonebinding globulins.

globulinuria (glob-yoo-lin-yoor-iă) *n.* the presence in the urine of globulins.

globus (gloh-bŭs) *n.* a spherical or globe-shaped anatomical structure, such as the *g. pallidus* (*see* basal ganglia). *g. pharyngeus* (formerly *g. hystericus*) the sensation of having a lump in the throat, which is sometimes related to gastro-oesophageal reflux and tends to be worse during stress.

glomangioma (glomus tumour) (gloh-man-ji-oh-mă) *n. see* glomus.

glomerular filtration rate (GFR) (glom-e-roo-ler) *n.* the rate at which substances are filtered from the blood of the glomeruli into the Bowman's capsules of the nephrons. It is calculated by measuring the clearance of specific sub-

glucagon

stances (e.g. creatinine) and is an index of renal function.

glomerulitis (glom-e-roo-ly-tis) *n.* any one of a variety of lesions of the glomeruli associated with acute or chronic kidney disease.

glomerulonephritis (glomerular nephritis, GN) (glom-e-roo-loh-ni-fry-tis) *n.* any of a group of kidney diseases involving the glomeruli (*see* glomerulus), usually thought to be the result of antibody-antigen reactions that localize in the kidneys because of their filtering function. *Acute nephritis* is marked by blood in the urine and fluid and urea retention. It may be related to a recent streptococcal throat infection and usually settles completely, with rapid return of normal kidney function. Other forms of nephritis present with chronic haematuria or with the nephrotic syndrome; children often eventually recover completely, but adults are more likely to progress to *chronic nephritis* and eventual kidney failure.

glomerulus (glom-e-roo-lŭs) *n.* (*pl.* **glomeruli**) **1.** the network of blood capillaries contained within the cuplike end (Bowman's capsule) of a nephron. It is the site of primary filtration of waste products from the blood into the kidney tubule. **2.** any other small rounded mass. —**glomerular** *adj.*

glomus (gloh-mŭs) *n.* (*pl.* **glomera**) a small communication between a tiny artery and a vein that is well supplied with sensory receptors. For example, glomera in the skin of the limbs are concerned with temperature regulation. *g. jugulare* a collection of paraganglion cells in close relation to the internal jugular

vein at its origin at the base of the skull.

glomus tumour *n.* **1.** a benign tumour arising from paraganglion cells of the vagus nerve in the neck (*see* paraganglioma). In the middle ear they are called *glomus tympanicum tumours*; around the jugular vein they are called *glomus jugulare tumours*. **2.** (**glomangioma**) a harmless but often painful tumour produced by malformation and overgrowth of a glomus, usually in the skin at the ends of the fingers or toes.

gloss- (glosso-) *prefix denoting* the tongue.

glossa (glos-ă) *n. see* tongue.

glossectomy (glos-ek-tŏmi) *n.* surgical removal of the tongue, an operation usually carried out for cancer in this structure.

glossitis (glos-I-tis) *n.* inflammation of the tongue.

glossodynia (glos-oh-**din**-iă) *n.* pain in the tongue.

glossopharyngeal nerve (glos-oh-fa-rin-**jee**-ăl) *n.* the ninth cranial nerve (IX), which supplies motor fibres to part of the pharynx and to the parotid salivary glands and sensory fibres to the posterior third of the tongue and the soft palate.

glossoplegia (glos-oh-**plee**-jiă) *n.* paralysis of the tongue.

glottis (glot-iss) *n.* the space between the two vocal folds. The term is often applied to the vocal folds themselves or to that part of the larynx associated with the production of sound.

gluc- (gluco-) *prefix denoting* glucose.

glucagon (gloo-kă-gon) *n.* a hormone, produced by the pancreas, that causes an increase in the blood sugar level. Glucagon is administered by injection to counteract diabetic hypoglycaemia.

glucagonoma (gloo-kǎ-gŏn-oh-mǎ) *n.* a pancreatic tumour that secretes glucagon and produces attacks of hypoglycaemia.

glucagon stimulation test *n.* a test for phaeochromocytomas not displaying typically high levels of plasma catecholamines. An intravenous bolus of glucagon is administered and the test is positive when there is a threefold increase in plasma catecholamine levels with a consequent rise in blood pressure.

glucocorticoid (gloo-koh-**kor**-ti-koid) *n.* any of a group of corticosteroids, including cortisone, that are essential for the utilization of carbohydrate, fat, and protein by the body. Naturally occurring and synthetic glucocorticoids have very powerful anti-inflammatory effects.

gluconeogenesis (gloo-koh-nee-oh-jen-i-sis) *n.* the biochemical process in which glucose is synthesized from non-carbohydrate sources, such as amino acids, when carbohydrate is not available in sufficient amounts in the diet.

glucose (dextrose) (gloo-kohz) *n.* a simple sugar containing six carbon atoms (a hexose). Glucose, an important source of energy, is one of the constituents of both sucrose and starch, both of which yield glucose after digestion. It is stored in the body in the form of glycogen. If the blood-glucose concentration falls below the normal level of around 5 mmol/l, neurological and other symptoms may result (*see* hypoglycaemia). If the blood-glucose level is

raised to 10 mmol/l, the condition of hyperglycaemia develops. This is a symptom of diabetes mellitus.

glucose-6-phosphate dehydrogenase deficiency *n.* a hereditary (X-linked) condition in which absence of the enzyme glucose-6-phosphate dehydrogenase (G6PD), which functions in carbohydrate metabolism, results in haemolysis, usually after exposure to oxidants (such as drugs) or infections. *See also* favism.

glucose tolerance test (oral glucose tolerance test) *n.* the standard diagnostic test for diabetes mellitus and the related condition, *impaired glucose tolerance* (IGT). Blood-sugar levels are measured after an overnight fast and again after oral administration of 75 g glucose. Diabetes is diagnosed if the fasting level is above 7.0 mmol/l and/or the two-hour level is above 11.1 mmol/l. IGT is diagnosed when the fasting level is below 7.0 mmol/l and the two-hour level is between 7.0 mmol/l and 11.1 mmol/l.

glucoside (gloo-koh-syd) *n. see* glycoside.

glucuronic acid (gloo-kewr-on-ik) *n.* a sugar acid derived from glucose. Glucuronic acid is an important constituent of chondroitin sulphate (found in cartilage) and hyaluronic acid (found in synovial fluid).

glue ear (gloo) *n.* a common condition in which viscous fluid accumulates in the middle ear, causing deafness. It is most frequently seen in children and is due to a malfunctioning of the Eustachian tube. Many cases resolve spontaneously; treatment, if required, consists of surgical incision of the eardrum (myringotomy), drainage of the fluid, and insertion of a grommet. Medical names: **otitis media with effusion, secretory otitis media**.

glutamic acid (glutamate) (gloo-**tam**-ik) *n. see* amino acid.

glutamic acid decarboxylase (GAD) *n.* a common enzyme that can provoke an autoimmune reaction against the beta cells of the pancreas progressing to type 1 diabetes mellitus.

glutamic oxaloacetic transaminase (GOT) *n. see* aspartate aminotransferase (AST).

glutamic pyruvic transaminase (GPT) *n. see* alanine aminotransferase (ALT).

glutaminase (gloo-tam-in-ayz) *n.* an enzyme, found in the kidney, that catalyses the breakdown of the amino acid glutamine to ammonia and glutamic acid: a stage in the production of urea.

glutamine (gloo-tă-meen) *n. see* amino acid.

gluten (gloo-těn) *n.* a mixture of the two proteins *gliadin* and *glutenin*. Gluten is present in wheat and rye and is important for its baking properties. Sensitivity to gluten leads to coeliac disease in children.

gluteus (gloo-tee-ŭs) *n.* one of three paired muscles of the buttocks (*g. maximus, g. medius,* and *g. minimus*). They are responsible for movements of the thigh. —**gluteal** *adj.*

glyc- (glyco-) *prefix denoting* sugar.

glycerin (glycerol) (glis-er-in) *n.* a clear viscous liquid obtained by hydrolysis of fats and mixed oils and produced as a by-product in the manufacture of soap. It is used as

an emollient in many skin preparations, as a laxative (particularly in the form of suppositories), and as a sweetening agent in the pharmaceutical industry.

glyceryl trinitrate (GTN, nitroglycerin) (glis-er-il try-ny-trayt) *n.* a drug that dilates blood vessels and is used to prevent and treat angina (*see* vasodilator). It is administered as tablets, a mouth spray, ointment, skin patches, or an injection. Trade names: **Glytrin Spray, Nitrolingual Pumpspray, Sustac, Transiderm-Nitro**.

glycine (gly-seen) *n. see* amino acid.

glycocholic acid (gly-koh-kol-ik) *n. see* bile acids.

glycogen (gly-koh-jěn) *n.* a carbohydrate consisting of branched chains of glucose units. Glycogen is the principal form in which carbohydrate is stored in the body (in liver and muscles); it may be readily broken down to glucose.

glycogenesis (gly-koh-jen-i-sis) *n.* the biochemical process, occurring chiefly in the liver and in muscle, by which glucose is converted into glycogen.

glycogenolysis (gly-koh-jě-nol-i-sis) *n.* a biochemical process, occurring chiefly in the liver and in muscle, by which glycogen is broken down into glucose.

glycolysis (gly-kol-i-sis) *n.* the conversion of glucose, by a series of ten enzyme-catalysed reactions, to lactic acid, with the production of energy in the form of ATP.

glycoprotein (gly-koh-proh-teen) *n.* one of a group of compounds consisting of a protein combined with a carbohydrate (such as galactose or mannose). Examples of glycoproteins are certain enzymes, hormones, and antigens.

glycoside (gly-koh-syd) *n.* a compound formed by replacing the hydroxyl group (–OH) of a sugar by another group. (If the sugar is glucose the compound is known as a *glucoside*.) Glycosides found in plants include some pharmacologically important products (such as digitalis).

glycosuria (gly-kohs-yoor-iă) *n.* the presence of glucose in the urine in abnormally large amounts. Glycosuria may be associated with diabetes mellitus, kidney disease, and some other conditions.

GN *n. see* glomerulonephritis.

gnath- (gnatho-) *prefix denoting* the jaw.

gnathoplasty (nath-oh-plasti) *n.* plastic surgery of the jaw.

GnRH *n. see* gonadotrophin-releasing hormone.

GnRH analogue *n. see* LHRH analogue.

goal (gohl) *n.* a statement of what the nursing intervention is intended to achieve, usually expressed in terms of the patient's expected behaviour. *See* behavioural objective, expected outcome.

goblet cell (gob-lit) *n.* a column-shaped secretory cell found in the epithelium of the respiratory and intestinal tracts. Goblet cells secrete the principal constituents of mucus.

goitre (goi-ter) *n.* a swelling of the neck due to enlargement of the thyroid gland. This may be due to lack of dietary iodine, which is necessary for the production of thyroid hormone: the gland enlarges in an attempt to increase the output of hormone. Autoimmune thyroiditis can be associated with goitre (see

Hashimoto's disease). *exophthalmic g.* (*Graves' disease*) *see* thyrotoxicosis. *sporadic g.* goitre due to simple overgrowth (hyperplasia) of the gland or to a tumour.

goitrogen (goi-troh-jen) *n.* any substance that causes goitre. —**goitrogenic** *adj.*

gold (gohld) *n.* (in pharmacology) any of several compounds of the metal gold, used in the treatment of rheumatoid arthritis. *Sodium aurothiomalate* (*Myocrisin*) is administered by intramuscular injection. *See also* auranofin.

Goldmann applanation tonometer (gohld-măn) *n. see* tonometer. [H. Goldmann (1899– 1991), Swiss ophthalmologist]

golfer's elbow (golf-erz) *n.* inflammation of the origin of the common flexor tendon on the medial epicondyle of the humerus, caused by overuse of the forearm muscles. Treatment is by rest, anti-inflammatory medication, or steroid injection. *Compare* tennis elbow.

Golgi apparatus (gol-ji) *n.* a collection of vesicles and folded membranes in a cell. It stores and later transports the proteins manufactured in the endoplasmic reticulum. [C. Golgi (1844–1926), Italian histologist]

Golgi cells *pl. n.* types of neurones (nerve cells) within the central nervous system. *Golgi type I neurones* have very long axons that connect different parts of the system; *Golgi type II neurones* have only short axons or sometimes none.

gomphosis (gom-foh-sis) *n.* a form of synarthrosis (immovable joint) in which a conical process fits into a socket.

gonad (goh-nad) *n.* a male or female reproductive organ, which produces the gametes. *See* ovary, testis.

gonadarche (goh-năd-ar-ki) *n.* the period during which the gonads begin to secrete sex hormones, so triggering puberty. The timing for this event is controlled by the pituitary gland; gonadarche occurs usually between the ages of 10 and 11 in girls and 11 and 12 in boys.

gonadorelin (gon-ă-doh-rel-in) *n.* a synthetic analogue of gonadotrophin-releasing hormone (*see* LHRH analogue), administered by intravenous injection to stimulate the production of pituitary gonadotrophins. It is used in the treatment of amenorrhoea and certain types of infertility.

gonadotrophin (gonadotrophic hormone) (gon-ă-doh-troh-fin) *n.* any of several hormones synthesized and released by the pituitary gland, such as follicle-stimulating hormone and luteinizing hormone, that act on the gonads to promote production of sex hormones and either sperm or ova. *See also* human chorionic gonadotrophin.

gonadotrophin-releasing hormone (GnRH) *n.* a peptide hormone produced in the hypothalamus and transported via the bloodstream to the pituitary gland, where it controls the synthesis and release of other hormones, the pituitary gonadotrophins. *GnRH analogue see* LHRH analogue.

gonagra (gon-ag-ră) *n.* gout in the knee.

goni- (gonio-) *prefix denoting* an anatomical angle or corner.

goniopuncture (goh-ni-oh-punk-cher) *n.* a rarely performed operation for congenital glaucoma (*see* buphthalmos) to enable fluid to be drawn from the eye. *See* goniotomy.

gonioscope (goh-ni-oh-skohp) *n.* a special lens used for viewing the structures around the edge of the anterior chamber of the eye (in front of the iris).

goniotomy (trabeculotomy) (goh-ni-ot-ŏmi) *n.* an operation for congenital glaucoma (*see* buphthalmos) in which a fine knife is used to make an incision into Schlemm's canal from within the eye. It is the first stage of goniopuncture.

gonococcus (gon-oh-kok-ŭs) *n.* (*pl.* **gonococci**) the causative agent of gonorrhoea: the bacterium *Neisseria gonorrhoeae*. —**gonococcal** *adj.*

gonocyte (gon-oh-syt) *n. see* germ cell.

gonorrhoea (gon-ŏ-ree-ă) *n.* a sexually transmitted disease, caused by the bacterium *Neisseria gonorrhoeae*, that affects the genital mucous membranes of either sex. Symptoms include pain on passing urine and discharge of gleet. In untreated cases, the infection may spread throughout the reproductive system, causing sterility; severe inflammation of the urethra in men can cause stricture. If a pregnant woman has gonorrhoea, her baby may contract ophthalmia neonatorum. Later complications can include arthritis, endocarditis, and infection of the eyes, causing conjunctivitis. Treatment with ciprofloxacin, ofloxacin, or cefotaxime is usually effective. —**gonorrhoeal** *adj.*

Goodpasture's syndrome (guud-pas-cherz) *n.* a haemorrhagic lung disorder, resulting in the coughing up of blood, associated with glomerulonephritis. [E. W. Goodpasture (1886–1960), US pathologist]

goose flesh *n.* the reaction of the skin to cold or fear. The blood vessels contract and the small muscle attached to the base of each hair follicle also contracts, causing the hairs to stand up: this gives the skin an appearance of plucked goose skin.

GOR *n.* see gastro-oesophageal reflux.

Gordh needle (gord) *n.* an intravenous needle with an expanded base containing a rubber diaphragm, used to administer repeated injections. [T. Gordh, Swedish anaesthetist]

gorget (gor-jit) *n.* an instrument formerly used in the operation for removal of stones from the bladder. It is a director or guide with a wide groove.

goserelin (gos-ĕ-rel-in) *n.* see LHRH analogue.

gouge (gowj) *n.* a curved chisel used in orthopaedic operations to cut and remove bone.

A gouge

gout (gowt) *n.* a disease in which a defect in purine metabolism causes an excess of uric acid and its salts (urates) to accumulate in the bloodstream and the joints respectively. It results in attacks of acute gouty arthritis and chronic destruction of the joints and deposits of urates

(tophi) in the skin and cartilage, especially of the ears. Treatment with uricosuric drugs or allopurinol can control the disease; acute attacks are treated with anti-inflammatory analgesics. *See also* podagra.

GPI *n.* see general paralysis of the insane.

Graafian follicle (grah-fi-ăn) *n.* a mature follicle in the ovary prior to ovulation, containing a large fluid-filled cavity that distends the surface of the ovary. The oocyte develops inside the follicle, attached to one side. [R. de Graaf (1641–73), Dutch physician and anatomist]

graded self-exposure (gray-did self-iks-**poh**-zher) *n.* a technique used in the behaviour therapy of phobias. A hierarchy of fears (increasingly fearful stimuli) is set up and the patients expose themselves to each level of the hierarchy in turn. Exposure continues until habituation occurs before proceeding to the next highest level of the hierarchy. The patient is then ultimately able to cope with the feared object or situation.

Graefe's knife (gray-fiz) *n.* a knife with a narrow sharply pointed blade, used in operations for the removal of cataract. [A. von Graefe (1928–70), German ophthalmologist]

graft (grahft) **1.** *n.* any organ, tissue, or object used for transplantation to replace a faulty part of the body. *bone g.* healthy bone used to fill a defect in a bone or to stimulate fracture healing. *corneal g. see* keratoplasty. *See also* skin (graft), transplantation. **2.** *vb.* to transplant an organ or tissue.

graft-versus-host **disease** **(GVHD)** *n.* a condition that occurs following bone marrow transplantation and sometimes blood transfusion, in which lymphocytes from the graft attack specific tissues in the host. The skin, gut, and liver are the most severely affected. Drugs that suppress the immune reaction (such as steroids and ciclosporin) and antibodies directed against lymphocytes reduce the severity of the tissue damage.

grain (grayn) *n.* a unit of mass equal to 1/7000 of a pound (avoirdupois). 1 grain = 0.0648 gram.

gram (gram) *n.* a unit of mass equal to one thousandth of a kilogram. Symbol: g.

-gram *suffix denoting a record; tracing.*

gramicidin (gram-i-sy-din) *n.* an antibiotic that acts against a wide range of bacteria. It is usually used in combination with other antibiotics or steroids in topical preparations for the treatment of skin, ear, and eye infections.

Gram's stain (gramz) *n.* a method of staining bacterial cells, used as a primary means of identification. The bacterial cells are stained with a violet dye, treated with decolorizer (e.g. alcohol), and then counterstained with red dye. *Gram-negative* bacteria lose the initial stain but take up the counterstain, so that they appear red microscopically. *Gram-positive* bacteria retain the initial stain, appearing violet microscopically. [H. C. J. Gram (1853–1938), Danish physician]

grand mal (major epilepsy) (gron mal) *n. see* epilepsy.

grand multiparity (grand multi-pa-riti) *n.* the condition of a woman who has had six or more previous pregnancies. Such women are more prone to the accidents of labour and to some of the diseases of pregnancy.

granular cast (gran-yoo-ler) *n.* a cellular cast derived from a kidney tubule. Such casts are shed from the kidney in certain kidney diseases, notably acute glomerulonephritis. Their presence in the urine indicates continued activity of the disease.

granulation (gran-yoo-**lay**-shŏn) *n.* the formation of a multicellular mass of tissue (*g. tissue*) in response to an injury: this is an essential part of the healing process. The tissue contains many new blood vessels and many fibroblasts.

granulocyte (gran-yoo-loh-syt) *n.* any of a group of white blood cells that contain granules in their cytoplasm. They can be subclassified into neutrophils, eosinophils, and basophils.

granulocytopenia (gran-yoo-loh-sy-toh-**pee**-niă) *n.* a reduction in the number of granulocytes in the blood. *See* neutropenia.

granuloma (gran-yoo-loh-mă) *n.* (*pl.* **granulomata** or **granulomas**) a localized collection of cells, produced in response to chronic infection, inflammation, or a foreign body, that is characterized by the presence of epithelioid histiocytes. *g. annulare* a chronic skin condition, of unknown cause, in which there is a ring or rings of closely set papules, principally on the hands and arms. If generalized, it may be associated with diabetes mellitus. *g. inguinale* a sexually transmitted disease caused by the bacterium *Calymmatobacterium granulomatis*, marked by a pimply rash on and around the genital organs, which develops into a granulomatous ulcer. *See also* pyogenic (granuloma). —**granulomatous** *adj.*

granulomatosis (gran-yoo-loh-mă-toh-sis) *n.* any condition marked by multiple widespread granulomata. *See also* Wegener's granulomatosis.

granulopoiesis (gran-yoo-loh-poi-ee-sis) *n.* the process of production of granulocytes, which normally occurs in the blood-forming tissue of the bone marrow. *See also* haemopoiesis.

graph- (**grapho-**) *prefix denoting* handwriting.

-graph *suffix denoting* an instrument that records.

grattage (grat-ahzh) *n.* the process of brushing or scraping the surface of a slowly healing ulcer or wound to remove granulation tissue, which may delay healing.

gravel (grav-ĕl) *n.* small stones formed in the urinary tract. The passage of gravel from the kidneys is usually associated with severe pain (ureteric colic) and may cause blood in the urine. *See also* calculus.

Graves' disease (exophthalmic goitre) (grayvz) *n. see* thyrotoxicosis. [R. J. Graves (1797– 1853), Irish physician]

gravid (grav-id) *adj.* pregnant.

Grawitz tumour (grah-vits) *n. see* hypernephroma. [P. A. Grawitz (1850–1932), German pathologist]

gray (gray) *n.* the SI unit of absorbed dose of ionizing radiation, being the absorbed dose when the energy per unit mass imparted to matter by ionizing radiation is 1 joule per kilogram. It has replaced the rad. Symbol: Gy.

green monkey disease *n. see* Marburg disease.

greenstick fracture (green-stik) *n. see* fracture.

grey matter (gray) *n.* the darker coloured tissues of the central nervous system, composed mainly of the cell bodies of neurones, branching dendrites, and glial cells. *Compare* white matter.

Grey Turner sign (gray ter-ner) *n.* a bluish bruiselike appearance around the flanks, which is seen in acute pancreatitis. [G. Grey Turner (1877–1951), British surgeon]

Griffith's types (grif-iths) *pl. n.* subdivisions of Lancefield group A streptococci (*see* Lancefield classification) on the basis of their agglutination reactions. [F. Griffith (1877– 1941), British bacteriologist]

gripe (gryp) *n.* severe abdominal pain (*see* colic).

griseofulvin (griz-i-oh-ful-vin) *n.* an antibiotic administered by mouth to treat fungal infections of the hair, skin, and nails, such as ringworm. Trade names: **Fulcin**, **Grisovin**.

grocer's itch (groh-serz) *n.* dermatitis of the hands caused by frequent contact with flour and sugar.

groin (groin) *n.* the external depression on the front of the body that marks the junction of the abdomen with either of the thighs. *See also* inguinal.

ground substance (grownd) *n. see* connective tissue.

group practice (groop) *n.* a partnership of two or more general practitioners who share such resources as premises and administrative and nursing staff. The premises from which they operate may be privately owned or a publicly owned health centre.

group therapy *n.* **1. (group psychotherapy)** psychotherapy involving at least two patients and a therapist. The patients are encouraged to understand and analyse their own and one another's problems. *See also* encounter group, psychodrama. **2.** therapy in which people with the same problem, such as alcoholism, meet and discuss together their difficulties and possible ways of overcoming them.

growth factor (grohth) *n.* a polypeptide that is produced by cells and stimulates them to proliferate. Some may be involved in the abnormal regulation of growth seen in cancer.

growth hormone (GH, somatotrophin) *n.* a hormone, synthesized and stored in the anterior pituitary gland, that promotes growth of the long bones in the limbs and increases protein synthesis (via somatomedin). Its release is controlled by the opposing actions of *growth-hormone releasing hormone* and somatostatin.

GSI *n. see* (genuine stress) incontinence.

GTN *n. see* glyceryl trinitrate.

guanethidine (gwahn-eth-i-deen) *n.* a drug that is administered by mouth to reduce high blood pressure (*see* sympatholytic). Trade name: **Ismelin**.

guanine (gwah-neen) *n.* one of the nitrogen-containing bases (*see* purine) that occurs in the nucleic acids DNA and RNA.

gubernaculum (gew-ber-**nak**-yoo-lŭm) *n.* (*pl.* **gubernacula**) either of a pair of fibrous strands of tissue

that connect the gonads to the inguinal region in the fetus.

Guillain-Barré syndrome (postinfective polyneuropathy) (gee-yan ba-ray) *n.* a disease of the peripheral nerves in which there is numbness and weakness in the limbs. It usually develops 10–20 days after a respiratory or gastrointestinal infection that provokes an allergic response in the peripheral nerves. [G. Guillain (1876–1961) and A. Barré (1880–1967), French neurologists]

guillotine (gil-ŏ-teen) *n.* **1.** a surgical instrument used for removing the tonsils. **2.** an encircling suture to control the escape of fluid or blood from an orifice or to close a gap.

A tonsil guillotine

guinea worm (ginn-i) *n.* a parasitic nematode worm, *Dracunculus medinensis*. The adult female lives in the connective tissues beneath the skin and releases its larvae into a large blister on the legs or arms. *See also* dracontiasis.

Gulf War syndrome (gulf wor) *n.* a variety of symptoms, mainly neurological (including chronic fatigue, dizziness, amnesia, digestive upsets, and muscle wasting), that have been attributed to exposure of armed forces personnel to chemicals (e.g. insecticides) used during the Gulf War (1991) or possibly to the effects of vaccines and tablets given to protect personnel against the anticipated threat of chemical and biological warfare during the conflict.

gullet (gul-it) *n. see* oesophagus.

gum (gum) *n.* (in anatomy) *see* gingiva.

GUM *n. see* genitourinary (medicine).

gumboil (gum-boil) *n.* the opening on the surface of the gum of a tract from a chronic abscess associated with the roots of a tooth. It may be accompanied by varying degrees of swelling, pain, and discharge.

gumma (gum-ă) *n.* a small soft tumour, characteristic of the tertiary stage of syphilis, that occurs in connective tissue, the liver, brain, testes, heart, or bone.

GUS *n.* genitourinary system. *See* genitourinary.

gustation (gus-tay-shŏn) *n.* the sense of taste or the act of tasting.

gustatory (gus-tă-ter-i) *adj.* relating to the sense of taste or to the organs of taste.

gut (gut) *n.* **1.** *see* intestine. **2.** *see* catgut.

Guthrie test (guth-ri) *n.* a blood test performed on all newborn babies at the end of the first week of life. It can detect several inborn errors of metabolism (including phenylketonuria), hypothyroidism, and cystic fibrosis (the last is not routinely offered). [R. Guthrie (1916–), US paediatrician]

gutta (gut-ă) *n.* (*pl.* **guttae**) (in pharmacy) a drop. Drops are the form in which many medicines are applied to the eyes and ears.

gutta-percha (gut-ă-per-chă) *n.* the juice of an evergreen Malaysian tree, which is hard at room temperature but becomes soft and elastic when heated in hot water. On cooling gutta-percha will retain any deformity imparted to it when hot; it is used in dentistry.

gutter splint (gut-er) *n.* a splint formed from a casting material, moulded to conform to the shape of the limb but not encircling it, in which the limb rests as in a gutter.

GVHD *n. see* graft-versus-host disease.

gyn- (gyno-, gynaec(o)-) *prefix* denoting women or the female reproductive organs.

gynaecology (gy-ni-kol-ŏji) *n.* the study of diseases of women and girls, particularly those affecting the female reproductive system. *Compare* obstetrics. —**gynaecological** *adj.* —**gynaecologist** *n.*

gynaecomastia (gy-ni-koh-mas-tiă) *n.* enlargement of the breasts in the male, due either to hormone imbalance or to hormone therapy.

gypsum (jip-sŭm) *n. see* plaster of Paris.

gyr- (gyro-) *prefix denoting* **1.** a gyrus. **2.** a ring or circle.

gyrus (jy-rŭs) *n.* (*pl.* **gyri**) a raised convolution of the cerebral cortex, between two sulci (clefts).

H *symbol for* hydrogen.

habit (hab-it) *n.* a constant, almost automatic, practice acquired by frequent repetition. **h. training** teaching psychiatric patients to relearn habits of personal hygiene by repetition and encouragement.

habitual abortion (hǎ-bit-yoo-ǎl) *n. see* abortion.

habituation (hǎ-bit-yoo-**ay**-shŏn) *n.*
1. (in psychology) a simple form of learning consisting of a gradual waning response by the subject to a continuous or repeated stimulus that is not associated with reinforcement. **2.** (in pharmacology) the condition of being psychologically dependent on a drug, following repeated consumption. It is marked by reduced sensitivity to its effects and a craving for the drug if it is withdrawn. *See also* dependence.

haem (heem) *n.* an iron-containing compound (a porphyrin) that combines with the protein globin to form haemoglobin.

haem- (haema-, haemo-, haemat(o)-) *prefix denoting* blood.

haemagglutination (heem-ǎ-gloo-tin-**ay**-shŏn) *n.* the clumping of red blood cells (*see* agglutination). It is caused by an antibody–antigen reaction of some viruses and other substances.

haemangioma (heem-an-ji-oh-mǎ) *n.* a benign tumour of blood vessels. It often appears on the skin as a type of birthmark (*see* naevus). *See also* angioma.

haemarthrosis (heem-arth-**roh**-sis) *n.* joint pain and swelling caused by bleeding into a joint. This may follow injury or may occur spontaneously in a disease of the blood, such as haemophilia.

haematemesis (heem-ǎ-tem-i-sis) *n.* the act of vomiting blood. The blood may have been swallowed but more often arises from bleeding in the oesophagus, stomach, or duodenum. Common causes are gastric and duodenal ulcers and oesophageal varices (varicose veins).

haematin (heem-ǎ-tin) *n.* a chemical derivative of haemoglobin formed by removal of the protein part of the molecule and oxidation of the iron atom from the ferrous to the ferric form.

haematinic (heem-ǎ-**tin**-ik) *n.* a drug that increases the amount of haemoglobin in the blood, e.g. ferrous sulphate and other iron-containing compounds. Haematinics are administered to prevent and treat anaemia due to iron deficiency, particularly during pregnancy.

haematocele (heem-ǎ-toh-seel) *n.* a swelling caused by leakage of blood into a cavity, especially that of the membrane overlying the front and sides of the testis. *parametric (pelvic) h.* a swelling near the uterus formed by the escape of blood, usually from a Fallopian tube in ectopic pregnancy.

haematocolpos (heem-ă-toh-**kol**-pos) *n.* the accumulation of menstrual blood in the vagina because the hymen lacks an opening. *See* cryptomenorrhoea.

haematocrit (heem-ă-toh-krit) *n. see* packed cell volume.

haematocyst (heem-ă-toh-sist) *n.* a cyst containing blood.

haematogenous (haematogenic) (heem-ă-toj-in-ŭs) *adj.* **1.** relating to the production of blood or its constituents. **2.** produced by, originating in, or carried by the blood.

haematology (heem-ă-**tol**-ŏji) *n.* the study of blood and blood-forming tissues and the disorders associated with them. —**haematological** (heem-ă-tŏ-**loj**-ik-ăl) *adj.* —**haematologist** *n.*

haematoma (heem-ă-**toh**-mă) *n.* an accumulation of blood within the tissues that clots to form a solid swelling. Injury, disease of the blood vessels, or a clotting disorder of the blood are the usual causative factors. *extradural h.* a haematoma caused by tearing of the middle meningeal artery, as a result of injury to the head. *intracerebral h.* a haematoma caused by bleeding into the brain resulting either from atherosclerosis of the cerebral arteries and high blood pressure or from severe head injury. *subdural h.* (SDH) a haematoma caused by tearing of the veins where they cross the space beneath the dura. *See also* perianal haematoma.

haematometra (heem-ă-toh-mee-tră) *n.* **1.** accumulation of menstrual blood in the uterus. **2.** abnormally copious bleeding in the uterus.

haematomyelia (heem-ă-toh-my-ee-liă) *n.* bleeding into the tissue of the spinal cord.

haematopoiesis (heem-ă-toh-poi-ee-sis) *n. see* haemopoiesis.

haematoporphyrin (heem-ă-toh-por-fi-rin) *n.* a type of porphyrin produced during the metabolism of haemoglobin.

haematosalpinx (haemosalpinx) (heem-ă-toh-sal-pinks) *n.* the accumulation of menstrual blood in the Fallopian tubes.

haematoxylin (heem-ă-**toks**-i-lin) *n.* a colourless crystalline compound extracted from logwood (*Haematoxylon campechianum*) and used in various histological stains.

haematozoon (heem-ă-toh-**zoh**-on) *n.* (*pl.* **haematozoa**) any animal parasite living in the blood.

haematuria (heem-a-**tewr**-ia) *n.* the passage of blood in the urine, which may be detected by the naked eye (*frank h.*), urine microscopy (*microscopic h.*), or urinalysis sticks ('*dipstix*' *h.*). Haematuria is associated with transitional cell carcinoma (the most common form of bladder cancer), kidney cancer, urinary-tract infections, stone disease, and some forms of glomerulonephritis.

haemin (heem-in) *n.* a chemical derivative of haemoglobin formed by removal of the protein part of the molecule, oxidation of the iron atom, and combination with an acid to form a salt. *Compare* haematin.

haemo- *prefix. see* haem-.

haemochromatosis (bronze diabetes, iron-storage disease) (heem-ŏ-kroh-mă-**toh**-sis) *n.*

a hereditary (autosomal recessive) disorder in which there is excessive absorption and storage of iron. This leads to damage of many organs, including the liver, pancreas, and endocrine glands. The main features are a bronze colour of the skin, diabetes, and liver failure. *Compare* haemosiderosis.

haemoconcentration (hee-moh-kon-sĕn-**tray**-shŏn) *n*. an increase in the proportion of red blood cells relative to the plasma, brought about by a decrease in the volume of plasma or an increase in the concentration of circulating red blood cells (*see* polycythaemia). *Compare* haemodilution.

haemocytometer (hee-moh-sy-**tom**-it-er) *n*. a special glass chamber of known volume into which diluted blood is introduced. The numbers of the various blood cells present are then counted visually, through a microscope.

haemodialysis (hee-moh-dy-**al**-i-sis) *n*. a technique of removing waste materials or poisons from the blood using the principle of dialysis. Haemodialysis is performed on patients whose kidneys have ceased to function; the process takes place in a *dialyser*.

haemodilution (hee-moh-dy-**lew**-shŏn) *n*. a decrease in the proportion of red blood cells relative to the plasma, brought about by an increase in the total volume of plasma. *Compare* haemoconcentration.

haemoglobin (Hb) (hee-moh-**gloh**-bin) *n*. a substance contained within the red blood cells (erythrocytes) and responsible for their colour, composed of the pigment haem linked to the protein globin. Haemo-globin is the medium by which oxygen is transported within the body. Blood normally contains 12–18 g/dl of haemoglobin. *See also* myo-haemoglobin, oxyhaemoglobin.

haemoglobinaemia (heem-ŏ-gloh-bin-ee-miǎ) *n*. the presence of haemoglobin in the blood plasma.

haemoglobinometer (heem-ŏ-gloh-bin-om-it-er) *n*. an instrument for determining the concentration of haemoglobin in a sample of blood.

haemoglobinopathy (heem-ŏ-gloh-bin-**op**-ǎ-thi) *n*. any of a group of inherited diseases, including thalassaemia and sickle-cell disease, in which there is an abnormality in the production of haemoglobin.

haemoglobinuria (heem-ŏ-gloh-bin-**yoor**-iǎ) *n*. the presence in the urine of free haemoglobin. The condition sometimes follows strenuous exercise. It is also associated with certain infectious diseases, ingestion of certain chemicals, and injury.

haemogram (hee-moh-gram) *n*. the results of a routine blood test, including an estimate of the blood haemoglobin level, packed cell volume, and blood count.

haemolysin (hi-mol-i-sin) *n*. *see* lysin.

haemolysis (hi-mol-i-sis) *n*. the destruction of red blood cells (erythrocytes). Within the body, haemolysis may result from poisoning, infection, or the action of antibodies; it may occur in mismatched blood transfusions. It usually leads to anaemia. *See also* laking.

haemolytic (hee-moh-**lit**-ik) *adj*. causing, associated with, or resulting from destruction of red blood cells (erythrocytes). *h. anaemia see* anaemia.

haemolytic disease of the newborn *n.* the condition resulting from destruction (haemolysis) of the red blood cells of the fetus by antibodies in the mother's blood passing through the placenta. This most commonly happens when the red blood cells of the fetus are Rh positive (*see* rhesus factor) but the mother's red cells are Rh negative. The fetal cells are therefore incompatible in her circulation and evoke the production of antibodies. This may result in very severe anaemia of the fetus or severe jaundice after birth. A blood test early in pregnancy enables the detection of antibodies in the mother's blood and the adoption of various precautions for the infant's safety. *See also* anti D.

haemolytic uraemic syndrome (HUS) *n.* a condition in which sudden rapid destruction of red blood cells (*see* haemolysis) causes acute renal failure due partly to obstruction of small arteries in the kidneys. The haemolysis also causes a reduction in the number of platelets, which can lead to severe haemorrhage. The syndrome may occur as a result of septicaemia following a respiratory or gastrointestinal infection (especially by pathogenic *Escherichia coli*), eclamptic fits in pregnancy (*see* eclampsia), or as a reaction to certain drugs.

haemopericardium (heem-ŏ-pe-ri-**kar**-diŭm) *n.* the presence of blood within the pericardium, which may result from injury, tumours, rupture of the heart, or a leaking aneurysm.

haemoperitoneum (heem-ŏ-pe-ri-

tŏn-ee-ŭm) *n.* the presence of blood in the peritoneal cavity, between the lining of the abdomen or pelvis and the membrane covering the organs within.

haemophilia (hee-moh-**fil**-iǎ) *n.* a hereditary disorder in which the blood clots very slowly, due to a deficiency of either of two coagulation factors: Factor VIII (antihaemophilic factor), causing *haemophilia A*; or Factor IX (Christmas factor), causing *haemophilia B* (Christmas disease). Prolonged bleeding follows any injury or wound, and in severe cases there is spontaneous bleeding into muscles and joints. Bleeding in haemophilia may be treated by administration of recombinant-DNA-derived Factor VIII or concentrated freeze-dried Factor VIII or Factor IX. Haemophilia is almost exclusively restricted to males: women can carry the disease without being affected themselves. —**haemophiliac** *n.* —**haemophilic** *adj.*

Haemophilus (hi-**mof**-i-lǔs) *n.* a genus of Gram-negative aerobic nonmotile parasitic rodlike bacteria frequently found in the respiratory tract. Most species are pathogenic. *H. influenzae* a species associated with acute and chronic respiratory infections: a common secondary cause of influenza infections and a primary cause of bacterial meningitis.

haemophthalmia (heem-off-**thal**-miǎ) *n.* bleeding into the vitreous humour of the eye: vitreous haemorrhage.

haemopneumothorax (heem-ŏ-new-moh-**thor**-aks) *n.* the presence of blood and air in the pleural cavity, usually as a result of injury. *See also* haemothorax.

haemopoiesis (haemato-poiesis) (hee-moh-poi-ee-sis) *n*. the process of production of blood cells and platelets which continues throughout life, replacing aged cells (which are removed from the circulation). In healthy adults, haemopoiesis is confined to the bone marrow. *See also* erythropoiesis, leucopoiesis, thrombopoiesis. —**haemopoietic** *adj*.

haemopoietin (hee-moh-poi-ee-tin) *n. see* erythropoietin.

haemoptysis (hi-mop-ti-sis) *n*. the coughing up of blood.

haemorrhage (bleeding) (hem-er-ij) *n*. the escape of blood from a ruptured blood vessel, externally or internally. Arterial blood is bright red and emerges in spurts, venous blood is dark red and flows steadily, while damage to minor vessels may produce only an oozing. Rupture of a major blood vessel such as the femoral artery can lead to the loss of several litres of blood in a few minutes, resulting in shock, collapse, and death, if untreated. *primary h.* haemorrhage occurring immediately after injury or surgery. *secondary h.* haemorrhage occurring some time after injury, usually due to sepsis. *See also* haematemesis, haematuria, haemoptysis, splinter haemorrhage.

haemorrhagic (hem-er-aj-ik) *adj*. associated with or resulting from blood loss. *See* haemorrhage.

haemorrhagic disease of the newborn *n*. a transient disorder of newborn infants in which prolonged bleeding may result from the slightest injury. It is caused by deficiency of vitamin K and therefore of prothrombin, which is necessary for blood clotting.

haemorrhoidectomy (hem-er-oid-ek-tŏmi) *n*. the surgical operation for removing haemorrhoids, which are tied and then excised. The operation is usually performed only for second- or third-degree haemorrhoids.

haemorrhoids (piles) (hem-er-oidz) *pl. n*. enlargement of the normal spongy blood-filled cushions in the wall of the anus (*internal h.*), usually a consequence of prolonged constipation or, occasionally, diarrhoea. The main symptom is bleeding. *external h.* prolapsed internal haemorrhoids or perianal haematomas. *first-degree h.* haemorrhoids that never appear at the anus but cause bleeding at the end of defecation. *second-degree h.* haemorrhoids that protrude beyond the anus as an uncomfortable swelling but return spontaneously. *third-degree h.* haemorrhoids that remain outside the anus and need to be returned by pressure. They often require surgery (*see* haemorrhoidectomy), especially if they become strangulated (producing severe pain and further enlargement).

haemosalpinx (hee-moh-sal-pinks) *n. see* haematosalpinx.

haemosiderosis (heem-ŏ-sid-er-oh-sis) *n*. the accumulation in various tissues of *haemosiderin*, an iron-storage compound normally found in the bone marrow, liver, and spleen.

haemostasis (hee-moh-stay-sis) *n*. the arrest of bleeding, involving the physiological processes of blood coagulation and the contraction of damaged blood vessels. The term is also applied to various surgical procedures used to stop bleeding.

haemostatic (styptic) (hee-moh-stat-ik) *n.* an agent that stops or prevents haemorrhage; for example, phytomenadione.

haemothorax (hee-moh-thor-aks) *n.* blood in the pleural cavity, usually due to injury.

HAI *n.* hospital-acquired infection (*see* nosocomial infection).

hair (hair) *n.* a threadlike keratinized outgrowth of the epidermis of the skin. The root of the hair, beneath the surface of the skin, is expanded at its base to form the bulb, which contains a matrix of dividing cells. As new cells are formed the older ones are pushed upwards and become keratinized to form the root and shaft. *h. follicle* a sheath of epidermal cells and connective tissue that surrounds the root of a hair. *h. papilla* a projection of the dermis that is surrounded by the base of the hair bulb. It contains the capillaries that supply blood to the growing hair.

hairball (hair-bawl) *n. see* trichobezoar.

hairy cell (hair-i) *n.* an abnormal white blood cell that has the appearance of an immature lymphocyte with fine hairlike cytoplasmic projections around the perimeter of the cell. It is found in a rare form of leukaemia (*h.-c. leukaemia*) most commonly occurring in young men.

half-life (hahf-lyf) *n.* **1.** the time taken for half the atoms of a radioactive isotope to decay: a measure of the radioactivity of the isotope. **2.** (in pharmacology) the time taken

for the body to excrete half a given amount of a drug.

halibut liver oil (hal-i-bŭt) *n.* an oil extracted from the liver of halibut. It is rich in vitamins A and D.

halitosis (hal-i-toh-sis) *n.* bad breath. Causes of temporary halitosis include recently eaten strongly flavoured food; other causes include mouth breathing, periodontal disease, and infective conditions of the nose, throat, and lungs.

hallucination (hă-loo-sin-ay-shŏn) *n.* a false perception of something that is not really there. Hallucinations may be provoked by psychological illness (such as schizophrenia) or physical disorders in the brain or they may be caused by drugs or sensory deprivation. *Compare* illusion.

Hallucinations Rating Scale (HRS) *n.* an 11-item scale to determine details of auditory hallucinations in patients.

hallucinogen (hă-loo-sin-ŏ-jen) *n.* a drug that produces hallucinations, e.g. cannabis and lysergic acid diethylamide. Hallucinogens were formerly used to treat certain types of mental illness. —**hallucinogenic** *adj.*

hallux (hal-ŭks) *n.* (*pl.* **halluces**) the big toe. *h. rigidus* painful stiffness of the joint between the big toe and the first metatarsal bone, usually resulting from osteoarthritis. *h. valgus* a deformity in which the big toe is displaced towards the other toes. It is usually associated with a bunion. *h. varus* displacement of the big toe away from the others.

halogen (hal-ŏ-jen) *n.* any one of the related elements fluorine, chlorine, bromine, or iodine.

haloperidol (hal-oh-**pe**-ri-dol) *n.* a butyrophenone antipsychotic drug that is administered by mouth or injection to relieve anxiety and tension in the treatment of schizophrenia and other psychiatric disorders. Trade names: **Haldol**, **Serenace**.

halothane (**hal**-oh-thayn) *n.* a potent general anaesthetic administered by inhalation. It is used for inducing and maintaining anaesthesia in all types of surgical operations. Trade name: **Fluothane**.

hamate bone (unciform bone) (**ham**-ayt) *n.* a hook-shaped bone of the wrist (*see* carpus). It articulates with the capitate and triquetral bones at the sides, with the lunate bone behind, and with the fourth and fifth metacarpal bones in front.

hammer (**ham**-er) *n.* (in anatomy) *see* malleus.

hammer toe *n.* a deformity of a toe, most often the second, caused by fixed flexion of the proximal interphalangeal joint, which produces extension of the joints distal and proximal to it. A corn often forms over the deformity, which may be painful.

hamstring (**ham**-string) *n.* any of the tendons at the back of the knee. *h. muscles* the biceps femoris, semitendinosus, and semimembranosus, attached by the hamstrings to their insertions in the tibia and fibula.

hand (hand) *n.* the terminal organ of the upper limb. It comprises the eight bones of the carpus, the five metacarpal bones, and the phalangeal bones plus the surrounding tissues.

handedness (**han**-did-nis) *n.* the preferential use of one hand, rather than the other, in voluntary actions. In right-handedness this correlates with the half of the brain that is dominant for speech: some 97% of right-handed people have left-hemisphere dominance for speech, while only 60% of left-handed people are right-hemisphere dominant for speech.

hand, foot, and mouth disease *n.* a self-limiting disease, mainly affecting young children, caused by Coxsackie virus A16. A feeling of mild illness is accompanied by mouth ulcers and blisters on the hands and feet.

handicap (**han**-di-kap) *n.* **1.** partial or total inability to perform a social, occupational, or other activity that the affected person wants to do. **2.** *see* mental handicap.

Hand-Schüller-Christian disease (hand shew-ler kris-chǎn) *n. see* Langerhans cell histiocytosis. [A. Hand (1868–1949), US paediatrician; A. Schüller (1874–1958), Austrian neurologist; H. A. Christian (1876–1951), US physician]

Hansen's bacillus (**han**-sĕnz) *n. see* Mycobacterium. [A. G. H. Hansen (1841–1912), Norwegian bacteriologist]

Hansen's disease *n. see* leprosy.

hantavirus (han-tǎ-vy-rŭs) *n.* a virus that infects rats, mice, and voles and causes disease in humans when the secretions or excreta of these rodents are inhaled or ingested. The symptoms, which vary according to the strain of the infecting virus, range from those of a mild influenza-like illness to serious kidney or lung damage.

haploid (monoploid) (**hap**-loid) *adj.* describing cells, nuclei, or organisms with a single set of unpaired chromosomes. In humans the gametes are haploid following meiosis. *Compare* diploid, triploid. —**haploid** *n.*

happy puppet syndrome (hap-i pup-it) *n. see* Angelman syndrome.

hapt- (**hapto-**) *prefix denoting* touch.

hapten (hap-těn) *n.* a substance that becomes antigenic by combining with and modifying the body's own proteins.

harelip (hair-lip) *n. see* cleft lip.

Harrison's sulcus (ha-ri-sŏnz) *n.* a depression on both sides of the chest wall of a child between the pectoral muscles and the lower margin of the ribcage. It develops in conditions in which the airways are partially obstructed or when the lungs are abnormally congested due to some congenital abnormality of the heart. [E. Harrison (1789–1838), British physician]

Harris's operation (ha-ris-ěz) *n.* an operation in which the prostate gland is removed through an incision above the pubic bone and through the bladder. *See* prostatectomy. [S. H. Harris (1880–1936), Australian surgeon]

Hartmann's pouch (hart-manz) *n.* a saclike dilatation of the gallbladder wall near its outlet; it is a common site for finding gallstones. [H. Hartmann (1860–1952), French surgeon]

Hartmann's solution *n.* a solution containing sodium, potassium, and calcium chlorides and sodium lactate, administered by infusion to treat dehydration. [A. Hartmann (1898–1964), US physician]

Hartnup disease (hart-nup) *n.* a rare hereditary defect in the ab-

sorption of the amino acid tryptophan, leading to mental retardation, thickening and roughening of the skin on exposure to light, and lack of muscular coordination. The condition is similar to pellagra. Treatment with nicotinamide is usually effective. [Hartnup family, in whom it was first reported]

Hashimoto's disease (hash-i-moh-tohz) *n.* chronic thyroiditis due to the formation of autoantibodies against normal thyroid tissue. Its features include a firm swelling of the thyroid and partial or total failure of secretion of thyroid hormones; often there are autoantibodies to other organs, such as the stomach. Women are more often affected than men and the condition often occurs in families. [H. Hashimoto (1881–1934), Japanese surgeon]

hashish (hash-eesh) *n. see* cannabis.

haustrum (how-strum) *n.* one of the pouches on the external surface of the colon.

HAV *n.* hepatitis A virus. *See* hepatitis.

Haversian canal (ha-ver-si-ăn) *n.* any one of the small canals that ramify throughout compact bone. *See also* bone. [C. Havers (1650–1702), English anatomist]

Haversian system *n. see* bone.

hay fever (hay) *n.* a form of allergy due to pollen, characterized by inflammation of the membrane lining the nose and sometimes of the conjunctiva (*vernal* or *allergic conjunctivitis*). The symptoms of sneezing, running or blocked nose, and watering eyes often respond to treatment with antihistamines. Medical name: **allergic rhinitis.**

Hb n. see haemoglobin.

HC n. head circumference.

HCG n. see human chorionic gonadotrophin.

HCV n. hepatitis C virus. See hepatitis.

HD n. see Huntington's disease.

HDU n. see high-dependency unit.

head (hed) n. **1.** the part of the body that contains the brain and the organs of sight, hearing, smell, and taste. **2.** the rounded portion of a bone, which fits into a groove of another to form a joint.

headache (hed-ayk) n. pain felt deep within the skull. Most headaches are caused by emotional stress or fatigue but some are symptoms of serious intracranial disease. See also cluster headache, migraine.

head injury (in-jeri) n. an injury usually resulting from a blow to the head and often associated with brain injury. It may result in contusion or – if the blood vessels in the head are torn – a haematoma. The level of consciousness of a patient following a head injury can be assessed using the Glasgow scoring system.

head tilt chin lift n. a manoeuvre for opening the airway of an unconscious patient. With the patient supine, the neck is extended and the chin simultaneously pulled gently upwards to pull the tongue away from the back of the pharynx. See also jaw thrust.

Heaf test (heef) n. a skin test to determine whether or not an individual is immune to tuberculosis, carried out before vaccination. A spring-loaded gun mounted with very short needles produces a circle of six punctures in the forearm through which tuberculin is introduced. If the test is positive a reaction causes the skin to become red and raised, indicating that the individual is immune. [F. R. G. Heaf (1895–1973), British physician]

healing (heel-ing) n. see intention.

Health and Safety Executive (HSE) (helth) n. (in Britain) a statutory body responsible for the health and safety of workers (including factory, office, and agricultural workers).

Health Authority n. a body through which the National Health Service is administered at district level. In many districts most of its functions have now been taken over by Primary Care Trusts.

health care n. see primary care, secondary care, tertiary care.

health-care assistant n. a support worker in a clinical area who works under the supervision of a registered practitioner who is accountable for the support worker's standards and activities. A healthcare assistant may be registered at level 1 or 2 of the National Council for Vocational Qualifications (NCVQ), having completed a recognized course. See also NCVQ, support worker.

health-care delivery n. the services provided by nurses and others in the health service.

health centre n. (in Britain) a building, owned or leased by a community trust or a Health Authority, that houses personnel and/or services from one or several sections of the National Health Service.

health education n. persuasive

methods used to encourage people to adopt lifestyles that the educators believe will improve health and to reject habits regarded as harmful to health.

Health Improvement Programme (HImP) n. a plan, developed by Primary Care Trusts and acute trusts, patient groups, and the voluntary sector, to improve health and health care at a local level.

Health of the Nation Outcome Scale (HoNOS) n. a 12-item scale, used in mental health care, that assesses risk behaviours, physical problems, deterioration or improvement in symptoms, and social functioning.

health promotion n. a programme of surveillance planned on a community basis to maintain the best possible health and quality of life of the members of that community. Programmes include health education, immunization, and screening tests.

Health Service Commissioner (Health Service Ombudsman) n. an official, responsible to Parliament, who is appointed to protect the interests of patients in relation to administration of and provision of health care by the National Health Service. The Commissioner can investigate complaints and allegations of maladministration by a Health Authority or trust and complaints involving the clinical judgment of medical practitioners.

health service manager n. an administrator with special training and skills in management who is concerned with running hospitals and other health services. Generally, the basic training for managers

is in disciplines other than health; however, doctors, nurses, and others may fill such posts, sometimes combining them with professional appointments.

health service planning n. balancing the needs of a community, assessed by such indices as mortality, morbidity, and disability, with the resources available to meet these needs in terms of medical manpower (ensuring the numbers in training grades meet but do not exceed future requirements for career grades) and technical resources, such as hospitals (capital planning), equipment, and medicines.

health visitor (public health nurse) n. (in Britain) a trained nurse with specialist qualifications in health promotion and public health. Most of the work of health visitors is focused on families with children under five years old but can be extended to other targeted groups (e.g. the elderly).

hearing aid (heer-ing ayd) n. a device to improve hearing. *analogue h. a.* a battery-powered aid, consisting of a miniature microphone, an amplifier, and a tiny loudspeaker (or a vibrator in some cases of conductive deafness), that usually fits behind or within the ear. *bone-anchored h. a.* (BAHA) a hearing aid for those with certain forms of conductive deafness in which the vibrator is a small titanium screw fixed into the bone of the skull behind the external ear. *digital h. a.* a device similar to an analogue hearing aid but with the addition of a digital-to-analogue converter and a tiny computer, which improves sound quality. *environmental h. a.* (*assistive listening device*) a device for assisting those with hearing difficulties, such as an amplified telephone, a door bell with a visible alarm, or a vibrating alarm clock. *implantable h. a.* a hearing aid in which a battery-powered device consisting of a microphone and electronic processing unit, fitted behind the ear, passes information to an electrical vibrator surgically attached to the ear ossicles.

hearing therapy (th'e-ră-pi) *n.* the support and rehabilitation of people with hearing difficulties, tinnitus, or vertigo. It includes teaching lipreading, advising on environmental hearing aids, and providing tinnitus retraining therapy.

heart (hart) *n.* a hollow muscular cone-shaped organ, lying between the lungs, with the apex directed downwards, forwards, and to the left. It is divided by a septum into separate right and left halves, each of which is divided into an upper atrium and a lower ventricle (see illustration). Deoxygenated blood is pumped to the lungs via the right atrium and ventricle; newly oxygenated blood is pumped out to the body via the left atrium and ventricle. The direction of blood flow within the heart is controlled by valves.

heart attack *n. see* myocardial infarction.

heart block *n.* a condition in which conduction of the electrical impulses generated by the sinoatrial node is impaired, so that the pumping action of the heart is slowed down. Heart block may be congenital or it may be due to heart disease, myocarditis, cardiomyopathy, and

semilunar valve — pulmonary artery

superior vena cava — aorta

inferior vena cava — pulmonary vein

right atrium — left atrium

tricuspid valve — bicuspid valve

chorda tendina (tendon)

right ventricle — left ventricle

septum —

direction of blood flow through the heart
→

Vertical section through the heart

disease of the valves. Symptoms may be abolished by the use of an artificial pacemaker. *first degree h. b.* heart block in which conduction between atria and ventricles is delayed. *second degree h. b.* heart block in which not all the impulses are conducted from the atria to the ventricles. *third degree h. b.* heart block in which no impulses are conducted and the ventricles beat at their own slow intrinsic rate (20–40 per minute).

heartburn (pyrosis) (hart-bern) *n.* discomfort or pain, usually burning in character, that is felt behind the breastbone. It may be accompanied by the appearance of acid or bitter fluid in the mouth and is usually caused by regurgitation of stomach contents into the gullet or by oesophagitis.

heart failure *n.* a condition in which the pumping action of either or both ventricles of the heart is inadequate. This results in back pressure of blood, with congestion of the lungs and liver, and oedema (*congestive h. f.*, CHF). There is a reduced flow of arterial blood from the heart, which in extreme cases results in peripheral circulatory failure (cardiogenic shock). Heart failure may result from any condition that overloads, damages, or reduces the efficiency of the heart muscle, such as coronary thrombosis or hypertension. Treatment consists of rest, a low salt diet, diuretic drugs (e.g. furosemide), and digitalis derivatives (e.g. digoxin).

heart-lung machine *n.* an apparatus for taking over temporarily the functions of both the heart and the lungs during heart surgery. It incorporates a pump, to maintain the circulation, and equipment to oxygenate the blood.

heater-probe (heet-er-prohb) *n.* a device that can be passed through an endoscope to apply controlled heat in order to coagulate a bleeding peptic ulcer.

heat exhaustion (heet) *n.* fatigue and collapse due to the low blood pressure and blood volume that result from loss of body fluids and salts after prolonged or unaccustomed exposure to heat.

heatstroke (sunstroke) (heet-strohk) *n.* raised body temperature (pyrexia), absence of sweating, and eventual loss of consciousness due to failure or exhaustion of the temperature-regulating mechanism of the body.

hebephrenia (hee-bi-free-niǎ) *n.* a form of schizophrenia. It is typically a chronic condition, and the most prominent features are disordered thinking; inappropriate emotions with thoughtless cheerfulness, apathy, or querulousness; and silly behaviour. It typically starts in adolescence or young adulthood. —**hebephrenic** *adj.*

Heberden's node (hee-ber-děnz) *n.* a bony thickening arising at the terminal joint of a finger in osteoarthritis. It is often inherited. [W. Heberden (1710–1801), British physician]

hebetude (heb-i-tewd) *n.* apathy and emotional dullness. This is not a symptom specific to any one condition; extreme degrees are found in schizophrenia and dementia.

hectic (hek-tik) *adj.* occurring regularly. *h. fever* a fever that typically develops in the afternoons, in cases of pulmonary tuberculosis.

hecto- *prefix denoting* a hundred.

heel (heel) *n.* the part of the foot that extends behind the ankle joint. *See* calcaneus.

Hegar's sign (hay-garz) *n.* an indication of pregnancy detectable between the 6th and 12th weeks: used before modern urine tests for pregnancy were available. If the fingers of one hand are inserted into the vagina and those of the other are placed over the pelvic cavity, the lower part of the uterus feels very soft compared with the body of the uterus above and the cervix below. [A. Hegar (1830–1914), German gynaecologist]

Heimlich manoeuvre (hym-lik) *n. see* abdominal thrusts. [H. J. Heimlich (1920–   ), US physician]

helc- (helco-) *prefix denoting* an ulcer.

Helicobacter (hel-i-koh-bak-ter) *n.* a genus of spiral and flagellated Gram-negative bacteria. *H. pylori* (formerly *Campylobacter pylori*) a species that occurs in the stomach and causes progressive gastritis. It is nearly always present in duodenal ulceration and usually in gastric ulceration, and has been implicated in lymphomas of the stomach. It can be eradicated using various combinations of antibiotics and antisecretory drugs.

helicopter-based emergency medical services (hel-i-kopt-er-bayst i-merj-ĕn-si) *pl. n. see* HEMS.

helio- *prefix denoting* the sun.

heliotherapy (hee-li-oh-th'e-ră-pi) *n.* the use of sunlight to promote healing; sunbathing.

helium (hee-li-ŭm) *n.* a colourless inert gas that is used in combination with oxygen in respiratory tests and therapy and to prevent decompression sickness in deep-sea divers. Symbol: He.

helix (hee-liks) *n.* the outer curved fleshy ridge of the pinna of the outer ear.

Heller's operation (hel-erz) *n. see* cardiomyotomy. [E. Heller (1877–1964), German surgeon]

Heller's test *n.* a test for the presence of protein (albumin) in the urine. [J. F. Heller (1813–71), Austrian pathologist]

HELLP syndrome (help) *n.* a form of severe pre-eclampsia affecting many body systems and characterized by *h*aemolysis, *e*levated *l*iver enzymes, and a *l*ow *p*latelet count (hence the name). It constitutes an emergency requiring prompt termination of the pregnancy.

helminth (hel-minth) *n.* any of the parasitic worms, including the flukes, tapeworms, and nematodes.

helminthiasis (hel-min-th'y-ă-sis) *n.* the diseased condition resulting from an infestation with parasitic worms (helminths).

helminthology (hel-min-thol-ŏji) *n.* the study of parasitic worms.

helper T-cell (help-er) *n. see* T-cell.

hemeralopia (hem-er-ă-loh-piă) *n. see* day blindness.

hemi- *prefix denoting* (in medicine) the right or left half of the body.

hemianopia (hemi-an-oh-piă) *n.* absence of half of the normal field of vision. *homonymous h.* hemianopia in which the same half of the visual field (right or left) is lost in both eyes.

hemiarthroplasty (hemi-arth-roh-plasti) *n.* replacement of the end of a bone on one side of a joint with a prosthesis (*see* arthroplasty). It is the treatment for some fractures of the hip and shoulder.

hemiballismus (hemi-bal-**iz**-mŭs) *n.* a violent involuntary movement usually restricted to one arm and primarily involving the proximal muscles. It is a symptom of disease of the basal ganglia.

hemicolectomy (hemi-koh-**lek**-tŏmi) *n.* surgical removal of about half the colon, usually the right section (*right* h.) with subsequent joining of the ileum to the transverse colon. This is performed for such diseases as Crohn's disease or cancer.

hemicrania (hemi-**kray**-niă) *n.* **1.** a headache affecting only one side of the head, usually migraine. **2.** absence of half of the skull in a developing fetus.

hemimelia (hemi-**mee**-liă) *n.* congenital absence or gross shortening (aplasia) of the distal portion of the arms or legs. *See also* ectromelia.

hemiparesis (hemi-pă-**ree**-sis) *n.* *see* hemiplegia.

hemiplegia (**hemiparesis**) (hemi-**plee**-jiă) *n.* paralysis of one side of the body. It is caused by disease of the opposite (contralateral) hemisphere of the brain.

hemisphere (hem-iss-**feer**) *n.* one of the two halves of the cerebrum, not in fact hemispherical but more nearly quarter-spherical.

hemlock (hem-lok) *n.* the plant *Conium maculatum*, found in Britain and central Europe. It is a source of the poisonous alkaloid coniine.

hemp (hemp) *n.* *see* cannabis.

HEMS *pl. n.* helicopter-based emergency medical services: a fast method for the provision of first aid and the rapid transport of the seriously injured (primary use) or the critically ill (secondary use) to a hospital.

Henderson's model (hen-der-sŏnz) *n.* a model for nursing that describes 14 components of basic nursing that define the unique function of the nurse, which is to act in the best interests of the patient when the patient lacks the ability to do so. *See also* nursing models. [V. Henderson (20th century), US nurse theorist]

Henle's loop (hen-liz) *n.* the part of a kidney tubule that forms a loop extending towards the centre of the kidney. It is surrounded by blood capillaries, which absorb water and selected soluble substances back into the bloodstream. [F. G. J. Henle (1809–85), German anatomist]

Henoch-Schönlein purpura (Schönlein-Henoch purpura, anaphylactoid purpura) (hen-ohk **shern**-lyn) *n.* a common and frequently recurrent form of purpura found especially (but not exclusively) in young children. It is characterized by red weals and a purple rash on the buttocks and lower legs due to bleeding into the skin from inflamed capillaries, together with arthritis, gastrointestinal symptoms, and (in some cases) nephritis. [E. H. Henoch (1820–1910), German paediatrician; J. L. Schönlein (1793–1864), German physician]

hepar (hee-par) *n.* the liver.

heparin (hep-er-in) *n.* an anticoagulant produced in liver cells, some white blood cells, and certain other sites, which acts by inhibiting the action of the enzyme thrombin in the final stage of blood coagulation. An extracted purified form of heparin is widely used for the prevention of blood coagulation both in patients with thrombosis and similar conditions and in blood collected for examination. *low-molecular-weight h.* a type of heparin used to prevent deep-vein thrombosis following surgery or during kidney dialysis. It is more readily absorbed and produces less risk of bleeding than standard preparations.

hepat- (hepato-) *prefix denoting* the liver.

hepatalgia (hep-ă-tal-jiă) *n.* pain in or over the liver. It is caused by liver inflammation or swelling.

hepatectomy (hep-ă-tek-tŏmi) *n.* the operation of removing the liver. *partial h.* the removal of one or more lobes of the liver; it may be carried out after severe injury or to remove a tumour localized in one part of the liver.

hepatic (hip-at-ik) *adj.* relating to the liver. *h. duct see* bile duct. *h. encephalopathy (portosystemic encephalopathy)* a condition in which brain function is impaired by the presence of toxic substances, absorbed from the colon, which are normally removed or detoxified by the liver. *h. flexure* the bend in the colon, just underneath the liver, where the ascending colon joins the transverse colon. *h. vein* one of several veins that drain blood from the liver directly into the inferior vena cava.

hepaticostomy (hip-at-i-kost-ŏmi) *n.* a surgical operation in which a temporary or permanent opening is made into the main duct carrying bile from the liver.

hepatitis (hep-ă-ty-tis) *n.* inflammation of the liver caused by viruses, toxic substances, or immunological abnormalities. *chronic h.* hepatitis that continues for months or years, eventually leading to cirrhosis, caused by persistent infection with a hepatitis virus or by autoimmune disease. *h. A (epidemic h.)* infectious hepatitis transmitted by contaminated food or drink. After an incubation period of 15–40 days, the patient develops fever and sickness. Yellow discoloration of the skin (*see* jaundice) appears about a week later and persists for up to three weeks. *h. B (formerly serum h.)* infectious hepatitis transmitted by infected blood or blood products contaminated hypodermic needles, blood transfusions, etc., by sexual contact, or by contact with other body fluids. Symptoms, which develop suddenly after an incubation period of 1–6 months, include headache, fever, chills, general weakness, and jaundice. *h. C (formerly non-A, non-B h.)* infectious hepatitis that has a mode of transmission similar to that of hepatitis B. *h. D* infectious hepatitis that occurs only with or after infection with hepatitis B and is associated with severe chronic hepatitis. *h. E* acute hepatitis caused by a virus transmitted by food or drink. *infectious h.* hepatitis caused by viruses, several types of which have been isolated as specific causes of the disease and can be detected by blood tests.

hepatization (hep-ă-ty-zay-shŏn) *n.* the conversion of lung tissue, which normally holds air, into a solid liver-like mass during the course of acute lobar pneumonia.

hepato- *prefix. see* hepat-.

hepatoblastoma (hep-ă-toh-blas-toh-mă) *n.* a malignant tumour of the liver occurring in children, made up of embryonic liver cells.

hepatocele (hip-at-oh-seel) *n.* a hernia of the liver.

hepatocellular (hep-ă-toh-**sel**-yoo-ler) *adj.* relating to or affecting the cells of the liver.

hepatocirrhosis (hep-ă-toh-si-roh-sis) *n.* cirrhosis of the liver. *See* cirrhosis.

hepatocyte (hip-at-oh-syt) *n.* the principal cell type in the liver: a large cell with many metabolic functions, including synthesis, storage, detoxification, and bile production.

hepatoma (hepatocellular carcinoma) (hep-ă-toh-mă) *n.* a malignant tumour of the liver, originating in mature liver cells. In Western countries it often develops in patients with cirrhosis, particularly after hepatitis B or C infection. The term hepatoma is often, though incorrectly, used to include malignant tumours arising in the bile duct (*see* cholangiocarcinoma).

hepatomegaly (hep-ă-toh-meg-ă-li) *n.* enlargement of the liver to such an extent that it can be felt below the rib margin. This may be due to congestion, inflammation, infiltration (e.g. by fat), or tumour.

hepatotoxic (hep-ă-toh-**toks**-ik) *adj.* damaging or destroying liver cells. Drugs such as paracetamol can be hepatotoxic at high doses or with prolonged use.

hept- (hepta-) *prefix denoting* seven.

hereditary (hi-red-it-er-i) *adj.*

transmitted from parents to their offspring; inherited.

heredity (hi-red-iti) *n.* the process that causes the biological similarity between parents and their offspring. Genetics is the study of heredity.

heredo- *prefix denoting* heredity.

Hering-Breuer reflexes (h'e-ring broi-er) *pl. n.* the reflexes that maintain the normal rhythm of inflation and deflation of the lungs. [K. E. K. Hering (1834–1918), German physiologist; J. Breuer (1842–1925), German physician]

hermaphrodite (her-maf-rŏ-dyt) *n.* an individual in which both male and female sex organs are present or in which the sex organs contain both ovarian and testicular cells. **—hermaphroditism** *n.*

hernia (her-niă) *n.* the protrusion of an organ or tissue out of the body cavity in which it normally lies. *diaphragmatic h.* the protrusion of an abdominal organ through the diaphragm into the chest cavity. *femoral h.* the protrusion of part of the bowel at the top of the thigh, through the point at which the femoral artery passes from the abdomen to the thigh. *hiatus h.* the most common type of diaphragmatic hernia, in which the stomach passes partly or completely into the chest cavity through the oesophageal opening. This hernia may be associated with gastro-oesophageal reflux. *incarcerated h.* a hernia that is swollen and fixed within its sac. *inguinal h.* (or *rupture*) the protrusion of a sac of peritoneum, containing fat or part of the bowel, through the lower abdominal wall. *irreducible h.* a hernia that cannot be returned to its normal site. *stran-*

gulated h. a hernia that is cut off from its blood supply, becoming painful and eventually gangrenous. *umbilical h.* (*exomphalos*) the protrusion of abdominal organs into the umbilical cord, due to a fault in embryonic development.

hernio- *prefix denoting* a hernia.

hernioplasty (her-ni-oh-plasti) *n.* the surgical operation to repair a hernia, in which the abnormal opening is sewn up and/or the weakness strengthened with suture material.

herniorrhaphy (her-ni-o-ră-fi) *n.* surgical repair of a hernia, which can be performed through a laparoscope.

herniotomy (her-ni-ot-ŏmi) *n.* an operation to repair a hernia that involves cutting the sac that contains it.

heroin (h'e-roh-in) *n.* a white crystalline powder derived from morphine but with a shorter duration of action. Like morphine it is a powerful narcotic analgesic whose abuse leads to dependence. *See also* diamorphine.

herpangina (herp-an-jy-nă) *n.* an acute viral infection, predominantly affecting children, that causes fever of sudden onset associated with acute ulceration of the soft palate and tonsillar area. It usually lasts 2–5 days.

herpes (her-peez) *n.* inflammation of the skin or mucous membranes caused by herpesviruses and characterized by collections of small blisters. Treatment is with aciclovir. *genital h.* a sexually transmitted disease, usually caused by *herpes simplex virus* (*HSV*) type II, that is characterized by painful blisters in the genital region. It may be recurrent and is extremely contagious as the blisters burst to release viruses that infect the sexual partner. *h. simplex* (*cold sore*) herpes that affects the lips or surrounding area, caused by HSV type I. *h. zoster* (*shingles*) herpes caused by the varicella-zoster virus, which also causes chickenpox. Following an attack of chickenpox, the virus lies dormant in the spinal cord and later migrates down a sensory nerve to affect the skin in a band. One side of the face or an eye (*ophthalmic zoster*) may be involved. Shingles may be chronically painful, especially in the elderly.

herpesvirus (her-peez-vy-rŭs) *n.* one of a group of DNA-containing viruses causing latent infections in humans and animals. The herpesviruses are the causative agents of herpes and chickenpox. *See also* cytomegalovirus, Epstein-Barr virus.

Herxheimer reaction *n. see* Jarisch-Herxheimer reaction.

hesitation (hez-i-tay-shŏn) *n.* (in urology) a delay between being ready to pass urine and the actual flow of urine. *See* lower urinary tract symptoms.

heter- (hetero-) *prefix denoting* difference; dissimilarity.

heterochromia (het-er-oh-kroh-miă) *n.* colour difference in the iris of the eye, which is usually congenital but is occasionally secondary to inflammation of the iris. —**heterochromic** *adj.*

heterogeneous (het-er-oh-jee-ni-ŭs) *adj.* having different properties or constituents. —**heterogeneity** (het-er-oh-jin-ay-iti) *n.*

heterogenous (het-er-oj-in-ŭs) *adj.* derived from a different source.

heterograft (het-er-oh-grahft) n. see xenograft.

heterologous (het-er-ol-ŏ-gŭs) adj. derived from a different species: describing tissue used for grafting, etc.

heterophoria (het-er-oh-for-iă) n. a tendency to squint. Under normal circumstances both the eyes work together, but if one eye is covered it will move out of alignment with the object the other eye is still viewing. When the cover is removed the eye immediately returns to its normal position. See also strabismus.

heterophyiasis (het-er-oh-fi-I-ă-sis) n. an infestation of the small intestine with the parasitic fluke Heterophyes heterophyes. Humans become infected on eating raw or salted fish that contains the larval stage of the fluke. Symptoms include abdominal pain and diarrhoea; if the eggs reach the brain, spinal cord, and heart they produce serious lesions.

heteropsia (het-er-op-siă) n. different vision in each eye.

heterosexuality (het-er-oh-seks-yoo-al-iti) n. the pattern of sexuality in which sexual behaviour and thinking are directed towards people of the opposite sex. —**heterosexual** adj., n.

heterosis (het-er-oh-sis) n. hybrid vigour: the increased sturdiness, resistance to disease, etc., of individuals whose parents are of different races or species.

heterotopia (**heterotopy**) (het-er-oh-toh-piă) n. the displacement of an organ or part of the body from its normal position.

heterotropia (het-er-oh-troh-piă) n. see strabismus.

heterozygous (het-er-oh-zy-gŭs)

adj. describing an individual in whom the members of a pair of genes determining a particular characteristic are dissimilar. See also allele. Compare homozygous. —**heterozygote** n.

hex- (**hexa-**) prefix denoting six.

hexachlorophene (**hexachlorophane**) (heks-ă-klor-ŏ-feen) n. a disinfectant similar to phenol, used as a dusting powder for the prevention and treatment of staphylococcal skin infections. Trade name: **Ster-Zac Powder**.

hexamine (heks-ă-meen) n. see methenamine.

hexose (heks-ohz) n. a simple sugar with six carbon atoms. Hexose sugars are the sugars most frequently found in food. The most important hexose is glucose.

HFEA n. see Human Fertilization and Embryology Authority.

Hg symbol for mercury.

HGP n. see Human Genome Project.

5-HIAA n. see 5-hydroxyindoleacetic acid.

hiatus (hy-ay-tŭs) n. an opening or aperture. For example, the diaphragm contains hiatuses for the oesophagus and aorta. h. hernia see hernia.

Hib vaccine (hib) n. a vaccine that gives protection against the bacterium Haemophilus influenzae type B, which is a common cause of meningitis in children under the age of two. The vaccine is given with the primary vaccines during the first year of life. See Appendix 8.

hiccup (hik-up) n. abrupt involuntary lowering of the diaphragm and closure of the sound-producing folds at the upper end of the trachea, producing a characteristic sound as the breath is drawn in. Hiccups, which usually occur repeatedly, may be caused by indigestion or more serious disorders, such as alcoholism. Medical name: **singultus**.

Hickman catheter (hik-măn) *n.* a fine plastic cannula usually inserted into the subclavian vein in the neck to allow administration of drugs and repeated blood samples. The catheter is tunnelled for several centimetres beneath the skin to prevent infection from entering the bloodstream. It is used most frequently in patients receiving long-term chemotherapy, particularly by infusion.

hidr- (hidro-) *prefix denoting* sweat.

hidradenitis suppurativa (hy-drad-ĕ-**ny**-tis sup-yoor-ă-**tee**-vă) *n.* a condition in which deep abscesses occur in the armpits, groin, and anogenital region. More common in women, it may be under androgen control.

hidrosis (hid-roh-sis) *n.* **1.** the excretion of sweat. **2.** excessive sweating.

hidrotic (hid-**rot**-ik) *n.* an agent that causes sweating. Parasympathomimetic drugs are hidrotics.

Higginson's syringe (hig-in-sŏnz) *n.* a rubber syringe with a bulb in the centre that is compressed to force liquid in one direction to irrigate a body cavity. [A. Higginson (1808–84), British surgeon]

high-dependency unit (HDU) (hy-di-pen-dăn-si) *n.* a unit in a hospital that offers specialist nursing care and monitoring to seriously ill patients. It provides greater care than is available on general wards but less than is given to patients in intensive care.

hilar cell tumour (hy-ler) *n.* an androgen-producing tumour of the ovary found in older women and often resulting in virilization. Such tumours tend to occur around the area of the ovary where the blood vessels enter (the hilum).

hilum (hy-lŭm) *n.* (*pl.* **hila**) a hollow situated on the surface of an organ, at which structures such as blood vessels and nerve fibres enter or leave it. —**hilar** *adj.*

HImP *n. see* Health Improvement Programme.

hindbrain (rhombencephalon) (hynd-brayn) *n.* the part of the brain comprising the cerebellum, pons, and medulla oblongata.

hindgut (hynd-gut) *n.* the back part of the embryonic gut, which gives rise to part of the large intestine, the rectum, bladder, and urinary ducts. *See also* cloaca.

hindquarter amputation (hynd-kwort-er) *n.* an operation involving removal of an entire leg and part or all of the pelvis associated with it. It is usually performed for soft tissue or bone sarcomas arising from the upper thigh, hip, or buttock. *Compare* forequarter amputation.

hinge joint (hinj) *n. see* ginglymus.

hip (hip) *n.* the region of the body where the thigh bone (femur) articulates with the pelvis: the region on each side of the pelvis. *h. bone* (*innominate bone*) a bone formed by the fusion of the ilium, ischium, and pubis. It articulates with the femur at the hip joint. *h. girdle see* pelvic girdle. *h. joint* the ball-and-socket joint between the head of the femur and the acetabulum (socket) of the ilium. *h. replacement* a surgical procedure for replacing a diseased hip joint with a prosthesis. *See also* arthroplasty.

hippocampal formation (hip-oh-kam-pål) *n*. a curved band of cortex lying within each cerebral hemisphere. It forms a portion of the limbic system and is involved in the complex physical aspects of behaviour governed by emotion and instinct.

hippocampus (hip-oh-**kam**-pŭs) *n*. a swelling in the floor of the lateral ventricle of the brain. It contains complex foldings of cortical tissue and is involved in the workings of the limbic system. —**hippocampal** *adj*.

Hippocratic oath (hip-ŏ-**krat**-ik) *n*. the oath formerly taken by a doctor to observe the code of behaviour and practice followed by the Greek physician Hippocrates (460–370 BC), called the 'Father of Medicine'.

Hirschsprung's disease (**heersh**-spruungz) *n*. a congenital condition in which the rectum and sometimes part of the lower colon have failed to develop a normal nerve network. The affected portion does not expand or conduct the contents of the bowel, which accumulate in and distend the upper section of the colon. *See also* megacolon. [H. Hirschsprung (1830–1916), Danish physician]

hirsutism (**herss**-yoo-tizm) *n*. the presence of coarse pigmented hair on the face, chest, upper back, or abdomen in a female as a result of hyperandrogenism (excessive production of androgen). *See also* virilization.

hirudin (hi-**roo**-din) *n*. an anticoagulant, present in the salivary glands of leeches and in certain snake venoms, that prevents blood coagulation by inhibiting the action of the enzyme thrombin.

Hirudo (hi-**roo**-doh) *n*. a genus of leeches. *See* leech.

hist- (histio-, histo-) *prefix denoting* tissue.

histamine (**hist**-ă-meen) *n*. a compound derived from the amino acid histidine, found in nearly all tissues of the body. Histamine causes dilation of blood vessels and contraction of smooth muscle; it is an important mediator of inflammation and is released in large amounts after skin damage, producing flushing, a flare, and a weal. Histamine is also released in anaphylactic reactions. *See also* anaphylaxis, antihistamine.

histidine (**hist**-i-deen) *n*. an amino acid from which histamine is derived.

histiocyte (**hist**-i-ŏ-syt) *n*. a fixed macrophage, i.e. one that is stationary within connective tissue.

histiocytoma (hist-i-oh-sy-**toh**-mă) *n*. a tumour that contains macrophages or histiocytes.

histiocytosis (hist-i-oh-sy-**toh**-sis) *n*. any of a group of diseases in which there are abnormalities in histiocytes due to abnormal storage of fats, as in Gaucher's disease; inflammatory disorders, as in Langerhans cell histiocytosis; or malignant proliferation of histiocytes.

histocompatibility (hist-oh-kŏm-pat-i-**bil**-iti) *n*. the form of compatibility that depends upon tissue components, mainly specific glycoprotein antigens in cell membranes. A high degree of histocompatibility is necessary for a tissue graft or organ transplant to be successful. —**histocompatible** *adj*.

histogenesis (hist-oh-**jen**-i-sis) *n.* the formation of tissues.

histoid (**hist**-oid) *adj.* **1.** resembling normal tissue. **2.** composed of one type of tissue.

histological grade (hist-oh-**loj**-ikǎl) *n.* the degree of differentiation of a tumour, such as a breast tumour.

histology (hiss-**tol**-ŏji) *n.* the study of the structure of tissues by means of special staining techniques combined with light and electron microscopy. —**histological** *adj.*

histolysis (hiss-**tol**-i-sis) *n.* disintegration of tissue.

histone (**hist**-ohn) *n.* a simple protein that combines with a nucleic acid to form a nucleoprotein.

histoplasmin (hist-oh-**plaz**-min) *n.* a preparation of antigenic material from a culture of the fungus *Histoplasma capsulatum*, used to test for the presence of histoplasmosis by subcutaneous injection.

histoplasmosis (hist-oh-plaz moh-sis) *n.* an infection caused by inhaling spores of the fungus *Histoplasma capsulatum*. The primary pulmonary form usually produces no symptoms or harmful effects. Occasionally, progressive histoplasmosis, which resembles tuberculosis, develops. The fungus may spread via the bloodstream to attack the liver, spleen, lymph nodes, or intestine. Symptomatic disease is treated with intravenous amphotericin.

histotoxic (hist-oh-**toks**-ik) *adj.* poisonous to tissues: applied to certain substances and conditions.

HIV (human immunodeficiency virus) *n.* a retrovirus responsible for AIDS. *HIV-1* the variety of HIV most common in Western countries. *HIV-2* the variety of HIV most common in Africa. *See also* HTLV.

hives (hyvz) *n. see* urticaria.

HLA system *n.* human leucocyte antigen system: a series of four gene families (termed A, B, C, and D) that code for polymorphic proteins expressed on the surface of most nucleated cells. Individuals inherit from each parent one gene (or set of genes) for each subdivision of the HLA system. If two individuals have identical HLA types, they are said to be histocompatible. Successful tissue transplantation requires a minimum number of HLA differences between donor and recipient tissues.

HMG *n. see* human menopausal gonadotrophin.

hobnail liver (hob-nayl) *n.* the liver of a patient with cirrhosis, which has a knobbly appearance caused by regenerating nodules separated by bands of fibrous tissue.

Hodgkin's disease (Hodgkin's lymphoma) (hoj-kinz) *n.* a malignant disease of lymphatic tissues – a form of lymphoma – usually characterized by painless enlargement of one or more groups of lymph nodes in the neck, armpits, groin, chest, or abdomen; the spleen, liver, bone marrow, and bones may also be involved. Treatment may include surgery, radiotherapy, drug therapy (using drugs such as procarbazine and prednisolone), or a combination of these. [T. Hodgkin (1798–1866), British physician]

hole in the heart (hohl) *n. see* septal defect.

holistic (hoh-**list**-ik) *adj.* describing an approach to patient care in which the physiological, psychological, and social factors of the patient's condition are taken into account, rather than just the diagnosed disease. The term is applied to a range of orthodox and unorthodox methods of treatment. *See also* complementary medicine.

holo- *prefix denoting* complete or entire.

holocrine (hol-ŏ-kryn) *adj.* describing a gland or type of secretion in which the entire cell disintegrates when the product is released.

Homans' sign (hoh-mănz) *n.* pain felt in the calf when the foot is flexed backwards: a sign of phlebothrombosis. [J. Homans (1877–1954), US physician]

home nurse (hohm) *n. see* district nurse.

homeo- (homoeo-) *prefix denoting* similar; like.

homeopathic (homoeopathic) (hoh-mi-ŏ-**path**-ik) *adj.* **1.** of or relating to homeopathy. **2.** infinitesimally small, as applied to the dose of a drug.

homeopathy (homoeopathy) (hoh-mi-**op**-ă-thi) *n.* a complementary therapy based on the theory that 'like cures like'. It involves treating a condition with a tiny dose of a substance that in larger doses would normally cause or aggravate that condition. The substance is diluted in purified water, then activated by shaking in an exact way. Homeopathy was developed by a German doctor, Samuel Hahnemann (1755–1843), in 1796. —**homeopathic** *adj.* —**homeopathist** *n.*

homeostasis (hoh-mi-oh-**stay**-sis) *n.* the physiological process by which the internal systems of the body are maintained at equilibrium, despite variations in the external conditions. —**homeostatic** *adj.*

homo- *prefix denoting* the same or common.

homocysteine (hoh-moh-**sis**-ti-een) *n.* a sulphur-containing amino acid that is an intermediate in the synthesis of cysteine. Elevated levels of homocysteine in the blood are a risk factor for vascular disease independent of diabetes, hypertension, elevated levels of cholesterol in the blood, and smoking. *See also* homocystinuria.

homocystinuria (hoh-moh-sis-tin-**yoor**-iă) *n.* an inborn error of metabolism caused by an enzyme deficiency resulting in an excess of homocysteine in the blood and the presence of homocystine (an oxidized form of cysteine) in the urine. Clinically affected individuals are mentally retarded, excessively tall with long fingers (due to overgrowth of bones), and have a tendency to form blood clots in the veins and arteries, leading to strokes.

homoeopathy (hoh-mi-op-ă-thi) *n. see* homeopathy.

homogenize (hŏ-**moj**-i-nyz) *vb.* to reduce material to a uniform consistency, e.g. by crushing and mixing. —**homogenization** *n.*

homogentisic acid (hoh-moh-jen-**tis**-ik) *n.* a product formed during the metabolism of the amino acids phenylalanine and tyrosine. In normal individuals homogentisic acid is oxidized by the enzyme *homogentisic acid oxidase*. In rare cases this enzyme is lacking and alcaptonuria results.

homograft (hom-ō-grahft) *n. see* allograft.

homoiothermic (hoh-moi-ō-therm-ik) *adj.* warm-blooded: able to maintain a constant body temperature independently of, and despite variations in, the temperature of the surroundings. *Compare* poikilothermic. —**homoiothermy** *n.*

homolateral (hoh-moh-lat-er-ăl) *adj. see* ipsilateral.

homologous (hoh-mol-ŏ-gŭs) *adj.* **1.** (in anatomy) describing organs or parts that have the same basic structure and evolutionary origin, but not necessarily the same function or superficial structure. *Compare* analogous. **2.** (in genetics) describing a pair of chromosomes of similar shape and size and having identical gene loci.

homonymous (hoh-mon-i-mŭs) *adj.* describing a visual defect in which the visual field to one side of the body is restricted in both eyes (*see* hemianopia).

homosexuality (hoh-moh-seks-ū-al-iti) *n.* a pattern of sexuality in which sexual behaviour and thinking are directed towards people of the same sex (*see also* lesbianism). Counselling can benefit people who are concerned about their sexual orientation. —**homosexual** *adj., n.*

homozygous (hoh-moh-zy-gŭs) *adj.* describing an individual in whom the members of a pair of genes determining a particular characteristic are identical. *See also* allele. *Compare* heterozygous. —**homozygote** *n.*

honeycomb lung (hun-i-kohm) *n.* the honeycomb pattern seen on X-ray at the later stages of chronic lung conditions, in which the lungs become less elastic and more fibrotic and are likely to progress to respiratory failure.

HoNOS *n. see* Health of the Nation Outcome Scale.

hook (huuk) *n.* a surgical instrument with a bent or curved tip, used to hold, lift, or retract tissue at operation.

hookworm (huuk-werm) *n.* either of two nematode worms, *Necator americanus* or *Ancylostoma duodenale*, which live as parasites in the human intestine. **h. disease** a condition resulting from an infestation of the small intestine by hookworms. Heavy hookworm infections may cause considerable damage to the wall of the intestine, leading to severe anaemia. Mebendazole is used in treatment.

hordeolum (hor-dee-ŏ-lum) *n. see* stye.

hormone (hor-mohn) *n.* a substance that is produced by an endocrine gland in one part of the body, passes into the bloodstream, and is carried to other (distant) organs or tissues, where it acts to modify their structure or function. Examples of hormones are corticosteroids, adrenaline, growth hormone, androgens, oestrogens, thyroid hormone, and insulin. *See also* pituitary gland.

hormone-binding globulins *pl. n.* a family of plasma proteins whose function is to bind free hormone molecules and thus reduce their function. Alterations in levels of the binding globulins, for example during pregnancy or ill health, can result in variations in assays of hormone levels in individuals.

hormone replacement therapy

(HRT) *n.* the use of female hormones for the relief of symptoms resulting from cessation of ovarian function, either at the time of the natural menopause or following surgical removal of the ovaries. Oestrogenic hormones may be prescribed orally, by subcutaneous implant, or transdermally (as skin patches or gel); a combination of progestogen with oestrogen is preferred if the woman has retained her uterus. HRT is also effective in preventing osteoporosis.

horn (horn) *n.* (in anatomy) a process, outgrowth, or extension of an organ or other structure. It is often paired.

Horner's syndrome (hor-nerz) *n.* a syndrome consisting of a constricted pupil, ptosis, and an absence of sweating over the affected side of the face. The symptoms are due to a disorder of the sympathetic nerves in the brainstem or cervical (neck) region. [J. F. Horner (1831–86), Swiss ophthalmologist]

horseshoe kidney (hors-shoo) *n.* an anatomical variation in kidney development whereby the lower poles of both kidneys are joined together. This usually causes no trouble but it may be associated with impaired drainage of urine from the kidney by the ureters.

Horton's syndrome (hor-t'nz) *n.* a severe headache caused by the release of histamine. [B. T. Horton (20th century), US physician]

hospice (hos-pis) *n.* an institution that specializes in the care of terminally ill patients, with emphasis on pain management and maintenance of psychological wellbeing to enable patients to face death with dignity.

hospital (hos-pi-t'l) *n.* an institution providing medical or psychiatric care and treatment of patients. *community h.* a small hospital, which may be staffed by general practitioners, providing care for patients for whom home care is not practicable. *day h.* a hospital at which patients are cared for during the day, returning home at night. *district general h.* a hospital that provides sufficient basic services for the population of a health district.

hospital-acquired infection (HAI) *n. see* nosocomial infection.

host (hohst) *n.* an animal or plant in or upon which a parasite lives. *intermediate h.* a host in which the parasite passes its larval or asexual stages. *definitive h.* a host in which the parasite develops to its sexual stage.

hourglass contraction (ow-er-glahs) *n.* constriction of an organ at its centre as a result of abnormal muscular contraction. Hourglass contraction may be a complication of labour, tending to trap the placenta in the upper part of the contracted uterus and possibly leading to excessive blood loss after delivery.

hourglass stomach *n.* a deformity of the stomach in which the 'waist' is constricted by fibrosis caused by a chronic peptic ulcer, producing an upper and a lower cavity separated by a narrow channel.

housemaid's knee (prepatellar bursitis) (howss-maydz) *n.* a fluid-filled swelling of the bursa in front of the kneecap, often resulting from frequent kneeling. *See also* bursitis.

HPV *n.* see human papillomavirus.

HR *n.* heart rate.

H₂-receptor antagonist *n.* see antihistamine.

HRS *n.* see Hallucinations Rating Scale.

HRT *n.* see hormone replacement therapy.

HSDU *n.* Hospital Sterilization and Disinfection Unit.

HSE *n.* see Health and Safety Executive.

HSV *n.* herpes simplex virus: *see* herpes.

5HT *n.* 5-hydroxytryptamine: *see* serotonin.

5HT₁ agonist *n.* a drug that stimulates serotonin receptors and is taken by mouth in the treatment of acute migraine for its effect of reversing the dilatation of blood vessels in the head that causes the headache. Such drugs include *sumatriptan* (Imigran), *almotriptan* (Almogran), *naratriptan* (Naramig), and *zolmitriptan* (Zomig).

HTLV (human T-cell lymphocytotrophic virus) *n.* a family of viruses that includes the AIDS virus, HTLV-III (or HIV). Other HTLV viruses may cause lymphomas and leukaemias.

human chorionic gonadotrophin (HCG) (hew-măn kor-i-on-ik) *n.* a hormone, similar to the pituitary gonadotrophins, that is produced by the placenta during pregnancy. Large amounts of HCG are excreted in the urine, and this is used as the basis for most pregnancy tests. HCG is given by injection to treat such conditions as de-

layed puberty, undescended testes, and premenstrual tension. *See also* triple marker test.

human chorionic somatomammotrophin (soh-mă-toh-mam-oh-**troh**-fin) *n.* see human placental lactogen.

Human Fertilization and Embryology Authority (HFEA) *n.* a body that controls and reviews research involving the use of embryos and issues licences for this research and for treatment in assisted conception. Children over the age of 18 can apply to the Authority for information concerning their ethnic and genetic background.

Human Genome Project (HGP) *n.* an international research project to elucidate the entire sequence of genes on all the human chromosomes. The human genome comprises some 3000 million nucleotide base pairs forming about 30,000 genes. A first draft of the sequence of these bases, along the length of each chromosome, was published in 2001. The HGP has already resulted in the identification of the genes associated with many hereditary disorders and revealed the existence of a genetic basis or component for many other diseases not previously known to have one.

human immunodeficiency virus *n.* see HIV.

human leucocyte antigen system *n.* see HLA system.

human menopausal gonadotrophin (HMG, menotrophin) *n.* a gonadotrophin combining the actions of follicle-stimulating hormone and luteinizing hormone, which is extracted from the urine of postmenopausal women and used to treat infertility caused by underactivity of the pituitary gland and to stimulate the ovaries in women undergoing fertility treatment. HMG is given by injection. Trade names: **Humegon, Menogon, Normegon, Pergonal**.

human papillomavirus (HPV) (pap-i-loh-mǎ-vy-rŭs) *n.* a virus – a member of the papovavirus group – that causes warts, including genital warts. Certain strains are considered to be causative factors in the development of anal and genital cancers, especially cervical cancer. HPV is one of the most common sexually transmitted infections.

human placental lactogen (human chorionic somatomammotrophin) (lak-tŏ-jěn) *n.* a protein hormone produced by the placenta during most but not all pregnancies. Its exact function remains obscure, but it seems to contribute to the development of diabetes in some pregnancies.

humectant (hew-mek-tănt) **1.** *n.* a substance that is used for moistening. **2.** *adj.* causing moistening.

humerus (hew-mer-ŭs) *n.* the bone of the upper arm. The head of the humerus articulates with the scapula at the shoulder joint. At the lower end of the shaft the trochlea articulates with the ulna and part of the radius.

humoral (hew-mer-ăl) *adj.* circulating in the bloodstream; humoral immunity requires circulating antibodies.

humour (hew-mer) *n.* a body fluid. *See* aqueous humour, vitreous humour.

hunger pain (hung-er) *n.* pain in the upper abdomen that is relieved by taking food. It is associated with a duodenal ulcer.

Hunner's ulcer (hun-erz) *n. see* interstitial cystitis. [G. L. Hunner (1868–1957), US urologist]

Hunter's syndrome (hunt-erz) *n.* a hereditary disorder caused by deficiency of an enzyme that results in the accumulation of protein–carbohydrate complexes and fats in the cells of the body. This leads to mental retardation, enlargement of the liver and spleen, and prominent coarse facial features (*gargoylism*). Medical name: **mucopolysaccharidosis type II**. [C. H. Hunter (1872–1955), US physician]

Huntington's disease (HD, Huntington's chorea) (hunting-tŏnz) *n.* a hereditary disease caused by a defect in a single gene that is inherited as an autosomal dominant characteristic, tending to

The humerus (posterior surface)

appear in half of the children of the parents with this condition. Symptoms, which begin to appear in early middle age, include unsteady gait and jerky involuntary movements (*see* chorea), accompanied later by behavioural changes and progressive dementia. [G. Huntington (1850–1916), US physician]

Hurler's syndrome (hoor-lerz) *n.* a hereditary disorder caused by deficiency of an enzyme that results in the accumulation of protein–carbohydrate complexes and fats in the cells of the body. This leads to severe mental retardation, enlargement of the liver and spleen, heart defects, deformities of the bones, and coarsening and thickening of the facial features (*gargoylism*). Medical name: **mucopolysaccharidosis type I**. [G. Hurler (1889–1965), Austrian paediatrician]

HUS *n. see* haemolytic uraemic syndrome.

Hutchinson's teeth (huch-in-sŏnz) *pl. n.* narrowed and notched permanent incisor teeth: a sign of congenital syphilis. [J. Hutchinson (1828–1913), British surgeon]

hyal- (hyalo-) *prefix denoting* **1.** glassy; transparent. **2.** hyalin. **3.** the vitreous humour of the eye.

hyalin (hy-ă-lin) *n.* a clear glassy material produced as the result of degeneration in certain tissues, particularly connective tissue and epithelial cells.

hyaline cartilage (hy-ă-lin) *n. see* cartilage.

hyaline membrane disease *n. see* respiratory distress syndrome.

hyalitis (hy-ă-ly-tis) *n.* inflammation of the vitreous humour of the

eye. *asteroid h. see* asteroid hyalosis.

hyaloid membrane (hy-ă-loid) *n.* the transparent membrane that surrounds the vitreous humour of the eye, separating it from the retina.

hyaluronidase (hy-ăl-yoor-on-i-dayz) *n.* an enzyme that increases the permeability of connective tissue. Hyaluronidase is found in the testes, in semen, and in other tissues.

hybrid (hy-brid) *n.* the offspring of a cross between two genetically unlike individuals. A hybrid, whose parents are usually of different species or varieties, is often sterile.

HYCOSY (hysterosalpingo-contrast sonography) *n.* an outpatient technique that tests for blocked Fallopian tubes. Using transvaginal ultrasonography and an echo contrast medium, flow along the tubes can be reliably visualized. *See also* Doppler ultrasound.

hydatid (hy-dă-tid) *n.* a bladder-like cyst formed in various human tissues following the growth of the larval stage of an *Echinococcus* tapeworm. *alveolar h.* an aggregate of small cysts, which enlarge by budding off external daughter cysts. *unilocular h.* a single large fluid-filled cyst, bound by a fibrous capsule, that gives rise internally to smaller daughter cysts. *See also* hydatid disease.

hydatid disease (hydatidosis, echinococciasis, echinococcosis) *n.* a condition resulting from the presence in the liver, lungs, or brain of hydatid cysts. Alveolar hydatids form malignant tumours; unilocular hydatids exert pressure as they grow and thereby damage surrounding tissues.

hydatidiform mole (hydatid mole, vesicular mole) (hy-da-tid-i-form) *n.* a collection of fluid-filled sacs that develop when the chorion degenerates in early pregnancy. The embryo dies, the uterus enlarges, and there is a discharge of pinkish liquid and cysts from the vagina. A malignant condition may subsequently develop (*see* chorionepithelioma).

hydatidosis (hy-da-tid-**oh**-sis) *n. see* hydatid disease.

hydr- (hydro-) *prefix denoting* water or a watery fluid.

hydraemia (hy-**dree**-miă) *n.* the presence in the blood of more than the normal proportion of water.

hydralazine (hy-**dral**-ă-zeen) *n.* a vasodilator administered by mouth or injection, usually in conjunction with diuretics, in the treatment of hypertension. Trade name: **Apresoline**.

hydramnios (hydramnion) (hy-**dram**-ni-ŏs) *n.* the presence of an abnormally large amount of amniotic fluid surrounding the fetus from about the 20th week of pregnancy.

hydrargyria (hy-drar-jy-riă) *n. see* mercurialism.

hydrarthrosis (hy-drar-**throh**-sis) *n.* swelling at a joint caused by excessive synovial fluid. The condition usually involves the knees and may be recurrent.

hydrate (hy-drayt) **1.** *vb.* to undergo treatment or impregnation with water. —**hydration** *n.* **2.** *n.* a chemical compound in which one or more molecules of water are combined with a molecule of another substance.

hydrocalycosis (hy-droh-kal-i-**koh**-sis) *n. see* caliectasis.

hydrocele (hy-droh-seel) *n.* the accumulation of watery liquid in a sac, usually the sac surrounding the testes. This condition is characterized by painless enlargement of the scrotum.

hydrocephalus (hy-droh-**sef**-ă-lŭs) *n.* an abnormal increase in the amount of cerebrospinal fluid within the ventricles of the brain. In childhood, before the sutures of the skull have fused, hydrocephalus makes the head enlarge. In adults, hydrocephalus raises the intracranial pressure, with consequent drowsiness and vomiting. Spina bifida may be associated with hydrocephalus in childhood.

hydrochloric acid (hy-drŏ-klor-ik) *n.* a strong acid present, in a very dilute form, in gastric juice. The secretion of excess hydrochloric acid by the stomach results in the condition hyperchlorhydria.

hydrochlorothiazide (hy-drŏ-klor-oh-th'y-ă-zyd) *n.* a thiazide diuretic administered by mouth to treat fluid retention (oedema) and high blood pressure.

hydrocortisone (hy-droh-**kor**-tiz-ohn) *n.* a pharmaceutical preparation of the steroid hormone cortisol. Hydrocortisone is used to treat adrenal failure (Addison's disease) and inflammatory, allergic, and rheumatic conditions (including rheumatoid arthritis, colitis, and eczema). It may be given by mouth, by injection, or in the form of a cream, ointment, or eye or ear drops.

hydrocyanic acid (prussic acid) (hy-droh-sy-an-ik) *n.* an intensely poisonous volatile acid that can cause death within a minute if inhaled. It smells of bitter almonds. *See* cyanide.

hydroflumethiazide (hy-droh-floo-meth-I-ă-zyd) *n.* a diuretic administered by mouth to treat fluid retention (oedema) and high blood pressure. Trade name: **Hydrenox**.

hydrogen (hy-drŏ-jĕn) *n.* a colourless gas that is combined with oxygen to form water (H_2O) and with various other molecules (chiefly carbon and oxygen) to form all organic compounds. Symbol: H. **h. ion concentration** *see* pH.

hydrogen peroxide (per-ok-syd) *n.* a colourless liquid used as a disinfectant for cleansing wounds and, diluted, as a deodorant mouthwash. Formula: H_2O_2.

hydrolysis (hy-drol-i-sis) *n.* any chemical reaction in which a compound and water react together to produce other compounds.

hydroma (hy-droh-mă) *n. see* hygroma.

hydrometer (hy-drom-it-er) *n.* an instrument for measuring the density or relative density of liquids. —**hydrometry** *n.*

hydrometra (hy-droh-mee-tră) *n.* an abnormal accumulation of watery fluid in the uterus.

hydronephrosis (hy-droh-ni-froh-sis) *n.* distension and dilatation of the pelvis of the kidney. This is due to an obstruction to the free flow of urine from the kidney. Surgical relief by pyeloplasty is advisable to avoid the back pressure atrophy of the kidney and the complications of infection and stone formation. —**hydronephrotic** *adj.*

hydropericarditis (hy-droh-pe-ri-kar-dy-tis) *n. see* hydropericardium.

hydropericardium (hy-droh-pe-ri-kar-di-ŭm) *n.* accumulation of a clear serous fluid within the membranous sac surrounding the heart. It occurs in many cases of pericarditis (*hydropericarditis*).

hydroperitoneum (hy-droh-pe-ri-tŏn-ee-ŭm) *n. see* ascites.

hydrophobia (hy-drŏ-foh-biă) *n. see* rabies.

hydrophthalmos (hy-drof-thal-mŏs) *n. see* buphthalmos.

hydropneumoperitoneum (hy-droh-new-moh-pe-ri-tŏn-ee-ŭm) *n.* the presence of fluid and gas in the peritoneal cavity.

hydropneumothorax (hy-droh-new-moh-thor-aks) *n.* air and fluid in the pleural cavity. An effusion of serous fluid commonly complicates a pneumothorax, and must be drained.

hydrops (hy-drops) *n.* an abnormal accumulation of fluid in body tissues or cavities. **corneal h.** the sudden painful accumulation of fluid in the cornea seen in keratoconus. It results in a sudden reduction of vision. *See also* hydrops fetalis, Ménière's disease (endolymphatic hydrops).

hydrops fetalis (fee-tah-lis) *n.* severe oedema that develops before birth. The excess fluid accumulates in the body cavities, especially in the peritoneal and pleural cavities. The most common cause is severe anaemia associated with haemolytic disease of the newborn. It can occur with a twin-to-twin transfusion.

hydrorrhachis (hy-dror-ră-kis) *n.* an abnormal accumulation of watery fluid in the space surrounding the spinal cord.

hydrosalpinx (hy-droh-**sal**-pinks) *n.* the accumulation of watery fluid in one of the Fallopian tubes, which becomes swollen.

hydrostatic accouchement (hy-droh-**stat**-ik) *n. see* accouchement.

hydrotherapy (hy-droh-th'e-ră-pi) *n.* the use of water in the treatment of disorders, now restricted in orthodox medicine to exercises in remedial swimming pools for the rehabilitation of arthritic or partially paralysed patients.

hydrothorax (hy-droh-**thor**-aks) *n.* fluid in the pleural cavity. *See also* hydropneumothorax.

hydrotubation (hy-droh-tew-**bay**-shŏn) *n.* the introduction of a fluid (usually a dye) through the cervix (neck) of the uterus under pressure to allow visualization, by laparoscopy, of the passage of the dye through the Fallopian tubes. It is used to test whether or not the tubes are blocked in the investigation of infertility.

hydroureter (hy-droh-yoor-ee-ter) *n.* an accumulation of urine in one of the ureters, usually resulting from obstruction of the ureter by a stone or a misplaced artery.

hydroxocobalamin (hy-droks-oh-koh-**bal**-ă-min) *n.* a cobalt-containing drug administered by injection to treat conditions involving vitamin B_{12} deficiency, such as pernicious anaemia. Trade names: **Cobalin-H**, **Neo-Cytamen**.

hydroxyapatite (hy-droks-i-ap-ă-tyt) *n.* **1.** the crystalline component of bones and teeth, consisting of a complex form of calcium phosphate.

2. a biocompatible ceramic material that is a synthetic form of natural hydroxyapatite. It is used to coat some joint replacement prostheses, which encourages bone to grow onto the implant, and is also used in some forms of middle-ear surgery.

hydroxycarbamide (hydroxyurea) (hy-droks-i-**kar**-bă-myd) *n.* a drug that prevents cell growth and is administered by mouth to treat some types of leukaemia. Hydroxycarbamide may lower the white cell content of the blood due to its effects on the bone marrow. Trade name: **Hydrea**.

hydroxychloroquine (hy-droks-i-**klor**-ŏ-kwin) *n.* a drug, similar to chloroquine, used mainly to treat lupus erythematosus and rheumatoid arthritis. Trade name: **Plaquenil**.

5-hydroxyindoleacetic acid (5-HIAA) (hy-droks-i-in-dohl-ă-see-tik) *n.* a metabolite of serotonin, the most common secretion product of carcinoid tumours (*see* argentaffinoma). Measured over 24 hours in the urine, this is the most reliable screening test for such tumours.

hydroxyprogesterone (hy-droks-i-proh-**jes**-ter-ohn) *n.* a synthetic female sex hormone (*see* progestogen) administered by injection to prevent miscarriage. Trade name: **Proluton**.

hydroxyproline (hy-droks-i-**proh**-leen) *n.* a compound, similar in structure to the amino acids, found only in collagen.

5-hydroxytryptamine (hy-droks-i **trip**-tă-meen) *n. see* serotonin.

hydroxyurea (hy-droks-i-yoor-ee-ă) *n. see* hydroxycarbamide.

hydroxyzine (hy-**droks**-i-zeen) *n.* an antihistamine drug with sedative properties, administered by mouth to relieve anxiety, tension, and agitation and to treat nausea and vomiting. Trade name: **Atarax**.

hygiene (hy-jeen) *n.* the science of health and the study of ways of preserving it, particularly by promoting cleanliness.

hygr- (hygro-) *prefix denoting* moisture.

hygroma (hydroma) (hy-**groh**-mă) *n.* a type of cyst. It may develop from a lymphangioma (*cystic h.*) or from the liquified remains of a subdural haematoma (*subdural h.*).

hygrometer (hy-**grom**-i-ter) *n.* an instrument for measuring the relative humidity of the atmosphere, i.e. the ratio of the moisture in the air to the moisture it would contain if it were saturated at the same temperature and pressure.

hymen (hy-měn) *n.* the membrane that covers the opening of the vagina at birth but usually perforates spontaneously before puberty.

hymenectomy (hy-měn-ek-tŏmi) *n.* surgical removal of the hymen to enlarge the vaginal opening.

hymenotomy (hy-měn-ot-ŏmi) *n.* incision of the hymen. This operation may be performed in cases of imperforate hymen. It is also carried out to alleviate dyspareunia (painful intercourse).

hyo- *prefix denoting* the hyoid bone.

hyoid bone (hy-oid) *n.* a small isolated U-shaped bone in the neck, below and supporting the tongue. It is held in position by muscles and ligaments between it and the styloid process of the temporal bone.

hyoscine (scopolamine) (hy-ŏ-seen) *n.* an anticholinergic drug that prevents muscle spasm. It is used in the treatment of gut spasm, to relax the uterus in labour, for preoperative medication, and for motion sickness. It is administered by mouth, injection, or skin patches. Trade names: **Buscopan, Scopoderm**.

hyp- (hypo-) *prefix denoting* **1.** deficiency, lack, or small size. **2.** (in anatomy) below; beneath.

hypaemia (hy-**pee**-miă) *n.* a decrease in the blood supply to an organ or tissue. *Compare* hyperaemia.

hypalgesia (hy-pal-**jeez**-iă) *n.* an abnormally low sensitivity to pain.

hyper- *prefix denoting* **1.** excessive; abnormally increased. **2.** (in anatomy) above.

hyperacidity (hy-per-ă-**sid**-iti) *n.* an abnormally increased concentration of acid, especially in the stomach (*see* hyperchlorhydria).

hyperactivity (hy-per-ak-**tiv**-iti) *n.* *see* hyperkinesia.

hyperacusis (hy-per-ă-**kew**-sis) *n.* abnormally acute hearing or painful sensitivity to sounds.

hyperadrenalism (hy-per-ă-**dren**-ă-lizm) *n.* overactivity of the adrenal glands. *See* Cushing's syndrome.

hyperaemia (hy-per-ee-miă) *n.* the presence of excess blood in the vessels supplying a part of the body. *active h.* (*arterial h.*) hyperaemia that occurs when the arterioles are relaxed and there is an increased blood flow. *passive h.* hyperaemia that occurs when the blood flow from the affected part is obstructed.

hyperaesthesia (hy-per-ees-**theez**-iă) *n.* excessive sensibility, especially of the skin.

hyperalgesia (hy-per-al-**jeez**-iă) *n.* an abnormal state of increased sensitivity to painful stimuli.

hyperandrogenism (hy-per-an-**droj**-in-izm) *n.* excessive secretion of androgen in women. It is associated with hirsutism, acne, sparse or infrequent menstruation (oligomenorrhoea), metrorrhagia, absent or infrequent ovulation, infertility, endometrial hyperplasia, hyperlipidaemia, hyperglycaemia, and hypertension. *See also* virilization.

hyperbaric (hy-per-**ba**-rik) *adj.* at a pressure greater than atmospheric pressure. *h. oxygenation* a technique for exposing a patient to oxygen at high pressure. It is used to treat compressed air illness, carbon monoxide poisoning, gas gangrene, and acute breathing difficulties.

hypercalcaemia (hy-per-kal-**see**-miă) *n.* the presence in the blood of an abnormally high concentration of calcium. It may be caused by excessive ingestion of vitamin D, overactivity of the parathyroid glands, or malignant disease. *idiopathic h.* congenital hypercalcaemia that is associated with mental retardation and heart defects. *Compare* hypocalcaemia.

hypercalcinuria (hypercalcuria) (hy-per-kal-sin-**yoor**-iă) *n.* the presence in the urine of an abnormally high concentration of calcium.

hypercapnia (hypercarbia) (hy-per-**kap**-niă) *n.* the presence in the blood of an abnormally high concentration of carbon dioxide.

hypercatabolism (hy-per-kă-**tab**-ŏl-izm) *n.* an abnormally increased rate of metabolic breakdown of substances in the body. *See* catabolism. —**hypercatabolic** *adj.*

hyperchloraemia (hy-per-klor-**ee**-miă) *n.* the presence in the blood of an abnormally high concentration of chloride.

hyperchlorhydria (hy-per-klor-**hy**-driă) *n.* a greater than normal secretion of hydrochloric acid by the stomach, usually associated with a duodenal ulcer.

hypercholesterolaemia (hy-per-kŏl-est-er-ol-**ee**-miă) *n. see* cholesterol.

hyperchromatism (hy-per-**kroh**-mă-tizm) *n.* the property of the nuclei of certain cells (for example, those of tumours) to stain more deeply than normal. —**hyperchromatic** *adj.*

hyperdactylism (polydactylism) (hy-per-**dak**-til-izm) *n.* the condition of having more than the normal number of fingers or toes.

hyperdynamia (hy-per-dy-**nay**-miă) *n.* excessive activity of muscles.

hyperemesis (hy-per-**em**-i-sis) *n.* severe vomiting. *h. gravidarum* severe vomiting during pregnancy. It starts in early pregnancy and may continue to produce marked dehydration and subsequent liver damage. Rarely, the condition may worsen in spite of active treatment; under such circumstances it may be necessary to terminate the pregnancy.

hyperextension (hy-per-iks-**ten**-shŏn) *n.* extension of a joint or limb beyond its normal limit.

hyperflexion (hy-per-**flek**-shŏn) *n.* excessive and forceful flexion of a limb or other part.

hyperglycaemia (hy-per-gly-**see**-

miă) *n.* an excess of glucose in the bloodstream. It may occur in a variety of diseases, most notably in diabetes mellitus.

hyperhidrosis (hyperidrosis) (hy-per-hy-**droh**-sis) *n.* excessive sweating, which may occur in certain diseases, such as fevers or thyrotoxicosis, or following the use of certain drugs, although more commonly there is no underlying cause.

hyperinsulinism (hy-per-**ins**-yoo-lin-izm) *n.* **1.** excessive secretion of the hormone insulin by the islet cells of the pancreas. **2.** metabolic disturbance due to administration of too much insulin.

hyperkalaemia (hy-per-kal-**ee**-miă) *n.* the presence in the blood of an abnormally high concentration of potassium, usually due to failure of the kidneys to excrete it. *See also* electrolyte.

hyperkeratosis (hy-per-ke-ră-**toh**-sis) *n.* thickening of the outer horny layer of the skin. It may occur as an inherited disorder, affecting the palms and soles.

hyperkinesia (hyperactivity) (hy-per-ki-**neez**-iă) *n.* a state of overactive restlessness in children. *See* attention-deficit/hyperactivity disorder. —**hyperkinetic** (hy-per-ki-**net**-ik) *adj.*

hyperlipidaemia (hyperlipaemia) (hy-per-lip-id-ee-miă) *n.* the presence in the blood of an abnormally high concentration of cholesterol and/or triglycerides in the form of lipoproteins.

hypermetropia (long-sightedness) (hy-per-mi-**troh**-piă) *n.* the condition in which parallel light rays are brought to a focus behind the retina when the accommodation

is relaxed. Normal vision can be restored by wearing spectacles with convex lenses (see illustration). *Compare* emmetropia, myopia.

focusing point is beyond the retina

Uncorrected

Corrected

convex lens converges light rays falling on the eye

Hypermetropia (long-sightedness)

hypermotility (hy-per-moh-**til**-iti) *n.* excessive movement or activity, especially of the stomach or intestine.

hypernatraemia (hy-per-nă-**tree**-miă) *n.* the presence in the blood of an abnormally high concentration of sodium. *See also* electrolyte.

hypernephroma (Grawitz tumour, renal cell carcinoma) (hy-per-ni-**froh**-mă) *n.* a malignant tumour of kidney cells. It may be present for some years before giving rise to symptoms, which include fever, loin pain, and blood in the urine. Treatment is by surgery but tumours are apt to recur locally or spread via the bloodstream.

hyperopia (hy-per-**oh**-piă) *n.* the usual US term for hypermetropia.

hyperosmolar non-ketotic diabetic coma (hy-per-oz-**moh**-ler) *n.* a coma induced by very poorly controlled diabetes mellitus in which the blood-sugar levels have become markedly high with severe dehydration but no excessive ketone production or acidosis.

hyperostosis (hy-per-os-**toh**-sis) *n.* excessive enlargement of the outer layer of a bone. It commonly affects the frontal bone of the skull (*h. frontalis*). *infantile cortical h.* (*Caffey's disease*) swelling of the long bones, jaw, and shoulder blade, associated with pain and fever, in infants under six months.

hyperparathyroidism (hy-per-pa-ră-**th'y**-roid-izm) *n.* overactivity of the parathyroid glands. *See* von Recklinghausen's disease.

hyperphagia (hy-per-**fay**-jiă) *n.* excessive overeating. *See* bulimia.

hyperpiesia (hy-per-py-ee-ziă) *n.* see hypertension.

hyperpituitarism (hy-per-pit-**yoo**-it-er-izm) *n.* overactivity of the pituitary gland, resulting in acromegaly or gigantism.

hyperplasia (hy-per-**play**-ziă) *n.* the increased production and growth of normal cells in a tissue or organ. *benign prostatic h. see* prostate gland. *See also* endometrial (hyperplasia). *Compare* hypertrophy, neoplasia.

hyperpnoea (hy-perp-**nee**-ă) *n.* an increase in the rate of breathing that is proportional to an increase in metabolism; for example, on exercise. *Compare* hyperventilation.

hyperpyrexia (hy-per-py-**reks**-iă)

n. a rise in body temperature above 106°F (41.1°C). *See* fever.

hypersecretion (hy-per-si-**kree**-shŏn) *n.* excessive secretion, as of hydrochloric acid by the stomach (*see* hyperchlorhydria).

hypersensitive (hy-per-**sen**-si-tiv) *adj.* prone to respond abnormally to the presence of a particular antigen, which may cause a variety of tissue reactions ranging from serum sickness to an allergy (such as hay fever) or, at the severest, to anaphylactic shock (*see* anaphylaxis). *See also* allergy, immunity. —**hypersensitivity** *n.*

hypersplenism (hy-per-**splen**-izm) *n.* a decrease in the numbers of red cells, white cells, and platelets in the blood resulting from destruction or pooling of these cells by an enlarged spleen.

hypertension (hy-per-**ten**-shŏn) *n.* high blood pressure, i.e. elevation of the arterial blood pressure above the normal range expected in a particular age group. Hypertension may be of unknown cause (*essential h.* or *hyperpiesia*). It may also result from disease (*secondary* or *symptomatic h.*), as of the kidneys (*renal h.*), endocrine system, or arteries. Complications that may arise from hypertension include atherosclerosis, heart failure, cerebral haemorrhage, and kidney failure. Most cases of hypertension depend upon long-term drug therapy to lower the blood pressure and maintain it within the normal range. The drugs used include thiazide diuretics, beta blockers, ACE inhibitors, and many others. *See also* portal hypertension, pulmonary (hypertension).

hyperthermia (hyperthermy)

(hy-per-**therm**-iă) *n.* **1.** exceptionally high body temperature (about 41°C or above). *See* fever. **2.** treatment of disease by inducing fever. *Compare* hypothermia.

hyperthyroidism (hy-per-**th'y**-roid-izm) *n.* overactivity of the thyroid gland, either due to a tumour, overgrowth of the gland, or Graves's disease. *apathetic h.* a condition seen in patients with thyrotoxicosis, characterized by slow atrial fibrillation and depressive illness. *See* thyrotoxicosis.

hypertonia (hypertonicity) (hy-per-**toh**-niă) *n.* exceptionally high tension in muscles.

hypertonic (hy-per-**tonn**-ik) *adj.* **1.** describing a solution that has a greater osmotic pressure than another solution. *See* osmosis. **2.** describing muscles that demonstrate an abnormal increase in tonicity.

hypertrichosis (hy-per-trik-**oh**-sis) *n.* excessive growth of hair.

hypertrophy (hypertrophia) (hy-**per**-trŏ-fi) *n.* increase in the size of a tissue or organ brought about by the enlargement of its cells rather than by cell multiplication. *Compare* hyperplasia.

hypertropia (hy-per-**troh**-piă) *n.* strabismus in which one eye looks upwards.

hyperuricaemia (lithaemia) (hy-per-yoor-i-**see**-miă) *n.* the presence in the blood of an abnormally high concentration of uric acid. *See* gout.

hyperuricuria (lithuria) (hy-per-yoor-ik-**yoor**-iă) *n.* the presence in the urine of an abnormally high concentration of uric acid.

hyperventilation (hy-per-ven-ti-lay-shŏn) *n.* breathing at an abnormally rapid rate at rest. This causes a reduction of the carbon dioxide concentration of the arterial blood, leading to dizziness, tingling in the lips and limbs, tetanic cramps in the hands, and tightness across the chest. *h. syndrome* prolonged hyperventilation, often of psychogenic origin, which may lead to loss of consciousness.

hypervitaminosis (hy-per-vit-ă-min-oh-sis) *n.* the condition resulting from excessive consumption of vitamins. The fat-soluble vitamins A and D are toxic if taken in excessive amounts.

hypervolaemia (hy-per-vŏ-lee-miă) *n.* an increase in the volume of circulating blood.

hyphaema (hy-fee-mă) *n.* a collection of blood in the chamber of the eye that lies in front of the iris.

hypn- (hypno-) *prefix denoting* **1.** sleep. **2.** hypnosis.

hypnagogic (hip-nă-goj-ik) *adj.* relating to the period immediately before falling asleep. *h. imagery* the production of vivid mental images just before falling asleep. *h. hallucination* a vivid and intense auditory or visual hallucination occurring at the beginning of sleep in 30–60% of patients with narcolepsy.

hypnosis (hip-noh-sis) *n.* a sleeplike state, artificially induced by a *hypnotist*, in which the mind is more than usually receptive to suggestion. Hypnotic suggestion has been used for a variety of purposes in medicine, for example as a cure for addiction and in other forms of psychotherapy.

hypnotherapy (hip-noh-**th'e**-ră-pi) *n.* any form of psychotherapy that utilizes hypnosis. —**hypnothera-pist** n.

hypnotic (soporific) (hip-**not**-ik) n. a drug that produces sleep by depressing brain function. Hypnotics include benzodiazepines (e.g. nitrazepam, lorazepam) and some sedative antihistamines (e.g. promethazine). They often cause hangover effects in the morning.

hypnotism (hip-**nŏ**-tizm) n. the induction of hypnosis.

hypo- prefix. see hyp-.

hypoaesthesia (hy-poh-ees-**theez**-iă) n. a condition in which the sense of touch is diminished. This may rarely be extended to include other forms of sensation.

hypocalcaemia (hy-poh-kal-**see**-miă) n. the presence in the blood of an abnormally low concentration of calcium. See tetany. Compare hypercalcaemia.

hypocapnia (hy-poh-**kap**-niă) n. see acapnia.

hypochloraemia (hy-poh-klor-**ee**-miă) n. the presence in the blood of an abnormally low concentration of chloride.

hypochlorhydria (hy-poh-klor-**hy**-driă) n. reduced secretion of hydrochloric acid by the stomach. See achlorhydria.

hypochlorite (hy-poh-**klor**-ryt) n. any salt of hypochlorous acid (chloric(I) acid; HClO). Hypochlorites have antiseptic and disinfectant properties, e.g. Milton (sodium hypochlorite).

hypochondria (hy-poh-**kon**-driă) n. preoccupation with the physical functioning of the body and with fancied ill health. In the most severe form there are delusions of ill health, usually due to underlying depression. —**hypochondriac** n. —**hypochondriacal** (hy-poh-kon-dry-ă-kăl) adj.

hypochondriasis (hypochondriacal disorder) (hy-poh-kon-dry-ă-sis) n. symptoms of hypochondria that have reached a level sufficient to be classified as a disorder.

hypochondrium (hy-poh-**kon**-dri-ŭm) n. the upper lateral portion of the abdomen, situated beneath the lower ribs. —**hypochondriac** adj.

hypochromic (hy-poh-**kroh**-mik) adj. **1.** deficient in pigmentation. **2.** (of red blood cells) deficient in haemoglobin.

hypocretin (hy-poh-**kree**-tin) n. a neuropeptide that originates in the hypothalamus. Low levels of hypocretin in the cerebrospinal fluid are found in most patients with narcolepsy and may also be found in patients who have suffered with stroke, brain tumours, head injuries, and infections of the nervous system.

hypodermic (hy-poh-**derm**-ik) adj. beneath the skin: usually applied to subcutaneous injections. The term is also applied to the syringe used for such injections.

hypofibrinogenaemia (fibrinogenopenia) (hy-poh-fi-brin-oh-jĕ-nee-miă) n. a deficiency of the clotting factor fibrinogen in the blood, which results in an increased tendency to bleed. It may occur as an inherited disorder or it may be acquired.

hypogammaglobulinaemia (hy-poh-gam-ă-glob-yoo-lin-ee-miă) n. a deficiency of the protein gammaglobulin in the blood, resulting in an increased susceptibility to infections. It may occur in a variety of inherited disorders or as an acquired defect.

hypogastrium (hy-poh-gas-triŭm) *n.* that part of the central abdomen situated below the region of the stomach. —**hypogastric** *adj.*

hypoglossal nerve (hy-poh-glos-ăl) *n.* the twelfth cranial nerve (XII), which supplies the muscles of the tongue and is therefore responsible for the movements of talking and swallowing.

hypoglycaemia (hy-poh-gly-see-miă) *n.* a deficiency of glucose in the bloodstream, causing muscular weakness and incoordination, mental confusion, and sweating. If severe it may lead to *hypoglycaemic coma.* Hypoglycaemia most commonly occurs in diabetes mellitus. It is treated by administration of glucose. *reactive h.* hypoglycaemia occurring after a meal, induced by excessive levels of insulin release from the pancreas. —**hypoglycaemic** (hy-poh-gly-see-mik) *adj.*

hypoglycaemic unawareness *n.* a serious condition in which a diabetic patient loses the earliest warning signs of an approaching hypoglycaemic episode and may thus suffer a severe attack, with confusion, seizures, or even coma and death. It is more common in longstanding diabetes and in those who experience many hypoglycaemic episodes.

hypohidrosis (hy-poh-hy-droh-sis) *n.* a reduction in sweating in the presence of an appropriate stimulus for sweating (such as heat). It may accompany disease or occur as a congenital defect.

hypoinsulinism (hy-poh-ins-yoo-

lin-izm) *n.* a deficiency of insulin due either to inadequate secretion of the hormone by the pancreas or to inadequate treatment of diabetes mellitus.

hypokalaemia (hy-poh-kal-ee-miă) *n.* the presence of abnormally low levels of potassium in the blood: occurs in dehydration. *See* electrolyte.

hypomania (hy-poh-may-niă) *n.* a mild degree of mania. Elated mood leads to faulty judgment; behaviour lacks the usual social restraints and the sexual drive is increased; speech is rapid and animated; the individual is energetic but not persistent and tends to be irritable. —**hypomanic** (hy-poh-man-ik) *adj., n.*

hypomenorrhoea (hy-poh-men-ŏ-ree-ă) *n.* the release of an abnormally small quantity of blood at menstruation.

hypomotility (hy-poh-moh-til-iti) *n.* decreased movement or activity, especially of the stomach or intestine.

hyponatraemia (hy-poh-nă-tree-miă) *n.* the presence in the blood of an abnormally low concentration of sodium: occurs in dehydration. *See* electrolyte.

hypoparathyroidism (hy-poh-pa-ră-th'y-roid-izm) *n.* subnormal activity of the parathyroid glands, causing a fall in the blood concentration of calcium and muscular spasms (*see* tetany).

hypopharynx (laryngopharynx) (hy-poh-fa-rinks) *n.* the part of the pharynx that lies below the level of the hyoid bone.

hypophysectomy (hy-pof-i-sek-tŏmi) *n.* the surgical removal or destruction (by radiotherapy) of the pituitary gland (hypophysis) in the brain.

hypophysis (hy-pof-i-sis) *n. see* pituitary gland.

hypopiesis (hy-poh-py-ee-sis) *n.* abnormally reduced blood pressure (*see* hypotension) in the absence of organic disease.

hypopituitarism (hy-poh-pit-yoo-it-er-izm) *n.* subnormal activity of the pituitary gland, causing dwarfism in childhood and a syndrome of impaired sexual function, pallor, and premature ageing in adult life (*see* Simmond's disease).

hypoplasia (hy-poh-play-ziă) *n.* underdevelopment of an organ or tissue. —**hypoplastic** (hy-poh-plast-ik) *adj.*

hypoplastic left heart *n.* a congenital heart disorder in which the left side of the heart, particularly the left ventricle, is underdeveloped. Affected babies usually develop severe heart failure within the first few days of life. Most babies die within the first few weeks, but milder cases may be amenable to surgery.

hypoplastic leukaemia *n.* a stage of leukaemia in which there is a decrease in the number of white cells, red cells, and platelets in the blood and reduced haemopoiesis in the bone marrow.

hypopnoea (hy-poh-nee-ă) *n.* an abnormal decrease in the rate and depth of breathing. *h. syndrome* a condition related to obstructive sleep apnoea, characterized by episodes of hypopnoea during sleep in which nasal airflow is between 30% and 50% of normal for more than 10 seconds.

hypoproteinaemia (hy-poh-proh-

ti-nee-miă) *n.* a decrease in the quantity of protein in the blood, resulting in oedema and increased susceptibility to infections. It may result from malnutrition, impaired protein production, or increased loss of protein from the body. *See also* hypogammaglobulinaemia.

hypoprothrombinaemia (hy-poh-proh-throm-bin-ee-miă) *n.* a deficiency of the clotting factor prothrombin in the blood, which results in an increased tendency to bleed.

hypopyon (hy-poh-pi-ŏn) *n.* pus in the chamber of the eye that lies in front of the iris.

hyposecretion (hy-poh-si-kree-shŏn) *n.* decreased secretion.

hyposensitive (hy-poh-sen-si-tiv) *adj.* less than normally responsive to the presence of antigenic material. *Compare* hypersensitive. —**hyposensitivity** *n.*

hyposensitization (hy-poh-sen-si-ty-zay-shŏn) *n. see* desensitization.

hypospadias (hy-poh-spay-di-ăs) *n.* a congenital abnormality in which the opening of the urethra is on the underside of the penis: either on the glans penis (*glandular h.*), at the junction of the glans with the shaft (*coronal h.*), or on the shaft itself (*penile h.*). *See* MAGPI operation.

hypostasis (hy-pos-tă-sis) *n.* accumulation of fluid or blood in a dependent part of the body in cases of poor circulation. *Hypostatic pneumonia* results from hypostatic congestion of the lung bases in debilitated patients who are confined to bed. —**hypostatic** (hy-poh-stat-ik) *adj.*

hyposthenia (hy-pos-th'ee-niă) *n.* a

state of physical weakness or abnormally low muscular tension.

hypotension (hy-poh-**ten**-shŏn) *n.* a condition in which the arterial blood pressure is abnormally low. It occurs after excessive fluid or blood loss. Other causes include myocardial infarction, pulmonary embolism, Addison's disease, severe infections, allergic reactions, arrhythmias, and acute abdominal conditions (e.g. pancreatitis). *orthostatic h.* temporary hypotension experienced when rising from a horizontal position.

hypothalamus (hy-poh-**thal**-ă-mŭs) *n.* the region of the forebrain in the floor of the third ventricle, linked with the thalamus above and the pituitary gland below. It contains several important centres controlling body temperature, thirst, hunger, and eating, water balance, and sexual function. It also functions as a centre for the integration of hormonal and autonomic nervous activity. —**hypothalamic** *adj.*

hypothenar (hy-poth i nar) *adj.* describing or relating to the fleshy prominent part of the palm of the hand below the little finger. *Compare* thenar.

hypothermia (hy-poh-**therm**-iă) *n.* **1.** accidental reduction of body temperature below the normal range. It is particularly liable to occur in babies and the elderly. **2.** deliberate lowering of body temperature for therapeutic purposes. This may be done during surgery, in order to reduce the patient's requirement for oxygen.

hypothyroidism (hy-poh-**th'y**-roid-izm) *n.* subnormal activity of the thyroid gland. If present at birth and untreated it leads to cretinism. In adult life it causes myxoedema. The condition can be treated by administration of thyroxine.

hypotonia (hy-poh-**toh**-niă) *n.* a state of reduced tension in muscle.

hypotonic (hy-poh-**tonn**-ik) *adj.* **1.** describing a solution that has a lower osmotic pressure than another solution. *See* osmosis. **2.** describing muscles that demonstrate diminished tonicity.

hypotony (hy-poh-toh-ni) *n.* a very low intraocular pressure, usually as a result of trauma or surgery to the eye.

hypotrichosis (hy-poh-trik-**oh**-sis) *n.* a condition in which less hair develops than normal.

hypotropia (hy-poh-**troh**-piă) *n.* strabismus in which one eye looks downwards.

hypoventilation (hy-poh-ven-ti-lay-shŏn) *n.* breathing at an abnormally shallow and slow rate, which results in an increased concentration of carbon dioxide in the blood.

hypovitaminosis (hy-poh-vit-ă-min-**oh**-sis) *n.* a deficiency of a vitamin caused either through lack of the vitamin in the diet or from an inability to absorb or utilize it.

hypovolaemia (oligaemia) (hy-poh-vŏ-lee-miă) *n.* a decrease in the volume of circulating blood. *See* shock.

hypoxaemia (hy-poks-ee-miă) *n.* reduction of the oxygen concentration in the arterial blood, recognized clinically by the presence of central and peripheral cyanosis.

hypoxia (hy-poks-iă) *n.* a deficiency of oxygen in the tissues. *See also* anoxia, hypoxaemia.

hyster- (hystero-) *prefix denoting* **1.** the uterus. **2.** hysteria.

hysterectomy (hiss-ter-ek-tŏmi) *n.* the surgical removal of the uterus, either through an incision in the abdominal wall (*abdominal h.*) or through the vagina (*vaginal h.*). *subtotal h.* removal of the body of the uterus, leaving the neck (cervix) in place. *total h.* removal of the entire uterus. *See also* Wertheim's hysterectomy.

hysteria (hiss-**teer**-iă) *n.* **1.** formerly, a neurosis whose principal features consist of emotional instability, repression, dissociation, physical symptoms, and vulnerability to suggestion. *conversion h.* see conversion disorder. *dissociative h.* see dissociative disorder. **2.** a state of great emotional excitement.

hysterical (hiss-**te**-ri-kăl) *adj.* **1.** describing symptoms characteristic of conversion disorder. **2.** describing a kind of personality disorder characterized by instability and shallowness of feelings.

hysteroptosis (hiss-ter-op-**toh**-sis) *n.* prolapse of the uterus. *See* prolapse.

hysterosalpingography (hiss-ter-oh-sal-ping-og-răfi) *n. see* uterosalpingography.

hysterosalpingosonography (hiss-ter-oh-sal-ping-oh-sonn-og-răfi) *n.* visualization of the Fallopian tubes by means of an ultrasound beam, usually directed via a vaginal probe, after a contrast medium has been passed through them via the cervix. *See also* (transvaginal) ultrasonography.

hysteroscope (uteroscope) (**hiss**-ter-oh-skohp) *n.* a tubular instrument with a light source for observing the interior of the uterus. *See also* endoscope.

hysterotomy (hiss-ter-**ot**-ŏmi) *n.* an operation for removal of the fetus by incision of the uterus through the abdomen before the 24th week of gestation; after this time the operation is called Caesarean section. Hysterotomy is now rarely performed.

hysterotrachelorrhaphy (hiss-ter-oh-trak-el-o-răfi) *n.* the operation of stitching a tear in the cervix of the uterus.

-iasis *suffix denoting* a diseased condition.

iatro- *prefix denoting* **1.** medicine. **2.** doctors.

iatrogenic (I-at-roh-**jen**-ik) *adj.* describing a condition that has resulted from treatment, as either an unforeseen or inevitable side-effect.

IBD *n. see* inflammatory bowel disease.

IBS *n. see* irritable bowel syndrome.

ibuprofen (I-bew-**proh**-fen) *n.* an anti-inflammatory drug (*see* NSAID), administered by mouth in the treatment of arthritic conditions. Trade names: **Brufen, Junifen.**

IC *n. see* inspiratory capacity.

ICD *n. see* International Classification of Diseases. *ICD-10* the latest version, published in 1992.

ichor (I-kor) *n.* a watery material oozing from wounds or ulcers.

ichthammol (ik-**tham**-ol) *n.* a sulphur-containing drug with antibacterial properties, used in the form of an ointment for treating certain skin diseases.

ichthyosis (ik-thi-**oh**-sis) *n.* any one of a group of genetically determined skin disorders in which there is abnormal scaling of the skin. Xeroderma is a very mild form of the disorder. *i. vulgaris* the most common form of the disease, which is inherited as an autosomal dominant condition.

ICP *n. see* intracranial (pressure).

ICSH (interstitial-cell-stimulating hormone) *n. see* luteinizing hormone.

ICSI (**ik**-si) *n.* intracytoplasmic sperm injection: a technique of assisted conception in some cases of male infertility in which a single spermatozoon is injected into the cytoplasm of an ovum in vitro. The fertilized ovum is then implanted into the uterus.

icterus (ik-**ter**-ŭs) *n. see* jaundice.

ictus (ik-**tŭs**) *n.* a stroke or any sudden attack. The term is often used for an epileptic seizure.

ICU *n. see* intensive care (unit).

id (Id) *n.* (in psychoanalysis) a part of the unconscious mind governed by the instinctive forces of libido and the death wish.

ID *adj. see* intradermal.

-id *suffix denoting* relationship or resemblance to.

IDDM *n.* insulin-dependent diabetes mellitus. *See* diabetes.

ideation (I-di-**ay**-shŏn) *n.* the process of thinking or of having imagery or ideas.

identical twins (I-den-**tik**-ăl) *pl. n. see* twins.

identification (I-den-ti-fi-**kay**-shŏn) *n.* (in psychological development) the process of adopting other people's characteristics more or less permanently. Identification with a parent is important in personality formation.

ideo- *prefix denoting* **1.** the mind or mental activity. **2.** ideas.

ideomotor (I-di-ō-moh-ter) *adj.* describing or relating to a motor action that is evoked by an idea. *i. apraxia* the inability to translate the idea of a complex behaviour into action.

idio- *prefix denoting* peculiarity to the individual.

idiopathic (idi-oh-*path*-ik) *adj.* denoting a disease or condition the cause of which is not known or that arises spontaneously. *i. thrombocytopenic purpura see* purpura. —**idiopathy** (idi-*op*-ă-thi) *n.*

idiosyncrasy (idi-oh-*sink*-răsi) *n.* an unusual and unexpected sensitivity exhibited by an individual to a particular drug or food. —**idiosyncratic** (idi-oh-sin-*krat*-ik) *adj.*

idiot savant (eed-yoh sa-*vahn*) *n.* an individual whose overall functioning is at the level of mental retardation but who has one or more special intellectual abilities that are advanced to a high level.

idioventricular (idi-oh-ven-*trik*-yoo-ler) *adj.* affecting or peculiar to the ventricles of the heart. *i. rhythm* the very slow beat of the ventricles under the influence of their own natural subsidiary pacemaker.

idoxuridine (I-doks-*yoor*-i-deen) *n.* an iodine-containing drug that inhibits the growth of viruses and is administered topically to treat herpes infections. Trade name: **Herpid**.

ifosfamide (I-fos-*fă*-myd) *n.* a cytotoxic drug used in the treatment of malignant disease, particularly sarcomas, testicular tumours, and lymphomas. It is administered intravenously by injection or infusion. Trade name: **Mitoxana**.

IGT *n.* impaired glucose tolerance (*see* glucose tolerance test).

IHD *n. see* ischaemic heart disease.

IL-2 *n. see* interleukin.

ile- (ileo-) *prefix denoting* the ileum.

ileal conduit (il-i-ăl) *n.* a segment of small intestine (ileum) used to convey urine from the ureters to the exterior into an appliance (*see also* urinary diversion). The ureters are implanted into an isolated segment of bowel, one end of which is brought through the abdominal wall to the skin surface.

ileal pouch (perineal pouch) *n.* a reservoir made from loops of ileum to replace a surgically removed rectum, avoiding the need for a permanent ileostomy.

ileectomy (ili-*ek*-tŏmi) *n.* surgical removal of the ileum or part of the ileum.

ileitis (ili-I-tis) *n.* inflammation of the ileum. It may be caused by Crohn's disease, tuberculosis, the bacterium *Yersinia enterocolitica*, or typhoid or it may occur in association with ulcerative colitis.

ileocaecal (ili-oh-*see*-kăl) *adj.* relating to the ileum and caecum. *i. valve* a valve at the junction of the small and large intestines consisting of two membranous folds that close to prevent the backflow of food from the colon and caecum to the ileum.

ileocaecocystoplasty (ili-oh-see-koh-*sis*-toh-plasti) *n.* an operation in which the dome of the bladder is removed by cutting across the bladder transversely or sagittally above the openings of the ureters; the dome is replaced by an isolated segment of caecum and terminal ileum. *See* cystoplasty.

ileocolitis (ili-oh-kŏ-ly-tis) *n.* inflammation of the ileum and the colon. The commonest causes are Crohn's disease and tuberculosis.

ileocolostomy (ili-oh-kŏ-lost-ŏmi) *n.* a surgical operation in which the ileum is joined to some part of the colon.

ileocystoplasty (ili-oh-sis-tohplasti) *n.* an operation in which the bladder is enlarged by an opened-out portion of small intestine. *See* cystoplasty.

ileoproctostomy (ili-oh-prok-tost-ŏmi) *n. see* ileorectal (anastomosis).

ileorectal (ili-oh-rek-t'l) *adj.* relating to the ileum and rectum. *i. anastomosis (ileoproctostomy)* a surgical operation in which the ileum is joined to the rectum, usually after surgical removal of the colon (*see* colectomy)

ileosigmoidostomy (ili-oh-sigmoid-ost-ŏmi) *n.* an operation in which an opening is created between the ileum and the sigmoid colon.

ileostomy (ili-ost-ŏmi) *n.* a surgical operation in which the ileum is brought through the abdominal wall to create an artificial opening (*stoma*) through which the intestinal contents can discharge, thus bypassing the colon. Various types of bag may be worn to collect the effluent.

ileum (il-iŭm) *n.* the lowest of the three portions of the small intestine (*see* intestine). It runs from the jejunum to the ileocaecal valve. —**ileal**, **ileac** *adj.*

ileus (il-i-ŭs) *n.* intestinal obstruction, usually obstruction of the small intestine (ileum). *paralytic* or *adynamic i.* functional obstruction of the ileum due to loss of peristalsis, which may be caused by abdominal surgery, spinal injuries, hypokalaemia, or peritonitis. Treatment consists of intravenous administration of fluid and nutrients and removal of excess stomach secretions by tube until peristalsis returns.

ili- (ilio-) *prefix denoting* the ilium.

iliac (il-i-ak) *adj.* relating to the ilium. *i. arteries* the arteries that supply most of the blood to the lower limbs and pelvic region. *i. fossa* a concave depression on the inside of the pelvis. The right iliac fossa provides space for the vermiform appendix. *i. veins* the veins draining most of the blood from the lower limbs and pelvic region.

iliacus (i-lee-ă-kŭs) *n.* a flat triangular muscle situated in the area of the groin. This muscle acts in conjunction with the psoas muscle to flex the thigh.

iliococcygeal (ili-oh-kok-sij-iăl) *adj.* relating to the ilium and the coccyx.

iliopsoas (ili-oh-soh-ăs) *n.* a composite muscle made up of the iliacus and psoas muscles, which have a common tendon.

ilium (il-iŭm) *n.* the haunch bone: a wide bone forming the upper part of each side of the hip bone (*see also* pelvis). —**iliac** *adj.*

illusion (i-loo-zhŏn) *n.* a false perception due to misinterpretation of the stimuli arising from an object. Illusions may occur in almost any psychiatric syndrome, especially depression. *Compare* hallucination. *optical i.* a perception that does not agree with the actual object in the external world. Optical illusions are produced by deceptive qualities of the stimulus and are in no way pathological.

IM *adj. see* intramuscular.

image (im-ij) *n.* **1.** (in physiology) an optical reproduction of an object formed on the retina when light is refracted through the eye. **2.** (in radiology) a representation of the structure of an organ, tissue, etc., produced by radiography and used by physicians in diagnosis and in monitoring the effects of treatment. *See* imaging. *i. intensifier* an electronic device that provides a TV image from an X-ray source. It amplifies the signal from the original image, giving a brighter picture, so that the radiation dose can be reduced. **3.** (in psychology) a mental representation resulting from thought rather than from sensory perception. *See* body image, imagery.

imagery (im-ij-er-i) *n.* the production of vivid mental representations by the normal processes of thought. *eidetic i.* the production of images of exceptional clarity, which may be recalled long after being first experienced.

imaging (im-ij-ing) *n.* the production of images of organs or tissues by a range of techniques. *See also* computerized tomography, crosssectional imaging, magnetic resonance imaging, real-time imaging, ultrasonography.

imago (i-may-goh) *n.* (in psychoanalysis) the internal unconscious representation of an important person in the individual's life, particularly a parent.

imatinib (i-mat-in-ib) *n.* a cytotoxic drug used in the treatment of adults with chronic myeloid leukaemia in which the Philadelphia chromosome is present, if interferon-alfa treatment fails or the disease is in a highly active phase. Trade name: **Glivec**.

imidazole (i-mid-ă-zohl) *n.* one of a group of chemically related antifungal drugs that are also effective against a wide range of bacteria; some (e.g. tiabendazole and mebendazole) are also used as anthelmintics. The group includes econazole, clotrimazole, ketoconazole, and miconazole.

imipramine (i-mip-ră-meen) *n.* a drug that is administered by mouth or injection to treat depression (*see* antidepressant). Trade name: **Tofranil**.

immersion foot (i-mer-shŏn) *n. see* trench foot.

immiscible (i-mis-ibŭl) *adj.* incapable of being mixed to form a homogeneous substance. Oil and water are immiscible.

immobilization (i-moh-bi-ly-zay-shŏn) *n.* the procedure of making a normally movable part of the body, such as a joint, immovable. This helps an infected, diseased, or injured tissue (bone, joint, or muscle) to heal.

immune (i-mewn) *adj.* protected against a particular infection by the presence of specific antibodies against the organisms concerned. *i. response* the reaction of the body to the presence of antigens (foreign tissues, bacteria, etc.), which are attacked and destroyed by antibodies. *See* antibody, antigen, immunity. *i. system* the organs and tissues responsible for immunity, including the thymus, bone marrow, lymph nodes, spleen, and tonsils. *See also* lymphoid tissue.

immunity (i-mewn-iti) *n.* the body's ability to resist infection, afforded by the presence of circulating antibodies and white blood cells. *active i.* immunity that arises when the body's own cells produce, and remain able to produce, appropriate antibodies following an attack of a disease or deliberate stimulation (*see* immunization). *cell-mediated i.* immunity resulting from the action of T-lymphocytes. *humoral i.* immunity resulting from the action of circulating antibodies produced by B lymphocytes. *natural* (or *innate*) *i.* immunity resulting from the activity of phagocytic cells, natural killer cells, and other mechanisms present before exposure to infection. *passive i.* temporary immunity that may be provided by injecting ready-made antibodies in antiserum taken from another person or an animal already immune. Babies have passive immunity, conferred by antibodies from the maternal blood and colostrum, to common diseases for several weeks after birth.

immunization (im-yoo-ny-**zay**-shŏn) *n.* the production of immunity by artificial means. Passive immunity may be conferred by the injection of an antiserum, but the production of active immunity calls for the use of a vaccine (*see* vaccination).

immuno- *prefix denoting* immunity or immunological response.

immunoassay (im-yoo-noh-**ass**-ay) *n.* any of various techniques for determining the levels of antigen and antibody in a tissue. *See* radioimmunoassay.

immunocompromised (im-yoo-noh-**kom**-prŏ-myzd) *adj.* describing patients in whom the immune response is reduced or defective due to immunosuppression. Such patients are vulnerable to opportunistic infections.

immunodeficiency (im-yoo-noh-di-**fish**-ĕn-si) *n.* deficiency in the immune response. This can be acquired, as in AIDS, but there are many varieties of primary immunodeficiency occurring as inherited disorders characterized by hypogammaglobulinaemia, defects in T-cell function, or both.

immunogenicity (im-yoo-noh-jĕn-**iss**-iti) *n.* the property that enables a substance to provoke an immune response, including foreignness (*see* antigen), size, route of entry into the body, dose, number and length of exposures to the antigen, and host genetic make-up.

immunoglobulin (Ig) (im-yoo-noh-**glob**-yoo-lin) *n.* one of a group of structurally related proteins (gammaglobulins) that act as antibodies.

immunological tolerance (im-yoo-nŏ-**loj**-ik-ăl) *n.* a failure of the body to distinguish between materials that are 'self', and therefore to be tolerated, and those that are 'not self', against which it mounts an immune response.

immunology (im-yoo-**nol**-ŏji) *n.* the study of immunity and all of the phenomena connected with the defence mechanisms of the body. —**immunological** *adj.*

immunosuppressant (im-yoo-noh-sŭ-**press**-ănt) *n.* a drug, such as azathioprine or cyclophosphamide, that reduces the body's resistance to infection and other foreign bodies by suppressing the immune system. Immunosuppressants are used to maintain the survival of organ and tissue transplants and to treat various autoimmune diseases. Ciclosporin is the immunosuppressant usually used in organ transplant recipients.

immunosuppression (im-yoo-noh-sŭ-**presh**-ŏn) *n.* suppression of the immune response, usually by disease (e.g. AIDS) or by drugs (e.g. steroids, azathioprine, ciclosporin). —**immunosuppressed** *adj.*

immunotherapy (im-yoo-noh-**th'e**-ră-pi) *n.* the prevention or treatment of disease using agents that may modify the immune response. It is a largely experimental approach, studied most widely in the treatment of leukaemias, melanoma, and hypernephroma.

immunotoxin (im-yoo-noh-**toks**-in) *n.* one of a new class of drugs undergoing clinical trials for the treatment of leukaemia. Immunotoxins combine monoclonal antibodies, which specifically target cancerous cells, with a highly toxic compound (such as ricin) that inhibits protein synthesis.

immunotransfusion (im-yoo-noh-trans-**few**-zhŏn) *n.* the transfusion of an antiserum to treat or give temporary protection against a disease.

impacted (im-**pak**-tid) *adj.* firmly wedged. *i. faeces* faeces that are so hard and dry that they cannot pass through the anus and require manual removal under an anaesthetic. *i. fracture see* fracture. *i. tooth* a tooth, usually a wisdom tooth, that cannot erupt into a normal position be-

cause it is obstructed by other tissues. —**impaction** *n.*

impaired glucose tolerance (IGT) (im-**paird**) *n. see* glucose tolerance test.

impairment (im-**pair**-mĕnt) *n. see* handicap.

impalpable (im-**palp**-ăbŭl) *adj.* describing a structure within the body that cannot be detected by feeling with the hand.

imperforate (im-**per**-fer-it) *adj.* lacking an opening. *i. anus (proctatresia)* partial or complete obstruction of the anus: a condition, discovered at birth, due to failure of the anus to develop normally in the embryo. Most mild cases of imperforate anus can be treated by a simple operation. *i. hymen* a condition in which the hymen completely closes the vagina and thus impedes the flow of menstrual blood.

impetigo (imp-i-**ty**-goh) *n.* a superficial bacterial infection of the skin, which usually responds to treatment with antibiotics. *bullous i.* impetigo caused by *Staphylococcus aureus*. It is characterized by blisters, is less contagious than the nonbullous form, and occurs at any age. *nonbullous i.* impetigo caused by *Staphylococcus aureus, Streptococcus* species, or both organisms; it mainly affects young children and is highly contagious, with yellowish-brown crusting.

implant (im-**plahnt**) *n.* a drug (such as a subcutaneous hormone implant), a prosthesis (such as an artificial hip), or a radioactive source (such as radium needles) that is put into the body. *breast i.* a prosthesis inserted subcutaneously to replace breast tissue that has been removed surgically during a simple mastectomy in the treatment of breast cancer or to augment existing breast tissue. The type of implant in current use is a silicone sac filled with silicone gel. **dental i.** a rigid structure that is embedded in the jawbone or under its periosteum to provide support for replacement teeth on a denture or a bridge. **heart i.** see artificial heart. **intraocular lens i.** a plastic lens placed inside the eye after cataract surgery. **osseointegrated i.** an implant that can be introduced into living bone without producing a foreign-body reaction (see osseointegration). See also cochlear implant.

implantation (im-plahn-tay-shŏn) n. **1.** (nidation) the attachment of the early embryo to the lining of the uterus, which occurs six to eight days after ovulation. **2.** the placing of a substance (e.g. a drug) or an object (e.g. an artificial pacemaker) within a tissue. **3.** the surgical replacement of damaged tissue with healthy tissue (see transplantation).

implementation (im-pli-men-tay-shŏn) n. the stage of the nursing process in which the patient's individual care plan is utilized and executed, in collaboration with other members of the health-care team.

implosion (im-ploh-zhŏn) n. see flooding.

impotence (im-pŏ-tĕns) n. inability in a man to have sexual intercourse. Impotence may be *erectile*, in which the penis does not become firm enough to enter the vagina, or *ejaculatory*, in which penetration occurs but there is no ejaculation of semen (orgasm).

impregnate (im-preg-nayt) vb. **1.**

to make pregnant. **2.** to saturate with another substance. —**impregnation** n.

impression (im-presh-ŏn) n. (in dentistry) a mould made of the teeth and surrounding soft tissues or of a toothless jaw. An impression is used in the construction of orthodontic appliances, restorations, and dentures.

impulse (im-puls) n. (in neurology) see nerve impulse.

IMV n. see intermittent mandatory ventilation.

in- (im-) prefix denoting **1.** not. **2.** in; within; into.

inaccessible (in-ak-ses-ibŭl) adj. (in psychiatry) unresponsive to words and similar stimuli: describing the mental state of certain patients, e.g. schizophrenics. —**inaccessibility** n.

inanition (in-ă-nish-ŏn) n. a condition of exhaustion caused by lack of nutrients in the blood. This may arise through starvation, malnutrition, or intestinal disease.

in articulo mortis (in ar-tik-yoo-loh mor-tis) Latin: at the moment of death.

inborn error of metabolism (in-born e-rer) n. any one of a group of inherited conditions in which there is a disturbance in either the structure, synthesis, function, or transport of protein molecules. Examples are phenylketonuria, homocystinuria, and hypogammaglobulinaemia.

inbreeding (in-breed-ing) n. the production of offspring by parents who are closely related. Compare outbreeding.

incarcerated (in-kar-ser-ayt-id) adj. confined or constricted so as to be immovable: applied particularly to a type of hernia.

incest (in-sest) *n.* sexual intercourse between close relatives, e.g. brother and sister or father and daughter.

incipient (in-sip-iĕnt) *adj.* coming into existence: describing a stage in a disease.

incision (in-sizh-ŏn) *n.* **1.** the surgical cutting of soft tissues, such as skin or muscle, with a knife or scalpel. *bladder neck i.* incision through the bladder neck and prostate to relieve lower urinary tract symptoms. **2.** the cut so made.

incisor (in-sy-zer) *n.* any of the four front teeth in each jaw, two on each side of the midline. *See also* dentition.

inclusion bodies (in-kloo-zhŏn) *pl. n.* particles occurring in the nucleus and cytoplasm of cells usually as a result of virus infection. Their presence can sometimes be used to diagnose such an infection.

inclusion conjunctivitis *n. see* conjunctivitis.

incompatibility (in-kŏm-pat-i-bil-iti) *n.* lack of compatibility. In cases of severe incompatibility, there are likely to be swift immune reactions to transplanted organs or tissues.

incompetence (in-kom-pi-tĕns) *n.* impaired function of the valves of the heart or veins, which allows backward leakage of blood. *See* aortic regurgitation, mitral incompetence, varicose veins.

incontinence (in-kon-ti-nĕns) *n.* **1.** the inappropriate involuntary passage of urine. *genuine stress i.* (*GSI*) incontinence in women for which a physical cause can be identified. *stress i.* the leak of urine on coughing and straining. It is common in women in whom the muscles of the pelvic floor are weakened after childbirth. *overflow i.* leakage from a full bladder, which occurs most commonly in elderly men with bladder outflow obstruction. *urge i.* leakage of urine that accompanies an intense desire to pass water with failure of restraint. *See also* enuresis. **2.** inability to control bowel movements (*faecal i.*). **3.** involuntary loss of faeces or flatus (*anal i.*).

incoordination (in-koh-or-din-ay-shŏn) *n.* (in neurology) an impairment in the performance of precise movements. Incoordination may result from a disorder in any part of the nervous system. *See* apraxia, ataxia, dyssynergia.

incubation (in-kew-bay-shŏn) *n.* **1.** the process of development of an egg or a culture of bacteria. **2.** the care of a premature baby in an incubator.

incubation period (latent period) *n.* the interval between exposure to an infection and the appearance of the first symptoms.

incubator (ink-yoo-bay-ter) *n.* a transparent container for keeping premature babies in controlled conditions and protecting them from infection. Other forms of incubator are used for cultivating bacteria and for hatching eggs.

incus (ink-ŭs) *n.* a small anvil-shaped bone in the middle ear that articulates with the malleus and the stapes. *See* ossicle.

independent nursing function (indi-pend-ĕnt) *n.* any aspect of nursing practice for which the nurse alone is responsible, acting on his or her own initiative and without instructions from any other discipline.

Inderal (in-der-al) *n. see* propranolol.

indican (in-di-kǎn) *n.* a compound excreted in the urine as a detoxification product of indoxyl.

indicanuria (in-di-kǎn-yoor-iǎ) *n.* the presence in the urine of an abnormally high concentration of indican. This may be a sign that the intestine is obstructed.

indication (indi-kay-shŏn) *n.* (in medicine) a strong reason for believing that a particular course of action is desirable. *Compare* contraindication.

indigenous (in-dij-in-ŭs) *adj.* occurring naturally in a particular area, region, or country. Certain diseases are indigenous to particular regions.

indigestion (indi-jes-chŏn) *n. see* dyspepsia.

indigo carmine (in-dig-oh **kar**myn) *n.* a blue dye that is administered by injection to test for kidney function.

indinavir (in-din-ǎ-veer) *n. see* protease inhibitor.

individualized nursing care (indi-vid-yoo-ǎ-lyzd) *n.* care that is planned to meet the particular needs of one patient, as opposed to a routine applied to all patients suffering from the same disease.

indole (in-dohl) *n.* a derivative of the amino acid tryptophan, excreted in the urine and faeces.

indolent (in-dŏl-ĕnt) *adj.* describing a disease process that is failing to heal or has persisted. The term is applied particularly to ulcers of skin or mucous membrane.

indometacin (indomethacin) (in-doh-**met**-ǎ-sin) *n.* an anti-inflammatory drug (*see* NSAID), administered by mouth or in suppositories in the treatment of arthritic conditions. Trade names: **Indocid, Indomod.**

indoramin (in-dor-ǎ-min) *n.* an alpha blocker drug used to treat high blood pressure. It is administered by mouth. Trade names: **Baratol, Doralese.**

indoxyl (in-doks-il) *n.* an alcohol derived from indole by bacterial action. It is excreted in the urine as indican.

induction (in-duk-shŏn) *n.* **1.** (in obstetrics) the artificial starting of childbirth, e.g. by injecting oxytocin or puncturing the amnion, when pregnancy has continued considerably beyond the expected date of birth or if there is a risk to the health of mother or infant. **2.** (in anaesthetics) initiation of anaesthesia. General anaesthesia is usually induced by intravenous injection of rapidly acting drugs, usually barbiturates (such as thiopental), into the bloodstream.

induration (in-dewr-ay-shŏn) *n.* abnormal hardening of a tissue or organ. *See also* sclerosis.

industrial disease (in-dus-tri-ǎl) *n.* an occupational disease associated with a particular industry or group of industries.

inertia (in-er-shǎ) *n.* (in physiology) sluggishness or absence of activity in certain smooth muscles. *uterine i.* inertia of the muscular wall of the uterus during labour, making the process excessively long. It may be present from the start of labour or it may develop because of exhaustion following strong contractions.

in extremis (in iks-**tree**-mis) Latin: at the point of death.

infant (**in**-fănt) *n.* a child incapable of any form of independence from its mother: usually, a child under one year of age, especially a newborn child. *i. mortality rate* the number of deaths of infants per 1000 live births in a given year. Included are the *neonatal mortality rate* (calculated from deaths occurring in the first four weeks of life) and *postneonatal mortality rate* (from deaths in the remainder of the first year).

infanticide (in-**fant**-i-syd) *n.* (in Britain) under the terms of the Infanticide Act 1938, the felony of child destruction by the natural mother within 12 months of birth when the balance of her mind is disturbed because she has not fully recovered from childbirth and/or lactation.

infantile (in-**făn**-tyl) *adj.* **1.** denoting conditions occurring in adults that are recognizable in childhood, e.g. poliomyelitis (*i. paralysis*). **2.** of, relating to, or affecting infants. *i. spasms* (*salaam attacks*) a rare but serious form of epilepsy that usually begins between three and eight months of age. It is characterized by involuntary flexing movements of the arms, legs, neck, and trunk. It may be arrested by treatment with antiepileptic drugs, corticosteroids, or ACTH.

infantilism (in-**fant**-il-izm) *n.* persistence of childlike physical or psychological characteristics into adult life.

infarct (in-**farkt**) *n.* a small localized area of dead tissue produced as a result of an inadequate blood supply.

infarction (in-**fark**-shŏn) *n.* the death of part or the whole of an organ that occurs when the artery carrying its blood supply is obstructed by a blood clot (thrombus) or an embolus. *See also* myocardial infarction.

infection (in-**fek**-shŏn) *n.* invasion of the body by harmful organisms (pathogens), such as bacteria, fungi, protozoa, rickettsiae, or viruses. The infective agent may be transmitted by a patient or carrier in airborne droplets or by direct contact; by animal or insect vectors; by ingestion of contaminated food or drink; or from an infected mother to the fetus. After an incubation period symptoms appear, usually consisting of either localized inflammation and pain or more remote effects. Treatment with drugs is usually effective against most infections, but there are few specific treatments for many common viral infections.

infectious disease (in-**fek**-shŭs) *n. see* communicable disease.

infectious mononucleosis *n. see* glandular fever.

inferior (in-**feer**-i-er) *adj.* (in anatomy) lower in the body in relation to another structure or surface.

inferiority complex (in-feer-i-o-**riti**) *n.* **1.** an unconscious exaggeration of feelings of inferiority, which is shown by compensatory behaviour, such as aggression. **2.** (in psychoanalysis) a complex said to result from the conflict between Oedipal wishes (*see* Oedipus complex) and the reality of the child's lack of power. This gives rise to repressed feelings of personal inferiority.

infertility (in-fer-**til**-iti) *n.* inability

in a woman to conceive or in a man to induce conception. *See also* sterility.

infestation (in-fes-**tay**-shŏn) *n.* the presence of animal parasites either on the skin or inside the body.

infibulation (in-fib-yoo-**lay**-shŏn) *n.* the most extensive form of female circumcision, involving excision of the clitoris, labia minora, and labia majora.

infiltration (in-fil-**tray**-shŏn) *n.* **1.** the abnormal entry of a substance (*infiltrate*) into a cell, tissue, or organ. Examples of infiltrates are blood cells, cancer cells, fat, or starch. **2.** the injection of a local anaesthetic solution into the tissues to cause local anaesthesia.

inflammation (in-flă-**may**-shŏn) *n.* the body's response to injury. *acute i.* the immediate defensive reaction of tissue to injury, which may be caused by infection, chemicals, or physical agents. It involves pain, heat, redness, swelling, and loss of function of the affected part. *chronic i.* the response that ensues when acute inflammation does not heal. —**inflammatory** (in-**flam**-ă-ter-i) *adj.*

inflammatory bowel disease (IBD) *n.* any of a group of inflammatory conditions of the intestine that include (among others) ulcerative colitis and Crohn's disease.

infliximab (in-**fliks**-i-mab) *n.* a monoclonal antibody used to treat severe cases of Crohn's disease and rheumatoid arthritis that have failed to respond to treatment with corticosteroids or immunosuppressants and antirheumatic drugs, respectively. It is administered by infusion. Trade name: **Remicade**.

influenza (in-floo-**en**-ză) *n.* a highly contagious virus infection that affects the respiratory system. Symptoms include headache, fever, loss of appetite, weakness, and general aches and pains. With bed rest and aspirin most patients recover, but a few go on to develop viral or bacterial pneumonia.

informed consent (in-**formd**) *n.* a legal requirement that physicians or researchers inform a patient undergoing surgery or invasive tests or a subject involved in a clinical trial of the nature, risks, and probable outcome of the treatment or research. The patient signs an agreement stating that he or she has been informed and accepts the treatment, surgery, or research protocol. Without informed consent, the physician or researcher is violating the patient's rights, regardless of whether the treatment is appropriate and successful.

infra- *prefix denoting* below.

infrared radiation (in-fră-**red**) *n.* the band of electromagnetic radiation that is longer in wavelength than the red of the visible spectrum and is responsible for the transmission of radiant heat. It may be used in physiotherapy to warm tissues, reduce pain, and improve circulation.

infundibulum (in-fun-**dib**-yoo-lŭm) *n.* any funnel-shaped channel or passage, particularly the hollow conical stalk that extends downwards from the hypothalamus and is continuous with the posterior lobe of the pituitary gland.

infusion (in-**few**-zhŏn) *n.* **1.** the slow injection of a substance, usually into a vein (*intravenous i.*, IVI).

This is a common method for replacing water, electrolytes, and blood products and is also used for the continuous administration of drugs or nutrition. *See also* drip. **2.** the process whereby the active principles are extracted from plant material by steeping it in boiling water (as in the making of tea). **3.** the solution produced by this process.

ingesta (in-**jes**-tă) *pl. n.* food and drink that is taken into the alimentary canal through the mouth.

ingestion (in-**jes**-chŏn) *n.* the process by which food is taken into the alimentary canal. It involves chewing and swallowing.

ingrowing toenail (in-**groh**-ing) *n.* a toenail whose free margin grows or is pressed into the skin at the side of the nail, causing inflammation.

inguinal (**ing**-win-ăl) *adj.* relating to or affecting the region of the groin (inguen). **i. canal** either of a pair of openings that connect the abdominal cavity with the scrotum in the male fetus. **i. hernia** *see* hernia. **i. ligament** (*Poupart's ligament*) a ligament in the groin that extends from the anterior superior iliac spine to the pubic tubercle. It is part of the aponeurosis of the external oblique muscle of the abdomen.

INH *n. see* isoniazid.

inhalation (in-hă-**lay**-shŏn) *n.* **1.** (**inspiration**) the act of breathing air into the lungs through the mouth and nose. *See* breathing. **2.** a gas, vapour, or aerosol breathed in for the treatment of conditions of the respiratory tract.

inhaler (in-**hay**-ler) *n.* a device for the administration of inhalations. **metered-dose i.** an inhaler designed to deliver the correct dose of an inhalation to the appropriate section of the airway.

inherent (in-**heer**-ĕnt) *adj.* inborn; innate.

inhibition (in-hib-**ish**-ŏn) *n.* **1.** (in physiology) the prevention or reduction of the functioning of an organ, muscle, etc., by the action of certain nerve impulses. **2.** (in psychoanalysis) an inner command that prevents one from doing something forbidden. **3.** (in psychology) a tendency not to carry out a specific action, produced each time the action is carried out.

inhibitor (in-**hib**-it-er) *n.* a substance that prevents the occurrence of a given process or reaction. *See also* MAO inhibitor.

injection (in-**jek**-shŏn) *n.* introduction into the body of drugs or other fluids by means of a syringe. Common routes for injection are into the skin (*intracutaneous* or *intradermal*); below the skin (*subcutaneous*); into a muscle (*intramuscular*), for drugs that are slowly absorbed; and into a vein (*intravenous*), for drugs to be rapidly absorbed. Enemas are also regarded as injections.

injury scoring system (injury severity scale, ISS) (in-jer-i) *n.* a system used, particularly in triage, for grading the severity of an injury. *See also* abbreviated injury scale.

inlay (**in**-lay) *n.* a substance or piece of tissue inserted within a tissue, generally to replace a defect.

innate (in-**ayt**) *adj.* describing a condition or characteristic that is present in an individual at birth and is inherited from his parents. *See also* congenital.

inner ear (in-er) *n. see* labyrinth.

innervation (in-er-vay-shŏn) *n.* the nerve supply to an area or organ of the body.

innominate artery (brachiocephalic artery) (in-om-in-it) *n.* a short artery originating as the first large branch of the aortic arch, which divides at the lower neck into the right common carotid and the right subclavian arteries.

innominate bone *n. see* hip (bone).

innominate vein (brachiocephalic vein) *n.* either of two veins, one on each side of the neck, formed by the junction of the external jugular and subclavian veins. The two veins join to form the superior vena cava.

INO *n. see* (internuclear) ophthalmoplegia.

ino- *prefix denoting* **1.** fibrous tissue. **2.** muscle.

inoculation (in-ok-yoo-lay-shŏn) *n.* the introduction of a small quantity of material, such as a vaccine, in the process of immunization: a more general name for vaccination.

inoculum (in-ok-yoo-lŭm) *n.* any material that is used for inoculation.

inorganic (in-or-gan-ik) *adj.* **1.** not of animal or vegetable origin. **2.** (in chemistry) describing or relating to compounds that do not contain carbon.

inositol (in-oh-sit-ol) *n.* a compound, similar to a hexose sugar, that is a constituent of some cell phospholipids; it is present in the bran of cereal grain. It is sometimes classified as a vitamin but it can be synthesized by most animals and there is no evidence that it is an essential nutrient in humans.

inositol triphosphate *n. see* second messenger.

inotropic (in-ŏ-trop-ik) *adj.* affecting the contraction of heart muscle. Such drugs as dobutamine and enoximone have positive inotropic action, stimulating heart muscle contractions. Beta-blocker drugs such as propranolol, have negative inotropic action.

in-patient (in-pay-shĕnt) *n.* a patient who is admitted to a bed in a hospital ward and remains there for a period of time for treatment, examination, or observation. *Compare* out-patient.

inquest (in-kwest) *n.* an official judicial enquiry into the cause of a person's death: carried out when the death is sudden or takes place under suspicious circumstances. *See also* autopsy.

insanity (in-san-iti) *n.* a degree of mental illness such that the affected individual is not responsible for his actions. The term is a legal rather than a medical one.

insect (in-sekt) *n.* a member of a large group of mainly land-dwelling arthropods. Insects of medical importance include various blood-sucking insects transmitting tropical diseases; lice, whose bites can cause intense irritation and bacterial infection; and flies, which transmit organisms causing diarrhoea and dysentery to food. *See also* myiasis.

insecticide (in-sekt-i-syd) *n.* a preparation used to kill destructive or disease-carrying insects. Some insect powders contain organic phosphorus compounds and fluorides; when ingested accidentally they may cause damage to the nervous system. The use of such compounds is generally under strict control. *See also* DDT.

insemination (in-sem-i-**nay**-shŏn) *n.* introduction of semen into the vagina. *See also* artificial insemination.

insertion (in-**ser**-shŏn) *n.* (in anatomy) the point of attachment of a muscle (e.g. to a bone) that is relatively movable when the muscle contracts. *Compare* origin.

insidious (in-**sid**-iŭs) *adj.* describing a disease that develops gradually and imperceptibly.

insight (**in**-syt) *n.* (in psychology) knowledge of oneself. The term is applied particularly to a patient's recognition that he or she has psychological problems; in this sense absence of insight is a feature of psychosis.

in situ (in **sit**-yoo) *adj.* **1.** in the natural or original position. **2.** describing a cancer that has not undergone metastasis to invade surrounding tissue.

insolation (in-soh-**lay**-shŏn) *n.* exposure to the sun's rays. *See also* heatstroke.

insomnia (in-**som**-niă) *n.* inability to fall asleep or to remain asleep for an adequate length of time. Insomnia may be associated with disease, but is more often caused by worry. *See also* fatal familial insomnia.

inspiration (in-spi-**ray**-shŏn) *n. see* inhalation.

inspiratory capacity (IC) (in-**spir**-ă-teri) *n.* the maximum volume of air that can be inspired after normal expiration.

inspissated (in-**spis**-ayt-id) *adj.* thickened or hardened by absorption or evaporation. *i. sputum* a

thick sputum produced in whooping cough, which is difficult to cough up.

instillation (in-stil-**ay**-shŏn) *n.* **1.** the application of liquid medication drop by drop, as into the eye. **2.** the medication applied in this way.

instinct (**in**-stinkt) *n.* **1.** a complex pattern of behaviour innately determined, which is characteristic of all individuals of the same species. **2.** an innate drive that urges the individual towards a particular goal.

institutionalization (in-sti-tyoo-shŏn-ăl-I-**zay**-shŏn) *n.* a condition produced by long-term residence in an unstimulating impersonal institution (such as some residential care homes). The individual adapts to the behaviour characteristic of the institution to such an extent that he or she is handicapped in other environments. The features often include apathy, dependence, and a lack of personal responsibility.

insufficiency (in-sŭ-**fish**-ĕn-si) *n.* inability of an organ or part, such as the heart or kidney, to carry out its normal function.

insufflation (in-suf-**lay**-shŏn) *n.* the act of blowing gas or a powder, such as a medication, into a body cavity.

insulin (**ins**-yoo-lin) *n.* a protein hormone, produced in the pancreas by the beta cells of the islets of Langerhans, that is important for regulating the amount of sugar (glucose) in the blood. Lack of this hormone gives rise to diabetes mellitus, in which large amounts of sugar are present in the blood and urine. This condition may be treated successfully by insulin injections. *analogue i.* an insulin medication that has a very fast onset of action and can be injected immediately before eating. *isophane i.* insulin combined with protamine, which reduces its rate of absorption from the injection site and hence prolongs its action in the bloodstream. *i. shock see* shock. *i. stress test* a test of anterior pituitary gland function involving the induction of a hypoglycaemic episode with injected insulin and subsequent measurements of plasma cortisol and growth hormone.

insulinase (ins-yoo-lin-ayz) *n.* an enzyme, found in such tissues as the liver and kidney, that is responsible for the normal breakdown of insulin in the body.

insulinoma (ins-yoo-lin-oh-mă) *n.* an insulin-producing tumour of the beta cells in the islets of Langerhans of the pancreas. Symptoms include sweating, faintness, and other features of hypoglycaemia (*see* Whipple's triad).

insult (in-sult) *n.* an injury or physical trauma.

Intal (in-tal) *n. see* cromoglicate.

integument (in-teg-yoo-měnt) *n.* **1.** the skin. **2.** a membrane or layer of tissue covering any organ of the body.

intelligence quotient (IQ) (in-tel-i-jěns kwoh-shěnt) *n.* an index of intellectual development. In childhood and adult life it represents intellectual ability relative to the rest of the population; in children it can also represent rate of development (mental age as a percentage of chronological age).

intelligence test *n.* a standardized assessment procedure for the determination of intellectual ability. The score produced is usually expressed as an intelligence quo-

tient. Scores on intelligence tests are used for such purposes as the diagnosis of mental retardation and the assessment of intellectual deterioration.

intensive care (intensive therapy) (in-ten-siv) *n.* specialized and monitored health care provided for critically ill and immediately postoperative patients by specialist multidisciplinary staff in a specially designed hospital unit (*i. c.* or *i. t. unit*, *ICU* or *ITU*). *neonatal i. c. unit* (*NICU*) a unit providing intensive care for preterm, very low-birth-weight, and seriously ill babies. *paediatric i. c. unit* (*PICU*) a unit providing intensive care for seriously ill children. *See also* coronary care.

intention (in-ten-shŏn) *n.* a process of healing. *first i.* healing in which the edges of a wound are brought together under aseptic conditions and granulation tissue forms. *second i.* healing in which the wound edges are separated and the cavity is filled with granulation tissue over which epithelial tissue grows from the wound edges. *third i.* healing in which the wound ulcerates, granulations are slow to form, and a scar forms at the wound site.

intention tremor *n. see* tremor.

inter- *prefix denoting* between.

intercalated (inter-kă-layt-id) *adj.* describing structures, tissues, etc., that are inserted or situated between other structures.

intercellular (inter-sel-yoo-ler) *adj.* situated or occurring between cells.

intercostal muscles (inter-kost'l) *pl. n.* muscles that occupy the spaces between the ribs and are responsible for controlling some of the movements of the ribs.

intercurrent (inter-ku-rĕnt) *adj.* going on at the same time: applied to an infection contracted by a patient who is already suffering from an infection or other disease.

interferon (inter-feer-on) *n.* a substance that is produced by cells infected with a virus and has the ability to inhibit viral growth. Particular interferons are effective only in the species that produces them. Preparations of human interferon produced by genetic engineering are used clinically in treating hepatitis B and C and certain cancers (*i. alfa*) and multiple sclerosis (*i. beta*).

interkinesis (inter-ky-nee-sis) *n.* **1.** the resting stage between the two divisions of meiosis. **2.** *see* interphase.

interleukin (inter-lew-kin) *n.* any of a family of 12 proteins that control aspects of haemopoiesis and the immune response. *interleukin 2 (IL-2)* an interleukin that stimulates T-lymphocytes to become natural killer cells. A recombinant form (*aldesleukin*, Proleukin), administered by subcutaneous injection, can be of benefit in the treatment of hypernephroma.

intermenstrual (inter-men-stroo-ăl) *adj.* between the menstrual periods.

intermittency (inter-mit-ĕn-si) *n.* a symptom in which the flow of urine is not continuous but stops and starts. *See* lower urinary tract symptoms.

intermittent claudication (inter-mit-ĕnt) *n. see* claudication.

intermittent fever *n.* a fever that rises, subsides, then returns again. *See* malaria.

intermittent mandatory ventilation (IMV) (man-dăt-eri) *n.* a form of assisted respiration in which the patient breathes at his or her normal rate but is assisted by a respirator set to deliver a fixed volume of air at a specified rate. IMV is often used to help patients to cease to rely on mechanical ventilation. *synchronized i. m. v. (SIMV)* intermittent mandatory ventilation synchronized with the patient's own efforts.

intermittent pneumatic compression (new-mat-ik) *n.* a technique to prevent thrombosis in bedridden patients. It uses an inflatable device that squeezes the calf when it inflates, preventing pools of blood forming behind the valves in the veins, thus mimicking the effects of walking.

intermittent self-catheterization (ISC, clean intermittent self-catheterization, CISC) *n.* a procedure in which the patient periodically passes a disposable catheter through the urethra into the bladder for the purpose of emptying it of urine. It is increasingly used in the management of patients of both sexes (including children) with chronic retention and large residual urine volumes, often due to neuropathic bladder. ISC may prevent back pressure and dilatation of the upper urinary tract with consequent infection and incontinence.

International Classification of Diseases (ICD) (inter-nash-ŏn-ăl) *n.* a list of all known diseases and syndromes published by the World Health Organization every ten years (approximately).

interoceptor (inter-oh-sep-ter) *n.*

any receptor organ composed of sensory nerve cells that respond to and monitor changes within the body, such as the stretching of muscles or the acidity of the blood.

interosseous (inter-oss-i-ŭs) *adj.* between two bones.

interparietal bone (inca bone, incarial bone) (inter-pă-ry-i-t'l) *n.* the bone lying between the parietal bones, at the back of the skull.

interphase (interkinesis) (inter-fayz) *n.* the period when a cell is not undergoing division (mitosis), during which activities such as DNA synthesis occur.

intersex (in-ter-seks) *n.* an individual who shows anatomical characteristics of both sexes. *See* hermaphrodite. —**intersexuality** *n.*

interstice (in-ter-stiss) *n.* a small space in a tissue or between parts of the body. —**interstitial** (inter-stish-ăl) *adj.*

interstitial cells (Leydig cells) *pl. n.* the cells interspersed between the seminiferous tubules of the testis. They secrete androgens in response to stimulation by luteinizing hormone.

interstitial-cell-stimulating hormone *n. see* luteinizing hormone.

interstitial cystitis *n.* a chronic nonbacterial inflammation of the bladder accompanied by an urgent desire to pass urine frequently and bladder pain; it is usually associated with an ulcer in the bladder wall (*Hunner's ulcer*). The cause is unknown and contracture of the bladder eventually occurs.

intertrigo (inter-try-goh) *n.* superficial inflammation of two skin surfaces that are in contact. It is caused by friction and sweat.

interventional radiology (interven-shŏn-ăl) *n. see* radiology.

intervertebral disc (inter-ver-tib-răl) *n.* the flexible plate of fibrocartilage that connects any two adjacent vertebrae in the backbone. The intervertebral discs act as shock absorbers, protecting the brain and spinal cord from the impact produced by running and other movements. *See also* prolapsed intervertebral disc.

intestinal flora (in-test-in-ăl) *pl. n.* bacteria normally present in the intestinal tract. Some are responsible for the synthesis of vitamin K.

intestinal glands *pl. n. see* Lieberkühn's glands.

intestinal juice *n. see* succus (entericus).

intestinal obstruction *n. see* obstruction.

intestine (bowel, gut) (in-test-in) *n.* the part of the alimentary canal that extends from the stomach to the anus. *large i.* the part that consists of the caecum, vermiform appendix, colon, and rectum. It is largely concerned with the absorption of water from the material passed from the small intestine. *small i.* the part of the intestine that consists of the duodenum, jejunum, and ileum. It is here that most of the processes of digestion and absorption of food take place. See illustration. —**intestinal** *adj.*

intima (tunica intima) (in-timă) *n.* **1.** the inner layer of the wall of an artery or vein. It is composed of a lining of endothelial cells and an elastic membrane. **2.** the inner layer of various other organs or parts.

intolerance (in-**tol**-er-ăns) *n.* the inability of a patient to tolerate a particular drug, manifested by various adverse reactions.

intoxication (in-toks-i-**kay**-shŏn) *n.* the symptoms of poisoning due to ingestion of any toxic material, including alcohol.

intra- *prefix denoting* inside; within.

intra-articular (intră-ar-**tik**-yoo-ler) *adj.* within or into a joint.

intracameral (intră-**kam**-ĕr-ăl) *adj.* within a chamber, such as the anterior or posterior chamber of the

villi

lacteal

smooth
muscle fibres

goblet cells

mucous
membrane

crypts of
Lieberkühn
(intestinal glands)

Paneth cells

muscularis
mucosa

blood vessel

circular
muscle layer

connective
tissue

longitudinal
muscle layer

serosa

mucosa

submucosa

myenteron

Longitudinal section through the ileum

eye. *i. anaesthesia* injection of an anaesthetic agent into the anterior chamber of the eye, usually during surgery.

intracellular (intră-sel-yoo-ler) *adj.* situated or occurring inside a cell or cells. Compare extracellular.

intracorneal (intră-korn-iăl) *adj.* within the cornea.

intracranial (intră-kray-ni-ăl) *adj.* within the skull. *i. pressure (ICP)* the normal pressure within the skull. Causes of raised intracranial pressure include haemorrhage, oedema, haematoma, brain tumours, and disturbances to the flow of cerebrospinal fluid.

intradermal (ID) (intră-derm-ăl) *adj.* within the skin. *i. injection* an injection that is made into the skin.

intradural (intră-dewr-ăl) *adj.* within or beneath the dura mater.

intramedullary (intră-mi-dul-er-l) *adj.* within the bone marrow.

intramuscular (IM) (intră-mus-kew-ler) *adj.* within a muscle. See also injection.

intraocular (intră-ok-yoo-ler) *adj.* of or relating to the area within the eyeball. *i. lens implant see* implant.

intraosseous (intră-oss-iŭs) *adj.* within a bone. *i. needle* a wide-bore needle for insertion directly into the bone marrow of (usually) the tibia in children, used only in emergencies to administer drugs and fluids to an unconscious patient when no other means of intravenous access can be gained.

intrastromal (intră-stroh-măl) *adj.* within the stroma, especially of the cornea.

intrathecal (intră-th'ee-kăl) *adj.* **1.** within the meninges of the spinal cord. **2.** within a sheath, e.g. a nerve sheath.

intrauterine (intră-yoo-teryn) *adj.* within the uterus. *i. contraceptive device see* IUCD. *i. growth retardation (IUGR)* the condition resulting in the birth of a baby whose birth weight is abnormally low in relation to its gestational age (i.e. *small for dates; SFD*). Causes include maternal disease (e.g. infection, malnutrition, high blood pressure, smoking, and alcoholism), poor socioeconomic conditions, multiple pregnancy (e.g. twins), and fetal disease. It may be associated with preterm birth. *i. system see* IUS.

intravascular (intră-vas-kew-ler) *adj.* within the blood vessels.

intravenous (IV) (intră-vee-nŭs) *adj.* into or within a vein. See also infusion, injection. *i. feeding see* nutrition. *i. urogram (IVU) see* urogram.

intraversion (intră-ver-shŏn) *n. see* introversion.

intra vitam (in-tră vy-tam) Latin: during life.

intravitreal (intră-vit-ri-ăl) *adj.* within the vitreous humour of the eye.

intrinsic (in-trin-sik) *adj.* exclusive to a part or body.

intrinsic factor *n.* a glycoprotein secreted in the stomach. The secretion of intrinsic factor is necessary for the absorption of vitamin B_{12}; a failure of secretion leads to a deficiency of the vitamin and the condition of pernicious anaemia.

intro- *prefix denoting* in; into.

introitus (in-troh-it-ŭs) *n.* (in anatomy) an entrance into a hollow organ or cavity.

introjection (intrŏ-jek-shŏn) *n.* (in

psychoanalysis) the process of adopting, or of believing that one possesses, the qualities of another person. This can be a form of defence mechanism. *See also* identification.

introspection (intrō-**spek**-shŏn) *n.* the study by an individual of his own mental processes, reactions, etc. —**introspective** *adj.*

introversion (intrō-**ver**-shŏn) *n.* **1.** (**intraversion**) an enduring personality trait characterized by interest in the self rather than the outside world. People high in introversion (*introverts*) tend to have a small circle of friends, like to persist in activities once they have started, and are highly susceptible to permanent conditioning. *Compare* extroversion. **2.** a turning inwards of a hollow organ (such as the uterus) on itself.

introvert (**in**-trō-vert) *n. see* introversion.

intubation (in-tew-**bay**-shŏn) *n.* the introduction of a tube into part of the body for the purpose of diagnosis or treatment. *gastric i.* intubation performed to remove a sample of the stomach contents for analysis or to administer drugs directly into the stomach. *tracheal i.* introduction of an endotracheal tube to maintain an airway in an unconscious or anaesthetized patient.

intumescence (in-tew-**mes**-ĕns) *n.* a swelling or an increase in the volume of an organ.

intussusception (in-tŭs-sŭ-**sep**-shŏn) *n.* the telescoping (*invagination*) of one part of the bowel into another, resulting in intestinal obstruction. It is most common in young children under the age of four. Symptoms include intermittent screaming and pallor, vomiting, and the passing of red jelly with the stools; if the condition does not receive prompt surgical treatment, shock from gangrene of the bowel may result.

inulin (**in**-yoo-lin) *n.* a carbohydrate with a high molecular weight that is filtered from the bloodstream by the kidneys. *i. clearance* a test of kidney function in which inulin is injected into the blood. By measuring the amount that appears in the urine over a given period, it is possible to calculate how much filtrate the kidneys are producing.

inunction (in-**unk**-shŏn) *n.* the rubbing in with the fingers of an ointment or liniment.

invagination (in-vaj-i-**nay**-shŏn) *n.* **1.** the infolding of the wall of a solid structure to form a cavity. **2.** *see* intussusception.

invasion (in-**vay**-zhŏn) *n.* **1.** the onset of a disease. **2.** the entry of bacteria into the body. **3.** the destruction of healthy tissue by a malignant tumour.

invasive (in-**vay**-ziv) *adj.* **1.** denoting tumours that spread into and destroy surrounding healthy tissue (*see* malignant). **2.** denoting a surgical or diagnostic procedure that involves penetration of the skin or underlying organs and tissues by needles or knives.

inversion (in-**ver**-shŏn) *n.* **1.** the turning inwards or inside-out of a part or organ: commonly applied to the state of the uterus after childbirth when its upper part is pulled through the cervical canal. **2.** a chromosome mutation in which a block of genes within a chromosome are in reverse order.

invertase (in-ver-tayz) *n.* an enzyme in intestinal juice that digest sugars.

in vitro (in vee-troh) Latin: describing biological phenomena that are made to occur outside the living body (traditionally in a test-tube).

in vitro fertilization (IVF) *n.* fertilization of an ovum outside the body, a technique used when a woman has blocked Fallopian tubes or some other impediment to the union of sperm and ovum in the reproductive tract. The woman is given hormone therapy causing a number of ova to mature at the same time (*see* superovulation). Several of them are then removed from the ovary through a laparoscope. The ova are mixed with spermatozoa from her partner and incubated in a culture medium until the blastocyst is formed. The blastocyst is then implanted in the mother's uterus and the pregnancy allowed to continue normally.

in vivo (in vee-voh) Latin: describing biological phenomena that occur within the bodies of living organisms.

involucrum (in-vŏ-loo-krŭm) *n.* a growth of new bone that sometimes surrounds a mass of infected and dead bone in osteomyelitis.

involuntary muscle (in-vol-ŭn-ter-i) *n.* muscle that is not under conscious control, such as the muscle of the gut, stomach, blood vessels, and heart. *See also* cardiac muscle, smooth muscle.

involution (in-vŏ-loo-shŏn) *n.* **1.** the shrinking of the uterus to its normal size after childbirth. **2.** atrophy of an organ in old age. —**involutional** (in-vŏ-loo-shŏn-ăl) *adj.*

involutional melancholia *n.* a severe depression, usually psychotic, appearing for the first time in the involutional period of middle life (approximately 40–55 for women, 50–65 for men). Characteristic features include agitation; delusions of ill-health, poverty, and sin; and preoccupations with death and loss. *See* manic-depressive psychosis.

iodine (I-ŏ-din) *n.* an element required in small amounts for healthy growth and development. The thyroid gland requires iodine to synthesize thyroid hormones; a deficiency of the element leads to goitre. *povidone-i.* an iodine-containing antiseptic and skin disinfectant. *radioactive i.* the radioactive isotope iodine-131, which is administered as a drink to shrink the thyroid gland in the treatment of hyperthyroidism. Symbol: I. *See also* Lugol's solution.

iodism (I-ŏ-dizm) *n.* iodine poisoning. The main features are a characteristic staining of the mouth and odour on the breath. Emergency treatment includes administration of starch or flour in water and lavage with sodium thiosulphate solution.

ion (I-ŏn) *n.* an atom or group of atoms that has lost one or more electrons, making it electrically charged and therefore more chemically active. *See* anion, cation, electrolyte.

ionization (I-ŏ-ny-zay-shŏn) *n.* **1.** the dissociation of a substance into ions. Some molecules ionize in solution (*see* electrolyte). **2.** *see* iontophoresis.

iontophoresis (ionization) (I-on-toh-fer-ee-sis) n. the technique of introducing through the skin, by means of an electric current, charged particles of a drug, so that it reaches a deep site. See also cataphoresis.

IOUS n. intraoperative ultrasound examination. See ultrasonography.

IPD n. intermittent peritoneal dialysis. See (peritoneal) dialysis.

ipecacuanha (ipi-kak-yoo-an-ă) n. a plant extract used in small doses, usually in the form of tinctures and syrups, as an expectorant to relieve coughing and to induce vomiting.

IPPV n. intermittent positive pressure ventilation. See positive pressure ventilation.

ipratropium (ip-ră-troh-piŭm) n. an anticholinergic drug used as a bronchodilator in the treatment of chronic reversible airways obstruction (see bronchospasm). It is administered by inhalation. Trade names: **Atrovent**, **Respontin**.

ipsilateral (ipselateral, homolateral) (ip-si-lat-er-ăl) adj. on or affecting the same side of the body. Compare contralateral.

IQ n. see intelligence quotient.

irbesartan (er-bess-ar-tan) n. see angiotensin II antagonist.

irid- (irido-) prefix denoting the iris.

iridectomy (i-ri-dek-tŏmi) n. an operation on the eye in which a part of the iris is removed.

iridocele (i-rid-oh-seel) n. the protrusion of part of the iris through a wound in the cornea.

iridocyclitis (i-ri-doh-sy-kly-tis) n. inflammation of the iris and ciliary body of the eye. See uveitis.

iridodialysis (i-ri-doh-dy-al-i-sis) n. a tear, caused by injury to the eye,

in the attachment of the iris to the ciliary body.

iridoplegia (i-ri-doh-plee-jiă) n. paralysis of the iris, which is usually associated with cycloplegia and results from injury, inflammation, or the use of pupil-dilating eye drops.

iridoptosis (i-ri-dop-tŏ-sis) n. prolapse of the iris.

iridotomy (i-ri-dot-ŏmi) n. an operation on the eye in which an incision is made in the iris using a knife or a YAG laser.

irinotecan (i-rin-oh-tee-kăn) n. a cytotoxic drug administered by intravenous infusion for treating advanced colorectal cancer. Trade name: **Campto**.

iris (I-ris) n. the part of the eye that regulates the amount of light that enters. It forms a coloured muscular diaphragm across the front of the lens; light enters through a central opening (the pupil). Contraction of different sets of muscles of the iris causes the pupil to dilate in dim light and to contract in bright light. *i. bombé* an abnormal condition of the eye in which the iris bulges forward towards the cornea.

iritis (I-ry-tis) n. inflammation of the iris. See uveitis.

iron (I-ŏn) n. an element essential to life. The body of an adult contains on average 4 g of iron, over half of which is contained in haemoglobin in the red blood cells. Iron is an essential component in the transfer of oxygen in the body; a deficiency of iron may lead to anaemia. Many preparations of iron are used to treat iron-deficiency anaemia. Symbol: Fe.

iron dextran n. a drug containing

iron and dextran, administered by intramuscular or intravenous injection to treat iron-deficiency anaemia. Trade name: **CosmoFer.**

iron lung *n. see* respirator.

iron-storage disease *n. see* haemochromatosis.

irradiation (i-ray-di-ay-shŏn) *n.* **1.** exposure of the body's tissues to ionizing radiation. The source may be background radiation, diagnostic X-rays, radiotherapy, or nuclear accidents. **2.** exposure of a substance or object to ionizing radiation. Irradiation of food with gamma rays to kill bacteria is a technique used in food preservation.

irreducible (i-ri-dew-sibŭl) *adj.* unable to be replaced in a normal position: applied particularly to a type of hernia.

irrigation (i-ri-gay-shŏn) *n.* the process of washing out a wound or hollow organ with a continuous flow of water or medicated solution. *whole-gut i.* washing out the entire intestinal tract as a prelude to surgery on the lower intestine.

irritability (i-ri-tă-bil-iti) *n.* (in physiology) the property of certain kinds of tissue that enables them to respond in a specific way to outside stimuli.

irritable bowel syndrome (IBS, spastic colon, mucous colitis) (i-ri-tă-bŭl) *n.* a common condition in which recurrent abdominal pain with constipation and/or diarrhoea continues for years without any general deterioration in physical health or detectable structural disease.

irritant (i-ri-tănt) *n.* any material that causes irritation of a tissue.

IRV *n. see* (inspiratory) reserve volume.

isch- (**ischo-**) *prefix denoting* suppression or deficiency.

ischaemia (isk-ee-miă) *n.* an inadequate flow of blood to a part of the body, caused by constriction or blockage of the blood vessels supplying it. —**ischaemic** (isk-ee-mik) *adj.*

ischaemic heart disease (IHD, coronary heart disease, CHD) *n.* a disease in which the supply of oxygen to the myocardium is inadequate, usually as a result of narrowing of the lumen of the coronary arteries by atheroma. The main symptom is chest pain of varying intensity. Untreated, it can lead to coronary thrombosis and myocardial infarction.

ischi- (**ischio-**) *prefix denoting* the ischium.

ischiorectal abscess (isk-i-oh-rek-t'l) *n.* an abscess in the space between the sheet of muscle that assists in control of the rectum and the pelvic bone. Symptoms are severe throbbing pain near the anus with swelling and fever; it may cause an anal fistula. Pus is drained from the abscess by surgical incision.

ischium (isk-iŭm) *n.* a bone forming the lower part of each side of the hip bone (*see also* pelvis). —**ischiac, ischial** *adj.*

ischuria (isk-yoor-iă) *n.* retention or suppression of the urine. *See* anuria, retention.

islets of Langerhans (I-lits ŏv lang-er-hans) *pl. n.* small groups of endocrine cells, scattered through the material of the pancreas, that secrete insulin, glucagon, and other hormones. *See also* alpha cells, beta cells, delta cells. [P. Langerhans (1847–88), German pathologist]

iso- *prefix denoting* equality, uniformity, or similarity.

isoantibody (I-soh-**an**-ti-bodi) *n.* an antibody that occurs only in some individuals of a species against the components of foreign tissues from an individual of the same species.

isoantigen (I-soh-**an**-ti-jĕn) *n.* an antigenic substance that occurs only in some individuals of a species.

isoimmunization (I-soh-im-yoo-ny-**zay**-shŏn) *n.* the development of antibodies (isoantibodies) within an individual against antigens from another individual of the same species.

isolation (I-sŏ-**lay**-shŏn) *n.* **1.** the separation of a person with an infectious disease from noninfected people. *See also* quarantine. **2.** (in surgery) the separation of a structure from surrounding structures by the use of instruments.

isolator (I-sŏ-**lay**-ter) *n.* a large transparent plastic bag in which a patient can be nursed or operated upon without the danger of contamination by infective agents.

isoleucine (I-soh-**loo**-seen) *n.* an essential amino acid. *See also* amino acid.

isometheptene (I-soh-meth-**ep**-teen) *n.* a sympathomimetic drug used in the treatment of migraine, in combination with paracetamol (as *Midrid*). It is administered by mouth.

isometric (I-soh-**met**-rik) *adj.* of or denoting muscular contraction that does not cause muscle shortening. *i. exercise see* exercise.

isomorphism (I-soh-**mor**-fizm) *n.*

the condition of two or more objects being alike in shape or structure.
—**isomorphic, isomorphous** *adj.*

isoniazid (isonicotinic acid hydrazide, INH) (I-soh-ny-ă-zid) *n.* a drug used in the treatment of tuberculosis, usually taken by mouth. Because tuberculosis bacteria soon become resistant to isoniazid, it is usually given in conjunction with other antibiotics.

isophane insulin (I-soh-fayn) *n. see* insulin.

isoprenaline (I-soh-**pren**-ă-leen) *n.* a sympathomimetic drug that stimulates the heart and is used to treat some heart conditions involving reduced heart activity. It is administered by injection. Trade name: **Saventrine**.

isosorbide dinitrate (I-soh-**sor**-byd dy-ny-trayt) *n.* a drug used for the treatment of angina (*see* vasodilator). It is administered orally, by injection, as a sublingual spray or tablets, or as a transdermal spray. Trade names: **Angitak, Cedocard, Isotard, Isoket, Isordil**.

isosthenuria (I-sos-thĕn-**yoor**-iă) *n.* inability of the kidneys to produce either a concentrated or a dilute urine. This occurs in the final stages of renal failure.

isotonic (I-soh-**ton**-ik) *adj.* **1.** describing solutions that have the same osmotic pressure. *See* osmosis. **2.** describing muscles that have equal tonicity. *i. exercise see* exercise.

isotope (I-sŏ-tohp) *n.* any one of the different forms of an element, having the same atomic number but different atomic weights. Radioactive isotopes decay into other isotopes or elements, emitting alpha, beta, or gamma radiation. Artificially produced radioactive isotopes are used extensively as tracers (*see also* gamma camera, scintigram) and in radiotherapy for the treatment of cancer.

isotretinoin (I-soh-tre-tin-oh-in) *n.* a drug related to vitamin A (*see* retinoid) and used in the treatment of severe acne that has failed to respond to other treatment. It is administered by mouth or topically. Trade names: **Isotrex, Roaccutane.**

ispaghula husk (iss-pag-yoo-lă husk) *n.* a bulking agent (*see* laxative) used to treat constipation, diverticulitis, and irritable bowel syndrome. It is administered by mouth. Trade names: **Fybogel, Konsyl, Isogel, Regulan.**

ISS *n. see* injury scoring system.

isthmus (iss-mŭs) *n.* a constricted or narrowed part of an organ or tissue.

itch (ich) *n.* discomfort or irritation of the skin, prompting the sufferer to scratch or rub the affected area. *See* pruritus.

-itis *suffix denoting* inflammation of an organ, tissue, etc.

itraconazole (I-tră-kon-ă-zohl) *n.* an antifungal drug that is administered by mouth or intravenous infusion to treat a wide variety of fungal infections, including candidosis and ringworm. Trade name: **Sporanox.**

ITU *n.* intensive therapy unit. *See* intensive care.

IUCD (intrauterine contraceptive device) *n.* a plastic or metal coil, spiral, or other shape, about 25 mm long, that is inserted into the cavity of the uterus to prevent conception. Its exact mode of action is unknown but it is thought to interfere with implantation of the embryo. *See also* postcoital (contraception).

IUGR *n. see* intrauterine (growth retardation).

IUS (intrauterine system) *n.* a removable hormonal contraceptive device that is inserted into the uterus. Consisting of a plastic T-shaped frame that carries a hormone (progestogen) in a sleeve around its stem, it provides a long-term method of contraception that is also reversible. Trade name: **Mirena.**

IV *adj. see* intravenous.

IVC *n. see* (inferior) vena cava.

ivermectin (I-ver-mek-tin) *n.* a drug administered by mouth in the treatment of onchocerciasis, creeping eruption, strongyloidiasis, and scabies. Trade name: **Mectizan.**

IVF *n. see* in vitro fertilization.

IVI *n. see* (intravenous) infusion.

IVU *n. see* (intravenous) urogram.

ixodiasis (iks-oh-dy-ă-sis) *n.* any disease caused by the presence of ticks.

Jj

Jacksonian epilepsy (jak-**sohn**-iăn) n. see epilepsy. [J. H. Jackson (1835–1911), British neurologist]

Jacquemier's sign (zhak-mi-ayz) n. a bluish or purplish coloration of the vagina: a possible indication of pregnancy. [J. M. Jacquemier (1806–79), French obstetrician]

jactitation (jak-ti-tay-shŏn) n. restless tossing and turning of a person suffering from a severe disease, frequently one with a high fever.

Jaeger test types (yay-gĕr) n. a card with text printed in type of different sizes, used for testing acuity of near vision. [E. R. Jaeger von Jastthal (1818–84), Austrian ophthalmologist]

jamais vu (zha-may-vew) n. one of the manifestations of temporal lobe epilepsy, in which there is a sudden feeling of unfamiliarity with everyday surroundings.

Jarisch-Herxheimer reaction (Herxheimer reaction) (yar-ish herks-hy-mer) n. exacerbation of the symptoms of syphilis that may occur on starting antibiotic therapy for the disease. The effect is transient and requires no treatment. [A. Jarisch (1850–1902), Austrian dermatologist; K. Herxheimer (1861–1944), German dermatologist]

jaundice (jawn-dis) n. a yellowing of the skin or whites of the eyes, indicating excess bilirubin in the blood. *haemolytic j.* jaundice that occurs when there is excessive destruction of red cells in the blood (*see* haemolysis). *hepatocellular j.* jaundice due to disease of the liver cells, such as hepatitis. *obstructive j.* jaundice that occurs when bile made in the liver fails to reach the intestine due to obstruction of the bile ducts (e.g. by gallstones) or to cholestasis. Medical name: **icterus**.

jaw (jaw) n. either the maxilla (upper jaw) or the mandible (lower jaw).

jaw thrust n. a manoeuvre for opening the airway of an unconscious patient. The flats of the hands are placed on the cheeks with the fingers hooked under the angles of the jaw so that the jaw can be pulled upwards to separate the tongue from the back of the pharynx. This method is particularly useful when spinal injury is suspected and movement of the neck is undesirable. *See also* head tilt chin lift.

JCA n. see juvenile chronic arthritis.

jejun- (jejuno-) *prefix denoting* the jejunum.

jejunal ulcer (ji-joo-năl) n. see peptic (ulcer), Zollinger-Ellison syndrome.

jejunectomy (ji-joo-**nek**-tŏmi) n. surgical removal of the jejunum or part of the jejunum.

jejunoileostomy (ji-joo-noh-ili-ost-ŏmi) n. an operation in which the jejunum is joined to the ileum (small intestine), when either the end of the jejunum or the beginning of the ileum has been removed or is to be bypassed.

jejunostomy (ji-joo-**nost**-ŏmi) *n.* a surgical operation in which the jejunum is brought through the abdominal wall and opened. It can enable the insertion of a catheter into the jejunum for short-term infusion of nutrients or other substances.

jejunotomy (ji-joo-**not**-ŏmi) *n.* a surgical incision into the jejunum in order to inspect the interior or remove something from within it.

jejunum (ji-**joo**-nŭm) *n.* part of the small intestine. It comprises about two-fifths of the whole small intestine and connects the duodenum to the ileum. —**jejunal** *adj.*

jerk (jerk) *n.* the sudden contraction of a muscle in response to a nerve impulse. *knee j. see* patellar reflex.

joint (joint) *n.* the point at which two or more bones are connected. The opposing surfaces of bone are lined with cartilaginous, fibrous, or soft (synovial) tissue. *See also* amphiarthrosis, diarthrosis, synarthrosis.

joule (jool) *n.* the SI unit of work or energy, equal to the work done when the point of application of a force of 1 newton is displaced through a distance of 1 metre in the direction of the force. Symbol: J. *See also* calorie.

jugular (jug-yoo-ler) *adj.* relating to or supplying the neck or throat. *j.*

vein any one of several veins in the neck. *j. venous pressure (JVP)* the blood pressure in the jugular veins, which gives an indication of the pressure in the right side of the heart. *internal j.* a very large paired vein running vertically down the side of the neck and draining blood from the brain, face, and neck into the subclavian vein.

jumper's knee (patellar tendinitis) (jump-erz) *n.* a form of tendinitis that occurs in athletes and dancers. Repeated sudden contracture of the quadriceps muscle at take-off causes inflammation of the attachment of the patellar tendon to the lower end of the patella.

junction (junk-shŏn) *n.* (in anatomy) the point at which two different tissues or structures are in contact. *See also* neuromuscular junction.

juvenile chronic arthritis (JCA, Still's disease) (joo-vĕ-nyl) *n.* any one of a group of conditions characterized by inflammation of the joints lasting longer than six weeks and occurring before the age of 16. JCA can affect either four or fewer joints (*pauciarticular JCA*) or more than four (*polyarticular JCA*).

juvenile polyp *n. see* polyp.

juxta- *prefix denoting* proximity to.

JVP *n. see* jugular (venous pressure).

Kk

K *symbol for* potassium.

Kahn reaction (kahn) *n.* a test for syphilis, in which antibodies specific to the disease are detected in a sample of the patient's blood by means of a precipitin reaction. This test is not as reliable as some. [R. L. Kahn (20th century), US bacteriologist]

kala-azar (visceral leishmaniasis, Dumdum fever) (kah-lă-ăzar) *n.* a tropical disease caused by the parasitic protozoan *Leishmania donovani*, which is transmitted to humans by sandflies. Symptoms include enlargement and subsequent lesions of the liver and spleen; anaemia; a low leucocyte count; weight loss; and irregular fevers.

Kallmann's syndrome (kalmänz) *n.* a familial condition that is the most common form of isolated gonadotrophin deficiency; it is combined with underdevelopment of the olfactory lobes, causing anosmia. [F. J. Kallmann (1897–1965), US geneticist]

kaolin (kay-ŏ-lin) *n.* a white clay that contains aluminium and silicon and is purified and powdered for use as an adsorbent. It is taken by mouth to treat chronic diarrhoea. Kaolin is also used in dusting powders and poultices.

Kaposi's sarcoma (kap-oh-siz) *n.* a malignant tumour arising from blood vessels in the skin and appearing as purple to dark brown plaques or nodules. It is common in Africa but rare in the Western world, except in patients with AIDS. The tumour evolves slowly; radiotherapy is the treatment of choice for localized lesions and chemotherapy may be of value in metastatic disease. *See* AIDS. [M. Kaposi (1837–1902), Austrian dermatologist]

Kartagener's syndrome (kartah-gay-nerz) *n.* a hereditary condition in which the heart and other internal organs lie on the opposite side of the body to the norm (i.e. the heart lies on the right; *see* dextrocardia); it is associated with chronic sinusitis and bronchiectasis. [M. Kartagener (1897–1975), German physician]

kary- (karyo-) *prefix denoting* a cell nucleus.

karyokinesis (ka-ri-oh-ky-nee-sis) *n.* division of the nucleus of a cell, which occurs during cell division before division of the cytoplasm (*cytokinesis*). *See* mitosis.

karyotype (ka-ri-ŏ-typ) **1.** *n.* the chromosome set of an individual or species described in terms of both the number and structure of the chromosomes. **2.** *n.* the representation of the chromosome set in a diagram. **3.** *vb.* to determine the karyotype of a cell, as by microscopic examination.

katathermometer (kat-ă-thĕr-mom-it-er) *n.* a thermometer used to measure the cooling power of the air surrounding it.

Kawasaki disease (mucocutaneous lymph node syndrome) (kah-wǎ-sah-ki) *n.* a condition of unknown cause affecting young children, usually less than five years old, and characterized by fever, conjunctivitis, a sore throat, and a generalized rash and reddening of the palms and soles. This is followed by peeling of the fingers and toes. The fever usually persists for 1–2 weeks. Approximately one-fifth of children develop myocarditis and aneurysms of the coronary arteries. Treatment involves aspirin therapy, and gammaglobulin has recently been shown to reduce the risk of coronary artery disease. [T. Kawasaki (20th century), Japanese physician]

Kayser-Fleischer ring (ky-zer fly-sher) *n.* a brownish-yellow ring in the outer rim of the cornea of the eye. It is a deposit of copper granules and is diagnostic of Wilson's disease. [B. Kayser (1869–1954), German ophthalmologist; B. Fleischer (1848–1904), German physician]

Kegel exercises (pelvic-floor exercises) (keg-ěl) *pl. n.* active rehabilitation of the pelvic-floor muscles, which leads to a cure in 50–80% of patients with stress incontinence. [A. H. Kegel (20th century), US gynaecologist]

Kehr's sign (kairz) *n.* pain in the left shoulder caused by irritation of the undersurface of the diaphragm by blood leaking from a ruptured spleen. The pain impulses are referred along the phrenic nerve. [H. Kehr (1862–1913), German surgeon]

Kell antigens (kel) *pl. n.* a group of antigens that may or may not be present on the surface of red blood cells, forming the basis of a blood group. This group is important in blood transfusion reactions. [Mrs Kell (20th century), patient in whom they were first demonstrated]

Keller's operation (kel-erz) *n.* a surgical operation to correct hallux valgus or hallux rigidus, in which the base of the first phalanx of the big toe is excised. [W. L. Keller (1874–1959), US surgeon]

keloid (kee-loid) *n.* an overgrowth of fibrous scar tissue following trauma to the skin. It does not resolve spontaneously but may be flattened by applied pressure or with injections of potent corticosteroids. Keloid formation is particularly common at certain sites, such as the breastbone or ear lobe.

kerat- (kerato-) *prefix denoting* **1.** the cornea. **2.** horny tissue, especially of the skin.

keratectasia (ke-rǎ-tek-tay-ziǎ) *n.* bulging of the cornea at the site of scar tissue (which is thinner than normal corneal tissue).

keratectomy (ke-rǎ-tek-tŏmi) *n.* an operation in which a part of the cornea is removed, usually a superficial layer. This procedure is now frequently done by an excimer laser, to correct refractive errors (*photorefractive k.*) or remove diseased tissue (*phototherapeutic k.*), or by an automated keratome (*automated lamellar k.*).

keratin (ke-rǎ-tin) *n.* one of a family of proteins that are the major constituents of the nails, hair, and the outermost layers of the skin.

keratinization (cornification) (ke-rǎ-tin-I-zay-shǒn) *n.* the process by which cells become horny due to the deposition of keratin within them. It occurs in the epidermis of the skin and associated structures (hair, nails, etc.).

keratinocyte (ke-rat-in-ō-syt) *n*. a type of cell that makes up 95% of the cells of the epidermis. Keratinocytes migrate from the deeper layers of the epidermis and are finally shed from the surface of the skin.

keratitis (ke-ră-ty-tis) *n*. inflammation of the cornea of the eye. The eye waters and is very painful and vision is blurred. It may be due to physical or chemical agents or result from infection. *disciform k.* inflammation within the cornea, usually as an immune response to viral infection, commonly herpes simplex virus. *interstitial k.* inflammation within the layers of the cornea caused by syphilis, leprosy, or tuberculosis.

keratoconjunctivitis (ke-ră-toh-kŏn-junk-ti-vy-tis) *n*. combined inflammation of the cornea and conjunctiva of the eye. *k. sicca* dryness of the cornea and conjunctiva due to deficient tear production, as occurs in Sjögren's syndrome, systemic lupus, systemic sclerosis, and sarcoidosis.

keratoconus (ke-ră-toh-koh-nŭs) *n*. conical cornea: an abnormal condition of the eye in which the cornea, instead of having a regular curvature, comes to a rounded apex towards its centre.

keratoglobus (megalocornea) (ke-ră-toh-gloh-bŭs) *n*. a congenital disorder of the eye in which the whole cornea bulges forward in a regular curve. *Compare* keratoconus.

keratolytic (ke-ră-toh-lit-ik) *n*. an agent, such as salicylic acid, that breaks down the outer horny layer of epidermis and is used for treating warts.

keratomalacia (ke-ră-toh-mă-lay-shiă) *n*. a progressive nutritional disease of the eye due to vitamin A deficiency. The cornea softens and may become perforated. *See also* xerophthalmia.

keratome (ke-ră-tohm) *n*. any instrument designed for cutting the cornea.

keratometer (ophthalmometer) (ke-ră-tom-it-er) *n*. an instrument for measuring the radius of curvature of the cornea. It is used for assessing the degree of abnormal curvature of the cornea in astigmatism. —**keratometry** *n*.

keratopathy (ke-ră-top-ă-thi) *n*. any disorder relating to the cornea.

keratoplasty (corneal graft) (ke-ră-toh-plasti) *n*. an eye operation in which any diseased parts of the cornea are replaced by clear corneal tissue from a donor.

keratoprosthesis (ke-ră-toh-prosth'ee-sis) *n*. an optically clear prosthesis that is implanted into the cornea to replace an area that has become opaque.

keratoscope (Placido's disc) (ke-ră-toh-skohp) *n*. an instrument for detecting abnormal curvature of the cornea. It consists of a black disc marked with concentric white rings. The examiner looks at the reflection of the rings in the patient's cornea; a cornea that is abnormally curved (for example in keratoconus) or scarred reflects distorted rings.

keratosis (ke-ră-toh-sis) *n*. a horny overgrowth of the skin. *actinic* (or *solar*) *k.* a red spot with a scaly surface, which may occasionally become malignant. These spots are found in older fair-skinned people who have been chronically overexposed to the sun. **seborrhoeic** *k.* (*basal-cell papilloma*) a superficial yellowish spot that never becomes malignant. Such spots occur especially on the trunk in middle age, slowly darkening and becoming warty over the years.

keratotomy (ke-ră-tot-ŏmi) *n.* an incision into the cornea. *arcuate k.* a curved incision in the periphery of the cornea to reduce astigmatism.

keratouveitis (ke-ră-toh-yoo-vi-I-tis) *n.* inflammation involving both the cornea (*see* keratitis) and the uvea (*see* uveitis).

kerion (keer-iŏn) *n.* an uncommon and severe form of tinea (ringworm) of the scalp consisting of a painful inflamed mass. It is caused by a fungus that usually infects animal species.

kernicterus (ker-nik-ter-ŭs) *n.* staining and subsequent damage of the brain by bile pigment (bilirubin), which may occur in severe cases of haemolytic disease of the newborn.

Kernig's sign (ker-nigz) *n.* a symptom of meningitis in which the patient is unable to extend his legs at the knee when the thighs are held at a right angle to the body. [V. Kernig (1840–1917), Russian physician]

ketamine (ket-ă-meen) *n.* a drug used to produce anaesthesia, mainly in children. It is administered by injection. Trade name: **Ketalar**.

ketoacidosis (kee-toh-asid-oh-sis) *n.* a life-threatening condition in which acidosis is accompanied by ketosis, such as occurs in diabetes mellitus (*diabetic k.*, *DKA*). Symptoms include nausea and vomiting, abdominal tenderness, confusion or coma, extreme thirst, and weight loss.

ketoconazole (kee-toh-kon-ă-zohl) *n.* an antifungal drug (*see* imidazole) that is used in the treatment of such fungal diseases as candidosis, histoplasmosis, and blastomycosis. It is taken by mouth. Trade name: **Nizoral**.

ketogenesis (kee-toh-jen-i-sis) *n.* the production of ketone bodies. These are normal products of lipid metabolism and can be used to provide energy.

ketogenic diet (kee-toh-jen-ik) *n.* a diet that promotes the formation of ketone bodies in the tissues, in which the principal energy source is fat rather than carbohydrate.

ketonaemia (kee-toh-nee-miă) *n.* the presence in the blood of ketone bodies.

ketone (kee-tohn) *n.* any of a group of organic compounds consisting of a carbonyl group (=CO) flanked by two alkyl groups. *k. bodies* (*acetone bodies*) the ketones acetoacetic acid, acetone, and β-hydroxybutyrate, produced during the metabolism of fats. *See also* ketosis.

ketonuria (acetonuria) (kee-tohn-yoor-iă) *n.* the presence in the urine of ketone bodies. This may occur in diabetes mellitus, starvation, or after persistent vomiting and results from the partial oxidation of fats.

ketoprofen (kee-toh-proh-fen) *n.* an anti-inflammatory drug (*see* NSAID) administered by mouth, injection, or topically to treat various arthritic and rheumatic diseases and to relieve pain. Trade names: **Orudis, Oruvail**.

ketosis (kee-toh-sis) *n.* raised levels of ketone bodies in the body tissues, resulting from an imbalance in fat metabolism. Ketosis may result in severe acidosis. *See also* ketonuria.

ketosteroid (kee-toh-steer-oid) *n.* a steroid that contains one or more ketone groups (–C=O). 17-ketosteroids (having the oxygen at carbon 17) are normally excreted in the urine; excess 17-ketosteroids in the urine indicates overactivity of the adrenal glands and gonads.

keyhole surgery (kee-hohl) *n. see* minimally invasive surgery.

kidney (kid-ni) *n.* either of the pair of organs responsible for the excretion of nitrogenous wastes, principally urea, from the blood (see illustration). The active units of the kidney are the nephrons, which filter the blood under pressure and then reabsorb water and selected substances back into the blood. The urine thus formed is conducted via the renal tubules to the ureter,

which leads to the bladder. *See also* haemodialysis, horseshoe kidney, renal (function tests).

Kienböck's disease (keen-berks) *n.* necrosis of the lunate bone of the wrist caused by interruption of its blood supply. It usually follows chronic stress to the bone or injury, often trivial. *See also* osteochondritis. [R. Kienböck (1871–1953), Austrian radiologist]

Kiesselbach's plexus (kees-ĕl-bahks) *n.* a collection of capillaries in the mucosa at the anterior part of the nasal septum. Nosebleeds frequently have their origin from this plexus. *See* epistaxis, Little's area. [W. Kiesselbach (1839–1902), German laryngologist]

killer cell (kil-er) *n. see* natural killer cell.

Killian's operation (kil-iănz) *n.* a surgical operation in which part of the frontal bone is removed to allow drainage of the frontal sinus (*see* paranasal sinuses), when this is filled with pus. [G. Killian (1860–1921), German otorhinolaryngologist]

Position of the kidneys

Section through a kidney

kilo- *prefix denoting* a thousand.

kilogram (kil-ō-gram) *n.* the SI unit of mass equal to 1000 grams. Symbol: kg.

Kimmelstiel-Wilson disease (kim-ĕl-steel wil-sŏn) *n.* a disease in which diabetes mellitus is associated with the nephrotic syndrome, which results from breakdown of the glomeruli of the kidneys. [P. Kimmelstiel (1900–70), German-born pathologist; C. Wilson (1906–), British physician]

kin- (kine-) *prefix denoting* movement.

kinaesthesia (kin-iss-theez-iă) *n.* the sense that enables the brain to be constantly aware of the position and movement of muscles in different parts of the body.

kinanaesthesia (kin-anis-theez-iă) *n.* inability to sense the positions and movements of parts of the body, with consequent disordered physical activity.

kinase (ky-nayz) *n.* **1.** an agent that can convert the inactive form of an enzyme (*see* proenzyme) to the active form. **2.** an enzyme that catalyses the transfer of phosphate groups.

kinematics (kin-i-mat-iks) *n.* the study of motion and the forces required to produce it. This includes the different forces at work during the movement of a single part of the body, and more complex movements such as running and climbing.

kineplasty (kin-i-plasti) *n.* a method of amputation in which the muscles and tendons of the affected limb are arranged so that they can be integrated with a specially made artificial replacement.

-kinesis *suffix denoting* movement.

kinetochore (ky-nee-toh-kor) *n. see* centromere.

King's model (kingz) *n.* a model for nursing based on the view that individuals function in social systems through interpersonal relationships. Nursing is seen as a process of action, reaction, interaction, and transaction in order to set and achieve goals that meet the care needs of the patient. *See also* nursing models. [I. King (1909–), US nurse theorist]

kinin (ky-nin) *n.* one of a group of naturally occurring polypeptides that are powerful vasodilators, which lower blood pressure and cause contraction of smooth muscle.

Kirschner's wire (keersh-nerz) *n.* a wire that can be inserted into a bone to exert skeletal traction or to fix fractures. [M. Kirschner (1879–1942), German surgeon]

kiss of life *n. see* mouth-to-mouth respiration.

Klebsiella (kleb-si-el-ă) *n.* a genus of Gram-negative rodlike nonmotile mostly lactose-fermenting bacteria found in the respiratory, intestinal, and urinogenital tracts of animals and humans.

Klebs-Loeffler bacillus (klebz-lerf-ler) *n. see* Corynebacterium. [T. Klebs (1834–1913) and F. A. J. Loeffler (1852–1915), German bacteriologists]

Kleine-Levin syndrome (klyn-lev-in) *n.* a rare episodic disorder characterized by periods (usually of a few days or weeks) in which sufferers eat enormously, sleep for most of the day and night, and may become more dependent or aggressive than normal. Between episodes they are usually quite unaffected. The disorder almost always resolves spontaneously. [W. Kleine (20th century), German neuropsychiatrist; M. Levin (20th century), US neurologist]

klepto- *prefix denoting* stealing.

kleptomania (kleptŏ-**may**-niă) *n.* a pathologically strong impulse to steal, often in the absence of any desire for the stolen object(s). It is sometimes associated with depression.

Klinefelter's syndrome (klyn-fel-terz) *n.* a genetic disorder in which there are three sex chromosomes, XXY, rather than the normal XX or XY. Affected individuals are apparently male, but have small testes, enlarged breasts, and absence of facial and body hair. [H. F. Klinefelter (1912–), US physician]

Klumpke's paralysis (kluump-kèz) *n.* a partial paralysis of the arm caused by injury to a baby's brachial plexus during birth. It results in weakness and wasting of the muscles of the hand. [A. Klumpke (1859–1927), French neurologist]

K-nail *n. see* Küntscher nail.

kneading (**need**-ing) *n. see* petrissage.

knee (nee) *n.* the hinge joint between the femur and the tibia. *k.-chest position see* genupectoral position. *k.-elbow position see* genucubital position. *k. jerk see* patellar reflex.

kneecap (nee-kap) *n. see* patella.

knock-knee (nok-nee) *n.* abnormal in-curving of the legs at the knees, resulting in a gap between the feet when the knees are in contact. Medical name: **genu valgum**.

Kocher manoeuvre (kok-er) *n.* a

method for reduction of a dislocated shoulder by manipulation. [E. T. Kocher (1841–1917), Swiss surgeon]

Koch's bacillus (koks) *n. see* Mycobacterium. [R. Koch (1843–1910), German bacteriologist]

Köhler's disease (ker-lerz) *n.* necrosis of the navicular bone of the foot (*see* osteochondritis). It occurs in children, causing pain and limping. [A. Köhler (1874–1947), German physician]

koilonychia (koi-loh-**nik**-iă) *n.* the development of brittle spoon-shaped nails, a common disorder that can occur with anaemia due to iron deficiency.

Koplik's spots (kop-liks) *pl. n.* small red spots with bluish-white centres that often appear on the mucous membranes of the mouth in measles. [H. Koplik (1858–1927), US paediatrician]

Korsakoff's syndrome (Korsakoff's psychosis) (kor-sak-offs) *n.* an organic disorder affecting the brain that results in impaired memory for recent events, disorientation for time and place, and confabulation. The commonest cause of the condition is alcoholism, especially when this has led to deficiency of thiamin (vitamin B₁). [S. S. Korsakoff (1854–1900), Russian neurologist]

kraurosis (kraw-roh-sis) *n.* shrinking of a body part, usually the vulva in elderly women (*k. vulvae*).

Krebs cycle (citric acid cycle) (krebz) *n.* a complex cycle of enzyme-catalysed reactions, occurring within the cells of all living animals, in which acetate is broken down to produce energy in the form of ATP and carbon dioxide. The cycle is the final step in the oxidation of carbohydrates, fats, and proteins. [Sir H. A. Krebs (1900–81), German-born biochemist]

Krukenberg tumour (kroo-kĕn-berg) *n.* a rapidly developing malignant growth in one or (more often) both ovaries. The tumour is secondary to a primary growth in the stomach or intestine. [F. E. Krukenberg (1871–1946), German pathologist]

krypton-81m (krip-ton) *n.* a radioactive gas that is the shortest-lived isotope in medical use (half-life 13 seconds). It can be used to investigate the ventilation of the lungs. *See also* rubidium-81.

KUB X-ray *n.* an abdominal plain X-ray film that is longer than normal to enable it to include the *k*idneys, *u*reters, and the entire *b*ladder.

Küntscher nail (K-nail) (koontsher) *n.* a long steel nail that is inserted down the long axis of a long bone, into the marrow, in order to fix a fracture. [G. Küntscher (1902–72), German orthopaedic surgeon]

Küntscher nail

Kupffer cells (kuup-fer) *pl. n.* phagocytic cells that line the sinusoids of the liver (*see* macrophage). They are particularly concerned with the formation of bile. [K. W. von Kupffer (1829–1902), German anatomist]

Kussmaul breathing (koos-mowl) *n.* the slow deep respiration associated with acidosis. [A. Kussmaul (1822–1902), German physician]

Kveim test (kvaym) *n.* a test used for the diagnosis of sarcoidosis. Tissue from a lymph node of a person suffering from the disease is injected intradermally; the development of a granuloma at the injection site indicates that the subject has sarcoidosis. [M. A. Kveim (20th century), Norwegian physician]

kwashiorkor (kwash-i-or-ker) *n.* a form of malnutrition due to a diet deficient in protein and energy-producing foods, common among young children in certain African tribes. The symptoms are oedema, loss of appetite, diarrhoea, general discomfort, and apathy; the child fails to thrive and there is usually associated gastrointestinal infection.

kymograph (ky-mŏ-grahf) *n.* an instrument for recording the flow and varying pressure of the blood within blood vessels. —**kymography** *n.*

kypho- *prefix denoting* a hump.

kyphos (ky-fos) *n.* a sharply localized anterior angulation of the spine, resulting in the appearance of a lump (the deformity of the traditional hunchback).

kyphoscoliosis (ky-foh-skoh-li-oh-sis) *n.* abnormal curvature of the spine both forwards and sideways: kyphosis combined with scoliosis.

kyphosis (ky-foh-sis) *n.* excessive outward curvature of the spine, causing hunching of the back, resulting in marked convexity when viewed from the side. It may result from bad posture or muscle weakness (*mobile k.*) or from diseases such as osteochondritis or ankylosing spondylitis (*fixed k.*). Treatment depends on the cause, and may include physiotherapy, bracing, and spinal osteotomy in severe cases. *See also* kyphos, kyphoscoliosis.

labetalol (la-bee-tǎ-lol) *n.* a combined alpha- and beta-blocking drug, sometimes found to be more effective in the treatment of high blood pressure than beta blockers. It is administered by mouth or intravenous infusion. Trade name: **Trandate**.

labia (lay-biǎ) *pl. n. see* labium.

labial (lay-bi-ǎl) *adj.* **1.** relating to the lips or to a labium. **2.** designating the surface of a tooth adjacent to the lips.

labile (lay-byl) *adj.* unstable. The term is applied to drugs and other chemicals that readily undergo change in solution, when subjected to heat, etc., and also to emotions when there are rapid mood swings.

labio- *prefix denoting* the lip(s).

labioplasty (cheiloplasty) (lay-bi-oh-plasti) *n.* surgical repair of injury or deformity of the lips (cleft lip).

labium (lay-bi-ŭm) *n.* (*pl.* **labia**) a lip-shaped structure, especially either of the two pairs of skin folds that enclose the vulva. The larger outer pair are known as the *labia majora* and the smaller inner pair the *labia minora*.

labour (lay-ber) *n.* the sequence of actions by which a baby and the afterbirth (placenta) are expelled from the uterus at childbirth (see illustration). Labour usually starts spontaneously about 280 days after conception, but it may be started by artificial means (*see* induction). In the first stage the muscular wall of the uterus begins contracting while the cervix expands. The amnion ruptures releasing amniotic fluid to the exterior. In the second stage the baby passes through the vagina, assisted by contractions of the abdominal muscles and conscious pushing by the mother. When the whole infant has been eased clear of the vagina, the umbilical cord is cut. In the final stage the placenta and membranes are pushed out by the continuing contraction of the uterus. *See also* Caesarean section.

labrum (lay-brŭm) *n.* (*pl.* **labra**) a lip or liplike structure; occurring, for example, around the margins of the acetabulum.

labyrinth (inner ear) (lab-er-inth) *n.* a convoluted system of cavities and ducts comprising the organs of hearing and balance. *bony l.* the bony canals and chambers, embedded in the petrous part of the temporal bone, that surround the membranous labyrinth. *membranous l.* the membranous canals and chambers comprising the semicircular canals, utricle, saccule, and cochlea.

labyrinthectomy (lab-er-inth-ek-tŏmi) *n.* a surgical procedure to ablate (*see* ablation) the structures of the labyrinth, usually performed for cases of severe Ménière's disease.

labyrinthitis (lab-er-inth-I-tis) *n.* see otitis (interna).

The mechanism of labour

laceration (las-er-ay-shŏn) *n.* a tear in the flesh producing a wound with irregular edges.

lacrimal (lak-rim-ăl) *adj.* relating to tears. *l. apparatus* the structures that produce and drain away fluid from the eye (see illustration). *l. bone* either of a pair of small rec-tangular bones that contribute to the orbits. *l. gland* the gland that se-cretes tears, which drain away through small openings (*puncta*) at the inner corner of the eye. *l. nerve* a branch of the ophthalmic nerve that supplies the lacrimal gland and conjunctiva.

lacrimation (lak-ri-**may**-shŏn) *n.* the production of excess tears; crying.

lacrimator (lak-rim-ay-ter) *n.* an agent that irritates the eyes, causing excessive secretion of tears.

lact- (lacti-, lacto-) *prefix denoting* **1.** milk. **2.** lactic acid.

lactalbumin (lak-tal-bew-min) *n.* a milk protein present in milk at a lower concentration than casein.

lactase (**lak**-tayz) *n.* an enzyme, secreted by the glands of the small intestine, that converts lactose (milk sugar) into glucose and galactose during digestion.

lactate (**lak**-tayt) **1.** *n.* any salt of lactic acid. **2.** *vb.* to secrete milk (*see* lactation).

lactation (lak-**tay**-shŏn) *n.* the secretion of milk by the mammary glands of the breasts, which usually begins at the end of pregnancy (*see also* colostrum) and is stimulated by the sucking of the baby at the nipple. Lactation is controlled by hormones (*see* prolactin, oxytocin); it stops when the baby is no longer breast-fed.

lacteal (**lak**-ti-ăl) *n.* a blind-ended lymphatic vessel that extends into a villus of the small intestine. Digested fats are absorbed into the lacteals.

lactic acid (lak-tik) *n.* a compound that forms in the cells as the end-product of glucose metabolism in the absence of oxygen (*see* glycolysis). Lactic acid (owing to its low pH) is an important food preservative.

lactic acidosis *n.* excessive plasma acidity due to an accumulation of lactic acid. This may be caused by a variety of illnesses, including heart failure or severe dehydration, or the accumulation of metformin used for treating type 2 diabetes mellitus, particularly when kidney failure is present.

lactiferous (lak-**tif**-er-ŭs) *adj.* transporting or secreting milk, as the ducts (*l. ducts*) of the breast.

lactifuge (lak-ti-fewj) *n.* a drug that reduces the secretion of milk. Some oestrogenic drugs have this effect.

Lactobacillus (lak-toh-bă-**sil**-ŭs) *n.* a genus of Gram-positive nonmotile rodlike bacteria that are capable of producing lactic acid from the fermentation of carbohydrates. They are found in fermenting animal and plant products, especially dairy products, and in the alimentary tract and vagina.

lactogenic hormone (lak-tŏ-**jen**-ik) *n. see* prolactin.

lactose (milk sugar) (lak-tohz) *n.* a sugar, consisting of one molecule of glucose and one of galactose, found only in milk. *l. intolerance* inability to absorb lactose, caused by

lacrimal gland
punctum
lacrimal canaliculus
lacrimal sac
nasal cavity
excretory ducts of lacrimal glands
nasolacrimal duct

The lacrimal apparatus

absence or low activity of the enzyme lactase.

lactosuria (lak-tohs-yoor-iǎ) n. the presence of lactose in the urine. This often occurs during pregnancy and breast-feeding or if the milk flow is suppressed.

lactulose (lak-tew-lohz) n. a disaccharide sugar that acts as a laxative. Administered by mouth, it remains intact until it reaches the colon. There it is split by bacteria into simpler sugars that help to retain water, thereby softening the stools. Trade names: **Duphalac**, **Lactugal**.

lacuna (lǎ-kew-nǎ) n. (pl. **lacunae**) (in anatomy) a small cavity or depression.

Laënnec's cirrhosis (la-en-neks) n. alcoholic cirrhosis: the commonest type of cirrhosis. [R. T. H. Laënnec (1781–1826), French physician]

laevo- prefix. see levo-.

laevocardia (lee-voh-kar-di-ǎ) n. the normal position of the heart, in which its apex is directed towards the left. Compare dextrocardia.

laking (layk-ing) n. the physical or chemical treatment of blood to abolish the structure of the red cells and thus form a homogeneous solution. Laking is an important preliminary step in the analysis of haemoglobin or enzymes present in red cells.

-lalia suffix denoting a condition involving speech.

lallation (lalling) (la-lay-shŏn) n. **1.** unintelligible speechlike babbling, as heard from infants. **2.** the immature substitution of one consonant for another (e.g. 'l' for 'r').

lambda (lam-dǎ) n. the point on the skull at which the lambdoidal and sagittal sutures meet.

lambdoidal suture (lam-doi-d'l)

n. the immovable joint between the parietal and occipital bones (see skull).

lambliasis (lam-bly-ǎ-sis) n. see giardiasis.

lamella (lǎ-mel-ǎ) n. (pl. **lamellae**) **1.** a thin layer, membrane, scale, or platelike tissue or part. **2.** a thin gelatinous medicated disc used to apply drugs to the eye. The disc is placed on the eyeball; the gelatinous material dissolves and the drug is absorbed.

lamina (lam-in-ǎ) n. (pl. **laminae**) a thin membrane or layer of tissue.

laminectomy (lam-in-ek-tŏmi) n. surgical cutting into the backbone to obtain access to the spinal cord. The operation is performed to remove tumours or prolapsed intervertebral discs or to relieve pressure on the spinal cord or roots.

lamivudine (lǎ-miv-yoo-deen) n. an antiviral drug administered by mouth for treating HIV infection and hepatitis B. Trade names: **Epivir**, **Zeffix**.

lamotrigine (lam-oh-try-geen) n. an anticonvulsant drug used in the control of epilepsy. Lamotrigine is administered by mouth. Trade name: **Lamictal**.

Lancefield classification (lans-feeld) n. a classification of the Streptococcus bacteria based on the presence or absence of antigenic carbohydrate on the cell surface. Species are classified into the groups A–S. Most species causing disease in humans belong to groups A, B, and D. [R. C. Lancefield (1895–1981), US bacteriologist]

lancet (lahn-sit) n. a broad two-edged surgical knife with a sharp point.

lancinating (lahn-sin-ayt-ing) *adj.* describing a sharp stabbing or cutting pain.

Landau reflex (land-ow) *n.* a reflex seen in normal babies from three months until one year, when it disappears. If the baby is held horizontally, face down, it will straighten its legs and back and try to lift up its head. The presence of this reflex beyond one year may indicate a developmental disorder.

Lange curve (lahng-ě) *n.* an obsolescent method of detecting excess globulins in the protein of the cerebrospinal fluid. It was useful in the diagnosis of neurosyphilis and multiple sclerosis but has been superseded by more specific tests. [F. A. Lange (20th century), German physician]

Langerhans cell histiocytosis (lang-er-hans) *n.* overgrowth of cells of the reticuloendothelial system. This includes disorders previously called *histiocytosis X*, including *eosinophilic granuloma*, *Hand-Schüller-Christian disease*, and *Letterer-Siwe disease*. [P. Langerhans (1847–88), German physician and anatomist]

Langer's lines (lahng-erz) *pl. n.* normal permanent skin creases. Incisions parallel to Langer's lines heal well and are less visible. [C. R. von E. Langer (1819–87), Austrian anatomist]

lanolin (lan-ŏ-lin) *n.* a fatty substance obtained from sheep's wool, used as an emollient and as a base for creams.

lanreotide (lan-ri-oh-tyd) *n.* an analogue of somatostatin that is administered by injection to treat acromegaly and hormone-secreting

neuroendocrine tumours. Trade name: **Somatuline**.

lanugo (lă-new-goh) *n.* fine hair covering the body and limbs of the human fetus.

laparo- *prefix denoting* the loins or abdomen.

laparoscope (peritoneoscope) (lap-er-ŏ-skohp) *n. see* laparoscopy.

laparoscopy (abdominoscopy, peritoneoscopy) (lap-er-os-kŏpi) *n.* examination of the abdominal structures by means of an illuminated tubular instrument (*laparoscope*). This is passed through a small incision in the wall of the abdomen after injecting carbon dioxide into the abdomen (pneumoperitoneum). In addition to being a diagnostic aid, it is used when taking a biopsy, aspirating cysts, and dividing adhesions. Surgery, including cholecystectomy, colectomy, and the occlusion of Fallopian tubes for sterilization, can also be performed through a laparoscope, using either a laser or diathermy to control bleeding (*see also* minimally invasive surgery). *laser l.* surgery performed through a laparoscope using a laser: used, for example, for collecting ova for in vitro fertilization. —**laparoscopic** *adj.*

laparotomy (lap-er-ot-ŏmi) *n.* a surgical incision into the abdominal cavity. The operation is done to examine the abdominal organs as a help to diagnosis.

lardaceous (lar-**day**-shŭs) *adj.* resembling lard: often applied to tissue infiltrated with the starchlike substance amyloid (*see* amyloidosis).

Lariam (la-ri-am) *n. see* mefloquine.

larva (lar-vă) n. (pl. **larvae**) the preadult or immature stage hatching from the egg of some animal groups, e.g. insects and nematodes, which may be markedly different from the sexually mature adult. *l. migrans see* creeping eruption. —**larval** adj.

laryng- (laryngo-) prefix denoting the larynx.

laryngeal (la-rin-jee-ăl) adj. relating to the larynx. *l. mask* an airway tube for insertion into the mouth of a patient requiring artificial ventilation and designed to fit into the throat over the top of the laryngeal opening. *l. reflex* a cough produced by irritating the larynx. *l. stroboscopy* a method of studying the movements of the vocal folds of the larynx by using stroboscopic light (controlled intermittent flashes) to slow or freeze the movement.

laryngectomy (la-rin-jek-tŏmi) n. surgical removal of the whole or a part (*partial l.*) of the larynx in the treatment of laryngeal carcinoma. *See also* electrolarynx.

laryngismus (la-rin-jiz-mŭs) n. closure of the vocal folds by sudden contraction of the laryngeal muscles, followed by a noisy indrawing of breath. It occurs in young children when a foreign body has lodged in the larynx or in croup; in the past it was associated with low-calcium rickets.

laryngitis (la-rin-jy-tis) n. inflammation of the larynx and vocal folds, due to infection or irritation. The voice becomes husky and is lost completely; breathing is harsh and difficult (*see* stridor); and the cough is painful. Obstruction of the airways may occasionally be serious, especially in children (*see* croup).

laryngofissure (lă-ring-oh-fish-er) n. a surgical operation to open the larynx, enabling access for further procedures.

laryngology (la-ring-ol-ŏji) n. the study of diseases of the larynx and vocal folds. —**laryngologist** n.

laryngomalacia (lă-ring-oh-mă-lay-shiă) n. a condition characterized by paroxysmal attacks of breathing difficulty and stridor. It occurs in small children and is caused by flaccidity of the structure of the larynx. It usually resolves spontaneously by the age of two years.

laryngopharynx (lă-ring-oh-fa-rinks) n. *see* hypopharynx.

laryngoscope (lă-ring-ŏ-skohp) n. a device consisting of a handle and a curved blade, fitted with a light, for moving the tongue and epiglottis aside in order to inspect the larynx. It is used to aid insertion of an endotracheal tube or for simple examination.

laryngoscopy (la-ring-os-kŏpi) n. examination of the larynx. This may be done indirectly using a small mirror or directly using a laryngoscope.

laryngospasm (lă-ring-oh-spazm) n. involuntary closure of the larynx, obstructing the flow of air to the lungs.

laryngostenosis (lă-ring-oh-sti-noh-sis) n. narrowing of the cavity of the larynx.

laryngotomy (la-ring-ot-ŏmi) n. surgical incision of the larynx. *inferior l.* surgical incision of the cricothyroid membrane beneath the larynx; a life-saving operation when there is obstruction to breathing at or above the larynx. *See* tracheostomy.

laryngotracheobronchitis (lă-ring-oh-trak-i-oh-brong-**ky**-tis) *n.* a severe and almost exclusively viral infection of the respiratory tract, especially of young children, in whom there may be a dangerous degree of obstruction either at the larynx (*see* croup) or bronchi.

larynx (**la**-rinks) *n.* the organ responsible for the production of vocal sounds, also serving as an air passage conveying air from the pharynx to the lungs. It is situated in the front of the neck, above the trachea. It is made up of a framework of nine cartilages, bound together by ligaments and muscles and lined with mucous membrane, and contains a pair of vocal folds. —**laryngeal** *adj.*

Cartilages of the larynx

- epiglottis
- hyoid bone
- thyroid cartilage
- arytenoid cartilage
- cricoid cartilage
- trachea

LASEK (lay-sek) *n.* laser *in situ* epithelial *k*eratomileusis: eye surgery used to correct both short sight and

long sight. A flap of corneal epithelium is raised, the surface of the cornea is reshaped using an excimer laser, and the epithelium is then replaced.

laser (**lay**-zer) *n.* a device that produces a very thin beam of light in which high energies are concentrated. In surgery, lasers can be used to operate on small areas of abnormality without damaging delicate surrounding tissue. They are used in eye surgery for cutting tissue (*YAG l.*), for photocoagulation of the retina (*argon l., diode l.*), and in operations on the cornea for correcting long- or short-sightedness (*excimer l.*). Lasers are also used to unblock coronary arteries narrowed by atheroma, to remove certain types of birthmark (*see* naevus), and in the treatment of cervical intraepithelial neoplasia (*see* CIN).

laser-assisted uvulopalatoplasty (LAUP) (yoov-yoo-loh-**pal**-a-toh-plasti) *n.* laser surgery to the palate, used in the treatment of obstructive sleep apnoea.

laser laparoscopy *n. see* laparoscopy.

LASIK (**lay**-sik) *n.* laser *in situ* keratomileusis; eye surgery used to correct both short sight and long sight. A thin corneal flap (epithelium and stroma) is raised, the surface of the cornea reshaped using an excimer laser, and the flap then replaced.

Lasix (**las**-iks) *n. see* furosemide.

Lassa fever (**las**-ă) *n.* a serious virus disease confined to Central West Africa. Symptoms include headache, high fever, and severe muscular pains; difficulty in swallowing often arises. Death from kidney or heart failure occurs in over

50% of cases. Treatment with plasma from recovered patients is the best therapy.

Lassar's paste (las-arz) *n.* an ointment containing zinc oxide, starch, and salicylic acid in a soft paraffin base, used in the treatment of eczema and similar skin diseases. [G. Lassar (1849–1907), German dermatologist]

latent heat (lay-tĕnt) *n.* the quantity of heat absorbed or released when a substance changes state (e.g. from solid to liquid or from liquid to vapour) without any change in temperature.

lateral (lat-er-ăl) *adj.* **1.** situated at or relating to the side of an organ or organism. **2.** (in anatomy) relating to the region or parts of the body that are furthest from the median plane. **3.** (in radiology) in the sagittal plane.

lateroversion (lat-er-oh-ver-shŏn) *n.* a turning or displacement of an organ, for example the uterus (*uterine l.*), to one side.

laudanum (lawd-nŭm) *n.* a hydroalcoholic solution containing 1% morphine, prepared from macerated raw opium. It was formerly widely used as a narcotic analgesic, taken by mouth.

laughing gas (lahf-ing) *n. see* nitrous oxide.

LAUP *n. see* laser-assisted uvulopalatoplasty.

Laurence-Moon-Biedl syndrome (lo-rĕns moon bee-d'l) *n.* an autosomal recessive condition involving obesity, short stature, mental retardation, retinitis pigmentosa, and, more variably, gonad failure. [J. Z. Laurence (1830–74), British ophthalmologist; R. C. Moon (1844–1914), US ophthalmologist; A. Biedl (1869–1933), Austrian physician]

lavage (lav-ahzh) *n.* washing out a body cavity, such as the colon or stomach, with water or a medicated solution. In cases of bowel obstruction the washing out can be done during the operation (*on-table l.*). *See also* bronchoalveolar lavage, diagnostic peritoneal lavage.

laxative (laks-ă-tiv) *n.* a drug used to treat constipation or to evacuate the bowel (e.g. before surgery). *bulk-forming l.* a laxative, such as methylcellulose, that encourages the passage of a softer or bulkier stool. *osmotic l.* a laxative, such as magnesium sulphate or lactulose, that acts by retaining water in the large bowel. *stimulant l.* (*cathartic, purgative*) a laxative, such as bisacodyl or senna, that stimulates or increases the frequency of bowel evacuation.

lazy eye (lay-zi) *n. see* amblyopia.

LBC *n. see* liquid-based cytology.

LDL *n.* low-density lipoprotein: *see* lipoprotein.

L-dopa *n. see* levodopa.

LE *n. see* lupus (erythematosus).

lead (led) *n.* a soft bluish-grey metallic element that forms several poisonous compounds. Acute lead poisoning causes abdominal pains, vomiting, diarrhoea, and sometimes encephalitis. In chronic poisoning a characteristic blue mark on the gums (*l. line*) is seen and the peripheral nerves are affected; there is also anaemia. Treatment is with edetate. The use of lead in paints is now strictly controlled. Symbol: Pb.

learning disability (learning

difficulty) (lern-ing) n. see mental handicap.

leather-bottle stomach (leth-er bot-t'l) n. see linitis plastica.

Leber's congenital amaurosis (lay-berz) n. a hereditary disease (inherited as an autosomal recessive inherited condition) causing severe visual loss in infants. [T. Leber (1840–1917), German ophthalmologist]

Leber's optic atrophy n. a rare hereditary disorder, affecting young males, that is characterized by rapid loss of central vision due to neuroretinal degeneration.

lecithin (les-i-thin) n. one of a group of phospholipids that are important constituents of cell membranes and are involved in the metabolism of fat by the liver. An example is *phosphatidylcholine*. *l-sphingomyelin ratio* (LS ratio) a measure of fetal lung maturity; an LS ratio below 2 indicates a higher risk of respiratory distress syndrome.

lecithinase (les-i-thin-ayz) n. an enzyme from the small intestine that breaks lecithin down into its constituents (i.e. glycerol, fatty acids, phosphoric acid, and choline).

leech (leech) n. a type of worm that possesses suckers at both ends of its body. Certain parasitic species suck blood from animals and humans, causing irritation and, occasionally, infection. Formerly widely used for bloodletting, the medicinal leech (*Hirudo medicinalis*) may now be used following microsurgery to restore patency to blocked or collapsed blood vessels.

leflunomide (lĕ-floo-nŏ-myd) n. an immunosuppressant drug administered by mouth to treat rheumatoid arthritis that has not responded to methotrexate or other antirheumatic drugs. Trade name: **Arava**.

Legg-Calvé-Perthes disease (Perthes disease, pseudocoxalgia) (leg kal-vay per-tĕz) n. necrosis of the head of the femur due to interruption of its blood supply (see osteochondritis). It occurs most commonly in boys between the ages of 5 and 10, and causes aching and a limp. [A. T. Legg (1874–1939), US surgeon; J. Calvé (1875–1954), French orthopaedist; G. C. Perthes (1869–1927), German surgeon]

legionnaires' disease (lee-jŏn-airz) n. an infection of the lungs caused by the bacterium *Legionella pneumophila*. Symptoms include malaise and muscle pain, succeeded by a fever, dry cough, chest pain, and breathlessness. Erythromycin provides the most effective therapy

legumin (lig-yoo-min) n. a protein (a globulin) obtained from the seeds of plants of the family Leguminosae, such as beans and peas.

Leininger's theory of transcultural nursing (lyn-in-gerz) n. see transcultural nursing.

leio- *prefix denoting* smoothness.

leiomyoma (ly-oh-my-oh-mă) n. a benign tumour of smooth muscle. Such tumours occur most commonly in the uterus (see fibroid) but can also arise in the digestive tract, walls of blood vessels, etc.

leiomyosarcoma (ly-oh-my-oh-sar-koh-mă) n. a malignant tumour of smooth muscle, most commonly found in the womb, stomach, small bowel, and at the base of the bladder.

Leishman-Donovan body

(leesh-măn don-ŏ-văn) *n. see* Leishmania. [Sir W. B. Leishman (1865–1926), British surgeon; C. Donovan (1863–1951), Irish physician]

Leishmania (leesh-may-niă) *n.* a genus of parasitic flagellate protozoans, several species of which cause disease in humans (*see* leishmaniasis). In humans, especially in kala-azar patients, the parasite is a small rounded structure called a *Leishman-Donovan body*, which is found within the cells of the lymphatic system, spleen, and bone marrow.

leishmaniasis (leesh-mă-ny-ă-sis) *n.* a disease, common in the tropics and subtropics, caused by parasitic protozoans of the genus *Leishmania*, which are transmitted by the bite of sandflies. *cutaneous l.* leishmaniasis that affects the tissues of the skin. *See* espundia, oriental sore. *visceral l.* leishmaniasis in which the cells of various internal organs are affected. *See* kala-azar.

lens (lenz) *n.* **1.** (in anatomy) the transparent crystalline structure situated behind the pupil of the eye. It helps to refract incoming light and focus it onto the retina. *See also* accommodation. **2.** (in optics) a piece of glass or other material shaped to refract rays of light in a particular direction. Lenses are worn to correct faulty eyesight. *l. implant* a plastic lens to replace a natural lens that has been removed because of cataract. *See also* dual focal lens, contact lenses, multifocal lens.

lenticular (len-tik-yoo-ler) *adj.* relating to or shaped like a lens.

lenticular nucleus (lentiform nucleus) *n. see* basal ganglia.

lentigo (len-ty-goh) *n.* (*pl.* **lentigi-**

nes) a flat dark brown spot found mainly in the elderly on skin exposed to light. *l. maligna (Hutchinson's l.)* a form of lentigo that occurs on the cheeks of the elderly. The spot is larger than 2 cm in diameter and has variable pigmentation; it is an early malignant melanoma that has not spread deeply.

leontiasis (lee-on-ty-ă-sis) *n.* a bilateral symmetrical hypertrophy of the bones of the face and cranium, said to resemble the appearance of a lion's head. It is a rare feature of untreated Paget's disease. Medical name: **leontiasis ossea**.

leproma (lep-roh-mă) *n.* a lump on the skin characteristic of leprosy.

leprosy (Hansen's disease) (lep-rŏ-si) *n.* a chronic disease, caused by the bacterium *Mycobacterium leprae*, that affects the skin, mucous membranes, and nerves. It is confined mainly to the tropics and is transmitted by direct contact. Symptoms mainly involve the skin and nerves. Leprosy should be treated with a combination of antibacterial drugs (including dapsone and rifampicin), to overcome the problem of resistance developing to a single drug, and reconstructive surgery can repair some of the damage caused by the disease. *indeterminate l.* a form of the disease in which the skin manifestations represent a combination of lepromatous and tuberculoid leprosy. *lepromatous* (or *multibacillary*) *l.* a contagious steadily progressive form of the disease characterized by the development of widely distributed lumps on the skin, thickening of the skin and nerves, and in serious cases by severe numbness of the

lethargy

skin, muscle weakness, and paralysis leading to disfigurement and deformity. Tuberculosis is a common complication. *paucibacillary l.* tuberculoid or indeterminate leprosy. *tuberculoid l.* a benign, often self-limiting, form of leprosy causing discoloration and disfiguration of patches of skin associated with localized numbness.

lept- (lepto-) *prefix denoting* **1.** slender; thin. **2.** small. **3.** mild; slight.

leptin (lep-tin) *n.* a protein, produced by white fat cells in adipose tissue, that acts on the brain and is involved in controlling the amount of white adipose tissue laid down in the body.

leptocyte (lep-toh-syt) *n.* a red blood cell (erythrocyte) that is wafer-thin and generally large in diameter, with the haemoglobin concentrated in a thin rim at the periphery. Leptocytes are seen in certain types of anaemia.

leptomeninges (lep-toh-min-in-jeez) *pl. n.* the inner two meninges: the arachnoid and pia mater.

leptomeningitis (lep-toh-men-in-jy-tis) *n.* inflammation of the leptomeninges. *See also* meningitis.

Leptospira (lep-toh-**spy**-ră) *n.* a genus of spirochaete bacteria, commonly bearing hooked ends. *L. icterohaemorrhagiae* a parasite that is the main causative agent of leptospirosis.

leptospirosis (Weil's disease) (lep-toh-spy-**roh**-sis) *n.* an infectious disease, caused by bacteria of the genus *Leptospira* (especially *L. icterohaemorrhagiae*), that is transmitted from rodents, dogs, and other mammals to humans. The disease

begins with a high fever and headache and may affect the liver (causing jaundice) or kidneys (resulting in renal failure); in some cases meningitis may develop.

leresis (ler-ee-sis) *n.* rambling speech, immature both in syntax and pronunciation. It is a feature of dementia.

Leriche's syndrome (lĕ-reesh-ĕz) *n.* a condition in males characterized by absence of penile erection combined with absence of pulses in the femoral arteries and wasting of the buttock muscles. It is caused by occlusion of the abdominal aorta and iliac arteries. [R. Leriche (1879–1956), French surgeon]

lesbianism (lez-bi-ăn-izm) *n.* a pattern of sexuality in which a woman is sexually attracted to, or engages in sexual behaviour with, another woman. *See* homosexuality. —**lesbian** *adj., n.*

Lesch-Nyhan disease (lesh-ny-hăn) *n.* a sex-linked hereditary disease caused by an enzyme deficiency resulting in overproduction of uric acid. Affected boys are mentally retarded and suffer from spasticity and gouty arthritis. They also have a compulsion for self-mutilation. [M. Lesch (1939–) and W. L. Nyhan Jr. (1926–), US physicians]

lesion (lee-zhŏn) *n.* a zone of tissue with impaired function as a result of damage by disease or wounding.

lethal gene (lee-thăl) *n.* a gene that, under certain conditions, causes the death of the individual carrying it. Lethal genes are usually recessive: an individual will die only if both parents carry the gene.

lethargy (leth-er-ji) *n.* mental and physical sluggishness: a degree of inactivity and unresponsiveness approaching or verging on the unconscious.

letrozole (let-rŏ-zohl) *n. see* aromatase inhibitor.

Letterer-Siwe disease (let-er-er sy-wē) *n. see* Langerhans cell histiocytosis. [E. Letterer (20th century) and S. A. Siwe (1897–1966), German physicians]

leuc- (leuco-, leuk-, leuko-) *prefix denoting* **1.** lack of colour; white. **2.** leucocytes.

leucine (loo-seen) *n.* an essential amino acid. *See also* amino acid.

leucocidin (loo-koh-sy-din) *n.* a bacterial exotoxin that selectively destroys white blood cells (leucocytes).

leucocyte (white blood cell, WBC) (loo-kŏ-syt) *n.* any blood cell that contains a nucleus. In health there are three major subdivisions: granulocytes, lymphocytes, and monocytes, which are involved in protecting the body against foreign substances and in antibody production. In disease, a variety of other types may appear in the blood.

leucocytolysis (loo-koh-sy-tol-i-sis) *n.* destruction of white blood cells.

leucocytosis (loo-koh-sy-toh-sis) *n.* an increase in the number of leucocytes in the blood. *See* basophilia, eosinophilia, lymphocytosis, monocytosis.

leucocytospermia (loo-koh-sy-toh-**sperm**-iă) *n.* the presence of excess white blood cells (leucocytes) in the semen (more than 1 million/ml). It has an adverse effect on fertility.

leucoderma (loo-koh-**der**-mă) *n.* loss of pigment in areas of the skin,

resulting in the appearance of white patches or bands.

leucolysin (loo-kol-i-sin) *n. see* lysin.

leucoma (loo-koh-mă) *n.* a white opacity in the cornea. Most leucomas result from scarring after corneal inflammation or ulceration.

leuconychia (loo-koh-nik-iă) *n.* white discoloration of the nails, which may be total or partial. The cause is unknown.

leucopenia (loo-koh-pee-niă) *n.* a reduction in the number of leucocytes in the blood. *See* eosinopenia, lymphopenia, neutropenia.

leucoplakia (loo-koh-**play**-kiă) *n. see* leukoplakia.

leucopoiesis (loo-koh-poi-ee-sis) *n.* the process of the production of leucocytes, which normally occurs in the blood-forming tissue of the bone marrow. *See also* granulopoiesis, haemopoiesis, lymphopoiesis, monoblast.

leucorrhoea (loo-kŏ-ree-ă) *n.* a whitish or yellowish discharge of mucus from the vaginal opening. An abnormally large discharge may indicate infection of the lower reproductive tract.

leucotomy (loo-kot-ŏmi) *n.* the surgical operation of interrupting the pathways of white nerve fibres within the brain: it involves stereotaxy to make selective lesions in small areas of the brain. The operation is occasionally used for intractable pain, severe depression, obsessional neurosis, and chronic anxiety. *prefrontal l.* (*lobotomy*) the original form of the operation, which involved cutting through the nerve fibres connecting the frontal lobe with the thalamus and the association fibres of the frontal lobe; it has now been abandoned.

leukaemia (loo-kee-miă) *n.* any of a group of malignant diseases in which increased numbers of certain immature or abnormal leucocytes are produced. This leads to increased susceptibility to infection, anaemia, and bleeding. Other symptoms include enlargement of the spleen, liver, and lymph nodes. Leukaemias may be *acute* or *chronic* depending on the rate of progression of the disease. They are also classified according to the type of white cell that is proliferating abnormally, as in *lymphocytic l.* or *monocytic l.* (*see also* hairy cell, lymphoblast, myeloblast, myeloid (leukaemia)). Leukaemias are treated with cytotoxic drugs, monoclonal antibodies, or (occasionally) radiotherapy.

leukoplakia (leucoplakia) (loo-koh-**play**-kiă) *n.* a thickened white patch on a mucous membrane, such as the mouth lining or vulva, that cannot be rubbed off. Occasionally leukoplakia can become malignant. *hairy l.* leukoplakia with a shaggy or hairy appearance, which is a marker of AIDS.

leukotriene receptor antagonist (loo-koh-**try**-een) *n.* one of a class of drugs that prevent the action of leukotrienes (chemicals involved in inflammatory reactions and the immune response) by blocking their receptors on cell membranes, such as those in the airways. These drugs are used in the treatment of asthma; they include *montelukast* (Singulair) and *zafirlukast* (Accolate), both of which are administered by mouth.

leuprorelin (loo-proh-**rel**-in) *n.* *see* LHRH analogue.

levator (li-**vay**-ter) *n.* **1.** a surgical instrument used for levering up displaced bone fragments in a depressed fracture of the skull. **2.** any muscle that lifts the structure into which it is inserted.

levo- (laevo-) *prefix denoting* **1.** the left side. **2.** (in chemistry) levorotation.

levobunolol (lee-voh-**boon**-ŏ-lol) *n.* a beta blocker used as eye drops in the treatment of glaucoma. Trade name: **Betagan**.

levodopa (L-dopa) (lee-voh-**doh**-pă) *n.* a naturally occurring amino acid (*see* dopa) administered by mouth to treat parkinsonism.

levodopa test *n.* a test of the ability of the pituitary to secrete growth hormone, in which levodopa is administered by mouth and plasma levels of growth hormone are subsequently measured (they should peak within the following hour).

levomepromazine (methotrimeprazine) (lee-voh-mě-**prohm**-ă-zeen) *n.* a phenothiazine antipsychotic drug that is used in the treatment of schizophrenia and to relieve tension, agitation, and pain in terminally ill patients. It is administered by mouth or injection. Trade name: **Nozinan**.

levonorgestrel (lee-voh-nor-**jest**-rĕl) *n.* a synthetic female sex hormone – a progestogen – used mainly in oral contraceptives, either in combination with an oestrogen or as a progestogen-only preparation. Trade names: **Microval, Norgeston, Norplant**.

levulosuria (lev-yoo-lohs-**yoor**-iă) *n.* *see* fructosuria.

Lewy bodies (loo-i) *pl. n.* abnormal proteins found in the nerve cells of the cerebral cortex and basal ganglia in patients with *cortical Lewy body disease*, which is characterized by a combination of parkinsonism and dementia. [F. H. Lewy (1885–1950), German neurologist]

Leydig cells (ly-dig) *pl. n.* see interstitial cells. [F. von Leydig (1821–1908), German anatomist]

Leydig tumour *n.* a tumour of the interstitial (Leydig) cells of the testis. Such tumours often secrete testosterone, which in prepubertal boys causes virilization.

LFTs *pl. n.* see liver function tests.

LGA *adj.* large for gestational age.

LH *n.* see luteinizing hormone.

Lhermitte's sign (lair-mits) *n.* a tingling shocklike sensation passing down the arms or trunk when the neck is flexed. It is a nonspecific indication of disease in the cervical (neck) region of the spinal cord. [J. Lhermitte (1877–1959), French neurologist]

LHRH analogue (GnRH analogue) *n.* any one of a group of analogues of *luteinizing hormone releasing hormone* (*LHRH*), which stimulates the release of luteinizing hormone from the pituitary gland (*see also* gonadotrophin-releasing hormone). They are used in the treatment of endometriosis, fibroids, and some types of female infertility. Two LHRH analogues, *goserelin* (Zoladex) and *leuprorelin* (Prostap), are administered subcutaneously in the treatment of advanced prostate cancer.

libido (lib-ee-doh) *n.* the sexual drive: the term is often used to refer to the intensity of sexual desires. In psychoanalytic theory, the libido is said to be one of the fundamental sources of energy for all mental life.

Librium (lib-riŭm) *n.* see chlordiazepoxide.

lice (lys) *pl. n.* see louse, pediculosis.

lichen (ly-kĕn) *n.* any of several types of skin disease. *l. planus* an extremely itchy skin disease of unknown cause. Shiny flat-topped mauve spots may occur anywhere but are characteristically found on the inside of the wrists. It may take the form of a white lacy pattern in the mouth, which usually produces no symptoms. *l. simplex chronicus* (*neurodermatitis*) thickened eczematous skin that develops at the site of constant rubbing, often at the nape of the neck (in women) or lower legs (in men). *l. sclerosus* a chronic disease affecting the anogenital area, especially in women, and characterized by sheets of ivory-white skin.

lichenification (ly-ken-i-fi-kay-shŏn) *n.* thickening of the epidermis with exaggeration of the normal creases. The cause is abnormal scratching or rubbing of the skin.

lichenoid (ly-kĕn-oid) *adj.* describing any skin disease that resembles lichen planus.

lidocaine (lignocaine) (ly-doh-kayn) *n.* a widely used local anaesthetic administered by injection or by direct application for minor surgery and dental procedures. For dental surgery it is normally used in combination with adrenaline. Lidocaine is also injected to treat conditions involving abnormal heart rhythm, particularly myocardial infarction. Trade name: **Xylocaine**.

Lieberkühn's glands (crypts of Lieberkühn, intestinal glands) (lee-ber-koonz) *pl. n.* simple tubular glands in the mucous membrane of the intestine. They are lined with columnar epithelium in which various types of secretory cells are found. [J. N. Lieberkühn (1711–56), German anatomist]

lien (ly-ĕn) *n. see* spleen.

lien- (lieno-) *prefix denoting the* spleen.

ligament (lig-ă-mĕnt) *n.* **1.** a tough band of white fibrous connective tissue that links two bones together at a joint. Ligaments are inelastic but flexible; they strengthen the joint and limit its movements to certain directions. **2.** a sheet of peritoneum that supports or links together abdominal organs.

ligation (li-gay-shŏn) *n.* the application of a ligature.

ligature (lig-ă-cher) *n.* any material – for example, nylon, silk, catgut, or wire – that is tied firmly round a blood vessel or duct to prevent bleeding, the passage of materials, etc.

light adaptation (lyt) *n.* reflex changes in the eye to enable vision either in normal light after being in darkness or in very bright light after being in normal light. *See* iris. *Compare* dark adaptation.

lightening (ly-t'n-ing) *n.* the sensation experienced, usually after the 36th week of gestation, by many pregnant women, particularly those carrying their first child, as the presenting part of the fetus enters the pelvis. This reduces the pressure on the diaphragm and the woman notices that it is easier to breathe. *Compare* engagement.

lightning pains (lyt-ning) *pl. n.* severe stabbing pains in the legs experienced in tabes dorsalis.

light reflex *n. see* pupillary reflex.

lignocaine (lig-nŏ-kayn) *n. see* lidocaine.

Likert scale (lik-ert) *n.* a tool used in questionnaires in which participants are asked to respond to statements on a scale ranging from "strongly agree" to "strongly disagree". [R. Likert (1903–81), US psychologist]

limbic system (lim-bik) *n.* a complex system of nerve pathways and networks in the brain that is involved in the expression of instinct and mood in activities of the endocrine and motor systems of the body. Among the brain regions involved are the amygdala, hippocampal formation, and hypothalamus.

limb lengthening (lim) *n.* an orthopaedic procedure for increasing the length of a limb (usually the leg). It involves division of the bone and the use of an external fixator to widen the gap between the divided ends. New bone is produced in the widening gap as the bone is stretched.

limbus (lim-bŭs) *n.* (in anatomy) an edge or border. *l. sclerae* the junction of the cornea and sclera of the eye.

limen (ly-men) *n.* (in anatomy) a border or boundary.

liminal (lim-in-ăl) *adj.* (in physiology) relating to the threshold of perception.

linac (ly-nak) *n. see* linear accelerator.

linctus (link-tŭs) *n.* a syrupy liquid

medicine, particularly one used in the treatment of irritating coughs.

linea (lin-iǎ) *n.* (*pl.* **lineae**) (in anatomy) a line, narrow streak, or stripe. *l. alba* a tendinous line, extending from the xiphoid process to the pubic symphysis, where the flat abdominal muscles are attached. *l. nigra* a pigmented line, seen on the abdomen in pregnancy, extending from the umbilicus to the pubis.

linear accelerator (linac) (lin-ier) *n.* a machine that accelerates particles to produce high-energy radiation, used in the treatment (radiotherapy) of malignant disease.

linezolid (lini-zoh-lid) *n.* an antibiotic that is active against Gram-positive bacteria, including MRSA, and is used to treat pneumonia and soft-tissue infections caused by these organisms. It is administered by mouth or intravenous infusion. Trade name: **Zyvox.**

lingual (ling-wǎl) *adj.* relating to, situated close to, or resembling the tongue (lingula).

lingula (ling-yoo-lǎ) *n.* a thin tonguelike projection of bone or other tissue.

liniment (lin-i-měnt) *n.* a medicinal preparation that is rubbed onto the skin or applied on a surgical dressing. Liniments often contain camphor and alcohol.

linitis plastica (leather-bottle stomach) (li-ny-tis plas-ti-kǎ) *n.* diffuse infiltration of the stomach submucosa with malignant tissue, producing rigidity and narrowing.

linoleic acid (lin-oh-lee-ik) *n. see* essential fatty acid.

linolenic acid (lin-oh-len-ik) *n. see* essential fatty acid.

lint (lint) *n.* a material used in sur-

gical dressings, made of scraped linen or a cotton substitute. It is usually fluffy one side and smooth the other.

liothyronine (ly-oh-th'y-rō-neen) *n.* a preparation of the thyroid hormone triiodothyronine, administered by mouth or injection to treat conditions of thyroid deficiency. Trade name: **Tertroxin.**

lip- (lipo-) *prefix denoting* **1.** fat. **2.** lipid.

lipaemia (lip-ee-miǎ) *n.* the presence in the blood of an abnormally large amount of fat, such as cholesterol.

lipase (steapsin) (lip-ayz) *n.* an enzyme, produced by the pancreas and the glands of the small intestine, that breaks down fats into glycerol and fatty acids during digestion.

lipid (lip-id) *n.* one of a group of naturally occurring compounds that are soluble in solvents such as chloroform or alcohol, but insoluble in water. Lipids are important dietary constituents. The group includes fats, steroids, phospholipids, and glycolipids.

lipidosis (lipoidosis) (lip-i-doh-sis) *n.* (*pl.* **-ses**) any disorder of lipid metabolism within the cells of the body.

lipoatrophy (lip-oh-at-rǒ-fi) *n.* an immune reaction to insulin injections close to the site of injection, resulting in localized hollowing of the fat tissue. It is rarely seen with more modern, highly purified, insulins.

lipochondrodystrophy (lip-oh-kon-droh-dis-trǒ-fi) *n.* multiple congenital defects affecting lipid (fat) metabolism, cartilage and bone, skin, and the major internal organs, leading to mental retardation, dwarfism, and deformities of the bones.

lipodystrophy (lip-oh-**dis**-trŏ-fi) *n.* any condition resulting in the loss of fat tissue from part or all of the body. It may be congenital or acquired later in life.

lipogenesis (lip-oh-**jen**-i-sis) *n.* the process by which glucose and other substances, derived from carbohydrate in the diet, are converted to fatty acids in the body.

lipohypertrophy (lip-oh-hy-**per**-trŏ-fi) *n.* a local build-up of fat tissue near the site of repeated insulin injections, which tends to alter the rate of absorption of further injections into the body. It is caused by the local action of the insulin, which promotes fat storage.

lipoid (**lip**-oid) *adj.* resembling a lipid.

lipoidosis (lip-oi-**doh**-sis) *n. see* lipidosis.

lipolysis (lip-**ol**-i-sis) *n.* the process by which lipids are broken down into their constituent fatty acids in the body by the enzyme lipase. —**lipolytic** *adj.*

lipoma (lip-**oh**-mă) *n.* (*pl.* **lipomas** or **lipomata**) a common benign tumour that is composed of well-differentiated fat cells.

lipomatosis (lip-oh-mă-**toh**-sis) *n.* **1.** the presence of an abnormally large amount of fat in the tissues. **2.** the presence of multiple lipomas.

lipoprotein (lip-oh-**proh**-teen) *n.* one of a group of compounds, found in blood plasma and lymph, each consisting of a protein (*see* apolipoprotein) combined with a lipid (cholesterol, a triglyceride, or a phospholipid). Lipoproteins are important for the transport of lipids in the blood and lymph. *high-density l.* (*HDL*) a type of lipoprotein that transports cholesterol from the tissues to the liver. *low-density l.* (*LDL*) a type of lipoprotein that is the main form in which cholesterol is transported in the bloodstream, from which it is taken into the cells by binding with LDL receptors. *very low-density l.* (*VLDL*) a type of lipoprotein that is the precursor of LDL.

liposarcoma (lip-oh-sar-**koh**-mă) *n.* a rare malignant tumour of fat cells. It is most commonly found in the thigh, usually in patients over the age of 30 years.

lipotropic (lip-oh-**trop**-ik) *adj.* describing a substance that promotes the transport of fatty acids from the liver to the tissues or accelerates the utilization of fat in the liver itself.

lipping (**lip**-ing) *n.* overgrowth of bone as seen in X-rays near a joint margin. This is a characteristic sign of degenerative or inflammatory joint disease, particularly osteoarthritis. *See also* osteophyte.

lipuria (adiposuria) (lip-**yoor**-iă) *n.* the presence of fat or oil droplets in the urine.

liquid-based cytology (LBC) (**lik**-wid) *n.* a new technology intended to improve the detection of cytological abnormalities, which has been heralded as a way forward for cervical screening. It provides uniformly well-fixed preparations that are free of inflammatory exudate and blood and seem easier to screen than conventional smears.

liquor (**lik**-er) *n.* (in pharmacy) any

solution, usually an aqueous solution.

Listeria (lis-teer-iǎ) *n.* a genus of Gram-positive aerobic motile rod-like bacteria that are parasites of warm-blooded animals. *L. monocytogenes* a species that, if transmitted to humans by eating infected animal products, may cause *listeriosis*, especially in the frail, ranging from influenza-like symptoms to meningoencephalitis. In pregnant women it may terminate the pregnancy or damage the fetus.

lith- (litho-) *prefix denoting* a calculus (stone).

-lith *suffix denoting* a calculus (stone).

lithaemia (lith-ee-miǎ) *n. see* hyperuricaemia.

lithiasis (lith-I-ǎ-sis) *n.* formation of stones (*see* calculus) in an internal organ.

lithium (lithium carbonate) (lith-iǔm) *n.* a drug given by mouth to prevent episodes of manic-depressive psychosis or to treat mania. Trade names: **Camcolit, Liskonum, Priadel.**

litholapaxy (lithotripsy) (lith-olǎ-paks-i) *n.* the operation of crushing a stone in the bladder, using an instrument called a *lithotrite*. The small fragments of stone can then be removed by irrigation and suction.

lithonephrotomy (lith-oh-ni-frot-ŏmi) *n.* surgical removal of a stone from the kidney. *See* nephrolithotomy, pyelolithotomy.

lithopaedion (lith-oh-pee-di-ŏn) *n.* a fetus that has died in the uterus or abdominal cavity and has become calcified.

lithotomy (lith-ot-ŏmi) *n.* the sur-

gical removal of a stone (calculus) from the urinary tract. *See also* nephrolithotomy, pyelolithotomy, ureterolithotomy.

lithotripsy (lith-ŏ-trip-si) *n.* **1.** the destruction of calculi (stones) by means of shock waves. *extracorporeal shock-wave l.* (ESWL) a technique for destroying calculi in the upper urinary tract; it uses a specialized machine (a *lithotripter*) for generating and transmitting the shock waves and localizing the stones. *electrohydraulic l.* (EHL) a technique for destroying urinary calculi in which an electrically generated shock wave is transmitted to the stone by a contact probe delivered via a nephroscope or ureteroscope. **2.** *see* litholapaxy.

lithotripter (lith-oh-trip-ter) *n. see* lithotripsy.

lithotrite (lith-ŏ-tryt) *n. see* litholapaxy.

lithuresis (lith-yoor-ee-sis) *n.* the passage of small stones or gravel in the urine.

lithuria (lith-yoor-iǎ) *n. see* hyperuricuria.

litmus (lit-mŭs) *n.* a pigment used as an indicator of acids and alkalis. In the presence of acids it turns red; with alkalis it turns blue.

litre (lee-ter) *n.* a unit of volume equal to the volume occupied by 1 kilogram of pure water at 4°C and 760 mmHg pressure.

Little's area (li-t'lz) *n.* the anterior region of the nasal septum (*see* nose), which is richly supplied with capillaries (*see* Kiesselbach's plexus) and is a common site from which nosebleeds arise. [J. L. Little (1836–85), US surgeon]

Little's disease *n.* a form of cerebral palsy involving both sides of the body and affecting the legs more severely than the arms. [W. J. Little (1810–94), British surgeon]

Litzmann's obliquity (lits-manz) *n. see* asynclitism. [K. C. T. Litzmann (1815–90), German obstetrician]

livedo (liv-ee-doh) *n.* a discoloured area or spot on the skin, often caused by local congestion of the circulation.

liver (liv-er) *n.* the largest gland of the body, weighing 1200–1600 g. Situated in the top right portion of the abdominal cavity, the liver has a number of important functions. It synthesizes bile, which drains into the gall bladder before being released into the duodenum. The liver

branch of hepatic portal vein

bile duct   sinusoids

central vein   portal area

lobule

liver cells

branch of hepatic artery

The microscopic structure of the liver

is an important site of metabolism of carbohydrates, proteins, and fats. It regulates the amount of blood sugar, removes excess amino acids, and stores and metabolizes fats. The liver also synthesizes fibrinogen, prothrombin, and heparin, and has an important role in the detoxification of poisonous substances.

liver function tests (LFTs) *pl. n.* blood tests carried out to assess the functioning of the liver. These include tests for serum proteins, serum bilirubin, alanine aminotransferase, and alkaline phosphatase.

livid (liv-id) *adj.* denoting a bluish colour of the skin, such as that produced locally by a bruise or of the general complexion in cyanosis.

living will (advance directive) (liv-ing) *n.* a statement signed by a person that outlines the degree of life-saving treatment desired in case of incapacitation. It enables terminally ill patients to refuse resuscitation in the event of cardiac arrest.

LMP *n.* (date of) last menstrual period.

Loa (loh-ă) *n.* a genus of parasitic nematode worms (*see* filaria). *L. loa* the eye worm, which lives in the tissues beneath the skin and causes loiasis.

lobe (lohb) *n.* a major division of an organ or part of an organ, especially one having a rounded form and often separated from other lobes by fissures or bands of connective tissue. —**lobar** *adj.*

lobectomy (loh-bek-tŏmi) *n.* the surgical removal of a lobe of an organ or gland, such as the lung, thyroid, or brain.

lobotomy (prefrontal leucot-

omy) (loh-bot-ŏmi) n. see leucotomy.

lobule (lob-yool) n. a subdivision of a part or organ, such as the liver or lung, that can be distinguished from the whole by boundaries, such as septa, that are visible with or without a microscope.

LOC n. level of consciousness.

localized (loh-kă-lyzd) adj. (of a lesion, eruption, etc.) restricted to a particular part of the body; not widespread.

lochia (lok-iă) n. the material eliminated from the uterus through the vagina after the completion of labour. The first discharge consists largely of blood (l. rubra). This is followed by a brownish mixture of blood and mucus (l. serosa), and finally a yellowish or whitish discharge containing microorganisms and cell fragments (l. alba). Each stage may last for several days. —**lochial** adj.

locked-in syndrome (lokt-in) n. a condition resulting from damage to the brainstem, in which the patient is conscious but unable to speak or to move any part of the body, except for blinking and upward eye movements, which permit signalling. Compare persistent vegetative state.

lockjaw (lok-jaw) n. see tetanus.

locomotor ataxia (loh-kŏ-moh-ter) n. see tabes dorsalis.

loculated (lok-yoo-layt-id) adj. divided into many cavities.

loculus (lok-yoo-lŭs) n. (in anatomy) a small space or cavity.

locum tenens (locum) (loh-kŭm teen-enz) n. a doctor who stands in temporarily for a colleague who is absent or ill.

locus (loh-kŭs) n. **1.** (in anatomy) a region or site. **2.** (in genetics) the region of a chromosome occupied by a particular gene.

lofepramine (loh-fep-ră-meen) n. a tricyclic antidepressant administered by mouth. Trade name: **Gamanil**.

log- (logo-) prefix denoting words; speech.

logopaedics (log-ŏ-pee-diks) n. the scientific study of defects and disabilities of speech and of the methods used to treat them; speech therapy.

-logy (-ology) suffix denoting field of study.

loiasis (loh-I-ă-sis) n. a disease, occurring in West and Central Africa, caused by the eye worm Loa loa. The adult worms live and migrate within the skin tissues, causing inflammation and swellings, and often migrate across the eyeball just beneath the conjunctiva, producing irritation and congestion. Loiasis is treated with diethylcarbamazine.

loin (loin) n. the region of the back and side of the body between the lowest rib and the pelvis.

Lomotil (lom-ŏ-til) n. see cophenotrope.

long-sightedness (long-syt-id-nis) n. see hypermetropia.

loop (loop) n. **1.** a bend in a tubular organ. **2.** one of the patterns of dermal ridges in fingerprints.

loperamide (loh-per-ă-myd) n. a drug used in the treatment of diarrhoea. It acts by reducing peristalsis of the digestive tract and is administered by mouth. Trade name: **Imodium**.

lopinavir (loh-pin-ă-veer) n. see protease inhibitor.

loprazolam (loh-praz-ŏ-lam) n. a

short-acting benzodiazepine drug that is administered by mouth for the treatment of insomnia.

loratidine (lŏ-rat-i-deen) *n.* a nonsedating antihistamine administered by mouth to treat allergic conditions, such as hay fever and urticaria. Trade name: **Clarityn**.

lorazepam (lor-az-ĕ-pam) *n.* a benzodiazepine administered by mouth to relieve moderate or severe anxiety and tension and to treat insomnia. Trade name: **Ativan**.

lordosis (lor-doh-sis) *n.* inward curvature of the spine. A certain degree of lordosis is normal in the lumbar and cervical regions of the spine. Exaggerated lordosis may occur in adolescence, through faulty posture or as a result of disease. *Compare* kyphosis.

losartan (loh-sar-tan) *n. see* angiotensin II antagonist.

lotion (loh-shŏn) *n.* a medicinal solution for external use. Lotions usually have a cooling, soothing, or antiseptic action.

Lou Gehrig's disease (loo gerigz) *n. see* (amyotrophic lateral) sclerosis. [Lou Gehrig (1903–41), US baseball player who suffered from it]

loupe (loop) *n.* a small magnifying hand lens used for examining the front part of the eye.

louse (lowss) *n.* (*pl.* **lice**) a small wingless bloodsucking insect that is an external parasite of humans and may transmit disease. Lice attach themselves to hair and clothing; they thrive in overcrowded and unhygienic conditions. *See also* pediculosis.

Løvset's manoeuvre (luv-setz) *n.* rotation and traction of the trunk of the fetus during a breech birth to facilitate delivery of the arms and the shoulders. [J. Løvset (20th century), Norwegian obstetrician]

low-density lipoprotein (LDL) (loh-**den**-siti) *n. see* lipoprotein.

lower urinary tract symptoms (LUTS) (loh-er) *pl. n.* symptoms occuring during urine storage, voiding, or immediately after, including frequency, urgency, nocturia, incontinence, hesitation, intermittency, terminal dribble, dysuria, and postmicturition dribble. These symptoms may be due to benign prostatic hyperplasia (*see* prostate gland), detrusor overactivity, excessive drinking, diuresis due to poorly controlled diabetes, or a urethral stricture.

low-molecular-weight heparin (loh-mŏ-lek-yoo-ler-wayt) *n. see* heparin.

lozenge (loz-inj) *n.* a medicated tablet containing sugar.

LP *n. see* lumbar (puncture).

LRTI *n.* lower respiratory tract infection.

LSD *n. see* lysergic acid diethylamide.

lubb-dupp (lub-dup) *n.* a representation of the normal heart sounds as heard through the stethoscope. The first coincides with closure of the mitral and tricuspid valves; the second with closure of the aortic and pulmonary valves.

lucid interval (loo-sid in-ter-văl) *n.* temporary recovery of consciousness after a blow to the head, before relapse into coma. It is a sign of intracranial arterial bleeding.

Ludwig's angina (luud-vigz) *n.* severe inflammation caused by bacterial infection of the floor of the mouth, resulting in massive swelling of the neck. [W. F. von Ludwig (1790–1865), German surgeon]

lues (loo-eez) *n.* a serious infectious disease such as syphilis.

Lugol's solution (loo-golz) *n.* an aqueous solution of iodine and potassium iodide used for treating thyrotoxicosis in emergencies. [J. G. A. Lugol (1786–1851), French physician]

lumbago (lum-bay-goh) *n.* pain in the lumbar region, of any cause or description. Severe lumbago, of sudden onset, can be due either to a slipped disc or to a strained muscle or ligament.

lumbar (lum-ber) *adj.* relating to the loin. *l. puncture* (*LP*) a procedure performed under local anaesthetic in which cerebrospinal fluid is withdrawn for diagnostic purposes by means of a hollow needle inserted into the subarachnoid space in the region of the lower back (usually between the third and fourth lumbar vertebrae). *See also* Queckenstedt test. *l. triangle* a weak area in the abdomen bounded by the iliac crest (below), the external oblique muscle (in front), and the erector spinae muscle (behind). *l. vertebrae* the five bones of the backbone that are situated between the thoracic vertebrae and the sacrum, in the lower part of the back. *See also* vertebra.

lumbo- *prefix denoting* the loin; lumbar region.

lumbosacral (lum-boh-say-krăl) *adj.* relating to the part of the spine composed of the lumbar vertebrae and the sacrum.

lumen (loo-min) *n.* **1.** the space within a tubular or saclike part. **2.**

the SI unit of luminous flux. Symbol: lm.

luminescence (loo-min-ess-ĕns) *n.* the emission of light from a substance after it has been irradiated. Fluorescence is a type of luminescence.

lumpectomy (lum-pek-tŏmi) *n.* an operation for breast cancer in which the tumour and surrounding breast tissue are removed: muscles, skin, and lymph nodes are left intact (*compare* mastectomy). The procedure, usually followed by radiation, is indicated for patients with a tumour less than 2 cm in diameter and who have no metastases to local lymph nodes or to distant organs.

lunate bone (loo-nayt) *n.* a bone of the wrist (*see* carpus). It articulates with the capitate and hamate bones in front, with the radius behind, and with the triquetral and scaphoid at the sides.

lung (lung) *n.* one of the pair of organs of respiration, situated in the chest cavity on either side of the

branch of pulmonary artery

terminal bronchiole

respiratory bronchiole

pulmonary vein

alveolar duct

alveoli

alveolar sacs

Details of the alveoli

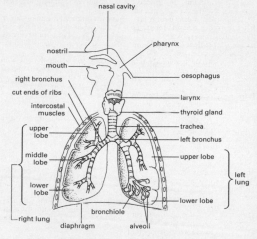

The lungs and main air passages

heart. The lungs communicate with the atmosphere through the trachea, which opens into the pharynx. The trachea divides into two bronchi, which enter the lungs and branch into bronchioles. These divide further and terminate in minute air sacs (alveoli), the sites of gaseous exchange. (See illustrations.) Atmospheric oxygen is absorbed and carbon dioxide from the blood of the pulmonary capillaries is released into the lungs (*see* (pulmonary) circulation).

lung cancer *n.* cancer arising in the epithelium of the air passages (*bronchial cancer*) or lung. It is strongly associated with cigarette smoking and exposure to industrial air pollutants (including asbestos). Treatment includes surgical removal of the affected lobe or lung, radiotherapy, and chemotherapy.

lunula (loon-yoo-lă) *n.* the whitish crescent-shaped area at the base of a nail.

lupus (loo-pŭs) *n.* any of several chronic skin diseases. *l. erythema-*

tosus (LE) an inflammatory auto-immune disease of connective tissue. In *systemic LE (SLE)* the skin and various internal organs are affected. Typically, there is a red scaly rash on the nose and cheeks; arthritis; and progressive damage to the kidneys. Often the heart, lungs, and brain are also affected. In a milder form, known as *discoid LE (DLE)*, only the skin is affected. LE is treated with corticosteroids or immunosuppressant drugs. *l. verrucosus* a rare tuberculous infection of the skin – commonly the arm or hand – typified by warty lesions. It occurs in those who have been reinfected with tuberculosis. *l. vulgaris* a tuberculous infection of the skin that often starts in childhood, with dark red patches on the nose or cheek. Unless treated with antituberculous drugs lupus vulgaris spreads, ulcerates, and causes extensive scarring.

lutein (loo-ti-in) *n.* the yellow pigment of the corpus luteum.

luteinizing hormone (LH) (loo-ti-i-nyz-ing) *n.* a hormone (*see* gonadotrophin), synthesized and released by the anterior pituitary gland, that stimulates ovulation, corpus luteum formation, progesterone synthesis by the ovary, and androgen synthesis by the testes. Also called: **interstitial-cell-stimulating hormone (ICSH)**.

luteo- *prefix denoting* **1.** yellow. **2.** the corpus luteum.

luteotrophic hormone (luteotrophin) (loo-ti-oh-trof-ik) *n. see* prolactin.

LUTS *pl. n. see* lower urinary tract symptoms.

luxation (luks-ay-shŏn) *n. see* dislocation.

LVF *n.* left ventricular failure. *See* heart failure.

Lyell's disease (ly-ĕlz) *n. see* staphylococcal scalded skin syndrome. [A. Lyell (20th century), British dermatologist]

Lyme disease (lym) *n.* a disease caused by a spirochaete, *Borrelia burgdorferi*, and transmitted by certain ticks of the genus *Ixodes*. Following a 3–32-day incubation period, a slowly extending red rash develops in approximately 75% of cases; intermittent symptoms include fever, malaise, headache and neck stiffness, and muscle and joint pains. Later, 60% of patients suffer intermittent attacks of arthritis, especially of the knees, each attack lasting months and recurring over several years. Treatment is with tetracycline or penicillin.

lymph (limf) *n.* the fluid present within the vessels of the lymphatic system, which is derived from the fluid that bathes the tissues. Lymph is similar in composition to plasma, but contains less protein and some cells, mainly lymphocytes. *l. node* one of a number of small swellings found at intervals along the lymphatic system. Groups of nodes occur in the groin and armpit, behind the ear, and in many other parts. They act as filters for the lymph and produce lymphocytes.

lymphaden- (lymphadeno-) *prefix denoting* lymph node(s).

lymphadenectomy (lim-fad-in-ek-tŏmi) *n.* surgical removal of lymph nodes.

lymphadenitis (lim-fad-in-I-tis) *n.* inflammation of lymph nodes, which become swollen, painful, and tender. The most commonly affected lymph nodes are those in the neck, in association with tonsillitis.

lymphadenoma (lim-fad-in-ohmǎ) n. an obsolete name for lymphoma.

lymphangi- (lymphangio-) prefix denoting a lymphatic vessel.

lymphangiectasis (lim-fan-ji-ektǎ-sis) n. dilatation of the lymphatic vessels, which is usually congenital. It may also be caused by obstruction of the lymphatic vessels (see lymphoedema).

lymphangiography (lymphography) (lim-fan-ji-og-rǎfi) n. X-ray examination of the lymphatic vessels and lymph nodes after a contrast medium has been injected into them (see angiography). Alternatively, the lymphatic system can be imaged using a gamma camera following the injection of a radioactive tracer.

lymphangioma (lim-fan-ji-oh-mǎ) n. a localized collection of distended lymphatic vessels, which may result in a large cyst in the neck or armpit (cystic hygroma).

lymphangioplasty (lim-fan-ji-ohplasti) n. the surgical creation of artificial lymph channels when the lymphatic vessels are obstructed.

lymphangiosarcoma (lim-fan-jioh-sar-koh-mǎ) n. a rare malignant tumour of the lymphatic vessels. It is most commonly seen in the arms of women who have had a mastectomy for breast cancer and may be induced by radiation.

lymphangitis (lim-fan-jy-tis) n. inflammation of the lymphatic vessels, which can be seen most commonly as red streaks in the skin

adjacent to a focus of streptococcal infection.

lymphatic (lim-fat-ik) **1.** n. a lymphatic vessel. See lymphatic system. **2.** adj. relating to or transporting lymph.

lymphatic system n. a network of vessels that conveys electrolytes, water, proteins, etc. – in the form of lymph – from the tissue fluids to the bloodstream. Lymph passes through fine capillaries into the lymphatic vessels, which have valves to prevent backflow of lymph. The lymphatics lead to two large channels – the *thoracic duct* and the *right lymphatic duct* – which return the lymph to the bloodstream via the innominate veins.

lympho- prefix denoting lymph or the lymphatic system.

lymphoblast (lim-foh-blast) n. an abnormal cell that is present in the blood and blood-forming organs in a type of leukaemia (*lymphoblastic leukaemia*). —**lymphoblastic** adj.

lymphocele (lim-foh-seel) n. a collection of lymph in the tissues, which follows injury to, or operations upon, lymph nodes or ducts.

lymphocyte (lim-foh-syt) n. a variety of white blood cell (leucocyte), present also in the lymph nodes, spleen, thymus gland, gut wall, and bone marrow. They are involved in immunity and can be subdivided into *B-lymphocytes* (or *B-cells*), which produce circulating antibodies, and *T-lymphocytes*, which are primarily responsible for cell-mediated immunity (see T-cell). —**lymphocytic** adj.

lymphocytopenia (lim-foh-sy-tohpee-niǎ) n. see lymphopenia.

lymphocytosis (lim-foh-sy-toh-sis)

n. an increase in the number of lymphocytes in the blood.

lymphoedema (lim-fee-**dee**-mă) *n.* an accumulation of lymph in the tissues, producing swelling; the legs are most often affected. It may be due to a congenital abnormality of the lymphatic vessels (as in Milroy's disease) or result from obstruction of the lymphatic vessels by a tumour, parasites, inflammation, or injury.

lymphogranuloma venereum (lim-foh-gran-yoo-**loo**-mă vi-**neer**-iŭm) *n.* a sexually transmitted disease that is caused by bacteria of the genus *Chlamydia* and is most common in tropical regions. An initial lesion on the genitals is followed by swelling and inflammation of the lymph nodes in the groin. Early treatment with sulphonamides or tetracyclines is usually effective.

lymphography (lim-**fog**-răfi) *n. see* lymphangiography.

lymphoid tissue (lim-foid) *n.* a tissue responsible for the production of lymphocytes and antibodies. It occurs in the form of the lymph nodes, tonsils, thymus, and spleen, and also as diffuse groups of cells. *See also* immune (system).

lymphokine (lim-foh-kyn) *n.* a substance produced by lymphocytes that has effects on other cells involved in the immune system. An example is interleukin 2 (IL-2).

lymphoma (lim-**foh**-mă) *n.* a malignant tumour of the lymph nodes, including Hodgkin's disease and other forms (*non-Hodgkin's l.*, *NHL*). Disease may be widespread, but in some cases is confined to a single area, which may be extranodal (such as the tonsil). Treatment is

with such drugs as chlorambucil or with combinations of cyclophosphamide, vincristine, and prednisolone. *See also* Burkitt's lymphoma.

lymphopenia (lymphocytopenia) (lim-foh-**pee**-niă) *n.* a decrease in the number of lymphocytes in the blood.

lymphopoiesis (lim-foh-poi-**ee**-sis) *n.* the process of the production of lymphocytes, which occurs in the bone marrow as well as in the lymph nodes, spleen, thymus gland, and gut wall.

lymphorrhagia (lim-fŏ-**ray**-jiă) *n.* the escape of the lymph from lymphatic vessels that have been injured.

lymphosarcoma (lim-foh-sar-**koh**-mă) *n.* a former name for non-Hodgkin's lymphoma.

lymphuria (limf-**yoor**-iă) *n.* the presence in the urine of lymph.

lyo- (**lysi-**, **lyso-**) *prefix denoting* lysis; dissolution.

lyophilization (ly-ofi-ly-**zay**-shŏn) *n.* preservation of biological material (e.g. plasma, serum, skin) by rapid freezing followed by dehydration.

lys- (**lysi-**, **lyso-**) *prefix denoting* lysis; dissolution.

lysergic acid diethylamide (LSD) (ly-**ser**-jik ass-id dy-eth-il-ay-myd) *n.* a psychedelic drug that is also a hallucinogen. It was formerly used to aid treatment of psychological disorders. Alterations in sight, hearing, and other senses occur, psychotic effects, depression, and confusion are common, and tolerance to the drug develops rapidly. Because of these toxic effects, LSD is no longer used clinically.

lysin (ly-sin) *n.* a specific complement-fixing antibody that is capable of bringing about the destruction (lysis) of whole cells. *Haemolysin* attacks red blood cells, *leucolysin* white cells, and a *bacteriolysin* bacterial cells.

lysine (ly-seen) *n.* an essential amino acid. *See also* amino acid.

lysis (ly-sis) *n.* **1.** the destruction of cells through damage or rupture of the plasma membrane, allowing escape of the cell contents. *See also* autolysis, lysozyme. **2.** gradual remission of the symptoms of a disease.

-lysis *suffix denoting* lysis; dissolution.

lysosome (ly-sŏ-sohm) *n.* a particle in the cytoplasm of cells that contains enzymes responsible for breaking down substances in the cell. Lysosomes are especially abundant in liver and kidney cells.

lysozyme (ly-sŏ-zym) *n.* an enzyme found in tears and egg white. It catalyses the destruction of the cell walls of certain bacteria.

Mm

maceration (mas-er-ay-shŏn) *n.* **1.** the softening of a solid by leaving it immersed in a liquid. **2.** (in obstetrics) the natural breakdown of a dead fetus within the uterus.

Mackenrodt's ligaments (mahk-ĕn-rohts) *pl. n.* *see* cardinal ligaments. [A. K. Mackenrodt (1859–1925), German gynaecologist]

macr- (macro-) *prefix denoting* large size.

macrocephaly (megalocephaly) (mak-roh-sef-ăli) *n.* abnormal largeness of the head. *Compare* microcephaly.

macrocheilia (mak-roh-ky-liă) *n.* hypertrophy of the lips: a congenital condition in which the lips are abnormally large. *Compare* microcheilia.

macrocyte (megalocyte) (mak-roh-syt) *n.* an abnormally large red blood cell (erythrocyte). *See also* macrocytosis. —**macrocytic** *adj.*

macrocytosis (mak-roh-sy-toh-sis) *n.* the presence of macrocytes in the blood. Macrocytosis is a feature of certain anaemias (known as *macrocytic anaemias*), including those due to deficiency of vitamin B_{12} or folic acid.

macrodactyly (mak-roh-dak-tili) *n.* abnormally large size of one or more of the fingers or toes.

macrogenitosoma (mak-roh-jen-it-oh-**soh**-mă) *n.* excessive bodily growth with marked enlargement of the genitalia.

macroglobulin (mak-roh-glob-yoo-lin) *n.* **1. (immunoglobulin M, IgM)** a protein of the globulin series that is present in the blood and functions as an antibody, forming an effective first-line defence against any bacteria that enter the bloodstream. *See also* immunoglobulin. **2.** an abnormal form of IgM produced by lymphoma cells or in other plasma-cell disorders.

macroglossia (mak-roh-glos-iă) *n.* an abnormally large tongue. It may be due to a congenital defect, to infiltration of the tongue with amyloid or a tumour, or to obstruction of the lymph vessels.

macrognathia (mak-roh-**nay**-thiă) *n.* a condition in which one or both jaws are unusually large.

macromelia (mak-roh-**mee**-liă) *n.* abnormally large size of the arms or legs. *Compare* micromelia.

macrophage (mak-roh-fayj) *n.* a large scavenger cell (*see* phagocyte) present in connective tissue and many major organs and tissues, including the bone marrow, spleen, lymph nodes, liver, and the central nervous system. *See also* histiocyte, reticuloendothelial system.

macropsia (mak-**rop**-siă) *n.* a condition in which objects appear larger than they really are. It is usually due to disease of the retina.

macroscopic (mak-roh-**skop**-ik) *adj.* visible to the naked eye. *Compare* microscopic.

macrosomia (mak-roh-soh-miă) n. abnormally large size. *fetal m.* large size in a baby associated with poorly controlled maternal diabetes; it is due to excessive production of fetal insulin and thence to increased deposition of glycogen in the fetus.

macrotia (mak-roh-tiă) n. a congenital deformity of the external ear in which the pinna is larger than normal.

macula (mak-yoo-lă) n. (*pl.* **maculae**) a small anatomical area that is distinguishable from the surrounding tissue. *m. lutea* the yellow spot on the retina at the back of the eye, which surrounds the greatest concentration of cones (*see* fovea). —**macular** (mak-yoo-ler) *adj.*

macular degeneration n. a group of conditions affecting the macula lutea of the eye, resulting in a reduction or loss of central vision. *age-related m. d.* (AMD, ARMD) the most common cause of blindness in the elderly. *Atrophic* or *dry AMD* results from chronic choroidal ischaemia: small blood vessels of the choroid, which lies beneath the retina, become constricted, reducing the blood supply to the macula. This gives rise to degenerative changes in the retinal pigment epithelium (RPE; *see* retina). *Wet AMD* is associated with the growth of abnormal new blood vessels under the retina, derived from the choroid (*see* choroidal) neovascularization). These can leak fluid and blood into the RPE, which further reduces macular function.

macule (mak-yool) n. a flat circumscribed area of skin or an area of altered skin colour (e.g. a freckle). *Compare* papule. —**macular** *adj.*

maculopapular (mak-yoo-loh-pap-yoo-ler) *adj.* describing a rash that consists of both macules and papules.

maculopathy (mak-yool-op-ă-thi) n. any abnormality of the macula lutea of the eye. *bull's-eye m.* the appearance of the macula in some toxic conditions (e.g. chloroquine toxicity) and in some hereditary disorders of the macula.

Madopar (mad-oh-par) n. *see* benserazide.

Madura foot (mă-dewr-ă) n. an infection of the tissues and bones of the foot producing chronic inflammation (mycetoma), occurring in the tropics. Medical name: **maduromycosis**.

Madurella (mad-yoo-rel-ă) n. a genus of widely distributed fungi. The species *M. grisea* and *M. mycetomi* cause the tropical infection Madura foot.

maduromycosis (mă-dewr-oh-my-koh-sis) n. *see* Madura foot.

MAG3 n. MercaptoAcetyltriGlycine: a tracer used in nuclear medicine, during renography, when labelled with technetium-99m. It enables the function and drainage of each kidney to be assessed, giving similar results to DTPA with a lower dose of ionizing radiation.

Magendie's foramen (ma-jen-deez) n. an opening in the roof of the fourth ventricle of the brain through which cerebrospinal fluid passes to the subarachnoid space. [F. Magendie (1783–1855), French physiologist]

magenta (mă-jen-tă) n. *see* fuchsin.

maggot (mag-ŏt) n. the wormlike larva of a fly, which occasionally infests human tissues (*see* myiasis).

Magill's forceps (mă-gilz) *n.* long angled forceps for use with a laryngoscope in removing foreign bodies from the mouth and throat of an unconscious patient. [Sir I. V. Magill (1888–1975), British anaesthetist]

magnesium (mag-nee-ziŭm) *n.* a metallic element essential to life. Magnesium is necessary for the proper functioning of muscle and nervous tissue. Symbol: Mg. *m. carbonate* a weak antacid used to relieve indigestion. *m. hydroxide* a magnesium salt used as an osmotic laxative and also as an ingredient in antacid preparations. *m. sulphate* a magnesium salt given in mixtures or enemas to treat constipation (*see* laxative). It is also administered by injection to treat magnesium deficiency. *m. trisilicate* a compound of magnesium with antacid and absorbent properties, used in the treatment of indigestion.

magnetic resonance imaging (MRI) (mag-net-ik) *n.* a diagnostic technique based on analysis of the absorption and transmission of high-frequency radio waves by the hydrogen in water molecules and other components of tissues placed in a strong magnetic field (*see* nuclear magnetic resonance). Using modern high-speed computers, this analysis can be used to produce images of the tissues in most parts of the body. It enables the noninvasive diagnosis and treatment planning of a wide range of diseases, including cancer, and guides interventional radiological procedures. MRI does not use potentially harmful ionizing radiation, such as X-rays, but should not be used in patients with metal clips or prostheses (e.g.

pacemakers) because the magnetic field may cause damage.

MAGPI operation (mag-py) *n.* *m*eatal *a*dvancement and *g*lanulo*p*lasty operation: a simple surgical procedure that is designed to correct minor to moderate degrees of coronal or subcoronal hypospadias. This single-stage operation corrects any associated minor degrees of chordee and transfers the urethral opening to the glans.

MAI complex *n.* a group of bacteria comprising *Mycobacterium avium* and *M. intracellulare*, which are responsible for opportunistic infections of the lung that mimic tuberculosis but are resistant to many antituberculosis drugs. These bacteria are particularly liable to cause superimposed infection in AIDS patients. *See* Mycobacterium.

mal (mal) *n.* illness or disease.

mal- *prefix denoting* disease, disorder, or abnormality.

malabsorption (mal-ăb-sorp-shŏn) *n.* a state in which absorption by the small intestine of one or more substances, such as fat, vitamins, or amino acids, is reduced. Symptoms (depending on the substances involved) include weight loss, diarrhoea, anaemia, swelling (oedema), and vitamin deficiencies. The commonest causes are coeliac disease, pancreatitis, cystic fibrosis, blind-loop syndrome, or surgical removal of a length of small intestine.

malacia (mă-lay-shiă) *n.* abnormal softening of a part, organ, or tissue, such as bone (*see* osteomalacia).

-malacia *suffix denoting* abnormal softening of a tissue.

maladie de Roger (Roger's disease) (ma-la-di dĕ ro-zhay) *n.* a form of congenital heart disease in which there is a small ventricular septal defect. It usually causes no symptoms. [H. L. Roger (1809–91), French physician]

malaise (mal-ayz) *n.* a general feeling of being unwell. The feeling may be accompanied by identifiable physical discomfort and may indicate the presence of disease.

malar bone (may-ler) *n. see* zygomatic bone.

malaria (ague, marsh fever, periodic fever, paludism) (mă-lair-iă) *n.* an infectious disease due to the presence of parasitic protozoa of the genus *Plasmodium* within the red blood cells. The disease is transmitted by the *Anopheles* mosquito and is confined mainly to tropical and subtropical areas. After an incubation period varying from 12 days to 10 months parasites invade, multiply within, and eventually destroy the red blood cells, releasing new parasites. This causes a short bout of shivering, fever, and sweating, and the loss of healthy red cells results in anaemia. When the next batch of parasites is released symptoms reappear. The interval between fever attacks varies in different types of malaria (*see* quartan fever, quotidian fever, tertian fever). Preventive and curative treatment relies on such drugs as chloroquine and proguanil. A vaccine is being tested.

malathion (mal-ă-th'y-on) *n.* an organophosphorous insecticide used to treat head and pubic lice and scabies. It is applied externally in the form of a lotion. Trade names: **Derbac-M, Prioderm, Suleo-M**.

malformation (mal-for-may-shŏn)

n. any variation from the normal physical structure, due either to congenital or developmental defects or to disease or injury.

malignant (mă-lig-nănt) *adj.* **1.** describing a tumour that invades and destroys the tissue in which it originates and can spread to other sites in the body via the bloodstream and lymphatic system. *See* cancer. **2.** describing any disorder that becomes life threatening if untreated. *Compare* benign.

malignant melanoma *n. see* melanoma.

malignant pustule *n. see* anthrax.

malingering (mă-ling-er-ing) *n.* pretending to be ill, usually in order to avoid work or to gain attention. It may be a sign of mental disorder (*see* Munchausen's syndrome).

malleolus (mal-lee-ŏ-lŭs) *n.* either of the two protuberances on each side of the ankle: at the lower end of the fibula (*lateral m.*) and at the lower end of the tibia (*medial m.*).

mallet finger (mal-it fing-er) *n.* a condition in which a finger (usually the index finger) is bent downwards at the tip, due to avulsion of the long extensor tendon from the bone.

malleus (mal-iŭs) *n.* a hammer-shaped bone in the middle ear that articulates with the incus and is attached to the eardrum. *See* ossicle.

Mallory bodies (mal-eri) *pl. n.* large irregular masses located in the hepatocytes of the liver. They are found in patients with alcoholic hepatitis, Wilson's disease, primary biliary cirrhosis, severe obesity, and hepatocellular carcinoma. [F. B. Mallory (1862–1941), US pathologist]

Mallory-Weiss syndrome (mal-eri-vys) *n*. tearing of the tissues around the junction of the oesophagus (gullet) and stomach as a result of violent vomiting or straining to vomit. It is associated with haematemesis and perforation of the oesophagus. [G. K. Mallory (1926–   ), US pathologist; S. Weiss (1899–1942), US physician]

malnutrition (mal-new-trish-ŏn) *n*. the condition caused by an improper balance between what an individual eats and what is required to maintain health. This can result from eating too little (*subnutrition* or *starvation*) but may also imply dietary excess or an incorrect balance of basic foodstuffs.

malocclusion (mal-ŏ-kloo-zhŏn) *n*. a condition in which there is an abnormal arrangement of the teeth, either within one jaw or in one jaw in relation to the other.

Malpighian body (mal-pig-iăn) *n*. the part of a nephron comprising the blood capillaries of the glomerulus and its surrounding Bowman's capsule. [M. Malpighi (1628–94), Italian anatomist]

Malpighian layer *n*. the stratum germinativum: one of the layers of the epidermis.

malposition (mal-pŏ-zish-ŏn) *n*. (in obstetrics) an abnormal position of the fetal head when this is the presenting part in labour, such that the diameter of the skull in relation to the pelvic opening is greater than normal. This is likely to result in a prolonged and complicated labour.

malpractice (mal-prak-tis) *n*. professional misconduct: treatment falling short of the standards of skill and care that can reasonably be expected from a qualified medical practitioner.

malpresentation (mal-prez-ĕn-tay-shŏn) *n*. the condition in which the presenting part of the fetus (*see* presentation) is other than the head.

malt (mawlt) *n*. a mixture of carbohydrates, predominantly maltose, produced by the breakdown of starch contained in barley or wheat grains. Malt is used for brewing and distilling; it has been used as a source of nutrients in wasting diseases.

Malta fever (mawl-tă) *n*. *see* brucellosis.

maltase (mawl-tayz) *n*. an enzyme, present in saliva and pancreatic juice, that converts maltose into glucose during digestion.

maltose (mawl-tohz) *n*. a sugar consisting of two molecules of glucose. Maltose is formed from the digestion of starch and glycogen.

malt-worker's lung *n*. a form of extrinsic allergic alveolitis seen in people who work with barley.

malunion (mal-yoon-yŏn) *n*. union of a fracture in an abnormal position. Osteotomy may be needed to correct the deformity.

mamilla (mă-mil-ă) *n*. *see* nipple.

mamma (mam-ă) *n*. *see* breast.

mammary gland (mam-er-i) *n*. the milk-producing gland of female mammals. *See* breast.

mammography (mam-og-răfi) *n*. X-ray examination of the female breast: used particularly to enable the early diagnosis of breast cancer. *See also* Forrest screening.

mammoplasty (mam-ŏ-plasti) *n*. plastic surgery of the breasts, in order to alter their shape or increase or decrease their size.

mammothermography (mam-oh-ther-**mog**-răfi) n. the technique of examining the breasts for the presence of abnormalities by thermography.

Manchester operation (man-ches-ter) n. see Donald-Fothergill operation.

mandible (man-dib-ŭl) n. the lower jawbone. It consists of a horseshoe-shaped body, the upper surface of which bears the lower teeth, and two vertical parts (rami). See also temporomandibular joint. —**mandibular** (man-dib-yoo-ler) adj.

mandibular advancement splint (MAS) n. an orthodontic device used to advance the mandible to improve the airway in the pharynx during sleep in the treatment of obstructive sleep apnoea.

manganese (mang-ă-neez) n. a greyish metallic element, the oxide of which, when inhaled by miners in underventilated mines, causes brain damage. It is a trace element. Symbol: Mn.

mania (may-niă) n. a state of mind characterized by excessive cheerfulness and increased activity. The mood is euphoric and changes rapidly to irritability. Thought and speech are rapid to the point of incoherence and the connections between ideas may be impossible to follow. Treatment is usually with drugs such as lithium or phenothiazines. See affective disorder, manic-depressive psychosis. —**manic** (man-ik) adj.

-mania suffix denoting obsession, compulsion, or exaggerated feeling for.

manic-depressive psychosis

(bipolar disorder) (man-ik-di-**pres**-iv) n. a severe mental illness that causes repeated episodes of depression, mania, or both. Treatment is with phenothiazine drugs for mania and with antidepressant drugs or electroconvulsive therapy for depression. Lithium and carbamazepine can prevent or reduce the frequency and severity of attacks, and the sufferer is usually well in the intervals between them.

manipulation (mă-nip-yoo-lay-shŏn) n. the use of the hands to produce a desired movement or therapeutic effect in part of the body.

mannitol (man-i-tol) n. a diuretic administered by intravenous infusion to supplement other diuretics in the treatment of fluid retention (oedema), to relieve pressure in brain injuries, and in the emergency treatment of glaucoma.

manometer (mă-nom-it-er) n. a device for measuring pressure in a liquid or gas. See also sphygmomanometer.

manometry (mă-nom-itri) n. measurement of pressures within organs of the body. The technique is used to record changes within fluid-filled chambers (e g, cerebral ventricles) or to indicate muscular activity in motile tubes, such as the oesophagus, rectum, or bile duct.

mantle (man-t'l) adj. (in radiotherapy) see treatment field.

Mantoux test (man-too) n. a test for immunity to tuberculosis. Tuberculin is injected beneath the skin and a patch of inflammation appearing in the next 48–72 hours indicates that a degree of immunity is present. [C. Mantoux (1877–1947), French physician]

manubrium (mă-**new**-bri-ŭm) *n.* (*pl.* **manubria**) **1.** the upper section of the breastbone (*see* sternum). It articulates with the clavicles and the first costal cartilage. **2.** the handle-like part of the malleus, attached to the eardrum. —**manubrial** *adj.*

MAO *n. see* monoamine oxidase.

MAO inhibitor (MAOI) *n.* any drug, such as phenelzine, that prevents the activity of the enzyme monoamine oxidase (MAO) in brain tissue and therefore affects mood. MAO inhibitors are antidepressants; their side-effects include interactions with other drugs and foods containing tyramine (e.g. cheese) to produce a sudden increase in blood pressure. *See also* moclobemide, selegiline.

maple syrup urine disease (aminoacidopathy) (may-pŭl si-rŭp) *n.* an inborn defect of amino acid metabolism causing an excess of valine, leucine, isoleucine, and alloisoleucine in the urine, which has an odour like maple syrup. Treatment is dietary; if untreated, the condition leads to mental retardation and death in infancy.

maprotiline (mă-**proh**-til-een) *n.* a drug administered by mouth to treat all types of depression, including that associated with anxiety (*see* antidepressant). It is administered by mouth and may cause drowsiness, dizziness, and tremor. Trade name: **Ludiomil**.

marasmus (mă-**raz**-mŭs) *n.* mixed deficiency of both protein and calories, resulting in severe wasting in infants. Body weight is below 60% of that expected for age; the infant looks 'old', has thin sparse hair, is pallid and apathetic, lacks skin fat,

and has subnormal temperature. The condition may be due to malabsorption, wrong feeding, metabolic disorders, repeated vomiting, diarrhoea, or disease.

marble-bone disease (mar-bŭl bohn) *n. see* osteopetrosis.

Marburg disease (green monkey disease) (mar-berg) *n.* a virus disease of vervet (green) monkeys transmitted to humans by contact with blood or tissues from an infected animal. Symptoms include fever, malaise, severe headache, vomiting, diarrhoea, and bleeding from mucous membranes. Treatment with antiserum and measures to reduce the bleeding are sometimes effective.

Marcus Gunn jaw-winking syndrome (mar-kŭs gun) *n.* a congenital condition characterized by drooping (ptosis) of one eyelid. On opening or moving the mouth, the droopy lid elevates momentarily, resembling a wink. [R. Marcus Gunn (1850–1909), British ophthalmologist]

Marfan's syndrome (mar-**fahnz**) *n.* an inherited disorder of connective tissue characterized by excessive height, abnormally long and slender fingers and toes (*arachnodactyly*), heart defects, and partial dislocation of the lenses of the eyes. [B. J. A. Marfan (1858–1942), French physician]

marijuana (ma-ri-**hwah**-nă) *n. see* cannabis.

Marion's disease (ma-ri-ŏnz) *n.* obstruction of the outlet of the bladder caused by enlargement of the muscle cells in the neck of the bladder. [J. B. C. G. Marion (1869–1960), French surgeon]

mastoid

Marjolin's ulcer (mar-*zhoh*-lanz) *n.* a carcinoma that develops at the edge of a chronic ulcer of the skin, usually a venous ulcer in the ankle region. [J. N. Marjolin (1780–1850), French surgeon]

marrow (**ma**-roh) *n. see* bone marrow.

marsupialization (mar-soo-piăl-Izay-shŏn) *n.* an operative technique for curing a cyst. The cyst is opened, its contents removed, and the edges then stitched to the skin incision.

MAS *n. see* mandibular advancement splint.

masculinization (mas-kew-lin-Izay-shŏn) *n.* development of excess body and facial hair, deepening of the voice, and increase in muscle bulk in a female due to a hormone disorder or to hormone therapy. *See also* virilism, virilization.

Maslow's hierarchy of human needs (**maz**-lohz) *n.* a listing of human needs in order of priority, from basic physiological needs (e.g. eating and drinking) to self-actualization. It is held that the individual does not consider meeting each level of need until the previous level has been at least partly satisfied. *See* self-actualization. [A. H. Maslow (1908–70), US psychologist]

masochism (mas-ŏ-kizm) *n.* sexual pleasure derived from the experience of pain. *See* sexual deviation. —**masochist** *n.* —**masochistic** *adj.*

massage (mas-**ahzh**) *n.* manipulation of the soft tissues of the body with the hands. Massage is used to improve circulation, prevent adhesions in tissues after injury, and reduce muscular spasm. *See also* effleurage, petrissage, tapotement.

masseter (ma-**see**-ter) *n.* a thick muscle in the cheek extending from the zygomatic arch to the outer corner of the mandible. It is important for mastication and acts by closing the jaws.

mast- (**masto-**) *prefix denoting* the breast.

mastalgia (mas-**tal**-jiă) *n.* pain in the breast.

mastatrophy (**mastatrophia**) (mas-**tat**-rŏfi) *n.* atrophy of the breasts.

mast cell (mahst) *n.* a large cell in connective tissue. Mast cells contain heparin, histamine, and serotonin, which are released during inflammation and allergic responses.

mastectomy (mas-**tek**-tŏmi) *n.* surgical removal of a breast. *radical m.* surgical removal of the breast with the skin and all the lymphatic tissue of the armpit. In modern surgical practice the underlying pectoral muscles are usually preserved. It is performed when breast cancer has spread to involve the lymph nodes. *simple m.* surgical removal of the breast retaining the skin and, if possible, the nipple. It is performed for extensive but not necessarily invasive tumours. *See also* lumpectomy.

mastication (mas-ti-**kay**-shŏn) *n.* the process of chewing food.

mastitis (mas-**ty**-tis) *n.* inflammation of the breast, usually caused by bacterial infection via damaged nipples. *cystic m.* chronic mastitis in which the breast feels lumpy due to the presence of cysts. *puerperal m.* acute mastitis that develops during the period of breast-feeding.

mastoid (**mas**-toid) *adj.* relating to the mastoid process. *m. antrum* an air-filled channel connecting the mastoid process to the cavity of the middle ear. *m. cells* air spaces in the mastoid process. *m. process* a nipple-shaped process on the temporal bone that extends downward and forward behind the ear canal.

mastoidectomy (mas-toi-dek-tŏmi) *n.* an operation to remove some or all of the mastoid cells when they have become infected (*see* mastoiditis) or invaded by cholesteatoma.

mastoiditis (mas-toi-dy-tis) *n.* inflammation of the mastoid process and antrum, usually caused by bacterial infection that spreads from the middle ear. *See* otitis (media).

masturbation (mas-ter-bay-shŏn) *n.* physical self-stimulation of the male or female external genital organs in order to produce sexual pleasure, which may result in orgasm.

materia medica (mă-teer-iă medik-ă) *n.* the study of drugs used in medicine and dentistry, including pharmacognosy, pharmacy, pharmacology, and therapeutics.

maternal deprivation (mă-ter-năl) *n.* the condition said to result if infants are deprived of the opportunity to form a close relationship with a single parental figure, who may or may not be the child's natural parent. It is characterized by distress and depression, leading to an inability to form lasting relationships.

maternal mortality rate *n.* the number of deaths due to complications of pregnancy, childbirth, and the puerperium expressed as a proportion of all births (i.e. including

stillbirths). The rate is usually expressed per 100,000 births.

matrix (may-triks) *n.* the substance of a tissue or organ in which more specialized structures are embedded.

mattress suture (mat-ris) *n.* a suture in which a loop is made on each side of the incision, which may be parallel with the incision (*horizontal m. s.*) or at right angles to it (*vertical m. s.*).

maturation (mat-yoor-ay-shŏn) *n.* the process of attaining full development.

maturity-onset diabetes of the young (MODY) (mă-tyoor-iti-on-set) *n. see* diabetes.

maxilla (maks-il-ă) *n.* (*pl.* maxillae) **1.** (loosely) the upper jaw. **2.** either of the pair of bones contributing to the upper jaw, the orbits, the nasal cavity, and the roof of the mouth (*see* palate). —**maxillary** (maks-il-er-i) *adj.*

maxillary sinus (maxillary antrum) *n. see* paranasal sinuses.

maxillofacial (maks-iloh-fay-shăl) *adj.* describing or relating to the region of the face, jaws, and related structures.

maximum breathing capacity (MBC) (maks-i-mǔm) *n.* the volume of gas exchanged per minute when breathing at maximum rate and depth.

MBC *n. see* maximum breathing capacity.

McArdle's disease (măk-ar-d'lz) *n.* an inborn error of metabolism in which a deficiency of the enzyme myophosphorylase prevents the breakdown of glycogen to lactate in exercising muscle. This results in fatigue, pain, and cramps in exer-

meconium

cising muscles. [B. McArdle (20th century), British biochemist]

McBurney's point (măk-ber-niz) *n.* the point on the abdomen that overlies the anatomical position of the appendix and is the site of maximum tenderness in acute appendicitis. [C. McBurney (1845–1913), US surgeon]

McGill Pain Questionnaire (MPQ) (mă-gil) *n.* an assessment tool that combines a list of questions about the nature and frequency of pain with a body-map diagram to pinpoint its location.

MCU *n.* see micturating cystourethrogram.

ME *n.* myalgic encephalomyelitis. See CFS/ME.

mean (arithmetic mean) (meen) *n.* the average of a group of observations calculated by adding their values and dividing by the number in the group.

measles (mee-zŭlz) *n.* a highly infectious virus disease that mainly affects children. Early symptoms are those of a cold accompanied by a high fever, and Koplik's spots may appear on the inside of the cheeks. On the third to fifth day a blotchy slightly elevated pink rash develops; it lasts 3–5 days. The patient is infectious throughout this period. In most cases the symptoms soon subside but patients are susceptible to pneumonia and middle ear infections. Medical names: **rubeola**, **morbilli**.

meat- (meato-) *prefix denoting* a meatus.

meatus (mee-ay-tŭs) *n.* (in anatomy) a passage or opening. *external auditory m.* the auditory canal: the passage leading from the

pinna of the outer ear to the eardrum. *nasal m.* one of three groovelike parts of the nasal cavity beneath each of the nasal conchae. *urethral m.* the external opening of the urethra.

mebendazole (mi-ben-dă-zohl) *n.* an anthelmintic drug used to get rid of roundworms, hookworms, threadworms, and whipworms. Trade name: **Vermox**. See also imidazole.

mechanism of labour (mek-ă-nizm) *n.* the sum of the forces that act to expel a fetus from the uterus together with those that resist its expulsion and affect its position during birth. See labour.

mechanotherapy (mek-ă-nohth'e-ră-pi) *n.* the use of mechanical equipment during physiotherapy to produce regularly repeated movements in part of the body.

Meckel's diverticulum (mek-ĕlz) *n.* see diverticulum. [J. F. Meckel (1781–1833), German anatomist]

meclozine (mek-lŏ-zeen) *n.* an antihistamine drug administered by mouth to prevent and treat nausea and vomiting, particularly in motion sickness, and also to relieve allergic reactions.

meconism (mek-oh-nizm) *n.* poisoning from the effects of eating or smoking opium or the products derived from it, especially morphine.

meconium (mi-koh-niŭm) *n.* the first stools of a newborn baby, which are sticky and dark green and composed of cellular debris, mucus, and bile pigments. *m. aspiration* a condition in which a baby inhales meconium into the lungs during delivery, which can cause plugs in the airway; the baby may become hypoxic. *m. ileus* obstruction of the ileum caused by thickened meconium in babies with cystic fibrosis.

media (tunica media) (meed-iă) *n.* **1.** the middle layer of the wall of a vein or artery. **2.** the middle layer of various other organs or parts.

medial (mee-di-ăl) *adj.* relating to or situated in the central region of an organ, tissue, or the body.

median (mee-di-ăn) *adj.* (in anatomy) situated in or towards the plane that divides the body into right and left halves.

mediastinitis (mee-di-asti-ny-tis) *n.* inflammation of the mediastinum, usually complicating a rupture of the oesophagus (gullet).

mediastinoscopy (mee-di-astinos-kŏpi) *n.* examination of the mediastinum, usually by means of an endoscope inserted through a small incision in the neck region. It can be used to assess the spread of intrathoracic tumours and for lymph node biopsy.

mediastinum (mee-di-ă-sty-nŭm) *n.* the space in the thorax between the two pleural sacs. The mediastinum contains the heart, aorta, trachea, oesophagus, and thymus gland.

medical (med-ik-ăl) *adj.* **1.** of or relating to the science or practice of medicine. **2.** of or relating to conditions that require the attention of a physician rather than a surgeon.

medical assistant *n.* a health service worker who is not a registered medical practitioner (often a nurse or an ex-serviceman with experience as a senior medical orderly) working in association with a doc-

tor to undertake minor treatments and preliminary assessments.

medical certificate *n.* a certificate stating a doctor's diagnosis of a patient's medical condition, disability, or fitness to work.

medical emergency team *n.* a designated team of doctors and senior nurses who attend to deteriorating patients in hospitals with the aim of preventing cardiac arrest or further deterioration. They also assess seriously ill patients with a view to admitting them to intensive care, high dependency, or coronary care units.

medical jurisprudence *n.* the study or practice of the legal aspects of medicine. *See* forensic medicine.

medical social worker *n.* a social worker employed to assist patients with domestic problems that may arise through illness.

medicated (med-i-kayt-id) *adj.* containing a medicinal drug: applied to lotions, soaps, sweets, etc.

medication (med-i-kay-shŏn) *n.* **1.** a substance administered by mouth, applied to the body, or introduced into the body for the purpose of treatment. *See also* premedication. **2.** treatment of a patient using drugs.

medicine (med-sin) *n.* **1.** the science or practice of the diagnosis, treatment, and prevention of disease. **2.** the science or practice of nonsurgical methods of treating disease. **3.** any drug or preparation used for the treatment or prevention of disease, particularly a preparation that is taken by mouth.

medicochirurgical (med-i-koh-kyr-rer-jik-ăl) *adj.* of or describing matters that are related to both medicine and surgery.

medicolegal (med-i-koh-**lee**-găl) *adj.* relating to the legal aspects of the practice of medicine.

Mediterranean fever (med-it-er-ay-ni-ăn) *n.* **1.** *see* brucellosis. **2.** *see* polyserositis.

medium (**meed**-iŭm) *n.* **1.** any substance, usually a broth, agar, or gelatin, used for the culture of microorganisms or tissue cells. **2.** *see* contrast medium.

medroxyprogesterone (med-roks-i-proh-**jes**-ter-ohn) *n.* a synthetic female sex hormone (*see* progestogen) administered by mouth or injection to treat menstrual disorders and certain cancers and in hormone replacement therapy. It is also given by depot injection as a long-term contraceptive. Trade names: **Depo-Provera, Farlutal, Provera.**

medulla (mi-**dul**-ă) *n.* **1.** the inner region of any organ or tissue, particularly the inner part of the kidney, adrenal glands, or lymph nodes. *m. oblongata* (*myelencephalon*) the extension within the skull of the upper end of the spinal cord, containing centres responsible for the regulation of the heart and blood vessels, respiration, salivation, and swallowing. **2.** the myelin layer of certain nerve fibres. —**medullary** *adj.*

medullated nerve fibre (myelinated nerve fibre) (med-ŭl-ayt-id) *n. see* myelin.

medulloblastoma (mi-dul-oh-blas-**toh**-mă) *n.* a malignant brain tumour that occurs during childhood and develops in the cerebellum. Symptoms include headaches,

dizziness, and unsteadiness; the flow of cerebrospinal fluid may become obstructed, causing hydrocephalus. Treatment involves surgery followed by radiotherapy.

mefenamic acid (me-fen-**am**-ik) *n.* an anti-inflammatory drug (*see* NSAID) administered by mouth to treat headache, toothache, rheumatic pain, and similar conditions. Trade name: **Ponstan.**

mefloquine (**mef**-loh-kween) *n.* a drug used in the prevention and treatment of malaria that is resistant to other drugs. It is administered by mouth but should not be taken during pregnancy, by psychiatric patients, or with beta blockers. Trade name: **Lariam.**

mega- *prefix denoting* **1.** large size or abnormal enlargement or distension. **2.** a million.

megacolon (meg-ă-koh-lŏn) *n.* dilatation, and sometimes lengthening, of the colon. It is caused by obstruction of the colon, Hirschsprung's disease, or longstanding constipation.

megakaryocyte (meg-ă-**ka**-ri-oh-syt) *n.* a cell in the bone marrow that produces platelets. *See also* thrombopoiesis.

megal- (megalo-) *prefix denoting* abnormal enlargement.

megaloblast (**meg**-ă-loh-blast) *n.* an abnormal form of erythroblast. Megaloblasts are unusually large and their nuclei fail to mature in the normal way; they are seen in the bone marrow in certain anaemias (*megaloblastic anaemias*) due to deficiency of vitamin B_{12} or folic acid. —**megaloblastic** *adj.*

megalocephaly (meg-ă-loh-**sef**-ăli) *n.* **1.** *see* macrocephaly. **2.** overgrowth and distortion of the skull bones (see leontiasis).

megalocyte (meg-ă-loh-syt) n. see macrocyte.

megalomania (meg-ă-loh-**may**-niă) n. delusions of grandeur. It may be a feature of a schizophrenic or manic illness or of cerebral syphilis.

-megaly suffix denoting abnormal enlargement.

megaureter (meg-ă-yoor-ee-ter) n. gross dilatation of the ureter. This occurs above the site of a long-standing obstruction in the ureter, which blocks the free flow of urine from the kidney.

megestrol (mi-jes-trohl) n. a synthetic female sex hormone (see progestogen) that is used in the treatment of metastatic breast cancer and metastatic endometrial cancer. Trade name: **Megace**.

meglitinides (meg-lit-in-ydz) pl. n. see oral hypoglycaemic drug.

megophthalmia (meg-off-thal-miă) n. an abnormally large eyeball.

meibomian cyst (my-boh-mi-ăn) n. see chalazion. [H. Meibom (1638–1700), German anatomist]

meibomian glands (tarsal glands) pl. n. small sebaceous glands that lie under the conjunctiva of the eyelids.

meibomianitis (my-boh-mi-ăn-I-tis) n. inflammation of the meibomian glands of the eyelids.

Meigs' syndrome (mIgz) n. the rare combination of a benign ovarian fibroma with ascites and a right-sided pleural effusion. [J. V. Meigs (1892–1963), US gynaecologist]

meiosis (reduction division) (my-oh-sis) n. a type of cell division that produces four daughter cells, each having half the number of

chromosomes of the original cell. It occurs before the formation of sperm and ova and the normal (diploid) number of chromosomes is restored after fertilization. Compare mitosis. —**meiotic** (my-ot-ik) adj.

Meissner's plexus (submucous plexus) (my-snerz) n. a fine network of parasympathetic nerve fibres in the wall of the alimentary canal, supplying the muscles and mucous membrane. [G. Meissner (1829–1905), German physiologist]

melaena (mi-lee-nă) n. black tarry faeces due to the presence of partly digested blood from higher up the digestive tract. It often occurs after vomiting blood (see haematemesis), having the same causes, but may be due to disease in the small intestine or upper colon, such as carcinoma or angiodysplasia. See also haemorrhagic disease of the newborn.

melan- (melano-) prefix denoting 1. black coloration. 2. melanin.

melancholia (mel-ăn-koh-liă) n. see depression, involutional melancholia.

melanin (mel-ă-nin) n. a dark-brown to black pigment occurring in the hair, the skin, and in the iris and choroid layer of the eyes.

melanism (melanosis) (mel-ăn-izm) n. an unusually pronounced darkening of body tissues caused by excessive production of the pigment melanin. Melanism may affect the skin after sunburn, during pregnancy, or in Addison's disease.

melanocyte (mel-ă-noh-syt) n. a cell within the epidermis of skin that produces melanin.

melanocyte-stimulating hormone (MSH) n. a hormone synthesized and released by the pituitary gland. In amphibians MSH brings about colour changes in the skin but its physiological role in humans is uncertain.

melanoma (malignant melanoma) (mel-ă-noh-mă) n. a highly malignant tumour of melanocytes. Such tumours usually occur in the skin (excessive exposure to sunlight is a contributory factor) but are also found in the eye and the mucous membranes. They may contain melanin or be free of the pigment (*amelanotic m.*). Superficial melanomas can often be successfully treated by surgical excision.

melanophore (mel-ă-noh-for) n. a cell that contains melanin.

melanoplakia (mel-ă-noh-play-kiă) n. pigmented areas of melanin in the mucous membrane lining the inside of the cheeks.

melanosis (mel-ă-noh-sis) n. **1.** see melanism. **2.** a disorder in the body's production of the pigment melanin. **3.** cachexia associated with the spread of the skin cancer melanoma. —**melanotic** adj.

melanuria (mel-ăn-yoor-iă) n. the presence of dark pigment in the urine. This may occur in some cases of melanoma; it may alternatively be caused by metabolic disease, such as porphyria.

melasma (mi-laz-mă) n. see chloasma.

melatonin (mel-ă-toh-nin) n. a hormone produced by the pineal gland in darkness but not in bright light. Melatonin is a derivative of serotonin, with which it works to regulate the sleep cycle.

melioidosis (mee-li-oi-doh-sis) n. a disease of wild rodents caused by the bacterium *Pseudomonas pseudo-*

mallei. It can be transmitted to humans, causing pneumonia, multiple abscesses, and septicaemia.

melphalan (mel-fă-lan) n. a drug administered by mouth or injection to treat various types of cancer, particularly myeloma but also including tumours of the breast and ovaries and Hodgkin's disease. Trade name: **Alkeran**.

membrane (mem-brayn) n. **1.** a thin layer of tissue surrounding an organ or tissue, lining a cavity, or separating adjacent structures or cavities. *See also* basement membrane, mucous membrane, serous membrane. **2.** the lipoprotein envelope surrounding a cell (*cell m.*). —**membranous** (mem-brăn-ŭs) adj.

membranous labyrinth n. see labyrinth.

men- (meno-) prefix denoting menstruation.

menarche (men-ar-ki) n. the start of the menstrual periods and other physical and mental changes associated with puberty. The menarche occurs when the reproductive organs become functionally active and may take place at any time between 10 and 19 years of age. *Compare* gonadarche.

Mendel's laws (men-d'lz) pl. n. rules of inheritance based on the breeding experiments of Gregor Mendel, which showed that the inheritance of characteristics is controlled by particles now known as genes. In modern terms they are as follows. (1) Each somatic cell of an individual carries two factors (genes) for every characteristic and each gamete carries only one. (2) Each pair of factors segregates independently of all other pairs at meiosis, so that the gametes show all possible combinations of factors. *See also* dominant, recessive. [G. J. Mendel (1822–84), Austrian monk]

Mendelson's syndrome (men-d'l-sŏnz) *n.* inhalation of regurgitated stomach contents by an anaesthetized patient, which may result in death from anoxia or cause extensive lung damage or pulmonary oedema with severe bronchospasm. It may be prevented by giving gastric-acid inhibitors (e.g. cimetidine, ranitidine) or sodium citrate before inducing anaesthesia. [C. L. Mendelson (1913–), US obstetrician]

Ménétrier's disease (may-nay-tri-ayz) *n.* a disorder in which gross enlargement (*see* hypertrophy) of the cells of the mucous membrane lining the stomach is associated with anaemia. [P. Ménétrier (1859–1935), French physician]

menidrosis (menhidrosis) (men-id-**roh**-sis) *n.* the production of sweat, sometimes containing blood, instead of the normal menstrual flow.

Ménière's disease (mayn-**yairz**) *n.* a disease of the inner ear characterized by episodes of deafness, buzzing in the ears (tinnitus), and vertigo. Symptoms last for several hours and between attacks the affected ear may return to normal. It is thought to be caused by the buildup of fluid in the inner ear and is treated by drugs or surgery. Medical name: **endolymphatic hydrops**. [P. Ménière (1799–1862), French physician]

mening- (meningo-) *prefix denoting* the meninges.

meninges (min-**in**-jeez) *pl. n.* (*sing.*

meninx) the three connective tissue membranes that line the skull and vertebral canal and enclose the brain and spinal cord: the dura mater, arachnoid mater, and pia mater. —**meningeal** *adj.*

meningioma (min-in-ji-**oh**-mă) *n.* a tumour arising from the meninges. It is usually slow-growing and produces symptoms by pressure on the underlying nervous tissue. Some meningiomas may behave in a malignant fashion and invade neighbouring tissues. Treatment of the majority of cases is by surgical removal if the tumour is accessible.

meningism (men-in-jizm) *n.* stiffness of the neck that is found in meningitis.

meningitis (men-in-**jy**-tis) *n.* an inflammation of the meninges due to viral, bacterial, or fungal infection. Meningitis causes an intense headache, fever, loss of appetite, intolerance to light and sound, rigidity of muscles, especially those in the neck (*see also* Kernig's sign), and in severe cases convulsions, vomiting, and delirium leading to death. Bacterial meningitis can be effectively treated with large doses of antibiotics administered as soon as possible after diagnosis. *See also* Hib vaccine, meningitis C vaccine. *meningococcal m.* a serious form of bacterial meningitis, caused by the meningococcus (most importantly, strains B and C), that can lead to widespread infection and *meningococcal septicaemia. pneumococcal m.* a form of bacterial meningitis caused by the pneumococcus.

meningitis C vaccine *n.* a vaccine that provides protection against the C strain of the bacterium *Neisseria meningitidis* (the meningococcus), which accounts for approximately 50% of all cases of meningococcal meningitis and tends to occur in clusters. The immunization is given to all babies with their primary immunizations at two, three, and four months (see Appendix 8). It can also be given as a single vaccine and is currently offered to everyone under the age of 24.

meningocele (min-ing-oh-seel) *n.* protrusion of the meninges through a gap in the spine. *See* neural tube defects.

meningococcus (min-ing-oh-kok-ŭs) *n.* (*pl.* **meningococci**) the bacterium *Neisseria meningitidis*, which can cause a serious form of septicaemia and is a common cause of meningitis. — **meningococcal** *adj.*

meningoencephalitis (min-ing-oh-en-sef-ă-ly-tis) *n.* inflammation of the brain and the meninges caused by bacterial, viral, or fungal infection.

meningoencephalocele (min-ing-oh-en-sef-ă-loh-seel) *n.* protrusion of the meninges and brain through a defect in the skull. *See* neural tube defects.

meningomyelocele (myelocele, myelomeningocele) (min-ing-oh-my-ĕ-loh-seel) *n.* protrusion of the meninges, spinal cord, and nerve roots through a gap in the spine, accompanied by paralysis of the legs and urinary incontinence. *See* neural tube defects.

meningovascular (min-ing-oh-vas-kew-ler) *adj.* relating to or affecting the meninges and the blood vessels that penetrate them to supply the underlying neural tissues.

meniscectomy (men-i-sek-tŏmi) *n.* surgical removal of a cartilage (meniscus) in the knee. This is carried out when the meniscus has been torn or is diseased. The operation can now be performed through an arthroscope.

meniscus (min-isk-ŭs) *n.* (in anatomy) a crescent-shaped structure, such as the fibrocartilaginous disc that divides the cavity of a synovial joint.

Menkes kinky-hair disease (men-kis) *n.* a genetic disorder characterized by severe mental retardation, seizures, poor vision, colourless fragile hair, and chubby red cheeks. Affected infants usually die before the age of three. [J. H. Menkes (1928–), US neurologist]

menopause (climacteric) (men-ŏ-pawz) *n.* the time in a woman's life when ovulation and menstruation cease and the woman is no longer able to bear children. The menopause can occur at any age between the middle thirties and the middle fifties, but occurs most commonly between 45 and 55; it can only be established in retrospect after 12 consecutive months of amenorrhoea. It is associated with a change in the balance of sex hormones in the body, which sometimes leads to hot flushes and other vasomotor symptoms, palpitations, and emotional disturbances. — **menopausal** *adj.*

menorrhagia (epimenorrhagia) (men-ŏ-ray-jiă) *n.* abnormally heavy bleeding at menstruation. Menorrhagia may be associated with hormonal imbalance (in which case it is described as *dysfunctional uterine bleeding*), pelvic inflammatory disease, tumours (especially fibroids in the pelvic cavity, endometriosis, or the presence of an IUCD.

MENS *pl. n.* multiple endocrine neoplasia syndromes, which involve tumour formation or hyperplasia in various combinations of endocrine glands. Type 1 (*Wermer's syndrome*) involves the parathyroid, pituitary, and pancreas, whereas type 2A (*Sipple's syndrome*) involves the thyroid medullary cells, the adrenal medulla (phaeochromocytoma), and the parathyroids. Type 2B is similar to 2A, but patients tend to resemble people with Marfan's syndrome and have multiple neuromas on their mucous membranes.

menses (men-seez) *n.* **1.** the blood and other materials discharged from the uterus at menstruation. **2.** *see* menstruation.

menstrual cycle (men-stroo-ǎl) *n.* the periodic sequence of events in sexually mature nonpregnant women by which an egg cell (ovum) is released from a follicle in the ovary at four-weekly intervals until the menopause (see illustration). The secretion of progesterone in the ruptured follicle causes the lining of the uterus (endometrium) to become thicker and richly supplied with blood in preparation for pregnancy. If the ovum is not fertilized the endometrium is shed at menstruation.

menstruation (menses) (menstroo-ay-shŏn) *n.* the discharge of blood and fragments of endometrium from the vagina at intervals of about four weeks in women of child-bearing age (*see* menarche, menopause). The normal duration of discharge varies from three to seven days. *anovular m.* discharge that takes place without previous release of an egg cell from the ovary. *vicarious m.* bleeding from a mucous membrane other than the endometrium when normal menstruation is due. *See also* amenor-

The menstrual cycle

rhoea, dysmenorrhoea, epimenorrhoea, hypomenorrhoea, menorrhagia, oligomenorrhoea.

mental¹ (men-t'l) *adj.* relating to or affecting the mind.

mental² *adj.* relating to the chin.

mental age *n.* a measure of the intellectual level at which an individual functions; for example, someone described as having a mental age of 6 years would be functioning at the level of an average 6-year-old child. *See also* intelligence quotient, intelligence test.

mental handicap *n.* delayed or incomplete intellectual development combined with some form of social malfunction, such as educational or occupational failure or inability to look after oneself. Good education alters the course of the handicap, for which the term *learning disability* (*or difficulty*) is often used.

Mental Health Acts *pl. n.* the Acts of Parliament governing the care of the mentally disordered They provide for compulsory admission when the mentally disordered put themselves or other people into danger, protection of the civil rights of patients, and for the *Mental Health Act Commission* to regulate aspects of the practice of psychiatry.

Mental Health Review Tribunal *n.* one of a number of tribunals, established under the Mental Health Act 1959 and now operating under the Mental Health Act 1983, to which applications may be made for the discharge from hospital of a person compulsorily detained there under provisions of the Act (*see* compulsory admission).

mental illness *n.* a disorder of one

or more of the functions of the mind, which causes suffering to the patient or others. Mental illness is broadly divided into psychosis, in which the capacity for appreciating reality is lost, and neurosis, in which insight is retained.

mental impairment *n.* (mostly in legal usage) the condition of significant or severe impairment of intellectual and social functioning associated with abnormally aggressive or seriously irresponsible behaviour.

mental retardation *n.* the state of those whose intellectual powers have failed to develop to such an extent that they are in need of care and protection and require special education. There are very many causes of mental retardation, including Down's syndrome, fragile-X syndrome, inherited metabolic disorders, brain injury, and gross psychological deprivation; some are preventable or treatable. *See also* mental handicap.

menthol (men-thol) *n.* a compound extracted from peppermint oil, used in inhalants to relieve cold symptoms, in ointments and liniments, and to relieve itching. Formula: $C_{10}H_{20}O$.

mento- *prefix denoting* the chin.

mentor (men-tor) *n.* a person with the experience and knowledge to fulfil the role of a trusted friend and adviser. The mentor guides, counsels, and supports a student or junior in a clinical or educational area. This role can be formal or informal.

mentum (men-tŭm) *n.* the chin.

mepacrine (mep-ă-kreen) *n.* a drug administered by mouth to treat various infestations, particularly giardiasis.

meprobamate (mi-proh-bă-mayt) *n.* a drug administered by mouth or injection to relieve anxiety and nervous tension (*see* anxiolytic).

meralgia paraesthetica (mi-ral-jiă pa-ris-thet-ik-ă) *n.* painful tingling and numbness felt over the outer surface of the thigh when the lateral cutaneous nerve is trapped as it passes through the muscular tissues of the groin.

mercaptopurine (mer-kap-tŏ-pewr-een) *n.* a drug that prevents the growth of cancer cells and is administered by mouth, chiefly in the treatment of some types of leukaemia (*see* antimetabolite). Trade name: **Puri-Nethol**.

mercurialism (hydrargyria) (mer-kewr-iă-lizm) *n.* mercury poisoning. Acute poisoning causes vomiting, diarrhoea, and kidney damage. Treatment is with dimercaprol. Chronic poisoning causes mouth ulceration, loose teeth, and intestinal and renal disturbances. Treatment is removing the patient from further exposure.

mercury (mer-kewr-i) *n.* a silvery metallic element that is liquid at room temperature. Its toxicity has caused a decline in the use of its compounds in medicine. The main use of mercury today is as a component of amalgam fillings in dentistry. Symbol: Hg. *See also* mercurialism, pink disease.

mes- (meso-) *prefix denoting* middle or medial.

mesaortitis (mes-ay-or-ty-tis) *n.* inflammation of the middle layer (media) of the wall of the aorta, generally the result of late syphilis.

mesarteritis (mes-ar-ter-I-tis) *n.* inflammation of the middle layer (media) of an artery, which is often combined with inflammation in all layers of the artery wall.

mescaline (mesk-ă-leen) *n.* an alkaloid present in the dried tops of the cactus *Lophophora williamsii* that produces inebriation and hallucinations when ingested.

mesencephalon (mes-en-sef-ă-lon) *n. see* midbrain.

mesentery (mes-ĕn-ter-i) *n.* a double layer of peritoneum attaching the stomach, small intestine, pancreas, spleen, and other abdominal organs to the posterior wall of the abdomen. —**mesenteric** (mes-ĕn-te-rik) *adj.*

mesial (mee-zi-ăl) *adj.* **1.** medial. **2.** relating to or situated in the median line or plane. **3.** designating the surface of a tooth towards the midline of the jaw.

mesmerism (mez-mer-izm) *n.* hypnosis based on the ideas of Franz Mesmer, sometimes employing magnets and a variety of other equipment. [F. A. Mesmer (1734–1815), Austrian physician]

mesna (mez-nă) *n.* a drug administered intravenously by injection or infusion to prevent the toxic effect of ifosfamide and cyclophosphamide on the bladder. It binds with the toxic metabolite acrolein in the urine.

mesoappendix (mes-oh-ă-pen-diks) *n.* the mesentery of the appendix.

mesocolon (mes-oh-koh-lon) *n.* the fold of peritoneum by which the colon is fixed to the posterior abdominal wall.

mesoderm (mes-oh-derm) *n.* the

middle germ layer of the early embryo. It gives rise to cartilage, muscle, bone, blood, kidneys, gonads and their ducts, and connective tissue. —**mesodermal** *adj.*

mesometrium (mes-oh-mee-tri-ŭm) *n.* the broad ligament of the uterus: a sheet of connective tissue that carries blood vessels to the uterus and attaches it to the abdominal wall.

mesomorphic (mes-oh-mor-fik) *adj.* describing a body type characterized by a well developed skeletal and muscular structure and a sturdy upright posture. —**mesomorph** *n.* —**mesomorphy** *n.*

mesonephros (Wolffian body) (mes-oh-nef-ross) *n.* kidney tissue that is functional only in the embryo. Its duct – the *mesonephric* (or *Wolffian*) *duct* – persists in males as the epididymis and vas deferens. —**mesonephric** *adj.*

mesosalpinx (mes-oh-sal-pinks) *n.* a fold of peritoneum that surrounds the Fallopian tubes. It is the upper part of the broad ligament that surrounds the uterus.

mesotendon (mes-oh-ten-dŏn) *n.* the delicate connective tissue membrane that surrounds a tendon.

mesothelioma (mes-oh-th'ee-li-oh-mǎ) *n.* a tumour of the pleura, peritoneum, or pericardium. The occurrence of pleural mesothelioma is often due to exposure to asbestos dust (*see* asbestosis).

mesothelium (mes-oh-th'ee-liŭm) *n.* the single layer of cells that lines serous membranes. It is derived from embryonic mesoderm. *Compare* epithelium.

mesovarium (mes-oh-vair-iŭm) *n.* the mesentery of the ovaries.

messenger RNA (mes-in-jer) *n.* a type of RNA that carries the information of the genetic code of the DNA from the cell nucleus to the ribosomes, where the code is translated into protein. *See* transcription, translation.

mestranol (mes-trǎ-nol) *n.* a synthetic female sex hormone (*see* oestrogen) that is used, in combination with a progestogen, to treat menopausal symptoms (*see* hormone replacement therapy) and as a constituent of oral contraceptive pills. Trade names: **Menophase, Norinyl-1**.

met- (meta-) *prefix denoting* **1.** distal to; beyond; behind. **2.** change; transformation.

metabolic syndrome X (met-ǎ-bol-ik) *n.* a common combination of insulin resistance with type 2 diabetes, obesity with fat distribution mainly around the waist, high blood pressure, hypercholesterolaemia, and early atherosclerosis.

metabolism (mi-tab-ŏl-izm) *n.* **1.** the sum of all the chemical and physical changes within the body and enable its continued growth and functioning. Metabolism involves the breakdown of complex organic constituents of the body (*see* catabolism) and the building up of complex substances from simple ones (*see* anabolism). *See also* basal metabolism. **2.** the sum of the biochemical changes undergone by a particular constituent of the body. —**metabolic** *adj.*

metabolite (mi-tab-ŏ-lyt) *n.* a substance that takes part in the process of metabolism.

metacarpal (met-ǎ-kar-pǎl) **1.** *adj.* relating to the metacarpus. **2.** *n.* any of the bones forming the metacarpus.

metacarpophalangeal (met-ă-kar-poh-fal-ăn-jee-ăl) *adj.* relating to the metacarpal bones and the phalanges, especially to the joints between these bones.

metacarpus (met-ă-kar-pŭs) *n.* the five bones of the hand that connect the carpus (wrist) to the phalanges (digits).

metamorphopsia (met-ă-mor-fop-siă) *n.* a condition in which objects appear distorted. It is usually due to a disorder of the retina affecting the macula.

metamorphosis (met-ă-mor-fŏ-sis) *n.* a structural change, especially the change from one developmental stage to another that occurs in certain animals (e.g. in amphibians from larval to adult form).

metaphase (met-ă-fayz) *n.* the second stage of mitosis and of each division of meiosis, in which the spindle forms and the chromosomes line up at the centre of the spindle, with their centromeres attached to the spindle fibres.

metaphysis (mi-taf-i-sis) *n.* the growing portion of a long bone that lies between the epiphyses and the diaphysis.

metaplasia (met-ă-play-ziă) *n.* an abnormal change in the nature of a tissue. *myeloid m.* the development of bone marrow elements in organs such as the spleen and liver. This may occur after bone marrow failure.

metaraminol (met-ă-ram-i-nol) *n.* a sympathomimetic drug that stimulates alpha receptors and is used as a vasoconstrictor to treat severe hypotension. It is administered by injection. Trade name: **Aramine**.

metastasis (mi-tas-tă-sis) *n.* (*pl.* **metastases**) the distant spread of disease, especially a malignant tumour, from its site of origin. This occurs by three main routes: (1) through the bloodstream; (2) through the lymphatic system; (3) across body cavities. —**metastatic** (met-ă-stat-ik) *adj.*

metastasize (mi-tas-tă-syz) *vb.* (of a malignant tumour) to spread by metastasis.

metatarsal (met-ă-tar-săl) **1.** *adj.* relating to the metatarsus. **2.** *n.* any of the bones forming the metatarsus.

metatarsalgia (met-ă-tar-sal-jiă) *n.* aching pain in the metatarsal bones of the foot. Repeated injury, arthritis, and deformities of the foot are common causes, and corrective footwear and insoles may be prescribed.

metatarsus (met-ă-tar-sŭs) *n.* the five bones of the foot that connect the tarsus (ankle) to the phalanges (toes).

meteorism (meet-i-er-izm) *n. see* tympanites.

-meter *suffix denoting* an instrument for measuring.

metformin (met-for-min) *n.* a biguanide drug that reduces blood sugar levels and is administered by mouth to treat noninsulin-dependent diabetes. Trade name: **Glucophage**. *See also* oral hypoglycaemic drug.

methadone (meth-ă-dohn) *n.* a potent narcotic analgesic drug administered by mouth or injection to relieve severe pain, as a linctus to suppress coughs, and to treat heroin addiction. Trade name: **Physeptone**.

methaemalbumin (met-heem-albew-min) *n.* a chemical complex of the pigment portion of haemoglobin (haem) with the plasma protein albumin. It is formed in the blood in conditions (e.g. blackwater fever) in which red blood cells are destroyed and free haemoglobin is released into the plasma.

methaemoglobin (met-hee-mō-gloh-bin) *n.* a substance formed when the iron atoms of haemoglobin have been oxidized from the ferrous to the ferric form (*compare* oxyhaemoglobin). Methaemoglobin cannot bind molecular oxygen and therefore cannot transport oxygen round the body.

methaemoglobinaemia (met-hee-mō-gloh-bin-ee-miǎ) *n.* the presence of methaemoglobin in the blood, which may result from ingestion of oxidizing drugs. Symptoms are fatigue, headache, dizziness and cyanosis.

methanol (meth-ǎ-nol) *n. see* methyl alcohol.

methenamine (hexamine) (meth-**en**-ǎ-meen) *n.* an antiseptic with a wide range of antibacterial activity, used to treat infections and inflammation of the urinary tract, such as cystitis. Trade name: **Hiprex**.

methicillin (meth-i-sil-in) *n.* a semisynthetic penicillin formerly used to treat infections caused by bacteria that destroy natural penicillin but now replaced by newer antibiotics. It is still used to test the drug sensitivity of staphylococci. *m.-resistant Staphylococcus aureus see* MRSA.

methionine (meth-I-ŏ-neen) *n.* a sulphur-containing essential amino acid. *See also* amino acid.

methotrexate (meth-oh-treks-ayt) *n.* a drug that interferes with cell growth and is administered by mouth or injection to treat various types of cancer, including leukaemia and breast cancer (*see* antimetabolite). Trade name: **Maxtrex**.

methotrimeprazine (meth-oh-try-mep-rǎ-zeen) *n. see* levomepromazine.

methoxamine (meth-oks-ǎ-meen) *n.* a sympathomimetic drug that causes blood vessels to be constricted and therefore raises blood pressure. It is administered by injection to maintain the blood pressure during surgical operations. Trade name: **Vasoxine**.

methyl alcohol (methanol) (mee-thyl) *n.* wood alcohol: an alcohol that is oxidized in the body much more slowly than ethyl alcohol and forms poisonous products. As little as 10 ml of pure methyl alcohol can produce permanent blindness, and 100 ml is likely to be fatal. *See also* methylated spirits.

methylated spirits (meth-il-ayt-id) *n.* a mixture consisting mainly of ethyl alcohol with methyl alcohol and petroleum hydrocarbons. It is used as a solvent, cleaning fluid, and fuel.

methylcellulose (mee-thyl-sel-yoo-lohz) *n.* a compound that absorbs water and is administered by mouth as a bulk laxative to treat constipation, to control diarrhoea, and in patients with a colostomy. Trade name: **Celevac**.

methyldopa (mee-thyl-doh-pa) *n.* a drug that is administered by mouth or injection to treat hypertension. Trade name: **Aldomet**.

methylphenidate (mee-thyl-**fen**-id-ayt) *n.* a drug, related to the amphetamines, that stimulates the central nervous system. It is administered by mouth to treat attention-deficit/hyperactivity disorder in children. Trade names: **Equasym**, **Ritalin**.

methylprednisolone (mee-thyl-pred-**nis**-ō-lohn) *n.* a glucocorticoid that is used in the treatment of inflammatory conditions, such as rheumatoid arthritis, rheumatic fever, and allergic states. It is administered by mouth, intravenously, and intramuscularly. Trade names: **Depo-Medrone**, **Medrone**, **Solu-Medrone**.

methyl salicylate *n.* oil of wintergreen: a liquid with counterirritant and analgesic properties, applied to the skin to relieve pain in lumbago, sciatica, and rheumatic conditions.

methysergide (meth-i-**ser**-jyd) *n.* a drug administered by mouth to prevent severe migraine attacks and to control diarrhoea associated with tumours in the digestive system. Trade name: **Deseril**.

metoclopramide (met-oh-**kloh**-pră-myd) *n.* a drug that antagonizes the actions of dopamine. It is administered by mouth or injection to treat nausea, vomiting, indigestion, heartburn, and flatulence. Trade names: **Gastromax**, **Maxolon**, **Primperan**.

metolazone (met-**oh**-lă-zohn) *n.* a diuretic administered by mouth to treat fluid retention (oedema) and high blood pressure. Trade name: **Metenix**.

metoprolol (met-oh-**proh**-lol) *n.* a drug that controls the activity of the heart (*see* beta blocker) and is administered by mouth to treat high blood pressure and angina. Trade names: **Betaloc**, **Lopresor**.

metr- (metro-) *prefix denoting* the uterus.

metralgia (mi-**tral**-jiă) *n.* pain in the uterus.

metre (mee-ter) *n.* the SI unit of length that is equal to 39.37 inches. Symbol: m.

metritis (mi-**try**-tis) *n.* inflammation of the uterus. *See also* endometritis, myometritis.

metronidazole (met-roh-**ny**-dă-zohl) *n.* a drug administered by mouth or in suppositories to treat infections of the urinary, genital, and digestive systems, such as trichomoniasis, amoebiasis, giardiasis, and acute ulcerative gingivitis. Trade names: **Flagyl**, **Metrozol**.

metropathia haemorrhagica (met-roh-**path**-iă hem-ŏ-rah-jik-ă) *n.* irregular episodes of bleeding from the uterus, without previous ovulation, due to excessive oestrogenic activity. It is associated with endometrial hyperplasia and usually with follicular cysts of the ovary.

metrorrhagia (met-roh-**ray**-jiă) *n.* bleeding from the uterus other than the normal menstrual periods. It may indicate serious disease and should always be investigated.

-metry *suffix denoting* measuring or measurement.

metyrapone (mi-ty-ră-pohn) *n.* a drug that interferes with the production of the hormones cortisol and aldosterone and is used in the treatment of Cushing's syndrome.

It is administered by mouth. Trade name: **Metopirone**.

mexiletine (meks-il-i-teen) *n.* an anti-arrhythmic drug used in the treatment or prevention of severe heart irregularity arising in the lower chambers (ventricles). It is administered by mouth. Trade name: **Mexitil**.

MI *n. see* myocardial infarction.

mianserin (mi-an-ser-in) *n.* a drug administered by mouth to relieve moderate or severe depression and anxiety.

Michel's clips (mee-shelz) *pl. n.* small metal clips used for suturing surgical wounds. [G. Michel (1875–1937), French surgeon]

miconazole (mi-kon-ă-zohl) *n.* a drug used to treat fungal infections, such as ringworm of the scalp, body, and feet, and candidosis. It is administered by mouth, intravenous injection, intravaginally, or topically. Trade names: **Daktarin, Gyno-Daktarin**.

micr- (micro-) *prefix denoting* **1.** small size. **2.** one millionth part.

microaneurysm (my-kroh-an-yoor-izm) *n.* a minute localized swelling of a capillary wall, which is found in the retina of patients with diabetic retinopathy.

microangiopathy (my-kroh-an-ji-op-ă-thi) *n.* damage to the walls of the smallest blood vessels. It may result from a variety of diseases, including diabetes mellitus, connective-tissue diseases, infections, and cancer.

microbe (my-krohb) *n. see* microorganism.

microbiology (my-kroh-by-ol-ŏji) *n.* the science of microorganisms. Microbiology in relation to medicine is concerned mainly with the isolation and identification of the microorganisms that cause disease. —**microbiological** *adj.* —**microbiologist** *n.*

microcephaly (my-kroh-sef-ăli) *n.* abnormal smallness of the head: a congenital condition in which the brain is not fully developed. *Compare* macrocephaly.

microcheilia (my-kroh-ky-liă) *n.* abnormally small size of the lips. *Compare* macrocheilia.

Micrococcus (my-kroh-kok-ŭs) *n.* a genus of spherical Gram-positive bacteria occurring in colonies. They are saprophytes or parasites. *M. tetragenus* a species that can cause arthritis, endocarditis, meningitis, or abscesses in tissues.

microcyte (my-kroh-syt) *n.* an abnormally small red blood cell (erythrocyte). *See also* microcytosis. —**microcytic** *adj.*

microcytosis (my-kroh-sy-toh-sis) *n.* the presence of microcytes in the blood. Microcytosis is a feature of certain anaemias (*microcytic anaemias*), including those due to iron deficiency.

microdactyly (my-kroh-dak-tili) *n.* abnormal smallness or shortness of the fingers.

microdiscectomy (my-kroh-disk-ek-tŏmi) *n.* surgical removal of all or part of a prolapsed intervertebral disc using an operating microscope. It is a form of minimally invasive surgery.

microdissection (my-kroh-dis-sek-shŏn) *n.* the process of dissecting minute structures under the microscope. Using this technique it is possible to dissect the nuclei of cells and even to separate individual chromosomes. *See also* microsurgery.

microdochectomy (my-kroh-dok-ek-tŏmi) *n.* an exploratory operation on the mammary ducts, usually to detect (or exclude) the presence of a suspected tumour (adenoma).

microdontia (my-kroh-**don**-tiă) *n.* a condition in which the teeth are unusually small.

microfilaria (my-kroh-fil-**air**-iă) *n.* (*pl.* **microfilariae**) the slender motile embryo of certain nematodes (*see* filaria). Microfilariae are commonly found in the circulating blood or lymph of patients suffering an infection with any of the filarial worms.

microglossia (my-kroh-**glos**-iă) *n.* abnormally small size of the tongue.

micrognathia (my-kroh-**nay**-thiă) *n.* a condition in which one or both jaws are unusually small.

microgram (my-kroh-gram) *n.* one millionth of a gram. Symbol: μg.

micrograph (photomicrograph) (my-kroh-graf) *n.* a photograph of an object viewed through a microscope. *electron m.* a micrograph that is photographed through an electron microscope. *light m.* a micrograph that is photographed through a light microscope.

micromanipulation (my-kroh-mă-nip-yoo-**lay**-shŏn) *n.* the manipulation of extremely small structures under the microscope, as in microdissection or microsurgery.

micromelia (my-kroh-**mee**-liă) *n.* abnormally small size of the arms or legs. *Compare* macromelia.

micrometastasis (my-kroh-mi-tas-tă-sis) *n.* (*pl.* **micrometastases**) a secondary tumour that is undetectable by clinical examination or diagnostic tests but is visible under the microscope.

micrometer (my-**krom**-it-er) *n.* an instrument for making extremely fine measurements of thickness or length.

micrometre (my-kroh-mee-ter) *n.* one millionth of a metre (10^{-6} m). Symbol: μm.

microorganism (microbe) (my-kroh-**or**-găn-izm) *n.* any organism too small to be visible to the naked eye. Microorganisms include bacteria, some fungi, mycoplasmas, protozoa, rickettsiae, and viruses.

microphthalmos (my-krof-**thal**-mos) *n.* a congenitally small eye, usually associated with a small eye socket.

micropsia (my-**krop**-siă) *n.* a condition in which objects appear smaller than they really are. It is usually due to disease of the retina.

microscope (my-krŏ-skohp) *n.* an instrument for producing a greatly magnified image of an object, which may be so small as to be invisible to the naked eye. *See also* electron microscope, operating microscope. —**microscopical** *adj.* —**microscopy** (my-kros-kŏ-pi) *n.*

microscopic (my-krŏ-skop-ik) *adj.* **1.** too small to be seen clearly without the use of a microscope. **2.** of, relating to, or using a microscope.

Microsporum (my-kroh-**spor**-ŭm) *n.* a genus of fungi causing tinea (ringworm). *See also* dermatophyte.

microsurgery (my-kroh-**ser**-jer-i) *n.* the branch of surgery in which extremely intricate operations are performed through highly refined operating microscopes using miniaturized precision instruments. The technique enables surgery of previously inaccessible parts of the eye, inner ear, spinal cord, and brain.

microtia (my-kroh-tiă) *n.* a congenital deformity of the external ear in which the pinna is small or absent. The ear canal may also be absent, giving a conductive deafness.

microtome (my-krŏ-tohm) *n.* an instrument for cutting extremely thin slices of material that can be examined under a microscope.

microvascular (my-kroh-vas-kew-ler) *adj.* involving small vessels. The term is often applied to techniques of microsurgery for reuniting small blood vessels (the same techniques are applied frequently to nerve suture).

microwave therapy (my-kroh-wayv) *n.* a form of diathermy using electromagnetic waves of extremely short wavelength.

micturating cystourethrogram (MCU) (mik-tewr-ayt-ing sist-oh-yoor-ee-throh-gram) *n.* an X-ray recording of the bladder and urethra taken during the voiding of water-soluble contrast material that has been previously inserted into the bladder. It demonstrates disorders of micturition.

micturition (mik-tewr-ish-ŏn) *n. see* urination.

midazolam (mid-az-oh-lam) *n.* a benzodiazepine drug used as a sedative for minor surgery, as a pre-medication, and to induce general anaesthesia. It is administered by injection. Trade name: **Hypnovel**.

midbrain (mesencephalon) (mid-brayn) *n.* the small portion of the brainstem, excluding the pons and the medulla, that joins the hindbrain to the forebrain.

middle ear (tympanic cavity)

(mi-d'l) *n.* the air-filled part of the ear that transmits vibrations from the eardrum to the inner ear via three small bones (*see* ossicle). It is connected to the pharynx by the Eustachian tube.

midgut (mid-gut) *n.* the middle portion of the embryonic gut, which gives rise to most of the small intestine and part of the large intestine.

midstream specimen of urine (MSU) (mid-streem) *n.* a specimen of urine that is subjected to examination for the presence of microorganisms. In order to obtain a specimen that is free of contamination, the periurethral area is cleansed and the patient is requested to discard the initial flow of urine before collecting the specimen in a sterile container.

midwife (mid-wyf) *n.* (in Britain) a registered nurse who, having undertaken an additional training, is qualified to attend professionally upon a woman during the antenatal, intranatal, and postnatal periods. *See also* community midwife. —**midwifery** (mid-wif-ri) *n.*

mifepristone (mi-fep-ris-tohn) *n.* a drug used to produce an abortion within the first 20 weeks of pregnancy: it acts by blocking the action of progesterone, which is essential for maintaining pregnancy. It is taken by mouth, followed after 36 hours by gemeprost intravaginally. Trade name: **Mifegyne**.

migraine (mee-grayn) *n.* a condition resulting from spasm and subsequent overdilatation of certain arteries in the brain, which causes a recurrent throbbing headache that characteristically affects one side of the head. The headache is often accompanied by prostration, nausea and vomiting, and photophobia. There is sometimes a preceding aura, consisting of visual disturbance or tingling and/or weakness of the limbs. —**migrainous** *adj.*

Mikulicz's disease (mik-oo-lich-iz) *n.* swelling of the lacrimal and salivary glands as a result of infiltration with lymphoid tissue. [J. von Mikulicz Radecki (1850–1905), Polish surgeon]

miliaria (mili-air-iă) *n. see* prickly heat.

miliary (mil-yer-i) *adj.* describing or characterized by very small nodules or lesions, resembling millet seed. *m. tuberculosis see* tuberculosis.

milium (mil-iŭm) *n.* (*pl.* **milia**) a white nodule in the skin, particularly on the face. Up to 2 mm in diameter, milia are tiny keratin cysts occurring just beneath the epidermis. Milia are commonly seen in newborn babies around the nose; they disappear without active treatment.

milk (milk) *n.* the liquid food secreted by female mammals from the mammary gland. Milk is a complete food in that it has most of the nutrients necessary for life: protein, carbohydrate, fat, minerals, and vitamins. Cows' milk is comparatively deficient in vitamins C and D. Human milk contains more sugar (lactose) and less protein than cows' milk.

milk rash *n.* a spotty red facial rash that is common during the first few months of life; it disappears without treatment.

milk sugar *n. see* lactose.

milk teeth *pl. n.* the primary teeth of young children. *See* dentition.

Miller-Abbott tube (mil-er ab-ŏt) *n.* a double-channel rubber tube used to relieve obstruction of the small intestine. One channel terminates in a balloon that is inflated when the tube reaches the duodenum; the other is used for suction of the obstructing material. [T. G. Miller (1886–1981) and W. O. Abbott (1902–43), US physicians]

milli- *prefix denoting* one thousandth part.

milliampere (mili-am-pair) *n.* one thousandth of an ampere (10^{-3} A). Symbol: mA.

milligram (mil-i-gram) *n.* one thousandth of a gram. Symbol: mg.

millilitre (mil-i-lee-ter) *n.* one thousandth of a litre. Symbol: ml.

millimetre (mil-i-mee-ter) *n.* one thousandth of a metre (10^{-3} m). Symbol: mm.

Milroy's disease (mil-roiz) *n.* congenital lymphoedema of the legs. *See* lymphoedema. [W. F. Milroy (1855–1942), US physician]

Milton (mil-tŏn) *n. Trademark.* a solution of sodium hypochlorite, used especially for sterilizing babies' feeding bottles.

mineralocorticoid (min-er-ăl-ohkor-ti-koid) *n.* any of a group of corticosteroids, such as aldosterone, that are necessary for the regulation of salt and water balance.

miner's elbow (my-nerz) *n.* inflammation of the bursa over the elbow, caused by pressure on the olecranon process.

minim (min-im) *n.* a unit of volume used in pharmacy, equivalent to one sixtieth part of a fluid drachm.

minimally invasive surgery

(min-i-măli) *n.* surgical intervention involving the least possible physical trauma to the patient, particularly surgery performed using an operating laparoscope or other endoscope (*see* laparoscopy) passed through a tiny incision; it is known popularly as *keyhole surgery*. Several types of abdominal surgery, including gall bladder removal (*see* cholecystectomy), are now commonly performed in this way.

minitracheostomy (min-i-tray-ki-ost-ōmi) *n.* temporary tracheostomy using a needle or fine-bore tube inserted through the skin.

minocycline (min-oh-sy-kleen) *n.* a tetracycline antibiotic active against a wide range of bacteria and against rickettsial infections, mycoplasmal pneumonia, and relapsing fever. It is administered by mouth or topically. Trade name: **Minoclin**.

minoxidil (min-oks-i-dil) *n.* a peripheral vasodilator used in the treatment of high blood pressure (hypertension) when other drugs are not effective; it is administered by mouth in conjunction with a diuretic. It is also applied to the scalp, in the form of a lotion, to restore hair growth. Trade names: **Loniten**, **Regaine**.

mio- *prefix denoting* **1.** reduction or diminution. **2.** rudimentary.

miosis (myosis) (my-oh-sis) *n.* constriction of the pupil. This occurs normally in bright light, but persistent miosis is most commonly caused by certain types of drugs used to treat glaucoma. *See also* miotic. *Compare* mydriasis.

miotic (myotic) (my-ot-ik) *n.* a drug, such as pilocarpine, that causes the pupil of the eye to contract.

miscarriage (mis-ka-rij) *n. see* abortion.

miso- *prefix denoting* hatred.

misophonia (mis-oh-foh-niă) *n.* dislike of or aversion to sound. *See* hyperacusis, phonophobia.

misoprostol (mis-oh-rŏ-stol) *n.* a prostaglandin drug administered by mouth for the prevention and treatment of peptic ulcer, especially when caused by nonsteroidal anti-inflammatory drugs (*see* NSAID). Trade names: **Cytotec**, **Napratec**.

missed case *n.* a person suffering from an infection in whom the symptoms and signs are so minimal that either there is no request for medical assistance or the doctor fails to make the diagnosis.

Misuse of Drugs Act 1971 *n.* (in the UK) an Act of Parliament that, together with the Misuse of Drugs Regulations 1985, restricts the prescription, dispensing, sale, and possession of dangerous drugs. These *controlled drugs* include the natural opiates and their synthetic substitutes, many stimulants (including amphetamine and cocaine), and hallucinogens such as LSD and cannabis.

mite (myt) *n.* a free-living or parasitic arthropod belonging to a group (Acarina) that also includes the ticks. Medically important mites include the many species causing dermatitis. **house-dust m.** a mite of the genus *Dermatophagoides*, the waste products of which produce an allergic response in susceptible people that is an important trigger for some forms of rhinitis and asthma.

mitochondrion (my-toh-kon-driŏn) n. (pl. **mitochondria**) a structure, occurring in varying numbers in the cytoplasm of every cell, that is the site of the cell's energy production. Mitochondria contain ATP and the enzymes involved in the cell's metabolic activities, and also their own DNA; mitochondrial genes are inherited through the female line. —mitochondrial adj.

mitomycin (my-toh-my-sin) n. an anthracycline antibiotic that inhibits the growth of cancer cells. It causes severe marrow suppression but is of use in the treatment of stomach and breast cancers. Trade name: **Mitomycin C Kyowa**.

mitosis (my-toh-sis) n. a type of cell division in which a single cell produces two genetically identical daughter cells. It is the way in which new body cells are produced for both growth and repair. Compare meiosis. —**mitotic** (my-tot-ik) adj.

mitoxantrone (mi-toks-an-trohn) n. a cytotoxic drug used in the treatment of certain cancers, including breast cancer, leukaemia, and lymphomas. Trade names: **Novantrone, Onkotrone**.

mitral incompetence (my-trăl) n. failure of the mitral valve to close, allowing a reflux of blood from the left ventricle of the heart to the left atrium. Its manifestations include breathlessness, atrial fibrillation, embolism, enlargement of the left ventricle, and a systolic murmur.

mitral stenosis n. narrowing of the opening of the mitral valve: a result of chronic scarring that follows rheumatic fever. Mild cases need no treatment, but severe cases are treated surgically by reopening the

stenosis (mitral valvotomy) or by inserting an artificial valve (mitral prosthesis).

mitral valve (bicuspid valve) n. a valve in the heart consisting of two cusps attached to the walls at the opening between the left atrium and left ventricle. It allows blood to pass from the atrium to the ventricle, but prevents any backward flow.

mittelschmerz (mit-ĕl-shmairts) n. pain in the lower abdomen experienced about midway between successive menstrual periods, i.e. at ovulation.

ml symbol for millilitre.

MLD n. minimal lethal dose: the smallest quantity of a toxic compound that is recorded as having caused death.

MMR vaccine n. a combined vaccine against measles, mumps, and German measles (rubella). It is currently recommended that this vaccine is given to all children between 13 and 15 months old, with a subsequent booster dose. See Appendix 8.

MND n. see motor neurone disease.

Mobitz type I and type II (moh-bitz) pl. n. types of abnormality on an electrocardiogram (ECG) tracing that indicate forms of heart block. [W. Mobitz (20th century), German cardiologist]

moclobemide (mok-loh-bi-myd) n. an antidepressant drug that reversibly inhibits the enzyme monoamine oxidase. It is less likely to cause the adverse effects associated with traditional MAO inhibitors. Trade name: **Manerix**.

modality (moh-dal-iti) n. **1.** a form of sensation, such as smell, hearing, tasting, or detecting temperature. **2.**

one form of therapy as opposed to another, such as the modality of physiotherapy contrasted with that of radiotherapy.

Modecate (mod-i-kayt) n. see fluphenazine.

modelling (mod-ēl-ing) n. a technique used in behaviour modification, whereby an individual learns a behaviour by observing someone else doing it.

modiolus (moh-dy-oh-lŭs) n. the conical central pillar of the cochlea in the inner ear.

MODS n. see multiple organ dysfunction syndrome.

MODY n. see maturity-onset diabetes of the young.

MOF n. see multi-organ failure.

Mogadon (mog-ă-don) n. see nitrazepam.

molar (moh-ler) n. the fourth or fifth tooth (in the primary dentition) or the sixth, seventh, or eighth tooth (in the permanent dentition) from the midline on each side of each jaw. See also dentition.

molarity (mol-a-ri-ti) n. the strength of a solution, expressed as the weight of dissolved substance in grams per litre divided by its molecular weight, i.e. the number of moles per litre.

mole¹ (mohl) n. the SI unit of amount of substance. One mole of a compound has a mass equal to its molecular weight expressed in grams. Symbol: mol.

mole² n. a nonmalignant collection of pigmented cells in the skin. Moles vary widely in appearance, being flat or raised, smooth or hairy. Changes in the shape, colour, etc., of moles in adult life may be an early

sign of malignant melanoma. Medical name: pigmented naevus.

molecular biology (mŏ-lek-yoo-ler) n. the study of the molecules that are associated with living organisms, especially proteins and nucleic acids.

molecule (mol-i-kewl) n. a particle consisting of two or more atoms held together by chemical bonds. It is the smallest unit of an element or compound capable of existing independently. —**molecular** adj.

molluscum contagiosum (mol-usk-ŭm kon-ta-joh-sŭm) n. a common disease of the skin, mainly affecting children. Characterized by papules less than 5 mm in diameter, each with a central depression, the disease is caused by a poxvirus and is spread by direct contact. Untreated, the papules disappear in 6–9 months.

mon- (mono-) prefix denoting one, single, or alone.

Mongolian blue spots (mong ohliăn) pl. n. blue-black pigmented areas seen at the base of the back and on the buttocks of babies. They are more common in dark-skinned babies and usually fade during the first year of life.

mongolism (mong-ŏ-lizm) n. see Down's syndrome.

Monilia (moh-nil-iă) n. the former name of the genus of yeasts now known as Candida.

moniliasis (mon-i-ly-ă-sis) n. an obsolete name for candidosis.

Monitor (mon-i-ter) n. see quality assurance (tool).

monitoring (mon-i-ter-ing) n. the periodic observation of a patient's condition, which may be by visual, manual, or automatic means.

monoamine oxidase (MAO)
(mon-oh-**ay**-meen) *n.* an enzyme that
catalyses the oxidation of a large variety of monoamines, including
adrenaline, noradrenaline, and
serotonin. Monoamine oxidase is
found in most tissues, particularly
the liver and nervous system. *See
also* MAO inhibitor.

monoblast (**mon**-oh-blast) *n.* the
earliest identifiable cell that gives
rise to a monocyte. It is normally
found in the blood-forming tissue of
the bone marrow but may appear in
the blood in certain diseases, most
notably in *acute monoblastic leukaemia.*

monochromat (mon-oh-**kroh**-mat)
n. a person who is completely col-
our-blind. The condition is probably
inherited.

monochromatic (mon-oh-krō-
mat-ik) *adj.* denoting radiation, especially light, of the same frequency
or wavelength.

monoclonal antibody (mon-oh-
kloh-năl) *n.* an antibody produced
artificially from a cell clone and
therefore consisting of a single type
of immunoglobulin. Monoclonal
antibodies are produced by fusing
antibody-forming lymphocytes from
mouse spleen with mouse myeloma
cells. The resulting hybrid cells multiply rapidly (like cancer cells) and
produce the same antibody as their
parent lymphocytes.

monocular (mon-**ok**-yoo-ler) *adj.*
relating to or used by one eye only.
Compare binocular.

monocyte (**mon**-oh-syt) *n.* a variety of white blood cell with a kid-
ney-shaped nucleus. Its function is
the ingestion of foreign particles,

such as bacteria and tissue debris.
—**monocytic** *adj.*

monocytosis (mon-oh-sy-**toh**-sis)
n. an increase in the number of
monocytes in the blood. Monocytosis occurs in a variety of diseases,
including monocytic leukaemias.

monodactylism (mon-oh-**dak**-til-
izm) *n.* the congenital absence of all
but one digit on each hand and foot.

monomania (mon-oh-**may**-niă) *n.*
the state in which a particular delusion or set of delusions is present in
an otherwise normally functioning
person. *See also* paranoia.

mononeuritis (mon-oh-newr-**I**-tis)
n. disease affecting a single peripheral nerve. *See* (peripheral) neuropathy.

mononuclear (mon-oh-**new**-kli-er)
adj. (of a cell) having one nucleus.

mononucleosis (mon-oh-new-kli-
oh-sis) *n.* the condition in which the
blood contains an abnormally high
number of mononuclear leucocytes
(monocytes and lymphocytes). *See*
glandular fever (infectious mononucleosis).

monoplegia (mon-oh-**plee**-jiă) *n.*
paralysis of one limb. —**mono-
plegic** *adj.*

monoploid (mon-ō-ploid) *adj. see*
haploid.

monorchism (mon-or-kizm) *n.* the
absence of one testis. This is usually
due to failure of one testicle to descend into the scrotum before birth.

monosaccharide (mon-oh-sak-ă-
ryd) *n.* a simple sugar having the
general formula $(CH_2O)_n$. The most
abundant monosaccharide is glucose.

monosomy (mon-ō-soh-mi) *n.* a
condition in which there is one
chromosome missing from the nor-

mal (diploid) set. *Compare* trisomy. —**monosomic** *adj.*

monozygotic twins (mon-oh-zy-got-ik) *pl. n. see* twins.

mons (monz) *n.* (in anatomy) a rounded eminence. *m. pubis* the mound of fatty tissue lying over the pubic symphysis.

montelukast (mon-ti-loo-kăst) *n. see* leukotriene receptor antagonist.

Montgomery's glands (mŏnt-gom-er-iz) *pl. n.* sebaceous glands on the areola surrounding the nipple of a woman's breast. They enlarge during pregnancy and their secretions lubricate and protect the breast during breast feeding. [W. F. Montgomery (1797–1859), Irish obstetrician]

Mooren's ulcer (moor ĕnz) *n.* a rare chronic progressive ulceration of the cornea, occurring in the elderly. It is typically very painful and difficult to control. [A. Mooren (1829–99), German ophthalmologist]

morbid (mor-bid) *adj.* diseased or abnormal; pathological.

morbidity (mor-bid-iti) *n.* the state of being diseased. *m. rate* the number of cases of a disease found to occur in a stated number of the population, usually given as cases per 100,000 or per million.

morbilli (mor-bil-I) *n. see* measles.

morbilliform (mor-bil-i-form) *adj.* describing a skin rash resembling that of measles.

morbus (mor-bŭs) *n.* disease. The term is usually used as part of the medical name of a specific disease.

moribund (mo-ri-bund) *adj.* dying.

morning sickness (mor-ning) *n.* nausea and vomiting during early pregnancy. *Compare* hyperemesis (gravidarum).

Moro reflex (startle reflex) (moh-roh) *n.* the normal reaction of a newborn baby to a sudden loud noise. The infant flings its arms and legs wide and appears to stiffen; the limbs are then drawn back into flexion. [E. Moro (1874–1951), German paediatrician]

morphine (mor-feen) *n.* a potent analgesic and narcotic drug administered by mouth or injection to relieve severe and persistent pain. Morphine causes feelings of euphoria; tolerance develops rapidly and dependence may occur.

morpho- *prefix denoting* form or structure.

morphoea (mor-fee-ă) *n.* a localized form of scleroderma characterized by firm ivory-coloured waxy plaques in the skin without any internal sclerosis.

morphogenesis (mor-foh-jen-i-sis) *n.* the development of form and structure of the body and its parts.

morphology (mor-fol-ŏji) *n.* the study of differences in form between species.

-morphous *suffix denoting* form or structure (of a specified kind).

Morquio-Brailsford disease (mor-kee-oh braylz-ferd) *n.* a defect of mucopolysaccharide metabolism that causes dwarfism with a kyphosis, knock-knee, and an angulated sternum. Intelligence is normal. [L. Morquio (1867–1935), Uruguayan physician; J. F. Brailsford (20th century), British radiologist]

mortality (mortality rate) (mor-tal-iti) *n.* the incidence of death in the population in a given period. *annual m. rate* the number of registered deaths in a year, multiplied by 1000 and divided by the population at the middle of the year. *See also* infant (mortality rate), maternal mortality rate.

mortification (mor-ti-fi-**kay**-shŏn) *n. see* necrosis.

morula (mo-roo-lă) *n.* an early stage of embryonic development formed by cleavage of the fertilized ovum. It consists of a solid ball of cells and is an intermediate stage between the zygote and blastocyst.

mosaicism (mŏ-**zay**-i-sizm) *n.* a condition in which the cells of an individual do not all contain identical chromosomes; there may be two or more genetically different populations of cells. —**mosaic** *adj.*

mosquito (mos-**kee**-toh) *n.* a small winged bloodsucking insect belonging to a large group – the Diptera. Female mosquitoes transmit the parasites responsible for several major infectious diseases, such as malaria. *See* Anopheles, Aëdes.

motile (**moh**-tyl) *adj.* being able to move spontaneously, without external aid: usually applied to a microorganism or a cell.

motions (**moh**-shŏnz) *pl. n.* the products of bowel evacuation.

motion sickness (travel sickness) (**moh**-shŏn) *n.* nausea, vomiting, and headache caused by motion during travel by sea, road, or air. The symptoms are due to overstimulation of the balance organs in the inner ear. Sedative antihistamine drugs are used for prevention and treatment.

motor cortex (**moh**-ter) *n.* the region of the cerebral cortex that is responsible for initiating nerve impulses that bring about voluntary activity in the muscles of the body.

motor nerve *n. see* nerve.

motor neurone *n.* one of the units (neurones) that goes to make up the nerve pathway between the brain and an effector organ, such as a skeletal muscle. **lower m.** a motor neurone that has a cell body in the spinal cord or brainstem and an axon that extends outwards to reach an effector. **upper m.** a motor neurone that has a cell body in the brain and an axon that extends into the spinal cord, where it ends in synapses.

motor neurone disease (MND) *n.* a progressive degenerative disease of the motor system occurring in middle age and causing muscle weakness and wasting. It primarily affects the cells of the anterior horn of the spinal cord, the motor nuclei in the brainstem, and the corticospinal fibres. Some forms of the disease are familial (inherited).

mould (mohld) *n.* any multicellular filamentous fungus that commonly forms a rough furry coating on decaying matter.

moulding (mohld-ing) *n.* the changing of the shape of an infant's head during labour, brought about by the pressures to which it is subjected when passing through the birth canal.

mountain sickness (mownt-in) *n. see* altitude sickness.

mouth-to-mouth respiration (mowth) *n.* emergency artificial respiration, performed mouth-to-mouth, by blowing air into the victim's lungs to inflate them and then allowing exhalation to occur automatically. It is commonly known as the *kiss of life*.

mouthwash (mowth-wosh) *n.* an aqueous solution with antiseptic, astringent, or deodorizing properties used for rinsing of the mouth and teeth. *m. test* a test for detecting carriers of single-gene defects (e.g. cystic fibrosis) in which cells from the buccal cavity are obtained from a saline mouthwash and their DNA is isolated and genetically analysed.

moxisylyte (thymoxamine) (moks-**i**-sy-lyt) *n.* an alpha blocker drug that causes peripheral blood vessels to dilate (*see* vasodilator). It is administered by mouth in the treatment of Raynaud's disease and similar conditions. Trade name: **Opilon**.

MPQ *n. see* McGill Pain Questionnaire.

MRI *n. see* magnetic resonance imaging.

MRSA *n.* methicillin- (or multiple-) resistant *Staphylococcus aureus*: an increasingly common dangerous bacterium that is resistant to many antibiotics and is responsible for outbreaks of infection in hospitals.

MS *n. see* multiple sclerosis.

MSA *n. see* multiple system atrophy.

MSH *n. see* melanocyte-stimulating hormone.

MSP *n. see* Munchausen's syndrome (by proxy).

MSU *n. see* midstream specimen of urine.

mucilage (mew-si-lij) *n.* (in pharmacy) a thick aqueous solution of a gum used as a lubricant in skin preparations, for the production of pills, and for the suspension of insoluble substances.

mucin (mew-sin) *n.* the principal constituent of mucus. Mucin is a glycoprotein.

muco- *prefix denoting* **1.** mucus. **2.** mucous membrane.

mucociliary transport (mew-koh-**sil**-i-er-i) *n.* the process by which cilia move a thin film of mucus from the upper and lower respiratory tracts towards the digestive tract. Particles of dust and microorganisms are trapped on the mucus and thereby removed from the respiratory tract.

mucocoele (mew-koh-seel) *n.* a space or organ distended with mucus. It may occur in the gall bladder when the exit duct becomes obstructed.

mucocutaneous (mew-koh-kew-tay-nius) *adj.* relating to or affecting mucous membrane and skin.

mucoid (mew-koid) *adj.* resembling mucus.

mucolytic (mew-koh-**lit**-ik) *n.* an agent, such as dornase alfa (*see* DNAse), that dissolves or breaks down mucus. Mucolytics are used to treat chest conditions involving excessive or thickened mucus secretions.

mucopolysaccharide (mew-koh-poli-**sak**-er-yd) *n.* one of a group of complex carbohydrates functioning mainly as structural components in connective tissue.

mucopolysaccharidosis (mew-koh-poli-sak-er-I-**doh**-sis) *n.* any one of a group of rare inborn errors of metabolism in which the storage of complex carbohydrates is disordered. *See* Hunter's syndrome, Hurler's syndrome.

mucoprotein (mew-koh-**proh**-teen) *n.* one of a group of proteins found in the globulin fraction of blood plasma. Mucoproteins are globulins combined with a carbohydrate group (an amino sugar).

mucopurulent (mew-koh-**pewr**-oo-

lĕnt) *adj.* containing mucus and pus. *See* mucopus.

mucopus (mew-koh-pus) *n.* a mixture of mucus and pus.

mucosa (mew-**koh**-să) *n. see* mucous membrane. —**mucosal** *adj.*

mucous membrane (mucosa) (mew-kŭs) *n.* the moist membrane lining many tubular structures and cavities, including the nasal sinuses, respiratory tract, gastrointestinal tract, biliary, and pancreatic systems. The surface layer of the membrane contains glands that secrete mucus.

mucoviscidosis (mew-koh-vis-i-doh-sis) *n. see* cystic fibrosis.

mucus (mew-kŭs) *n.* a viscous fluid secreted by mucous membranes. Mucus acts as a protective barrier over the surfaces of the membranes, as a lubricant, and as a carrier of enzymes. —**mucous** *adj.*

MUGA scan (multiple-gated acquisition scan) (mug-ă) *n.* a technique used in nuclear medicine for studying left-ventricular function and wall motion of the heart by injecting the patient's red cells with radioactive technetium-99m to form an image of the blood pool within the heart at specific points in the cardiac cycle, using an ECG, gamma camera, and computer.

Müllerian duct (mew-leer-iăn) *n. see* paramesonephric duct. [J. P. Müller (1801–58), German physiologist]

multi- *prefix denoting* many; several.

multifactorial (multi-fak-tor-iăl) *adj.* describing a condition, such as spina bifida, that is believed to have resulted from the interaction of genetic factors, usually polygenes,

with an environmental factor or factors.

multifocal lens (multi-foh-kăl) *n.* a lens in which the power (*see* dioptre) of the lower part gradually increases towards the lower edge. The wearer can see clearly at any distance by lowering or raising the eyes to look through an appropriate part of the lens.

multigravida (multi-**grav**-id-ă) *n.* a woman who has been pregnant at least twice.

multi-organ failure (multiple-organ failure, MOF) (multi-organ) *n.* the terminal stage of serious illness.

multipara (mul-**tip**-er-ă) *n.* a woman who has given birth to a live child after each of at least two pregnancies. *See also* grand multiparity.

multiple myeloma (mul-ti-**pŭl**) *n. see* myeloma.

multiple organ dysfunction syndrome (MODS) *n.* a common cause of death following severe injury, overwhelming infection, or immune deficiency states.

multiple personality disorder *n.* a psychiatric disorder in which the affected person has two or more distinct, and often contrasting, personalities. As each personality assumes dominance, it determines attitudes and behaviour and usually appears to be unaware of the other personality (or personalities). The condition is thought to be a late result of child abuse.

multiple sclerosis (MS, disseminated sclerosis) *n.* a chronic disease of the nervous system affecting young and middle-aged adults. The myelin sheaths surrounding nerves in the brain and spinal cord are damaged, which affects the function of the nerves involved. The course of the illness is usually characterized by recurrent relapses followed by remissions but a small proportion of patients run a chronic progressive course. Symptoms include ataxia, abnormal eye movements (e.g. nystagmus), dysarthria, spastic weakness, and retrobulbar neuritis.

multiple system atrophy (MSA) *n.* a condition that results from degeneration of brain cells in the basal ganglia (resulting in parkinsonism), the cerebellum, and the pyramidal system and degeneration of cells in the autonomic nervous system.

multisystem (multi-sis-tĕm) *adj.* describing a disease that affects many systems of the body.

mummification (mum-i-fi-kay-shŏn) *n.* the conversion of dead tissue into a hard shrunken mass, chiefly by dehydration.

mumps (mumps) *n.* a common virus infection mainly affecting children. Symptoms appear 2–3 weeks after exposure: fever, headache, and vomiting may precede a typical swelling of the parotid salivary glands. The infection may spread to other salivary glands and to the pancreas, brain, and testicles (*see* orchitis). *See also* MMR vaccine. Medical name: **infectious parotitis**.

Munchausen's syndrome (muunch-how-zĕnz) *n.* a mental disorder in which the patient persistently tries to obtain hospital treatment, especially surgery, for an illness that is nonexistent: an extreme form of malingering. *M. s. by proxy* (*MSP*) a condition in which the patient inflicts harm on others (often children) in order to attract medical attention. [Baron von Munchausen, a fictional character who told exaggerated stories]

murmur (mer-mer) *n.* a noise, heard with the aid of a stethoscope, that is generated by turbulent blood flow within the heart or blood vessels produced by damaged valves, septal defects, narrowed arteries, or arteriovenous communications. *continuous m.* murmur heard throughout systole and diastole. *diastolic m.* murmur heard during diastole. *innocent m.* heart murmur heard in normal individuals. *systolic m.* murmur heard during systole.

Murphy's sign (mer-fiz) *n.* an indication of an inflamed gall bladder: continuous pressure over the gall bladder will cause the patient to catch his breath just before the peak of inhalation. [J. B. Murphy (1857–1916) US surgeon]

muscae volitantes (mus-kee voli-tan-teez) *pl. n.* black spots seen floating before the eyes usually due to the presence of opacities in the vitreous humour as it becomes more fluid with age.

muscarine (musk-er-in) *n.* a highly poisonous alkaloid occurring in certain mushrooms, such as fly agaric (*Amanita muscaria*).

muscle (mus-ŭl) *n.* a tissue whose cells have the ability to contract, producing movement or force. The major functions of muscles are to produce movements of the body and of structures within it and to alter pressures or tensions of internal organs. There are three types of muscle (*see* cardiac muscle, smooth mus-bundle of muscle fibres

- epimysium
- single muscle fibre
- perimysium
- endomysium
- tendon

A voluntary muscle in transverse section (left) and in longitudinal section at its junction with a tendon (right)

cle, striated muscle). See illustration. —**muscular** (mus-kew-ler) *adj.*

muscle relaxant *n.* an agent that reduces tension in voluntary muscles. Drugs such as baclofen and diazepam are used to relieve skeletal muscular spasms. Other drugs, e.g. atracurium besilate, gallamine, and suxamethonium, are used to relax voluntary muscles during the administration of anaesthetics in surgical operations.

muscular dystrophy *n.* a group of muscle diseases, marked by weakness and wasting of selected muscles, in which there is a recognizable pattern of inheritance. The affected muscle fibres degenerate and are replaced by fatty tissue. The most common form is *Duchenne muscular dystrophy*, which is nearly always restricted to boys and usually begins before the age of four. The child has a waddling gait and lordosis of the lumbar spine. The calf muscles – and later the shoulders and upper limbs – often become firm and bulky. *See also* Becker

muscular dystrophy, dystrophia myotonica (myotonic dystrophy).

muscularis (mus-kew-lar-is) *n.* a muscular layer of the wall of a hollow organ (such as the stomach) or a tubular structure (such as the ureter or intestine).

musculo- *prefix denoting* muscle.

musculocutaneous nerve (mus-kew-loh-kew-**tay**-niŭs) *n.* a nerve of the brachial plexus that supplies some muscles of the arm and the skin of the lateral part of the forearm.

musculoskeletal (mus-kew-loh-skel-i-t'l) *adj.* relating to both the muscles and the bones.

mushroom (mush-room) *n.* the spore-producing body of various fungi. Great care must be taken in identifying edible mushrooms, as many species are poisonous, including *Amanita phalloides* (death cap) and *A. muscaria* (fly agaric).

mustine (nitrogen mustard) (must-een) *n. see* chlormethine.

mutant (mew-tănt) *n.* **1.** an individual in which a mutation has occurred, especially when the effect of the mutation is visible. **2.** a characteristic showing the effects of a mutation. —**mutant** *adj*.

mutation (mew-tay-shŏn) *n*. a change in the amount or structure of the genetic material (DNA) of a cell, or the change this causes in a characteristic of the individual. A mutation affecting developing sex cells can be inherited. Mutations may occur spontaneously or be caused by external agents (e.g. radiation or certain viruses).

mutism (mewt-izm) *n*. inability or refusal to speak; dumbness. Innate speechlessness most commonly occurs in those who have been totally deaf since birth (*deaf m.*). Mutism may also result from brain damage (*see* aphasia) or be caused by depression or psychological trauma. —**mute** *adj.*, *n*.

my- (**myo-**) *prefix denoting* muscle.

myalgia (my-al-jiă) *n*. pain in the muscles. —**myalgic** (my-al-jik) *adj*.

myalgic encephalomyelitis (myalgic encephalopathy, ME) *n. see* CFS/ME.

myasthenia (my ăs-th'een-iă) *n*. weakness of the muscles. *m. gravis* a chronic disease marked by abnormal fatigability and weakness of selected muscles, initially those around the eyes, mouth, and throat, resulting in drooping of the upper eyelid (ptosis), double vision, dysarthria, and dysphagia. It is an autoimmune disease in which the ability of the neurotransmitter acetylcholine to induce muscular contraction is impaired. Treatment with anticholinesterase drugs and surgical removal of the thymus in patients under the age of 45 lessen the severity of the symptoms.

Steroid therapy or plasma exchange may be used to treat the more severely affected patients.

myc- (**myco-**, **mycet(o)-**) *prefix denoting* a fungus.

mycelium (my-see-liŭm) *n*. (*pl.* **mycelia**) the tangled mass of fine branching threads that make up the feeding and growing part of a fungus.

mycetoma (my-si-toh-mă) *n*. a chronic inflammation of tissues caused by a fungus. *See* Madura foot.

Mycobacterium (my-koh-bak-teer-iŭm) *n*. a genus of rodlike aerobic Gram-positive bacteria. Several species are responsible for opportunistic infections of the lung (*see* MAI complex). *M. leprae* (*Hansen's bacillus*) the species that causes leprosy. *M. tuberculosis* (*Koch's bacillus*) the species that causes tuberculosis.

mycology (my-kol-ŏji) *n*. the science of fungi. *See also* microbiology. —**mycologist** *n*.

mycoplasma (my-koh-plaz-mă) *n*. one of a group of minute non-motile microorganisms that lack a rigid cell wall and hence display a variety of forms. The species *Mycoplasma pneumoniae* causes atypical pneumonia. The group also includes the *pleuropneumonia-like organisms* (*PPLO*).

mycosis (my-koh-sis) *n*. any disease caused by a fungus, including actinomycosis, aspergillosis, cryptococcosis, rhinosporidiosis, ringworm, and sporotrichosis.

mycosis fungoides (fung-oid-eez) *n*. a variety of reticulosis confined to the skin, with plaques and later nodules infiltrated with T-lymphocytes.

It progresses very slowly and can be treated initially with topical corticosteroids.

Mycota (my-koh-ta) *n.* *see* decenoic acid.

mydriasis (mid-ry-ă-sis) *n.* widening of the pupil, which occurs normally in dim light. The commonest cause of prolonged mydriasis is drug therapy (*see* mydriatic) or injury to the eye. *See also* cycloplegia. *Compare* miosis.

mydriatic (mid-ri-at-ik) *n.* a drug, such as atropine or phenylephrine, that causes the pupil of the eye to dilate.

myectomy (my-ek-tŏmi) *n.* a surgical operation to remove part of a muscle.

myel- (myelo-) *prefix denoting* **1.** the spinal cord. **2.** bone marrow. **3.** myelin.

myelencephalon (my-ĕl-en-sef-ă-lon) *n.* *see* medulla (oblongata).

myelin (my-ĕ-lin) *n.* a complex material formed of protein and phospholipid that is laid down as a sheath around the axons of certain neurones, known as *myelinated* (or *medullated*) *nerve fibres*.

myelination (my-ĕ-lin-ay-shŏn) *n.* the process in which myelin is laid down as an insulating layer around the axons of certain nerves.

myelitis (my-ĕ-ly-tis) *n.* **1.** an inflammatory disease of the spinal cord. The most usual kind (*transverse m.*) most often occurs during the development of multiple sclerosis. The inflammation spreads across the tissue of the spinal cord, resulting in paralysis of the legs and lower trunk. **2.** inflammation of the bone marrow. *See* osteomyelitis.

myeloblast (my-ĕ-loh-blast) *n.* the earliest identifiable cell that gives rise to a granulocyte. It is normally found in the blood-forming tissue of the bone marrow, but may appear in the blood in a variety of diseases, most notably in *acute myeloblastic leukaemia*. *See also* granulopoiesis. —**myeloblastic** *adj.*

myelocele (my-ĕ-loh-seel) *n.* *see* meningomyelocele.

myelocyte (my-ĕ-loh-syt) *n.* an immature form of granulocyte. It is normally found in the blood-forming tissue of the bone marrow, but may appear in the blood in a variety of diseases, including infections, infiltrations of the bone marrow, and certain leukaemias. *See also* granulopoiesis.

myelofibrosis (my-ĕ-loh-fy-broh-sis) *n.* a chronic but progressive disease characterized by fibrosis of the bone marrow, which leads to anaemia; enlargement of the spleen; and the presence of myeloid tissue in abnormal sites, such as the spleen and liver. Its cause is unknown.

myelography (my-ĕ-log-răfi) *n.* a specialized method of X-ray examination to demonstrate the spinal canal that involves injection of a radiopaque contrast medium into the subarachnoid space. The X-rays obtained are called *myelograms*.

myeloid (my-ĕ-loid) *adj.* **1.** like, derived from, or relating to bone marrow. *m. leukaemia* a variety of leukaemia in which the type of blood cell that proliferates abnormally originates in the blood-forming tissue of the bone marrow. *See also* Philadelphia chromosome. *m. tissue* a tissue in the bone marrow in which the various classes of blood

myoclonus

cells are produced. *See* haemopoiesis. **2.** resembling a myelocyte. **3.** relating to the spinal cord.

myeloma (multiple myeloma, myelomatosis) (my-ĕ-loh-mă) *n.* a malignant disease of the bone marrow, characterized by two or more of the following: (1) the presence of an excess of abnormal malignant plasma cells in the bone marrow; (2) lytic deposits in the bones, giving the appearance of holes on X-rays; (3) the presence in the serum of an abnormal gammaglobulin, usually IgG (*see* paraprotein). The patient may complain of tiredness due to anaemia and of bone pain and may develop pathological fractures. Treatment is usually with drugs, such as melphalan or cyclophosphamide, with local radiotherapy to particular areas of pain. *See also* plasmacytoma.

myelomalacia (my-ĕ-loh-mă-lay-shiă) *n.* softening of the tissues of the spinal cord, most often caused by an impaired blood supply.

myelomatosis (my-ĕ-loh-mă-toh-sis) *n. see* myeloma.

myelomeningocele (my-ĕ-loh-min-ing-oh-seel) *n. see* meningomyelocele.

myelosuppression (my-ĕ-loh-sŭ-presh-ŏn) *n.* a reduction in blood-cell production by the bone marrow. It commonly occurs after chemotherapy and may result in anaemia, infection, and abnormal bleeding (*see* thrombocytopenia, neutropenia). —**myelosuppressive** *adj.*

myenteron (my-en-ter-on) *n.* the muscular layer of the intestine, consisting of a layer of circular muscle inside a layer of longitudinal mus-

cle. These muscles are used in peristalsis. —**myenteric** (my-en-te-rik) *adj.*

myiasis (my-ă-sis) *n.* an infestation of a living organ or tissue by maggots. Treatment of external myiases involves the destruction and removal of maggots followed by the application of antibiotics to wounds and lesions.

myo- *prefix. see* my-.

myoblast (my-oh-blast) *n.* a cell that develops into a muscle fibre. —**myoblastic** *adj.*

myocardial infarction (MI) (my-oh-kar-di-ăl) *n.* death of a segment of heart muscle, which follows interruption of its blood supply (*see* coronary thrombosis). The patient experiences sudden severe chest pain, which may spread to the arms and throat. The main danger is that of ventricular fibrillation, which accounts for most of the fatalities. Other complications include heart failure, rupture of the heart, phlebothrombosis, pulmonary embolism, pericarditis, shock, mitral incompetence, and perforation of the septum between the ventricles.

myocarditis (my-oh-kar-dy-tis) *n.* acute or chronic inflammation of the heart muscle. It may be seen alone or as part of endomyocarditis.

myocardium (my-oh-kar-diŭm) *n.* the middle of the three layers forming the wall of the heart (*see also* endocardium, epicardium). It is composed of cardiac muscle and forms the greater part of the heart wall. —**myocardial** *adj.*

myocele (my-oh-seel) *n.* protrusion of a muscle through a rupture in its sheath.

myoclonus (my-oh-kloh-nŭs) *n.*

a sudden spasm of the muscles. Myoclonus is a major feature of some progressive neurological illnesses with extensive degeneration of brain cells. *nocturnal m.* spasm of the muscles on falling asleep, which occurs in normal individuals. —**myoclonic** (my-oh-**klon**-ik) *adj.*

myocyte (my-oh-syt) *n.* a muscle cell.

myodynia (my-oh-**din**-iă) *n.* pain in the muscles.

myofibrosis (my-oh-fy-**broh**-sis) *n.* the replacement of muscle tissue by fibrous tissue, with consequent loss of muscle function.

myogenic (my-oh-**jen**-ik) *adj.* originating in muscle: applied to the inherent rhythmicity of contraction of some muscles (e.g. cardiac muscle), which does not depend on neural influences.

myoglobin (my-oh-**gloh**-bin) *n. see* myohaemoglobin.

myoglobinuria (my-oh-gloh-bin-yoor-iă) *n. see* myohaemoglobinuria.

myogram (my-ŏ-gram) *n.* a recording of the activity of a muscle. *See* electromyography.

myograph (my-ŏ-graf) *n.* an instrument for recording the activity of muscular tissues. *See* electromyography.

myohaemoglobin (myoglobin) (my-oh-hee-moh-**gloh**-bin) *n.* an iron-containing protein, resembling haemoglobin, found in muscle cells. Like haemoglobin it contains a haem group, which binds reversibly with oxygen, and so acts as an oxygen reservoir within the muscle fibres.

myohaemoglobinuria (myo-globinuria)** (my-oh-hee-moh-gloh-bin-yoor-iă) *n.* the presence in the urine of the pigment myohaemoglobin.

myokymia (my-oh-**ky**-miă) *n.* prominent quivering of a few muscle fibres. It is a benign condition. *See also* fasciculation.

myology (my-ol-ŏji) *n.* the study of the structure, function, and diseases of the muscles.

myoma (my-oh-mă) *n.* a benign tumour of muscle. It may originate in smooth muscle (*see* leiomyoma) or in striated muscle.

myomectomy (my-oh-**mek**-tŏmi) *n.* an operation in which benign tumours (fibroids) are removed from the muscular wall of the uterus.

myometritis (my-oh-mi-**try**-tis) *n.* inflammation of the myometrium.

myometrium (my-oh-**mee**-tri-ŭm) *n.* the muscular tissue of the uterus, which surrounds the endometrium. It is composed of smooth muscle that undergoes small regular spontaneous contractions.

myoneural junction (my-oh-**newr**-ăl) *n. see* neuromuscular junction.

myopathy (my-**op**-ă-thi) *n.* any disease of the muscles. The myopathies are usually subdivided into those that are inherited (*see* muscular dystrophy) and those that are acquired. All are typified by weakness and wasting of the muscles, which may be associated with pain and tenderness.

myopia (short-sightedness) (my-**oh**-piă) *n.* the condition in which parallel light rays are brought to a focus in front of the retina. The condition is corrected by wearing spectacles with concave lenses and can now be treated surgically. *Compare* emmetropia, hypermetropia. —**myopic** (my-**op**-ik) *adj.*

Myopia (short-sightedness)

myoplasm (my-oh-plazm) *n. see* sarcoplasm.

myoplasty (my-oh-plasti) *n.* the plastic surgery of muscle, in which part of a muscle is used to repair tissue defects or deformities in the vicinity of the muscle.

myosarcoma (my-oh-sar-koh-mă) *n.* a malignant tumour of muscle. *See also* leiomyosarcoma, rhabdomyosarcoma.

myosin (my-oh-sin) *n.* the most abundant protein in muscle fibrils, having the important properties of elasticity and contractility. *See* striated muscle.

myosis (my-oh-sis) *n. see* miosis.

myositis (my-oh-sy-tis) *n.* any of a group of muscle diseases in which inflammation and degenerative changes occur. Polymyositis is the most commonly occurring example. *m. ossificans* the formation of bone in a muscle that occurs after dislocations or fractures, especially around the elbow.

myotactic (my-oh-tak-tik) *adj.* relating to the sense of touch in muscles. *m. reflex see* stretch reflex.

myotic (my-ot-ik) *n. see* miotic.

myotomy (my-ot-ŏmi) *n.* the dissection or surgical division of a muscle. *See also* cardiomyotomy.

myotonia (my-oh-toh-niă) *n.* a disorder of the muscle fibres that results in abnormally prolonged contractions. It is a feature of a hereditary condition starting in infancy or early childhood (*m. congenita*) and of a form of muscular dystrophy (dystrophia myotonica).

myotonic (my-oh-ton-ik) *adj.* **1.** relating to muscle tone. **2.** relating to myotonia.

myotonus (my-oh-toh-nŭs) *n.* **1.** a tonic muscular spasm. **2.** muscle tone.

myringa (mi-ring-ă) *n.* the eardrum (*see* tympanic membrane).

myringitis (mi-rin-jy-tis) *n.* inflammation of the eardrum, often due to a viral infection.

myringoplasty (**tympano-plasty**) (mi-ring-oh-plasti) *n.* surgical repair of a perforated eardrum by grafting.

myringotome (mi-**ring**-oh-tohm) *n.* a surgical knife used to pierce the eardrum in myringotomy.

myringotomy (mi-ring-ot-ŏmi) *n.* incision of the eardrum to create an artificial opening, either to allow infected fluid to drain from the middle ear in acute otitis media or to re-move fluid in glue ear and permit the insertion of a grommet.

myx- (myxo-) *prefix denoting* mucus.

myxoedema (miks-i-**dee**-mǎ) *n.* **1.** a dry firm waxy swelling of the skin and subcutaneous tissues found in patients with underactive thyroid glands (*see* hypothyroidism). **2.** the clinical syndrome due to hypothyroidism in adult life, including coarsening of the skin, intolerance to cold, weight gain, and mental dullness. *m. coma* a life-threatening condition due to severe hypothyroidism, often precipitated by an acute event, such as surgery, prolonged exposure to cold, infection, trauma, or sedative drugs. —**myxoedematous** *adj.*

myxofibroma (miks-oh-fy-**broh**-mǎ) *n.* a benign tumour of fibrous tissue that contains myxomatous elements or has undergone mucoid degeneration.

myxoid cyst (**miks**-oid) *n.* a small cyst containing a thick sticky fluid.

It develops over the end joint of a finger or toe and should not be cut out, because the cyst is usually in communication with the underlying joint.

myxoma (miks-**oh**-mǎ) *n.* a benign gelatinous tumour of connective tissue. *atrial m.* a tumour of the heart, usually of the left side, arising from the septum dividing the two upper chambers. Symptoms may include fever, lassitude, joint pains, and sudden loss of consciousness. —**myxomatous** *adj.*

myxosarcoma (miks-oh-sar-**koh**-mǎ) *n.* a sarcoma containing mucoid material.

myxovirus (**miks**-oh-vy-rǔs) *n.* one of a group of RNA-containing viruses that are associated with various diseases in animals and humans. The *orthomyxoviruses* cause diseases of the respiratory tract, most notably influenza. The related *paramyxoviruses* include the respiratory syncytial virus (RSV) and the agents causing measles, mumps, and parainfluenza.

Nn

N *symbol for* nitrogen or newton.

Na *symbol for* sodium.

nabilone (nab-i-lohn) *n.* a drug related to cannabis, administered by mouth to control severe nausea and vomiting caused by anticancer drugs. Trade name: **Cesamet**.

nabothian follicle (nabothian cyst, nabothian gland) (nă-boh-thi-ăn) *n.* one of a number of cysts on the cervix of the uterus. The sacs, which contain mucus, form when the ducts of the glands in the cervix are blocked by a new growth of epithelium over an area damaged because of infection. [M. Naboth (1675–1721), German anatomist]

nadolol (nad-ŏ-lol) *n.* a beta blocker administered by mouth for the treatment of angina pectoris and high blood pressure (hypertension). Trade name: **Corgard**.

Naegele rule (nay-gi-li) *n.* a method used to estimate the probable date of the onset of labour: nine months and seven days are added to the date of the first day of the last menstrual period. A correction is required if the woman does not have 28-day menstrual cycles. [F. K. Naegele (1777–1851), German obstetrician]

Naegele's obliquity *n. see* asynclitism.

naevus (nee-vŭs) *n.* (*pl.* **naevi**) a birthmark: a clearly defined malformation of the skin, present at birth. *capillary n.* (*port-wine stain*) a permanent purplish discoloration, composed of small blood vessels, that may occur anywhere but usually appears on the upper half of the body. Laser treatment can reduce the discoloration. Occasionally it may be associated with a malformation of blood vessels over the brain, for example in the Sturge-Weber syndrome. *strawberry n.* (*strawberry mark*) a raised red lump, composed of small blood vessels, usually appearing on the face and growing rapidly in the first month of life. It slowly resolves and spontaneously disappears between the ages of five and ten. *See also* mole[2].

Naga sore (nah-gă) *n. see* tropical ulcer.

NAI *n. see* nonaccidental injury.

nail (nayl) *n.* a horny structure, composed of keratin, formed from the epidermis on the dorsal surface of each finger and toe. Growth of the nail occurs at the end of the nail root, behind the exposed nail, by division of the germinative layer of the underlying epidermis. Anatomical name: **unguis**.

nalidixic acid (nal-i-diks-ik) *n.* a quinolone antibiotic active against various bacteria and administered by mouth to treat infections of the urinary and digestive systems. Trade names: **Negram, Uriben**.

naloxone (nal-oks-ohn) *n.* a drug

that is a specific antidote to morphine and similar narcotic drugs. It is administered by intravenous or subcutaneous injection. As it is short-acting, repeated doses may be necessary. Trade name: **Narcan**.

naltrexone (nal-treks-ohn) *n.* a narcotic antagonist drug used in the maintenance treatment of heroin- and other opiate-dependent patients. It is administered by mouth. Trade name: **Nalorex**.

nandrolone (nan-droh-lohn) *n.* a synthetic male sex hormone with anabolic effects. It is administered by injection in the treatment of aplastic anaemia. Trade name: **Deca-Durabolin**.

nano- *prefix denoting* **1.** extremely small size. **2.** one thousand-millionth part (10^{-9}).

nanometre (nan-oh-mee-ter) *n.* one thousand-millionth of a metre (10^{-9} m). One nanometre is equal to 10 angstrom. Symbol: nm.

nanophthalmos (nan-off-thal-mŏs) *n.* a congenitally small eye in which all the structures are proportionally reduced.

nape (nayp) *n. see* nucha.

napkin rash (nappy rash) (nap-kin) *n.* a red skin rash within the napkin area, usually caused by chemical irritation (ammoniacal dermatitis) or fungal infection with *Candida*. Ammoniacal dermatitis is caused by skin contact with wet soiled nappies; treatment involves exposure to air, application of barrier creams, and frequent nappy changes. Candidal nappy rash is treated with antifungal creams. Other causes of napkin rash include eczema and psoriasis.

naproxen (nă-proks-ĕn) *n.* an anal-

gesic drug that also reduces inflammation and fever (*see* NSAID). It is administered by mouth to treat rheumatoid arthritis, ankylosing spondylitis, and gout. Trade names: **Naprosyn, Nycopren**.

naratriptan (na-ră-trip-tan) *n. see* 5HT₁ agonist.

narcissism (nar-sis-izm) *n.* an excessive involvement with oneself and one's self-importance. In Freudian terms it is a state in which the ego has taken itself as a love object. An extreme degree of narcissism may be a symptom of schizophrenia or personality disorder. —**narcissistic** *adj.*

narco- *prefix denoting* narcosis; stupor.

narcoanalysis (nar-koh-ă-nal-i-sis) *n.* a type of psychotherapy during which the patient is in a relaxed or sleeplike state induced by drugs.

narcolepsy (nar-kŏ-lep-si) *n.* an extreme tendency to fall asleep in quiet surroundings or when engaged in monotonous activities. The patient can be woken easily and is immediately alert. It is often associated with cataplexy, sleep paralysis, and hallucinations at the beginning or end of sleep. —**narcoleptic** *adj., n.*

narcosis (nar-koh-sis) *n.* a state of diminished consciousness or complete unconsciousness caused by the use of narcotic drugs. The body's normal reactions to stimuli are diminished and the body may become sedated or completely anaesthetized.

narcotic (nar-kot-ik) *n.* a drug that relieves pain and also induces stupor and insensibility. The term is used particularly for morphine and other derivatives of opium (*see* opiate) but is also applied to other drugs that depress brain function (e.g. general anaesthetics and hypnotics).

nares (nair-eez) *pl. n.* (*sing.* **naris**) openings of the nose. **external** (or *anterior*) *n.* the nostrils, which lead from the nasal cavity to the outside. **internal** (or *posterior*) *n.* (*choanae*) the openings leading from the nasal cavity into the pharynx.

nasal (nay-zǎl) *adj.* relating to the nose. *n. bone* either of a pair of narrow oblong bones that together form the bridge and root of the nose. *n. cavity* the space inside the nose that lies between the floor of the cranium and the roof of the mouth. *n. concha* (*turbinate bone*) any of three thin scroll-like bones that form the sides of the nasal cavity.

naso- *prefix denoting* the nose.

nasogastric (NG) (nay-zoh-gas-trik) *adj.* relating to the nose and stomach. *n. tube* a tube inserted into the stomach through the nose (*see* intubation).

nasolacrimal (nay-zoh-lak-ri-mǎl) *adj.* relating to the nose and the lacrimal (tear-producing) apparatus. *n. duct* the duct that drains the tears away from the lacrimal apparatus into the inferior meatus of the nose.

nasopharyngeal airway (nay-zoh-fǎ-**rin**-ji-ǎl) *n.* a curved tube to be slotted down one nostril of an unconscious patient, to sit behind the tongue, to create a patent airway. *See also* oropharyngeal airway.

nasopharynx (postnasal space, rhinopharynx) (nay-zoh-fa-rinks) *n.* the part of the pharynx that lies above the level of the junc-

tion of the hard and soft palates. It connects the nasal cavity to the oropharynx. —**nasopharyngeal** *adj.*

nates (nay-teez) *pl. n.* the buttocks. —**natal** (nay-t'l) *adj.*

National Council for Vocational Qualifications (nash-ŏn-ǎl) *n. see* NCVQ.

National Health Service (NHS) *n.* (in the UK) a comprehensive service offering therapeutic and preventive medical and surgical care, including the prescription and dispensing of medicines, spectacles and medical and dental appliances. Exchequer funds pay for the services of doctors, nurses, and other professionals, as well as residential costs in NHS hospitals, and meet a substantial part of the cost of the medicines and appliances.

National Institute of Clinical Excellence (NICE) *n.* a special health authority that aims to promote high-quality treatment and cost-effectiveness of treatments and services. It defines the standards of care to be provided by the NHS, providing guidance and advice on best clinical practice and aiming to reduce geographical variations in care.

national service frameworks (NSF) *pl. n.* national standards of care published for a variety of conditions (the first were for coronary heart disease and mental health), which are designed to improve the quality of care and reduce variations in standards of care.

natriuretic (nay-tri-yoor-et-ik) *n.* an agent that promotes the excretion of sodium salts in the urine. Most diuretics are natriuretics.

natural childbirth (nach-ĕr-ăl) *n.* labour and delivery that relies largely on the efforts of the mother alone, with the minimum of medical intervention.

natural killer cell *n.* a type of lymphocyte that can kill virus-infected cells and cancerous cells and mediates rejection of bone-marrow grafts. These cells are a part of natural immunity.

naturopathy (nay-cher-**op**-ă-thi) *n.* a system of medicine that relies upon the use of only 'natural' substances for the treatment of disease, rather than drugs.

nausea (naw-ziă) *n.* the feeling that one is about to vomit, as experienced in seasickness. Actual vomiting often occurs subsequently.

navel (**nay**-věl) *n. see* umbilicus.

navicular bone (nă-**vik**-yoo-ler) *n.* a boat-shaped bone of the ankle (*see* tarsus) that articulates with the three cuneiform bones in front and with the talus behind.

NBM *n.* nothing (or nil) by mouth.

NCVQ *n.* (in the UK) National Council for Vocational Qualifications: a body set up by the government to achieve a coherent national framework for vocational qualifications in England, Wales, and Northern Ireland. Five levels of *National Vocational Qualification* (*NVQ*) are currently accredited by the council.

NDU *n.* (in the UK) Nursing Development Unit: a centre for creative nursing managed directly by nurses, who are responsible for controlling the budget and appointing staff. The unit can be based in hospital or the community in either the public or the private sector. NDUs are committed to practising research-based patient-centred care.

nearthrosis (nee-arth-**roh**-sis) *n. see* pseudarthrosis.

nebula (**neb**-yoo-lă) *n.* a faint opacity of the cornea that remains after an ulcer has healed.

nebulizer (**neb**-yoo-ly-zer) *n.* an instrument used for applying a liquid in the form of a fine spray.

NEC *n. see* necrotizing enterocolitis.

Necator (ni-**kay**-ter) *n.* a genus of parasitic nematodes that live in the small intestine (*see* hookworm). *N. americanus* the species that infests humans.

neck (nek) *n.* **1.** a narrowed region of the body connecting the head to the trunk. It contains the cervical vertebrae. **2.** any other constricted region of an organ or part, such as the narrow section of the femur between the head and shaft. *See* cervix.

necro- *prefix denoting* death or dissolution.

necrobiosis (nek-roh-by-**oh**-sis) *n.* a gradual process by which cells lose their function and die.

necrology (nek-**rol**-ŏji) *n.* the study of the phenomena of death, involving determination of the moment of death and the different changes that occur in the tissues of the body after death.

necrophilism (**necrophilia**) (nek-**rof**-il-izm) *n.* sexual attraction to corpses. *See also* sexual deviation. —**necrophile** (**nek**-roh-fyl) *n.*

necropsy (**nek**-rop-si) *n. see* autopsy.

necrosis (**mortification**) (nek-**roh**-sis) *n.* the death of some or all of the cells in an organ or tissue, caused by disease, physical or chemical injury, or interference with

the blood supply (*see* gangrene).
—**necrotic** *adj.*

necrospermia (nek-roh-**sper**-miă) *n.* the presence of either dead or motionless spermatozoa in the semen. *See* infertility.

necrotizing enterocolitis (NEC) (nek-rŏ-tyz-ing) *n.* a serious disease affecting the bowel during the first three weeks of life; it is much more common in preterm babies. The abdomen distends and blood and mucus appear in the stools; the bowel may perforate.

necrotizing fasciitis *n.* bacterial infection of the layer of fascia beneath the skin by *Streptococcus* Type A. There is tissue necrosis and toxin production causing shock and organ failure. The elderly and those who have recently undergone surgery are particularly vulnerable to the infection, which requires prompt treatment with antibiotics and excision of the involved tissue.

nedocromil (ned-oh-**kroh**-mil) *n.* a drug used to prevent asthma attacks and treat allergic conjunctivitis. It is administered by metered-dose aerosol inhaler or as eye drops. Trade names: **Rapitil, Tilade**.

needle (nee-d'l) *n.* a slender sharp-pointed instrument. Needles used for sewing up tissue during surgery are equipped with an eye for threading suture material or have the suture material fused onto them. Hollow needles are used to inject substances into the body, to obtain specimens of tissue (*see* puncture), or to withdraw fluid from a cavity. *intraosseous n. see* intraosseous. *See also* stop needle.

needle-stick injury *n.* a common accidental injury to the fingers and hands of nurses and doctors by contaminated injection needles. It can result in transmitted infections (e.g. hepatitis, AIDS).

needling (need-ling) *n.* a form of capsulotomy in which a sharp needle is used to make a hole in the capsule surrounding the lens of the eye. This technique has now largely been replaced by use of the YAG laser.

needs deprivation *n.* an unhealthy state said to exist if an individual is unable to meet basic human needs.

negativism (neg-ă-tiv-izm) *n.* uncooperative or obstructive behaviour. *active n.* negativism in which the individual does the opposite of what he or she is asked. This is usually associated with other features of catatonia. *passive n.* negativism in which the person fails to cooperate, occurring in schizophrenia and depression.

Neisseria (ny-seer-iă) *n.* a genus of spherical Gram-negative aerobic nonmotile bacteria characteristically grouped in pairs. *N. gonorrhoeae* (the gonococcus) the species that causes gonorrhoea, found within pus cells of urethral and vaginal discharge. *N. meningitidis* (the meningococcus) the species that causes meningococcal meningitis. Meningococci are found within pus cells of infected cerebrospinal fluid and blood or in the nasal passages of carriers.

nelfinavir (nel-fin-ă-veer) *n. see* protease inhibitor.

nematode (roundworm) (nem-ă-tohd) *n.* any one of a large group of worms having an unsegmented cylindrical body, tapering at both ends. Some nematodes, including hookworms, filariae, pinworms, and guinea worms, are parasites of humans.

neo- *prefix denoting* new or newly formed.

neoadjuvant chemotherapy (nee-oh-**aj**-oo-vănt) *n.* chemotherapy given before (usually) surgical treatment of a primary tumour with the aim of improving the results of surgery or radiotherapy and preventing the development of metastases. *Compare* adjuvant therapy.

neocerebellum (nee-oh-se-ri-bel-ŭm) *n.* the middle lobe of the cerebellum, excluding the pyramid and uvula.

neologism (ni-ol-ŏ-jizm) *n.* (in psychiatry) the invention of words to which meanings are attached. It may be a symptom of a psychotic illness, such as schizophrenia.

neomycin (nee-oh-**my**-sin) *n.* an aminoglycoside antibiotic used to treat infections caused by a wide range of bacteria, mainly those affecting the skin, ears, and eyes. It is usually applied in creams or drops with other antibiotics, but can also be given by mouth.

neonatal intensive care unit (NICU) (nee-oh-**nay**-t'l) *n.* see intensive care.

neonatal mortality rate *n.* see infant (mortality rate).

neonatal screening *n.* screening tests carried out on newborn babies to detect diseases that appear in the neonatal period, such as phenylketonuria (*see* Guthrie test). Early detection enables treatment to be instigated before irreversible damage occurs to the baby.

neonate (nee-oh-nayt) *n.* an infant

at any time during the first 28 days of life. The word is particularly applied to infants just born or in the first week of life. —**neonatal** *adj.*

neoplasia (nee-oh-**play**-ziă) *n.* the formation of abnormal cells. *See also* CIN, MENS, prostatic intraepithelial neoplasia. *Compare* hyperplasia. —**neoplastic** (nee-oh-**plast**-ik) *adj.*

neoplasm (nee-oh-plazm) *n.* any new and abnormal growth: a benign or malignant tumour. —**neoplastic** *adj.*

neosphincter (nee-oh-sfink-ter) *n.* a substituted muscle or an implant for an absent or ineffective sphincter (*see* artificial sphincter).

neostigmine (nee-oh-**stig**-meen) *n.* an anticholinesterase drug used mainly to diagnose and treat myasthenia gravis and as an antidote to some muscle-relaxant drugs. It is administered by mouth or injection.

neovascularization (nee-oh-vas-kew-ler-I-**zay**-shŏn) *n.* the abnormal formation of new and fragile blood vessels, usually in response to ischaemia. **choroidal n.** the growth of abnormal vessels, derived from the choroid, to form a *choroidal neovascular membrane* in the space below the retinal pigment epithelium (*see* retina). This occurs, for example, in macular degeneration and diabetic retinopathy.

nephr- (nephro-) *prefix denoting* the kidney(s).

nephralgia (ni-**fral**-jiă) *n.* pain in the kidney, which is felt in the loin and can be caused by a variety of kidney complaints.

nephrectomy (ni-**frek**-tŏmi) *n.* surgical removal of a kidney. *radical n.* removal of the entire organ together with its surrounding fat and the adjacent adrenal gland, performed for cancer of the kidney.

nephritis (Bright's disease) (ni-**fry**-tis) *n.* inflammation of the kidney. Nephritis is a nonspecific term used to describe a condition resulting from a variety of causes. *See* glomerulonephritis.

nephroblastoma (Wilms' tumour) (nef-roh-blas-**toh**-mă) *n.* a malignant tumour arising from the embryonic kidney and found in young children (usually between the ages of three and eight). In some cases it is associated with a chromosome abnormality, when aniridia and other abnormal features are present. Treatment is by nephrectomy followed by chemotherapy.

nephrocalcinosis (nef-roh-kal-si-**noh**-sis) *n.* the presence of calcium deposits in the kidneys. This can be caused by excess calcium in the blood, due to overactivity of the parathyroid glands, or it may result from an underlying abnormality of the kidney.

nephrocapsulectomy (nef-roh-kaps-yoo-**lek**-tŏmi) *n.* surgical removal of the fibrous capsule around a kidney.

nephrolithiasis (nef-roh-lith-**I**-ă-sis) *n.* the presence of stones in the kidney (*see* calculus). Such stones can cause pain and blood in the urine, but they may produce no symptoms.

nephrolithotomy (nef-roh-lith-**ot**-ŏmi) *n.* the surgical removal of a stone from the kidney by an incision into the kidney substance. *percutaneous n.* nephrolithotomy that is performed via a nephroscope

passed into the kidney through a tract from the skin surface.

nephrology (ni-**frol**-ŏji) *n.* the branch of medicine concerned with the study, investigation, and management of diseases of the kidney. *See also* urology. —**nephrologist** *n.*

nephroma (ni-**froh**-mă) *n.* a tumour of the kidney.

nephron (**nef**-ron) *n.* the active unit of excretion in the kidney (see illus-

A single nephron

tration). Blood is filtered through the glomerulus into the Bowman's capsule so that water, nitrogenous waste, and many other substances pass into the renal tubule. Here most of the substances are reabsorbed back into the blood, the remaining fluid (urine) passing into the collecting duct, which drains into the ureter.

nephropathy (ni-frop-ă-thi) *n.* disease of the kidney. *diabetic n.* progressive damage to the kidneys seen in some people with long-standing diabetes mellitus.

nephropexy (nef-roh-peks-i) *n.* an operation to fix a mobile kidney. The kidney is fixed to the twelfth rib and adjacent posterior abdominal wall.

nephroptosis (nef-rop-toh-sis) *n.* abnormal descent of a kidney into the pelvis on standing. If this is accompanied by pain and obstruction to free drainage of urine by the kidney, nephropexy may be advised.

nephrosclerosis (nef-roh-skleer-oh-sis) *n.* hardening of the arteries and arterioles of the kidneys.

nephroscope (nef-roh-skohp) *n.* an instrument (*see* endoscope) that is used for examining the interior of the kidney (*nephroscopy*). It is usually passed into the renal pelvis through a track from the skin surface after needle nephrostomy and dilatation of the tract over a guide wire. The nephroscope allows the passage of instruments under direct vision to remove calculi (*see* nephrolithotomy) or disintegrate them by ultrasound probes or electrohydraulic shock waves (*see* lithotripsy).

nephrosis (ni-froh-sis) *n.* (in pathology) degenerative changes in the epithelium of the kidney tubules. The term is sometimes used loosely for the nephrotic syndrome.

nephrostomy (ni-frost-ŏmi) *n.* drainage of urine from the kidney by a tube (catheter) passing through the kidney via the skin surface. This is commonly used as a temporary procedure after operations on the kidney.

nephrotic syndrome (ni-frot-ik) *n.* a condition in which there is great loss of protein in the urine, reduced levels of albumin in the blood, and generalized oedema. It can be caused by a variety of disorders, most usually glomerulonephritis.

nephrotomy (ni-frot-ŏmi) *n.* surgical incision into the substance of the kidney. This is usually undertaken to remove a kidney stone (*see* nephrolithotomy).

nephrotoxic (nef-roh-toks-ik) *adj.* liable to cause damage to the kidneys. Nephrotoxic drugs include aminoglycoside antibiotics, sulphonamides, and gold compounds.

nephroureterectomy (ureteronephrectomy) (nef-roh-yoor-i-ter-ek-tŏmi) *n.* surgical removal of a kidney together with its ureter. This operation is performed for cancer of the kidney pelvis or ureter.

nerve (nerv) *n.* a bundle of nerve fibres enclosed in a connective tissue sheath (see illustration). *motor n.* a nerve that transmits impulses from the brain or spinal cord to the muscles and glands. *sensory n.* a nerve that transmits impulses inwards from the sense organs to the brain and spinal cord.

nerve block *n.* a method of producing anaesthesia in part of the body by blocking the passage of pain impulses in the sensory nerves supplying it. A local anaesthetic, such as lidocaine, is injected into the tissues in the region to be anaesthetized. *See also* ring block.

nerve cell *n. see* neurone.

nerve ending *n.* the final part (terminal) of one of the branches of a nerve fibre, where a neurone makes contact either with another neurone or with a muscle or gland cell.

nerve entrapment syndrome (in-**trap**-mĕnt) *n.* any syndrome resulting from pressure on a nerve from surrounding structures. Examples include the carpal tunnel syndrome and meralgia paraesthetica.

nerve fibre *n.* the long fine process that extends from the cell body of a neurone and carries nerve impulses. Bundles of nerve fibres running together form a nerve.

nerve gas *n.* any gas that disrupts the normal functioning of nerves and thus of the muscles they supply.

nerve impulse *n.* the electrical activity in the membrane of a neurone that is the means by which information is transmitted within the nervous system along the axons of the neurones.

nerve regeneration *n.* the growth of new nerve tissue, which occurs at a very slow rate (1–2 mm per day) after a nerve has been severed and is often partially or totally incomplete. *See also* axonotmesis, neurotmesis.

nervous breakdown (ner-vŭs brayk-down) *n.* a lay term applied to a range of emotional crises varying from a brief attack of 'hysterical' behaviour to a major psychoneurotic illness with severe long-term effects on the life of the sufferer. The term is also sometimes used as a euphemism for a frank psychiatric illness, such as schizophrenia.

nervous system *n.* the vast network of cells specialized to carry information (in the form of nerve impulses) to and from all parts of the body in order to bring about bodily activity. *See* autonomic nervous system, central nervous system, peripheral nervous system.

Nesbit's operation (nez-bits) *n.* an operation originally devised to surgically straighten a congenitally curved penis but now more frequently employed to correct the penile curvature caused by Peyronie's disease. [R. M. Nesbit (20th century), US surgeon]

neurilemma
myelin sheath
nerve fibre
endoneurium
epineurium
perineurium

fascicle
(a group
of fibres)

Transverse section through a
nerve

nesidioblastosis (nes-idi-oh-blas-toh-sis) *n.* a rare condition of childhood in which abnormal cells in the pancreas secrete a selection of hormones (including insulin) in an uncontrolled manner. This causes a variety of problems, including recurrent hypoglycaemia.

nettle rash (ne-t'l) *n. see* urticaria.

Neuman's model (new-mǎnz) *n.* a systems model for nursing that can be interpreted to include various social and physiological systems. The goal of nursing is seen as maintaining equilibrium within these systems, which should lead to the 'whole' person being restored to health. *See also* nursing models. [B. Neuman (1924–), US nurse theorist]

neur- (**neuro-**) *prefix denoting* nerves or the nervous system.

neural (newr-ǎl) *adj.* relating to a nerve or nerves. *n. arch see* vertebra.

neuralgia (newr-al-jǎ) *n.* a severe burning or stabbing pain often following the course of a nerve. *postherpetic n.* intense debilitating pain felt at the site of a previous attack of shingles. *trigeminal n.* (*tic douloureux*) neuralgia in which brief paroxysms of searing pain are felt in the distribution of one or more branches of the trigeminal nerve in the face.

neural tube *n.* a hollow tube of tissue in the embryo from which the brain and spinal cord develop. It is formed when two edges of a groove in a plate of primitive neural tissue (*neural plate*) come together and fuse.

neural tube defects *pl. n.* a group of congenital abnormalities involving defects in the spine or skull caused by failure of the neural tube to form normally. They include spina bifida, in which the bony arches of the spine fail to close, and more severe defects of bone fusion involving herniation of neural tissue and consequent mental and physical disorders, such as meningocele, meningomyelocele, and meningoencephalocele.

neurapraxia (newr-ǎ-praks-iǎ) *n.* temporary loss of nerve function resulting in tingling, numbness, and weakness. It is usually caused by compression of the nerve.

neurasthenia (newr-ǎs-th'ee-niǎ) *n.* a set of psychological and physical symptoms, including fatigue, irritability, headache, and dizziness. It can be caused by organic damage, such as a head injury, or it can be due to neurosis. —**neurasthenic** *adj., n.*

neurectasis (newr-ek-tǎ-sis) *n.* the surgical procedure for stretching a peripheral nerve.

neurectomy (newr-ek-tŏmi) *n.* the surgical removal of the whole or part of a nerve.

neurilemma (**neurolemma**) (newr-i-lem-ǎ) *n.* the sheath of the axon of a nerve fibre. The neurilemma of a medullated fibre contains myelin. —**neurilemmal** *adj.*

neurilemmoma (**neurinoma**) (newr-i-lem-oh-mǎ) *n.* a benign slow-growing tumour that arises from the neurilemma of a nerve fibre.

neurinoma (newr-i-noh-mǎ) *n. see* neurilemmoma.

neuritis (newr-I-tis) *n.* a disease of the peripheral nerves showing the pathological changes of inflammation. The term is also used in a less precise sense as an alternative to neuropathy. *See also* retrobulbar neuritis.

neuroanatomy (newr-oh-ă-**nat**-ŏmi) *n.* the study of the structure of the nervous system.

neuroblast (**newr**-oh-blast) *n.* any of the nerve cells of the embryo that give rise to neurones.

neuroblastoma (newr-oh-blas-**toh** mă) *n.* a malignant tumour, usually of childhood, composed of embryonic nerve cells. It may originate in any part of the sympathetic nervous system, most commonly in the medulla of the adrenal gland.

neurocranium (newr-oh-**kray**-niŭm) *n.* the part of the skull that encloses the brain.

neurodermatitis (newr-oh-derm-ă-**ty**-tis) *n.* see lichen (simplex chronicus).

neuroendocrine system (newr-oh-**end**-ŏ-kryn) *n.* the system of dual control of certain activities of the body by means of both nerves and circulating hormones. It can give rise to *neuroendocrine tumours*, which secrete active hormones. *See* neurohormone, neurosecretion.

neuroepithelioma (newr-oh-epith'ee-li-**oh**-mă) *n.* a malignant tumour of the retina of the eye. It is a form of glioma and may spread into the brain if not treated early.

neuroepithelium (newr-oh-epith'ee-liŭm) *n.* a type of epithelium associated with organs of special sense. It contains sensory nerve endings and is found in the retina, the membranous labyrinth, and the taste buds. —**neuroepithelial** *adj.*

neurofibroma (Schwannoma) (newr-oh-fy-**broh**-mă) *n.* a benign tumour growing from the fibrous coverings of a peripheral nerve.

neurofibromatosis (von Recklinghausen's disease) (newr-oh-fy-broh-mă-**toh**-sis) *n.* a congenital disease, typified by numerous neurofibromas. Tumours may occur in the spinal canal, where they may press on the spinal cord. The tumours sometimes (but rarely) become malignant, giving rise to *neurofibrosarcomas*.

neurogenesis (newr-oh-**jen**-i-sis) *n.* the growth and development of nerve cells.

neurogenic (newr-oh-**jen**-ik) *adj.* **1.** caused by disease or dysfunction of the nervous system. **2.** arising in nervous tissue. **3.** caused by nerve stimulation.

neuroglia (newr-**og**-liă) *n.* see glia.

neurohormone (newr-oh-**hor**-mohn) *n.* a hormone, such as vasopressin or noradrenaline, that is produced within specialized nerve cells and is secreted from the nerve endings into the circulation.

neurohypophysis (newr-oh-hy-**pof**-i-sis) *n.* see pituitary gland.

neurolemma (newr-oh-**lem**-ă) *n.* see neurilemma.

neuroleptic (newr-oh-**lep**-tik) *n.* any drug that induces an altered state of consciousness, such as an antipsychotic drug.

neurology (newr-**ol**-ŏji) *n.* the study of the structure, functioning, and diseases of the nervous system (including the brain, spinal cord, and all the peripheral nerves). —**neurological** *adj.* —**neurologist** *n.*

neuroma (newr-oh-**mă**) *n.* any tumour derived from cells of the nervous system, now usually categorized more specifically (e.g.

neurofibroma, neurilemmoma).

acoustic n. a slow-growing benign tumour of the sheath of the vestibular nerve. It progresses to cause tinnitus and hearing loss.

neuromuscular junction (myoneural junction) (newr-oh-mus-kew-ler) *n.* the meeting point of a motor nerve fibre and the muscle fibre that it supplies. It consists of a minute gap across which a neurotransmitter must diffuse from the nerve to trigger contraction of the muscle.

neuromyelitis optica (Devic's disease) (newr-oh-my-ĕ-ly-tis op-tik-ă) *n.* a condition that is closely related to multiple sclerosis. Typically there is a transverse myelitis, producing paralysis and numbness of the limbs and trunk below the inflamed spinal cord, and retrobulbar (optic) neuritis affecting both optic nerves.

neurone (nerve cell) (newr-ohn) *n.* one of the basic functional units of the nervous system: a cell specialized to transmit electrical nerve impulses and so carry information from one part of the body to another (see illustration). Impulses enter the neurone through branches of the dendrites and are carried away from the cell body through the axon (nerve fibre). They are transmitted to adjacent neurones or to effector organs through minute gaps (*see* synapse, neuromuscular junction). *See also* motor neurone.

neuropathic bladder *n.* a malfunctioning bladder due to partial or complete interruption of its nerve supply. Causes include injury to the spinal cord, spina bifida, mul-

tiple sclerosis, and diabetic neuropathy.

neuropathy (newr-op-ă-thi) *n.* disease of one or more of the peripheral nerves, usually causing weakness and numbness. *diabetic n.* neuropathy seen in some people with long-standing diabetes, most commonly affecting the legs. *peripheral n.* (*polyneuritis, polyneuropathy*) neuropathy affecting sensory and/or motor nerves and

Types of neurone:
motor (left) and sensory (right)

tending to start in the fingers and toes and progress proximally. Causes include diabetes, alcohol, certain drugs, infections (e.g. HIV), and Charcot-Marie-Tooth disease. —**neuropathic** (newr-oh-**path**-ik) *adj.*

neurophysiology (newr-oh-fiz-i-ol-ŏji) *n.* the study of the complex chemical and physical changes that are associated with the activity of the nervous system.

neuroplasty (**newr**-oh-plasti)*n.* reconstructive surgery for damaged or severed peripheral nerves.

neuropsychiatry (newr-oh-si-ky-ă-tri) *n.* the branch of medicine concerned with the psychiatric effects of disorders of neurological function or structure. It investigates the relationship between demonstrable brain changes and the resulting effects on the mind.

neurorrhaphy (newr-o-răfi) *n.* the operation of suturing a cut nerve.

neurosecretion (newr-oh-si-**kree**-shŏn) *n.* any substance produced within, and secreted by, a nerve cell. Important examples are the hormone-releasing factors produced by the cells of the hypothalamus.

neurosis (newr-**oh**-sis) *n.* (*pl.* **neuroses**) any long-term mental or behavioural disorder in which contact with reality is retained and the condition is recognized by the sufferer as abnormal. A neurosis essentially features anxiety or behaviour exaggeratedly designed to avoid anxiety. Defence mechanisms against anxiety take various forms and may appear as phobias, obsessions, compulsions, or sexual dysfunctions. Behaviour therapy seems effective in some cases. In accordance with a recent classification, the disorders formerly included under the neuroses have been renamed *anxiety disorders*. *See also* anxiety, conversion disorder, depression, dissociative disorder, obsession. —**neurotic** (newr-**ot**-ik) *adj.*

neurosurgery (newr-oh-**ser**-jer-i) *n.* the surgical or operative treatment of diseases of the brain and spinal cord.

neurosyphilis (newr-oh-**sif**-i-lis) *n.* syphilis affecting the nervous system.

neurotmesis (newr-ot-**mee**-sis) *n.* an injury in which a nerve is severed. Nerve regeneration is slow.

neurotomy (newr-**ot**-ŏmi) *n.* the surgical procedure of severing a nerve.

neurotoxic (newr-oh-**toks**-ik) *adj.* poisonous or harmful to nerve cells.

neurotransmitter (newr-oh-tranz-**mit**-er) *n.* a chemical substance, such as acetylcholine, noradrenaline, dopamine, or serotonin, that is released from nerve endings to transmit impulses across synapses to other nerves and across the minute gaps between the nerves and the muscles or glands that they supply.

neurotrophic (newr-oh-**trof**-ik) *adj.* relating to the growth and nutrition of neural tissue in the body.

neurotropic (newr-oh-**trop**-ik) *adj.* growing towards or having an affinity for neural tissue. The term may be applied to viruses, chemicals, or toxins.

neutropenia (new-troh-**pee**-niă) *n.* a decrease in the number of neutrophils in the blood. Neutropenia may occur in a wide variety of diseases, including aplastic anaemias, agranulocytosis, and acute leukae-mias, and after chemotherapy or radiotherapy. It results in an increased susceptibility to infections.

neutrophil (new-trŏ-fil) *n.* a variety of granulocyte distinguished by the presence in its cytoplasm of fine granules that stain purple with Romanowsky stains. It is capable of ingesting and killing bacteria and provides an important defence against infection.

newton (new-t'n) *n.* the SI unit of force, equal to the force required to impart to 1 kilogram an acceleration of 1 metre per second per second. Symbol: N.

nexus (neks-ŭs) *n.* (in anatomy) a connection or link.

NG *adj. see* nasogastric.

NGU *n. see* (nongonococcal) urethritis.

NHL *n. see* (non-Hodgkin's) lymphoma.

NHS *n. see* National Health Service.

NHS Direct *n.* a 24-hour nurse-led telephone helpline providing health-care advice and information on a variety of medical problems. There is also an NHS Direct online service available via the Internet, which provides a guide to treating many medical conditions.

NHSTA *n.* (in the UK) National Health Service Training Authority: a statutory body established in 1983 to identify training needs, formulate, coordinate, and develop national policies and standards, and provide and arrange for the provision of training programmes, courses, and research to cover all health professionals working in the NHS.

NHS walk-in centre *n.* a medical centre offering free and fast access to health-care advice and treatment. Centres provide guidance on how to utilize NHS services as well as advice on minor injuries and illnesses.

niacin (ny-ă-sin) *n. see* nicotinic acid.

nicardipine (ni-kar-di-peen) *n.* a calcium antagonist used to treat long-term angina. It is administered by mouth. Trade name: **Cardene**.

NICE *n. see* National Institute of Clinical Excellence.

niclosamide (ni-kloh-să-myd) *n.* an anthelmintic drug used to remove tapeworms. It is administered by mouth and is relatively free of side effects. Trade name: **Yomesan**.

nicorandil (nik-or-and-il) *n. see* potassium-channel activator.

nicotinamide (nik-ŏ-tin-ă-myd) *n.* a B vitamin: the amide of nicotinic acid.

nicotine (nik-ŏ-teen) *n.* a poisonous alkaloid derived from tobacco, responsible for the dependence of regular smokers on cigarettes. In small doses nicotine has a stimulating effect on the autonomic nervous system. Large doses cause paralysis of the autonomic ganglia.

nicotinic acid (niacin) (nik-ŏ-tin-ik) *n.* a B vitamin. Nicotinic acid is required in the diet but can also be formed in small amounts in the body from the essential amino acid tryptophan. A deficiency of the vitamin leads to pellagra. Good sources of nicotinic acid are meat, yeast extracts, and some cereals.

nictitation (nik-ti-tay-shŏn) *n.* exaggerated and frequent blinking or winking of the eyes.

NICU *n.* neonatal intensive care unit: *see* intensive care.

nidation (ny-**day**-shŏn) *n. see* implantation.

nidus (**ny**-dŭs) *n.* a place in which bacteria have settled and multiplied because of particularly suitable conditions: a focus of infection.

Niemann-Pick disease (nee-man pik) *n.* a rare inherited disease of phospholipid metabolism in which sphingomyelin and lecithin accumulate in the bone marrow, spleen, and lymph nodes. It is characterized by enlargement of the liver and the spleen and by physical and mental retardation. [A. Niemann (1880–1921), German paediatrician; F. Pick (1868–1935), German physician]

nifedipine (ny-**fed**-i-peen) *n.* a calcium antagonist used in the treatment of angina, hypertension, and Raynaud's phenomenon. It is administered by mouth; side-effects include dizziness, headache, and nausea. Trade names: **Adalat, Coracten, Nifopress, Slofedine.**

night blindness (nyt) *n.* the inability to see in dim light or at night. It is due to a disorder of the rods in the retina and can result from dietary deficiency of vitamin A. Its manifestations may progress to include xerophthalmia and keratomalacia. Night blindness may be caused by other retinal diseases, e.g. retinitis pigmentosa. Medical name: **nyctalopia.** *Compare* day blindness.

night sweat *n.* copious sweating during sleep. Night sweats may be an early indication of tuberculosis, AIDS, or other disease.

night terror *n.* the condition in which a young child, soon after falling asleep, starts screaming and

appears terrified. The attack ceases when the child wakes up fully and is never remembered.

nihilistic (ny-i-lis-tik) *adj.* (in psychiatry) describing or relating to the state of patients who believe that they and things about them do not exist.

nipple (mamilla, papilla) (nip-ŭl) *n.* the protuberance at the centre of the breast. In females the milk ducts open at the nipple.

Nissl granules (nis-ŭl) *pl. n.* collections of dark-staining material, containing RNA, seen in the cell bodies of neurones on microscopic examination. [F. Nissl (1860–1919) German neuropathologist]

nit (nit) *n.* the egg of a louse. The eggs of head lice are firmly cemented to the hair; those of body lice are fixed to the clothing.

nitrates (**ny**-trayts) *pl. n.* a class of drugs used as coronary vasodilators for the treatment and prevention of angina attacks. They include glyceryl trinitrate, isosorbide dinitrate, and isosorbide mononitrate.

nitrazepam (ny-**traz**-ĕ-pam) *n.* a benzodiazepine drug administered by mouth to treat insomnia and sleep disturbances. Trade name: **Mogadon.**

nitric acid (**ny**-trik) *n.* a strong corrosive mineral acid, the concentrated form of which is capable of producing severe burns of the skin. Swallowing the acid leads to intense burning pain and ulceration of the mouth and throat. Treatment is by immediate administration of alkaline solutions. Formula: HNO_3.

nitric oxide *n.* an important gaseous mediator that is involved in the manifestations of sepsis and septic shock. Formula: NO.

nitrofurantoin (ny-troh-fewr-**ant**-oh-in) *n.* a drug administered by mouth to treat bacterial infections of the urinary system. Trade names: **Furadantin, Macrodantin.**

nitrogen (**ny**-trŏ-jĕn) *n.* a gaseous element and a major constituent of air (79%). Nitrogen is an essential constituent of proteins and nucleic acids and is obtained by humans in the form of protein-containing foods. Nitrogenous waste is excreted as urea. Liquid nitrogen is used to freeze some specimens before pathological examination. Symbol: N.

nitrogen balance *n.* the relationship between the nitrogen taken into the body and that excreted, denoting the balance between the manufacture and breakdown of the body mass. A negative nitrogen balance, when excretion exceeds intake, is usual after injury or operations as the energy requirements of the body are met disproportionately from endogenous sources.

nitrogen mustard *n. see* chlormethine.

nitroglycerin (ny-troh-**glis**-er-in) *n. see* glyceryl trinitrate.

nitroprusside (ny-troh-**prus**-syd) *n.* a cyanide-containing drug used in the emergency treatment of high blood pressure. Given by controlled infusion into a vein, its effects and level in the blood must be closely monitored.

nitrous oxide (**ny**-trŭs) *n.* a colourless gas used as an anaesthetic with good analgesic properties. A mixture of nitrous oxide and oxygen is administered by inhalation for some dental procedures and in childbirth. Because it tends to excite the patient when used alone, nitrous oxide was formerly known popularly as *laughing gas*. Formula: N_2O.

nizatidine (ny-**zat**-i-deen) *n.* an H_2-receptor antagonist (*see* antihistamine) used to treat gastric and duodenal ulcers and prevent their recurrence and to treat gastrooesophageal reflux disease. It is administered by mouth or infusion. Trade names: **Axid, Zinga.**

nm *symbol for* nanometre.

NMC *n. see* Nursing and Midwifery Council.

NMR *n. see* nuclear magnetic resonance.

Nocardia (noh-**kar**-diǎ) *n.* a genus of rodlike or filamentous Gram-positive nonmotile bacteria found in the soil. *N. asteroides* the species that causes nocardiosis. *N. madurae* the species associated with the disease Madura foot.

nocardiosis (noh-kar-di-**oh**-sis) *n.* a disease caused by bacteria of the genus *Nocardia*, primarily affecting the lungs, skin, and brain, resulting in the formation of abscesses.

noci- *prefix denoting* pain or injury.

nociceptive (noh-si-**sep**-tiv) *adj.* describing nerve fibres, endings, or pathways that are concerned with the condition of pain.

nociceptor (noh-si-**sep**-ter) *n.* a receptor that responds to the stimuli responsible for the sensation of pain. Nociceptors may be interoceptors, responding to such stimuli as inflammation, or exteroceptors, sensitive to heat, etc.

noct- (nocti-) *prefix denoting* night.

noctambulation (nok-tam-bew-lay-shŏn) *n. see* somnambulism.

nocturia (nokt-yoor-iă) *n.* the passage of urine at night. Nocturia usually occurs in elderly people, since the normal rhythm of making less urine at night is lost with age.

nocturnal enuresis (nok-ter-năl) *n. see* enuresis.

node (nohd) *n.* a small swelling or knot of tissue. *See* atrioventricular node, lymph node, sinoatrial node. **n. of Ranvier** one of the gaps that occur at regular intervals in the myelin sheath of medullated nerve fibres, between adjacent Schwann cells. [L. A. Ranvier (1835–1922), French pathologist]

nodule (nod-yool) *n.* a small swelling or aggregation of cells.

noma (noh-mă) *n.* a gangrenous infection of the mouth that spreads to involve the face. It is a severe form of ulcerative gingivitis that is usually found in debilitated or undernourished individuals.

nonaccidental injury (NAI) (non-aks-i-**den**-t'l) *n.* injury inflicted on babies and young children; the perpetrator is usually an adult – often a parent or step-parent. Known colloquially as the *battered baby syndrome*, it is most commonly seen in babies aged six months or less. It usually takes the form of bruising, particularly on the face; bite marks; burns or scalds, particularly cigarette burns; and bone injuries, especially spiral fractures of the long bones in the limbs and skull fractures. Internal injuries may be fatal. Careful examination often reveals several injuries of different ages, indicating long-term abuse. NAI usually has serious consequences for the child, including failure to thrive and behavioural problems.

non compos mentis (non kompŏs men-tis) *adj.* Latin: mentally incapable of managing one's own affairs.

noninvasive (non-in-vay-siv) *adj.* **1.** denoting techniques of investigation or treatment that do not involve penetration of the skin by needles or knives. **2.** denoting tumours that do not spread into surrounding tissues (*see* benign).

nonmaleficence (non-mal-ef-i-sĕns) *n.* (in health care) the duty to avoid harming the interests of others.

Nonne's syndrome (cerebellar syndrome) (non-ĕz) *n.* a form of cerebellar ataxia. *See* ataxia. [M. Nonne (1861–1959), German neurologist]

nonsteroidal anti-inflammatory drug (non-steer-oi-d'l) *n. see* NSAID.

Noonan's syndrome (noo-nănz) *n.* an autosomal dominant condition of males who have all or some of the physical features of Turner's syndrome in females but normal sex chromosomes. It is often associated with a low testosterone level and sometimes with reduced sperm production. Other features include cardiovascular defects. [J. Noonan (1921–), US paediatrician]

noradrenaline (norepinephrine) (nor-ă-dren-ă-lin) *n.* a hormone, closely related to adrenaline, secreted by the medulla of the adrenal gland and also released as a neurotransmitter by sympathetic nerve endings. Among its many actions are constriction of small blood vessels leading to an increase in blood pressure, increase in the rate and depth of breathing, and relaxation of the smooth muscle in intestinal walls.

norepinephrine (nor-epi-**nef**-rin) *n. see* noradrenaline.

norethisterone (nor-eth-ist-er-ohn) *n.* a synthetic female sex hormone (*see* progestogen) administered by mouth to treat menstrual disorders, including amenorrhoea. Its main use, however, is in oral contraceptives and hormone replacement therapy. Trade names: **Micronor, Primolut N**, etc.

norfloxacin (nor-**floks**-ă-sin) *n.* a quinolone antibiotic used for treating urinary-tract infections. Trade name: **Utinor**.

normalization (nor-mă-ly-**zay**-shŏn) *n.* (in psychiatry) the process of making the living conditions of people with mental handicap as similar as possible to those of people who are not handicapped. This includes moves to living outside institutions and encouragement to cope with work, pay, social life, sexuality, and civil rights.

normo- *prefix denoting* normality.

normoblast (nor-moh-blast) *n.* a nucleated cell that forms part of the series giving rise to the red blood cells and is normally found in the blood-forming tissue of the bone marrow. *See also* erythroblast, erythropoiesis.

normocyte (nor-moh-syt) *n.* a red blood cell of normal size. —**normocytic** *adj.*

normotensive (nor-moh-ten-siv) *adj.* describing the state in which the arterial blood pressure is within the normal range. *Compare* hypertension, hypotension.

nortriptyline (nor-**trip**-ti-leen) *n.* a tricyclic antidepressant drug that is administered by mouth to relieve all types of depression. Trade name: **Allegron**.

nose (nohz) *n.* the organ of olfaction, which also acts as an air passage that warms, moistens, and filters the air on its way to the lungs. It consists of a triangular cartilaginous projection in the front of the face that contains the nostrils (*see* nares). It leads to the nasal cavity, which is lined with mucous membrane containing olfactory cells.

nosebleed (nohz-bleed) *n. see* epistaxis.

noso- *prefix denoting* disease.

nosocomial infection (hospital-acquired infection, HAI) (nos-oh-**koh**-mi-ăl) *n.* an infection whose development is favoured by a hospital environment, such as one acquired by a patient during a hospital visit or one developing among hospital staff. Such infections include fungal and bacterial infections and are aggravated by the reduced resistance of individual patients.

nosology (nos-ol-ŏji) *n.* the naming and classification of diseases.

nostrils (nos-trilz) *pl. n. see* nares.

notch (noch) *n.* (in anatomy) an indentation, especially one in a bone.

notifiable disease (noh-ti-fy-ăbŭl) *n.* a disease that must be reported to the Health Authorities in order that speedy control and preventive action may be undertaken if necessary. In Great Britain such diseases include diphtheria, dysentery, food poisoning, infective jaundice, malaria, measles, polio-myelitis, tuberculosis, typhoid, and whooping cough.

NPF *n. see* nurse prescribers' formulary.

NSAID (nonsteroidal anti-inflammatory drug) *n.* any one of a large group of drugs that are used for pain relief, particularly in rheumatic disease associated with inflammation. NSAIDs act by inhibiting the enzymes controlling the formation of prostaglandins, which are important mediators of inflammation. They include aspirin, azapropazone, diflunisal, ibuprofen, ketoprofen, and naproxen. Adverse effects include gastric bleeding and ulceration. *See also* COX 2 inhibitor.

NSF *pl. n. see* national service frameworks.

NSU *n. see* (nonspecific) urethritis.

nucha (new-kǎ) *n.* the nape of the neck.

nuchal (new-kǎl) *adj.* relating to the nape of the neck. *n.* fold of skin at the back of the neck of the fetus. *n. thickness scanning* an ultrasound screening test performed during pregnancy at 10–14 weeks of gestation that examines the thickness of the nuchal fold as an aid to the prenatal diagnosis of chromosomal defects. The thicker the nuchal fold, the higher the risk of the baby having a chromosomal defect. *See also* ultrasound marker.

nucle- (nucleo-) *prefix denoting* a cell nucleus.

nuclear magnetic resonance (NMR) *n.* the absorption and emission of high-frequency radio waves by the nuclei of certain elements when placed in a strong magnetic field. The strongest signal is obtained from hydrogen atoms, which are abundant in the water and organic molecules in the body. NMR has important applications in noninvasive diagnostic techniques. *See* magnetic resonance imaging.

nuclear medicine *n.* the use of radionuclides (especially technetium-99m) as tracers to study the structure and function of organs of the body, often using a gamma camera. *See also* cardiology.

nuclease (new-kli-ayz) *n.* an enzyme that catalyses the breakdown of nucleic acids by cleaving the bonds between adjacent nucleotides.

nucleic acid (new-klee-ik) *n.* either of two organic acids, DNA or RNA, present in the nucleus and in some cases the cytoplasm of all living cells.

nucleolus (new-kli-oh-lŭs) *n.* (*pl.* **nucleoli**) a dense spherical structure within the cell nucleus that disappears during cell division. The nucleolus contains RNA for the synthesis of ribosomes.

nucleoprotein (new-kli-oh-proh-teen) *n.* a compound that occurs in cells and consists of nucleic acid and protein tightly bound together.

nucleoside (new-kli-ŏ-syd) *n.* a compound that consists of a nitrogen-containing base (a purine or pyrimidine) linked to a sugar.

nucleotide (new-kli-ŏ-tyd) *n.* a compound that consists of a nitrogen-containing base (a purine or pyrimidine) linked to a sugar and a phosphate group. Nucleic acids are long chains of linked nucleotides.

nucleus (new-kli-ŭs) *n.* (*pl.* **nuclei**) **1.** the part of a cell that contains the genetic material, DNA. The nucleus also contains RNA, most of which is located in the nucleolus. **2.** an anatomically and functionally distinct mass of nerve cells within the brain or spinal cord. **3.** the central part of the lens of the eye, which is harder than the outer cortex.

nucleus pulposus (pul-poh-sŭs) *n.* the central part of an intervertebral disc, which consists of a soft pulpy material.

nullipara (nul-ip-er-ǎ) *n.* a woman who has never given birth to an infant capable of survival.

nurse (ners) *n.* a person who has completed a programme of basic nursing education and is qualified and authorized in his or her country to practise nursing. In Britain, the Nursing and Midwifery Council is the registering statutory body and is responsible for the regulation of these professions in the interest of the public. Students of nursing undertake a three-year course to qualify as a *registered n.* (*RN*; adult health, child health, mental health, or learning disabilities). Before 1989 training culminated in qualification as a *first-level n.*, leading to registration either as a *registered general n.* (*RGN*), *mental n.* (*RMN*), *sick children's n.* (*RSCN*), or a *n. for the mentally handicapped* (*RNMH*), or as a *second-level n.* See district nurse, enrolled nurse, first-level nurse, health visitor, midwife, nurse practitioner, occupational health nurse, practice nurse, school nurse, second-level nurse.

nurse practitioner *n.* a nurse specialist with advanced skills in physical diagnosis, psychosocial assessment, and management of patients' needs in primary care. A key member of the health-care team, a nurse practitioner can be based in a group practice or a health centre. Patients may present to the nurse or be referred to her for direct consultation about health problems. The nurse practitioner has the authority to prescribe drugs and other treatments within agreed policies.

nurse prescribers' formulary (NPF) *n.* a formulary from which nurses who have completed an appropriate course are required to prescribe. It covers a limited range of drugs that relate to an individual specialist practice area.

Nursing and Midwifery Council (NMC) *n.* a body that superseded the UKCC in April 2002. It combines the functions of the old UKCC and the National Boards (England, Scotland, Wales, and Northern Ireland), having a regulatory role for both professional issues and education.

nursing audit (ners-ing) *n.* the process of collecting information from nursing reports and other documented evidence about patient care and assessing the quality of care by the use of quality assurance programmes. *See* quality assurance, performance indicators.

nursing intervention *n.* an act to implement the care plan as part of the nursing process. *See* planning.

nursing models *pl. n.* abstract frameworks, linking facts and phenomena, that assist nurses to plan nursing care, investigate problems related to clinical practice, and study the outcomes of nursing actions and interventions. Most nursing models are of North American origin but some have gained acceptance in the UK and are used in conjunction with the nursing process. *See* Casey's model, Henderson's model, King's model, Neumann's model, Orem's model, Peplau's model, Roper, Logan, and Tierney model, Roy's model.

nursing process *n.* an individualized problem-solving approach to nursing care. It involves four stages: assessment (of the patient's problems), planning (how to resolve them), implementation (of the plans), and evaluation (of their success).

nursing standard *n.* a measure or measures by which nursing care can be judged or compared; the measures used are agreed upon by common consent. Standards for an agreed level of care for a particular purpose should be derived and set with the participation of all those involved. *See also* quality circle.

nutation (new-**tay**-shŏn) *n.* the act of nodding the head.

nutrient (**new**-tri-ĕnt) *n.* a substance that must be consumed as part of the diet to provide a source of energy, material for growth, or substances for regulating growth or energy production. Nutrients include carbohydrates, proteins, fats, vitamins, and certain minerals, including the trace elements.

nutrition (new-**trish**-ŏn) *n.* **1.** the study of food in relation to the physiological processes that depend on its absorption by the body. The science of nutrition includes the study of diets and deficiency diseases. **2.** the intake of nutrients and their subsequent absorption and assimilation by the tissues. Patients who cannot be fed in a normal way can be given either nutrients by tubes into the intestines (*enteral feeding*)

or a nutrient solution that does not require digesting by infusion into a vein (*parenteral feeding*). **total parenteral** *n.* (*TPN*) the provision of all the essential nutrients to a patient by parenteral feeding.

nyct- (nycto-) *prefix denoting* night or darkness.

nyctalopia (nik-tă-**loh**-piă) *n. see* night blindness.

nyctohemeral (nik-toh-**hem**-er-ăl) *adj.* denoting a cyclical event occurring both in the day and the night.

nyctophobia (nik-toh-**foh**-biă) *n.* extreme fear of the dark. It is common in children and not unusual in normal adults.

nympho- *prefix denoting* **1.** the labia minora. **2.** female sexuality.

nymphomania (nim-fŏ-**may**-niă) *n.* an extreme degree of sexual promiscuity in a woman. —**nymphomaniac** *adj.*, *n.*

nystagmus (nis-**tag**-mŭs) *n.* rapid involuntary movements of the eyes that may be from side to side, up and down, or rotatory. Nystagmus may be congenital and associated with poor sight; it also occurs in disorders of the part of the brain responsible for eye movements and in disorders of the organ of balance in the ear.

nystatin (**nis**-tă-tin) *n.* an antifungal drug used especially to treat yeast infections, such as candidosis. It is formulated, often in combination with other drugs, as a cream or ointment for skin infections, as tablets for oral and intestinal infections, as pessaries or suppositories for vaginal or anal infections, or as eye drops for eye infections. Trade name: **Nystan**.

Oo

O *symbol for* oxygen.

OAE *pl. n. see* otoacoustic emissions.

oat-cell carcinoma (small-cell lung cancer) (oht-sel) *n.* carcinoma of the bronchus associated with the presence of oat cells (small cells with darkly staining nuclei). Oat-cell carcinoma is usually related to smoking and accounts for about one-quarter of bronchial carcinomas. It can be cured in its early stages by chemotherapy and radiotherapy.

obesity (oh-beess-iti) *n.* the condition in which excess fat has accumulated in the body, mostly in the subcutaneous tissues. Clinical obesity is considered to be present when a person has a body mass index of 30 or over. *See also* leptin. —**obese** *adj.*

objective (ŏb-jek-tiv) **1.** *n.* (in microscopy) the lens or system of lenses in a light microscope that is nearest to the object under examination and furthest from the eyepiece. **2.** *n. see* behavioural objective. **3.** *adj.* existing independently of a patient's perception: applied particularly to the signs of a disease.

obligate (ob-lig-ayt) *adj.* describing an organism that is restricted to one particular way of life. *Compare* facultative.

obscure auditory dysfunction (ŏb-skyoor) *n.* hearing difficulty, especially in noisy environments, in an individual with a normal audiogram. Treatment includes hearing therapy. In the USA it is known as *central auditory processing disorder.*

obsession (ŏb-sesh-ŏn) *n.* a recurrent thought, feeling, or action that is unpleasant and provokes anxiety but cannot be got rid of. Although an obsession dominates the person, he (or she) realizes its senselessness and struggles to expel it. Obsessions are a feature of *obsessive-compulsive disorder* (OCD, formerly known as *obsessional neurosis*); they can be treated with behaviour therapy and also with psychotherapy and anxiolytic drugs. *See also* neurosis. —**obsessional** *adj.*

obsessive-compulsive disorder (ŏb-ses-iv kŏm-pul-siv) *n. see* obsession.

obstetrics (ŏb-stet-riks) *n.* the branch of medical science concerned with the care of women during pregnancy, childbirth, and the period of about six weeks following the birth. *Compare* gynaecology. —**obstetrical** *adj.* —**obstetrician** (ob-stit-rish-ăn) *n.*

obstruction (ŏb-struk-shŏn) *n.* the condition of being blocked, which may affect any tubular organ or structure. *intestinal o.* blockage of the intestines, producing symptoms of vomiting, distension, and abdominal pain; failure to pass flatus or faeces (complete constipation) is usual. The causes may be acute (e.g. hernia) or chronic (e.g. tumours,

Crohn's disease). **—obstructive** (ŏb-**struk**-tiv) *adj.*

obstructive sleep apnoea *n. see* sleep apnoea.

obturation (ob-tewr-**ay**-shŏn) *n.* obstruction of a body passage, usually by impaction of a foreign body, thickened secretions, or hard faeces

obturator (**ob**-tewr-ay-ter) *n.* **1.** a wire or rod within a cannula or hollow needle for piercing tissues or fitting aspirating needles. **2.** a removable form of denture that both closes a defect in the palate and also restores the dentition. **3.** (*o. muscle*) either of two muscles that cover the outer surface of the anterior wall of the pelvis and are responsible for lateral rotation of the thigh and movements of the hip. *o. foramen* a large opening in the hip bone, below and slightly in front of the acetabulum. *See also* pelvis.

obtusion (ŏb-**tew**-zhŏn) *n.* the weakening or blunting of normal sensations. This may be associated with disease.

occipital bone (ok-**sip**-i-t'l) *n.* a saucer-shaped bone of the skull that forms the back and part of the base of the cranium. At the base of the occipital are two condyles that articulate with the first (atlas) vertebra of the backbone. Between the condyles is the foramen magnum.

occipito-anterior (ok-sip-i-toh-an-**teer**-i-er) *adj.* describing the position of a baby at the time of delivery in which the back of the head is towards the front of the mother's pelvis.

occipito-posterior (ok-sip-i-toh-pos-**teer**-i-er) *adj.* describing the position of a baby at the time of deliv-

ery in which the back of the head is towards the mother's backbone.

occiput (**oks**-ip-ut) *n.* the back of the head. **—occipital** *adj.*

occlusion (ŏ-**kloo**-zhŏn) *n.* **1.** the closing or obstruction of a hollow organ or part. **2.** (in dentistry) the relation of the upper and lower teeth when they are in contact. *See also* malocclusion.

occult (ŏ-**kult**) *adj.* not apparent to the naked eye; not easily detected. *o. blood* blood present in such small quantities, for example in the faeces, that it can only be detected microscopically or by chemical testing.

occupational disease (ok-yoo-**pay**-shŏn-ăl) *n.* any one of various specific diseases to which workers in certain occupations are particularly prone. Examples include the various forms of pneumoconiosis, cataracts in glassblowers, decompression sickness in divers, and infectious diseases contracted from animals by farm workers, such as woolsorter's disease (*see* anthrax). *See also* industrial disease, prescribed disease.

occupational health nurse *n.* (in the UK) a nurse who has undergone a specialized course of study (full or part time) in the health care of people at work. An occupational health nurse is responsible for promoting a high degree of physical and mental health in industrial and commercial settings and in the NHS.

occupational therapy *n.* the treatment of physical and psychiatric conditions through specific activities in order to help people reach their maximum level of function and independence in all aspects of daily life.

OCD *n.* obsessive–compulsive disorder (*see* obsession).

oct- (octa-, octi-, octo-) *prefix denoting* eight.

octreotide (ok-tri-oh-tyd) *n.* an analogue of somatostatin that is administered by injection to treat acromegaly and hormone-secreting neuroendocrine tumours. Trade name: **Sandostatin**.

ocular (ok-yoo-ler) *adj.* of or concerned with the eye or vision. *o. pemphigoid see* pemphigoid.

oculo- *prefix denoting* the eye(s).

oculogyric (ok-yoo-loh-**jy**-rik) *adj.* causing or concerned with movements of the eye.

oculomotor (ok-yoo-loh-**moh**-ter) *adj.* concerned with eye movements. *o. nerve* the third cranial nerve (III), which supplies muscles in and around the eye, including those responsible for altering the size of the pupil and those that turn the eyeball in different directions.

oculonasal (ok-yoo-loh-**nay**-zăl) *adj.* concerned with the eye and nose.

oculoplastics (ok-yoo-loh-**plast**-iks) *n.* a surgical specialty concerned with reconstructive and cosmetic surgery around the eye (including the orbit, eyelids, lacrimal apparatus, and other accessory structures).

oculoplethysmography (ok-yoo-loh-pleth-iz-**mog**-răfi) *n.* measurement of the pressure inside the eyeball. A rising or above-normal pressure is an important indication of the presence of glaucoma.

o.d. (omni die) Latin: daily, used as a direction in prescriptions.

odont- (odonto-) *prefix denoting* a tooth.

odontalgia (od-on-**tal**-jiă) *n.* toothache.

odontoid process (od-ont-oid) *n.* a toothlike process from the upper surface of the axis vertebra.

odontology (od-on-**tol**-ŏji) *n.* the study of the teeth.

odontoma (od-on-**toh**-mă) *n.* an abnormal mass of calcified dental tissue, usually representing a developmental abnormality.

-odynia *suffix denoting* pain in (a specified part).

odynophagia (od-i-noh-**fay**-jiă) *n.* a sensation of pain behind the sternum as food or fluid is swallowed; particularly, the burning sensation experienced by patients with oesophagitis when hot, spicy, or alcoholic liquid is swallowed.

oedema (ee-**dee**-mă) *n.* excessive accumulation of fluid in the body tissues: popularly known as *dropsy*. The resultant swelling may be local, as with an injury or inflammation, or more general. In generalized oedema there may be collections of fluid within the chest cavity, abdomen (*see* ascites), or within the air spaces of the lung (*pulmonary o.*). It may result from heart or kidney failure, cirrhosis of the liver, acute nephritis, the nephrotic syndrome, starvation, allergy, or certain drugs. Diuretics are administered to get rid of the excess fluid. *angio-o. see* urticaria. *subcutaneous o.* oedema that commonly occurs in the legs and ankles; the swelling subsides with rest and elevation of the legs. —**oedematous** *adj.*

Oedipus complex (ee-dip-ŭs) *n.* repressed sexual feelings of a child for its opposite-sexed parent, combined with rivalry towards the same-sexed parent: in Freudian psychoanalytic theory, this is said to be a normal stage of development. Arrest of development at the Oedipal stage is said to be responsible for sexual deviations and other neurotic behaviour.

oesophag- (oesophago-) *prefix* denoting the oesophagus.

oesophageal ulcer (ee-sof-ă-jee-ăl) *n.* a peptic ulcer in the oesophagus, which is associated with reflux oesophagitis.

oesophageal varices *pl. n.* dilated veins in the lower oesophagus due to portal hypertension. These veins may rupture and bleed, resulting in haematemesis. Bleeding may be arrested by a compression balloon, by sclerotherapy, by applying elastic bands via an endoscope, or by intravenous infusions of vasopressin or somatostatin.

oesophagectomy (ee-sof-ă-jek-tŏmi) *n.* surgical removal of part or the whole of the oesophagus.

oesophagitis (ee-sof-ă-jy-tis) *n.* inflammation of the oesophagus. *corrosive o.* oesophagitis caused by the ingestion of caustic acid or alkali. *infective o.* oesophagitis caused by infection with *Candida* or, more rarely, by viruses. It is common in AIDS patients. *reflux o.* the commonest form of oesophagitis, caused by frequent regurgitation of acid and peptic juices from the stomach. It may be associated with a hiatus hernia. The main symptoms are heartburn, regurgitation of bitter fluid, and sometimes difficulty in swallowing; complications include bleeding, narrowing (stricture) of

the oesophageal canal, and ulceration.

oesophagocele (ee-sof-ă-goh-seel) *n.* protrusion of the lining (mucosa) of the oesophagus through a tear in its muscular wall.

oesophagogastroduodenoscopy (OGD) (ee-sof-ă-goh-gas-troh-dew-ŏ-di-**nos**-kŏpi) *n.* endoscopic examination of the upper alimentary tract using a fibreoptic or video instrument. *See also* gastroscope.

oesophagoscope (ee-sof-ă-goh-skohp) *n.* an illuminated optical instrument that is used to inspect the interior of the oesophagus, dilate its canal, obtain material for biopsy, or remove a foreign body. —**oesophagoscopy** (ee-sof-ă-gos-kŏ-pi) *n.*

oesophagostomy (ee-sof-ă-gost-ŏmi) *n.* a surgical operation in which the oesophagus is opened onto the neck It is usually performed after operations on the throat as a temporary measure to allow feeding.

oesophagotomy (ee-sof-ă-got-ŏmi) *n.* surgical opening of the oesophagus in order to inspect its interior or to remove or insert something.

oesophagus (ee-sof-ă-gŭs) *n.* the gullet: a muscular tube, about 23 cm long, that extends from the pharynx to the stomach. It is lined with mucous membrane, whose secretions lubricate food as it passes from the mouth to the stomach. —**oesophageal** *adj.*

oestradiol (ees-tră-dy-ol) *n.* the major female sex hormone produced by the ovary. *See* oestrogen.

oestriol (ees-tri-ol) *n.* one of the female sex hormones produced by the ovary. *See* oestrogen.

oestrogen (ees-trŏ-jĕn) *n.* one of a group of steroid hormones (including oestriol, oestrone, and oestradiol) that control female sexual development. Oestrogens are synthesized mainly by the ovary; small amounts are also produced by the adrenal cortex, testes, and placenta. Naturally occurring and synthetic oestrogens are administered by mouth or injection to treat amenorrhoea, menopausal symptoms (*see* hormone replacement therapy), and androgen-dependent cancers, and to inhibit lactation. Synthetic oestrogens are a major constituent of oral contraceptives. —**oestrogenic** *adj.*

oestrone (ees-trohn) *n.* one of the female sex hormones produced by the ovary. *See* oestrogen.

ofloxacin (oh-floks-ă-sin) *n.* a quinolone antibiotic used to treat infections of the genitourinary and respiratory tracts, skin, and eye. It is administered by mouth, injection, or as eye drops. Trade names: **Exocin, Tarivid.**

OGD *n. see* oesophagogastroduodenoscopy.

ohm (ohm) *n.* the SI unit of electrical resistance, equal to the resistance between two points on a conductor when a constant potential difference of 1 volt applied between these points produces a current of 1 ampere. Symbol: Ω.

-oid *suffix denoting* like; resembling.

ointment (oint-mĕnt) *n.* a greasy preparation, which may or may not contain a medication, applied to the skin or mucous membranes.

olecranon process (oh-lek-ră-

non) *n.* the large process of the ulna that projects behind the elbow joint.

oleic acid (oh-lee-ik) *n. see* fatty acid.

oleo- *prefix denoting* oil.

oleum (oh-li-ŭm) *n.* (in pharmacy) an oil.

olfaction (ol-fak-shŏn) *n.* **1.** the sense of smell. **2.** the process of smelling. Sensory cells in the mucous membrane that lines the nasal cavity are stimulated by the presence of chemical particles dissolved in the mucus. —**olfactory** (ol-fak-ter-i) *adj.*

olfactory nerve *n.* the first cranial nerve (I): the special sensory nerve of smell. Fibres of the nerve run upwards from smell receptors in the nasal mucosa and join to form the olfactory tract to the brain.

olig- (oligo-) *prefix denoting* **1.** few. **2.** a deficiency.

oligaemia (ol-ig-ee-miă) *n. see* hypovolaemia.

oligodactylism (ol-i-goh-dak-tilizm) *n.* the congenital absence of some of the fingers and toes.

oligodipsia (ol-i-goh-dip-siă) *n.* a condition in which thirst is diminished or absent.

oligohydramnios (ol-i-goh-hy-dram-ni-os) *n.* a condition in which the amount of amniotic fluid bathing a fetus during pregnancy is abnormally small (0–200 ml in the third trimester).

oligomenorrhoea (ol-i-goh-men-ŏ-ree-ă) *n.* sparse or infrequent menstruation.

oligospermia (ol-i-goh-sper-miă) *n.* the presence of less than the normal amount of spermatozoa in the semen (*see* seminal analysis). In oligospermia there are less than 20 million spermatozoa per ml with poor motility and often including many bizarre and immature forms. It is a cause of male infertility.

oliguria (ol-ig-yoor-iă) *n.* the production of an abnormally small volume of urine. This may be a result of copious sweating, kidney disease, oedema, loss of blood, diarrhoea, or poisoning.

olive (ol-iv) *n.* a smooth oval swelling in the upper part of the medulla oblongata on each side. It contains a mass of nerve cells, mainly grey matter (*olivary nucleus*). —**olivary** *adj.*

Ollier's disease (ol-i-ayz) *n.* see dyschondroplasia. [L. L. X. E. Ollier (1830–1900), French surgeon]

-ology *suffix. see* -logy.

olsalazine (ol-sal-ă-zeen) *n.* a salicylate preparation used to treat mild ulcerative colitis. It is administered by mouth. Trade name: **Dipentum**.

o.m. (omni mane) *Latin:* in the morning, used as a direction in prescriptions.

om- (omo-) *prefix denoting* the shoulder.

-oma *suffix denoting* a tumour.

omentectomy (oh-men-tek-tŏmi) *n.* the removal of all or part of the omentum.

omentum (epiploon) (oh-men-tŭm) *n.* a double layer of peritoneum attached to the stomach and linking it with other abdominal organs. *great o.* a highly folded portion of the omentum that covers the intestines in an apron-like fashion. It acts as a heat insulator and prevents friction between abdominal organs. *lesser o.* a portion of the omentum

that links the stomach with the liver. —**omental** *adj.*

omeprazole (oh-mep-ră-zohl) *n.* a drug used to treat gastric and duodenal ulcers and the Zollinger-Ellison syndrome (*see* proton-pump inhibitor). Administered by mouth, it is long-acting and need only be taken once a day. Trade name: **Losec**.

omphal- (omphalo-) *prefix denoting* the navel or umbilical cord.

omphalitis (om-fă-ly-tis) *n.* inflammation of the navel, especially in newborn infants.

omphalocele (om-fă-loh-seel) *n.* an umbilical hernia.

omphalus (om-fă-lŭs) *n.* see umbilicus.

o.n. (omni nocte) *Latin:* at night, used as a direction in prescriptions.

Onchocerca (onk-oh-ser-kă) *n.* a genus of parasitic worms (*see* filaria) occurring in central Africa and central America. *O. volvulus* the cause of onchocerciasis.

onchocerciasis (onk-oh-ser-ky-ă-sis) *n.* a tropical disease of the skin and underlying connective tissue caused by the parasitic worm *Onchocerca volvulus.* Fibrous nodular tumours grow around the adult worms in the skin; the migration of the larvae into the eye can cause total or partial blindness (*river blindness*). Ivermectin is used in treatment.

onco- *prefix denoting* **1.** a tumour. **2.** volume.

oncogene (onk-oh-jeen) *n.* a gene in viruses and mammalian cells that can cause cancer; it results from the mutation of a normal gene and is capable of both initiation and continuation of malignant transformation of normal cells. Oncogenes probably produce peptides (growth factors) regulating cell division that, under certain conditions, become uncontrolled and may transform a normal cell to a malignant state.

oncogenesis (onk-oh-jen-i-sis) *n.* the development of a new abnormal growth (a benign or malignant tumour).

oncogenic (onk-oh-jen-ik) *adj.* describing a substance, organism, or environment that is known to be a causal factor in the production of a tumour. Some viruses are oncogenic. *See also* carcinogen.

oncology (onk-ol-ŏji) *n.* the study and practice of treating tumours. It is often subdivided into medical, surgical, and radiation oncology. —**oncologist** *n.*

oncolysis (onk-ol-i-sis) *n.* the destruction of tumours and tumour cells. This may occur spontaneously or, more usually, in response to treatment with drugs or radiotherapy.

oncometer (onk-om-it-er) *n. see* plethysmography.

oncotic (onk-ot-ik) *adj.* **1.** characterized by a tumour or swelling. **2.** relating to an increase in volume or pressure.

ondansetron (on-dan-si-tron) *n.* a drug used to control severe nausea and vomiting, especially when this is caused by chemotherapy and radiotherapy. Trade name: **Zofran**.

onomatomania (on-oh-mat-oh-may-niă) *n.* the repeated intrusion of a specific word or a name into a person's thoughts: a form of obsession.

ontogeny (on-toj-ĕ-ni) *n.* the history of the development of an indi-

vidual from the fertilized egg to maturity.

onych- (onycho-) *prefix denoting* the nail(s).

onychogryphosis (on-i-koh-grif-oh-sis) *n.* thickening and lateral curvature of a nail, usually the big toenail.

onycholysis (on-i-kol-i-sis) *n.* separation or loosening of part or all of a nail from its bed. The condition may occur in psoriasis and in fungal infections of the skin and nail bed or it may be caused by drugs.

onychomycosis (on-i-koh-my-koh-sis) *n.* fungus infection of the nails caused by dermatophytes or *Candida*. The nails become yellow, opaque, and thickened. *See also* tinea.

O'nyong nyong fever (jointbreaker fever) (oh-n'yong-n'yong) *n.* an East African disease caused by an arbovirus and transmitted by mosquitoes of the genus *Anopheles*. Symptoms include rigor, severe headache, an irritating rash, fever, and pains in the joints.

oo- *prefix denoting* an egg; ovum.

oocyte (oh-ŏ-syt) *n.* a cell in the ovary that undergoes meiosis to form an ovum. *See* oogenesis.

oocyte donation *n.* the transfer of oocytes from one woman to another. It allows the recipient, who is unable to ovulate, to achieve a normal pregnancy.

oogenesis (oh-ŏ-jen-i-sis) *n.* the process by which mature ova are produced in the ovary (see illustration). Primordial germ cells multiply to form oogonia, which start their first meiotic division to become oocytes in the fetus and complete it at ovulation. Fertilization stimulates the completion of the second meiotic division, which produces a mature ovum.

Oogenesis

oogonium (oh-ŏ-goh-niŭm) *n.* (*pl.* **oogonia**) a cell produced at an early stage in the formation of an ovum. *See* oogenesis.

oophor- (oophoro-) *prefix denoting* the ovary.

oophorectomy (ovariectomy) (oh-ŏ-fŏ-**rek**-tŏmi) *n.* surgical removal of an ovary.

oophoritis (ovaritis) (oh-ŏ-fŏ-**ry**-tis) *n.* inflammation of an ovary, either on the surface or within the organ. Oophoritis may be associated with infection of the Fallopian tubes (*see* salpingitis) or the lower part of the abdominal cavity.

oophoropexy (oh-off-ŏ-roh-peks-i) *n.* the stitching of a displaced ovary to the wall of the pelvic cavity.

oophorosalpingectomy (oh-off-ŏ-roh-sal-pin-jek-tŏmi) *n.* surgical removal of an ovary and its associated Fallopian tube.

opacity (ŏ-pas-iti) *n.* **1.** lack of transparency. **2.** an opaque area, as occurs in the lens of the eye in cataract.

operating microscope (op-er-ayt-ing) *n.* a binocular microscope commonly used in microsurgery. The field of operation is illuminated through the objective lens by a light source within the microscope.

operculum (oh-per-kew-lŭm) *n.* (*pl.* **opercula**) a plug of mucus that blocks the cervical canal of the uterus in a pregnant woman. When the cervix begins to dilate at the start of labour, the operculum, slightly stained with blood, comes away as a discharge ('show').

operon (op-er-on) *n.* a group of closely linked genes that regulate the production of enzymes in bacteria.

ophthalm- (ophthalmo-) *prefix denoting* the eye or eyeball. Examples: *ophthalmectomy* (surgical removal of); *ophthalmorrhexis* (rupture of).

ophthalmia (off-thal-miă) *n.* inflammation of the eye, particularly the conjunctiva (*see* conjunctivitis). *o. neonatorum* a form of conjunctivitis occurring in newborn infants, who contract the disease as they pass through an infected birth canal. The two most common infections are gonorrhoea and *Chlamydia*. Unless both mother and baby are treated (with antibiotics), the infection may cause permanent eye disease. *sympathetic o.* a granulomatous uveitis affecting all parts of the uveal tract of both eyes that may develop after trauma or (more rarely) eye surgery.

ophthalmic (off-thal-mik) *adj.* concerned with the eye.

ophthalmitis (off-thal-my-tis) *n.* inflammation of the eye. *See* conjunctivitis, uveitis.

ophthalmologist (off-thal-mol-ŏ-jist) *n.* a doctor who specializes in the diagnosis and treatment of eye diseases.

ophthalmology (off-thal-mol-ŏji) *n.* the branch of medicine that is devoted to the study and treatment of eye diseases. —**ophthalmological** *adj.*

ophthalmometer (off-thal-mom-it-er) *n. see* keratometer.

ophthalmoplegia (off-thal-moh-plee-jiă) *n.* paralysis of the muscles of the eye. It may accompany exophthalmos due to thyrotoxicosis. *external o.* ophthalmoplegia affecting the muscles that move the eye. *internal o.* ophthalmoplegia affecting the iris and ciliary muscle. *internuclear o.* ophthalmoplegia due to a lesion in the brainstem, seen in patients with multiple sclerosis or stroke.

ophthalmoscope (off-thal-mŏ-skohp) *n.* an instrument for examining the interior of the eye (see illustration). —**ophthalmoscopy** (off-thal-mos-kŏ-pi) *n.*

ophthalmotomy (off-thal-mot-ŏmi) *n.* the operation of making an incision in the eyeball.

ophthalmotonometer *n. see* tonometer.

-opia *suffix denoting* a defect of the eye or of vision.

opiate (oh-piăt) *n.* one of a group of drugs derived from opium. Syn-

thetic drugs with similar effects are called *opioids*, a term often used to include both the natural and synthetic drugs. This group includes apomorphine, codeine, diamorphine (heroin), morphine, and papaverine. They depress the central nervous system and are used to relieve pain, suppress coughing, and stimulate vomiting. *See also* narcotic.

opioid (oh-pi-oyd) *n. see* opiate.

opisth- (opistho-) *prefix denoting* **1.** dorsal; posterior. **2.** backwards.

opisthorchiasis (op-iss-thor-ky-ă-sis) *n.* a condition caused by the presence of the parasitic fluke *Opisthorchis* in the bile ducts. Heavy infections can damage the tissues of the bile duct and liver and may progress to cirrhosis. The disease is treated with chloroquine.

Opisthorchis (op-iss-thor-kis) *n.* a

disc for changing lenses

An ophthalmoscope

genus of parasitic flukes occurring in E Europe and parts of SE Asia. The adult flukes, which live in the bile ducts, can cause opisthorchiasis.

opisthotonos (op-iss-thot-oh-nŏs) *n.* the position of the body in which the head, neck, and spine are arched backwards. It is assumed involuntarily by patients with tetanus and strychnine poisoning

opium (oh-piŭm) *n.* an extract from the poppy *Papaver somniferum*, which has analgesic and narcotic action due to its content of morphine. It has the same uses and side-effects as morphine and prolonged use may lead to dependence. *See also* opiate.

opponens (oh-poh-nenz) *n.* one of a group of muscles in the hand that bring the digits opposite to other digits. *o. pollicis* the principal muscle causing opposition of the thumb.

opportunistic (op-er-tew-nis-tik) *adj.* denoting a disease that occurs when the patient's immune system is impaired by, for example, an infection, another disease, or drugs. The infecting organism rarely causes the disease in healthy persons. Opportunistic infections, such as *Pneumocystis carinii* pneumonia and those caused by *Mycobacterium* (*see* MAI complex), are common in patients with AIDS.

-opsia *suffix denoting* a condition of vision.

opsoclonus (op-soh-kloh-nŭs) *n.* a series of erratic eye movements in any direction, which is seen in people with disease of the cerebellum.

opsonin (op-sŏn-in) *n.* a serum complement component that attaches itself to invading bacteria and appar-ently makes them more susceptible to phagocytosis.

opt- (opto-) *prefix denoting* vision or the eye.

optic (op-tik) *adj.* concerned with the eye or vision. *o. atrophy* degeneration of the optic nerve. *o. chiasma* (*o. commissure*) the X-shaped structure formed by the two optic nerves as nerve fibres from the nasal side of the retina of each eye cross over to join fibres from the lateral side of the retina of the opposite eye (*see* illustration). *o. disc* (*o. papilla*) the start of the optic nerve, where nerve fibres from the rods and cones leave the eyeball. *See* blind spot. *o. nerve* the second cranial nerve (II), which is responsible for vision. It passes into the skull

The optic chiasma

behind the eyeball to reach the optic chiasma, after which the visual pathway continues to the occipital lobe. *o. neuritis see* retrobulbar neuritis.

optician (op-tish-ăn) *n.* a person who either makes and fits glasses (*dispensing o.*) or who can both test people for glasses and dispense glasses (*ophthalmic o.* or *optometrist*).

opticokinetic (op-tik-oh-ky-net-ik) *adj.* relating to the movements of the eye.

optometer (refractometer) (op-tom-it-er) *n.* an instrument for measuring the refraction of the eye.

optometrist (op-tom-i-trist) *n. see* optician.

optometry (op-tom-itri) *n.* the practice of testing the visual acuity of eyes and prescribing lenses to correct defects of vision.

oral (or-ăl) *adj.* **1.** relating to the mouth. **2.** taken by mouth: applied to medicines, etc.

oral contraceptive *n.* the Pill: a preparation, consisting of one or more synthetic female sex hormones, taken by women to prevent conception. Most oral contraceptives are combined pills, consisting of an oestrogen, which blocks the normal process of ovulation, and a progestogen, which acts on the pituitary gland to block the normal control of the menstrual cycle.

oral hypoglycaemic drug (oral antidiabetic drug) (hy-poh-gly-see-mik) *n.* one of the group of drugs that reduce the level of glucose in the blood and are taken by mouth for the treatment of noninsulin-dependent (type 2) diabetes mellitus. They include the sulphonylurea drugs; metformin (a biguanide); acarbose (an alpha-glucosidase inhibitor); the *meglitinides* (e.g. repaglinide), which stimulate insulin release; and the *thiazolidinediones* (e.g. pioglitazone), which reduce the body's resistance to insulin.

oral rehydration therapy (ORT) (ree-hy-dray-shŏn) *n.* the administration of an isotonic solution of various sodium salts, potassium chloride, glucose, and water to treat acute diarrhoea, particularly in children. In developing countries it is the mainstay of treatment for cholera. Preparations in clinical use include *Dioralyte* and *Rehidrat*.

orbicularis (or-bik-yoo-lar-iss) *n.* either of two circular muscles of the face. *o. oculi* the muscle around each orbit that is responsible for closing the eye. *o. oris* the muscle around the mouth that closes and compresses the lips.

orbit (or-bit) *n.* the cavity in the skull that contains the eye. It is formed from parts of the frontal, sphenoid, zygomatic, lacrimal, ethmoid, palatine, and maxillary bones. —**orbital** *adj.*

orbitotomy (or-bit-ot-ŏmi) *n.* surgical removal of part of the orbital bones to gain access to the orbital space.

orchi- (orchido-, orchio-) *prefix* denoting the testis or testicle.

orchidalgia (or-kid-al-jiă) *n.* pain in the testicle, often due to a varicocele, orchitis, or torsion of the testis.

orchidectomy (or-kid-ek-tŏmi) *n.* surgical removal of a testis, usually to treat germ-cell tumours of the testis, such as seminoma and teratoma, which are malignant tumours of the testis.

orchidometer (or-kid-**om**-it-er) *n.* a calliper device for measuring the size of the testicles. *Prader o.* a collection of testicle-shaped beads of different sizes, each of known volume, for direct comparison to and sizing of the testicles, enabling the precise charting of testicular growth.

orchidopexy (or-kid-oh-peks-i) *n.* the operation of mobilizing an undescended testis in the groin and fixing it in the scrotum.

orchidotomy (or-kid-ot-ŏmi) *n.* an incision into the testis, usually done to obtain biopsy material for histological examination.

orchis (or-kis) *n.* the testis or testicle.

orchitis (or-ky-tis) *n.* inflammation of the testis. This causes pain, redness, and swelling of the scrotum, and may be associated with inflammation of the epididymis (*epididymo-orchitis*). The condition is usually caused by infection spreading down the vas deferens but can develop in mumps (*mumps o.*).

orciprenaline (or-si-pren-ă-leen) *n.* a sympathomimetic drug used as a bronchodilator to relieve bronchitis and asthma. It is administered by mouth. Trade name: **Alupent**.

Orem's model (or-ĕmz) *n.* a model for nursing based on the self-care deficit theory of nursing, in which patients are seen as able, when they are well, to initiate and perform activities on their own behalf, in order to maintain life, health, and wellbeing. Infants, children, the elderly, the disabled, and the ill may require assistance or complete care with

these activities. *See also* nursing models. [D. Orem (1914–), US nurse theorist]

orf (orf) *n.* an infectious disease of sheep and goats caused by a parapoxvirus. Those bottle-feeding infected lambs may develop a painful nodule on the fingers or hands; it resolves spontaneously.

organ (or-găn) *n.* a part of the body, composed of more than one tissue, that forms a structural unit responsible for a particular function (or functions). *o. of Corti* (spiral o.) the sense organ of the cochlea, which converts sound signals into nerve impulses that are transmitted to the brain via the cochlear nerve. [A. Corti (1822–88), Italian anatomist]

organelle (or-gă-nel) *n.* a structure within a cell that is specialized for a particular function.

organic (or-gan-ik) *adj.* **1.** relating to any or all of the organs of the body. *o. disorder* a disorder associated with changes in the structure of an organ or tissue. *Compare* functional disorder. **2.** describing chemical compounds containing carbon, found in all living systems.

organism (or-găn-izm) *n.* any living thing, which may consist of a single cell (*see* microorganism) or a group of differentiated but interdependent cells.

organo- *prefix denoting* organ or organic.

orgasm (or-gazm) *n.* the climax of sexual excitement.

oriental sore (Baghdad boil, Delhi boil, Aleppo boil, (or-i-en-t'l) *n.* a skin disease, occurring in tropical and subtropical Africa and Asia, caused by the parasitic protozoan *Leishmania tropica*. The disease takes the form of a slow-healing open sore or ulcer, which sometimes becomes secondarily infected with bacteria.

orientation (or-i-en-tay-shŏn) *n.* (in psychology) awareness of oneself in time, space, and place. Orientation may be disturbed in such conditions as organic brain disease, toxic drug states, and concussion.

orifice (o-ri-fis) *n.* an opening in an anatomical part. *See* ostium.

origin (o-ri-jin) *n.* (in anatomy) **1.** the point of attachment of a muscle that remains relatively fixed during contraction of the muscle. *Compare* insertion. **2.** the point at which a nerve or blood vessel branches from a main nerve or blood vessel.

orlistat (or-lis-tat) *n.* a drug that reduces the absorption of fat in the stomach and small intestine by inhibiting the action of pancreatic lipases. It is administered by mouth to treat clinical obesity; side-effects include the production of copious oily stools and flatulence. Trade name: **Xenical**.

ornithine (or-ni-theen) *n.* an amino acid produced in the liver as a by-product during the conversion of ammonia to urea.

ornithosis (or-ni-thoh-sis) *n. see* psittacosis.

oro- *prefix denoting* the mouth.

oropharyngeal airway (o-roh-fă-rin-ji-ăl) *n.* a curved tube designed to be placed in the mouth of an unconscious patient, behind the tongue, to create a patent airway. *See also* nasopharyngeal airway.

oropharynx (o-roh-fa-rinks) *n.* the part of the pharynx that lies between the level of the junction of the hard and soft palates above and the hyoid bone below. It contains the tonsils. —**oropharyngeal** *adj.*

orphenadrine (or-fen-ă-dreen) *n.* a drug that relieves spasm in muscle; it is administered by mouth or injection to treat all types of parkinsonism. Trade names: **Biorphen**, **Disipal**,

ORT *n. see* oral rehydration therapy.

ortho- *prefix denoting* **1.** straight. **2.** normal.

orthodontics (orthŏ-don-tiks) *n.* the branch of dentistry concerned with the growth and development of the face and jaws and the treatment of irregularities of the teeth by means of various *orthodontic appliances.* —**orthodontic** *adj.*

orthokeratology (orthŏ-ke-ră-tol-ŏji) *n.* the use of contact lenses designed to reshape the cornea in the treatment of refractive errors, such as myopia (short sight).

orthopaedics (orthŏ-pee-diks) *n.* the science or practice of correcting deformities caused by disease of or damage to the bones and joints of the skeleton. —**orthopaedic** *adj.*

orthopnoea (or-thop-nee-ă) *n.* breathlessness that prevents the patient from lying down, so that he or she has to sleep propped up in bed or sitting in a chair. —**orthopnoeic** *adj.*

orthoptics (or-thop-tiks) *n.* the practice of using nonsurgical methods, particularly eye exercises, to treat abnormalities of vision and of coordination of eye movements (most commonly strabismus and amblyopia). —**orthoptist** *n.*

orthoptoscope (or-thop-toh-skohp) *n. see* amblyoscope.

orthosis (or-thoh-sis) *n.* a surgical appliance that exerts external forces on part of the body to support joints or correct deformity.

orthostatic (ortho-stat-ik) *adj.* relating to the upright position of the body: used when describing this posture or a condition caused by it.

orthotics (or-thot-iks) *n.* the science and practice of fitting surgical appliances to assist weakened joints.

Ortolani manoeuvre (or-toh-lah-ni mă-noo-ver) *n.* a test for congenital dislocation of the hip in which, with the baby lying supine and the pelvis steadied with one hand, the examiner attempts to relocate a dislocated hip by gently abducting the hip while simultaneously pushing upwards on the greater trochanter. If the hip is dislocated, it will relocate with a detectable and sometimes audible clunk. [M. Ortolani (20th century), Italian orthopaedic surgeon]

os^1 (oss) *n.* (*pl.* **ossa**) a bone.

os^2 *n.* (*pl.* **ora**) the mouth or a mouthlike part.

OSA (OSAS) *n.* see (obstructive) sleep apnoea (syndrome).

osche- (oscheo-) *prefix denoting* the scrotum.

oscillation (oss-i-lay-shŏn) *n.* a regular side-to-side movement; vibration.

oscilloscope (oss-il-ŏ-skohp) *n.* a cathode-ray tube designed to display electronically a wave form corresponding to the electrical data fed into it. Oscilloscopes are used to provide a continuous record of many different measurements, such as the activity of the heart and brain. *See* electrocardiography, electroencephalography.

osculum (osk-yoo-lŭm) *n.* (in anatomy) a small aperture.

Osgood-Schlatter disease (Schlatter's disease) (oz-guud shlat-er) *n.* inflammation and swelling at the site of insertion of the main quadriceps tendon at the top of the tibia (the tibial tubercle), just below the knee (*see* apophysitis, osteochondritis). It is common in adolescence and results from excessive physical activity. [R. B. Osgood (1873–1956), US orthopaedist; C. Schlatter (1864–1934), Swiss surgeon]

-osis *suffix denoting* **1.** a diseased condition. **2.** any condition. **3.** an increase or excess.

Osler's nodes (ohss-lerz) *pl. n.* small tender swellings in or beneath the skin at the ends of the fingers and toes, seen in subacute bacterial endocarditis. [Sir W. Osler (1849–1919), Canadian physician]

osm- (osmo-) *prefix denoting* **1.** smell or odour. **2.** osmosis or osmotic pressure.

osmolality (oz-moh-lal-iti) *n.* the osmotic pressure of a substance expressed in terms of osmoles of substance per kg of water. *Compare* osmolarity.

osmolarity (oz-moh-la-riti) *n.* the osmotic pressure of a substance expressed in terms of osmoles of substance per kg of solution.

osmole (oz-mohl) *n.* a unit of osmotic pressure equal to the molecular weight of a solute in grams divided by the number of ions or other particles into which it dissociates in solution.

osmoreceptor (oz-moh-ri-sep-ter) *n.* a group of cells in the hypothalamus that monitor blood concentration.

osmosis (oz-**moh**-sis) *n*. the passage of a solvent from a less concentrated solution to a more concentrated solution through a semipermeable membrane. In living organisms, the process of osmosis plays an important role in controlling the distribution of water. —**osmotic** (oz-**mot**-ik) *adj*.

osmotic pressure *n*. the pressure by which water is drawn into a solution through a semipermeable membrane; the more concentrated the solution, the greater its osmotic pressure.

osseointegration (oss-i-oh-in-ti-**gray**-shŏn) *n*. the process by which certain materials, such as titanium, may be introduced into living bone without producing a foreign-body reaction. This allows a very tight and strong joint between the two structures. Osseointegration is used, for example, to fix some dental implants and bone-anchored hearing aids.

osseous (oss-iŭs) *adj*. bony: applied to the bony parts of the inner ear.

ossicle (oss-i-kŭl) *n*. a small bone. *auditory o.* any of the three small bones (the incus, malleus, and stapes) in the middle ear.

ossification (osteogenesis) (oss-i-fi-**kay**-shŏn) *n*. the formation of bone, which takes place in three stages by the action of osteoblasts. A meshwork of collagen fibres is deposited in connective tissue, followed by the production of a cementing polysaccharide. Finally the cement is impregnated with minute crystals of calcium salts. The os-

teoblasts become enclosed within the matrix as osteocytes.

ost- (oste-, osteo-) *prefix denoting* bone.

ostectomy (oss-**tek**-tŏmi) *n*. the surgical removal of a bone or a piece of bone. *See also* osteotomy.

osteitis (osti-I-tis) *n*. inflammation of bone, due to infection, damage, or metabolic disorder. *o. deformans see* Paget's disease. *o. fibrosa cystica* the characteristic cystic changes that occur in bones during long-standing hyperparathyroidism.

osteo- *prefix. see* ost-.

osteoarthritis (osteoarthrosis) (osti-oh-arth-**ry**-tis) *n*. a degenerative disease of joints resulting from wear of the articular cartilage, which may lead to secondary changes in the underlying bone. The joints are painful and stiff, with restricted movement. The condition may be primary or may result from abnormal load to the joint or damage to the cartilage from inflammation or trauma. Treatment consists of analgesics, reducing the load to the joint (e.g. by weight loss), or surgery (osteotomy, arthrodesis, or arthroplasty).

osteoarthropathy (osti-oh-arth-**rop**-ă-thi) *n*. any disease of the bone and cartilage adjoining a joint.

osteoarthrosis (osti-oh-arth-**roh**-sis) *n*. *see* osteoarthritis.

osteoarthrotomy (osti-oh-arth-**rot**-ŏmi) *n*. surgical excision of the bone adjoining a joint.

osteoblast (oss-ti-oh-blast) *n*. a cell, originating in the mesoderm of the embryo, that is responsible for the formation of bone. *See also* ossification.

osteochondritis (osti-oh-kon-dry-tis) *n.* **1.** necrosis of a bone due to interruption of its blood supply, which causes it to fragment and collapse before undergoing revascularization. *See* Kienböck's disease, Köhler's disease, Legg-Calvé-Perthes disease. **2.** inflammation of an apophysis from the pull of the attached tendon. *See* Osgood-Schlatter disease, Sever's disease. *o. dissecans* separation of a small fragment (or fragments) of bone and cartilage from the surface of a joint, most frequently the knee, with resulting pain, swelling, and limitation of movement.

osteochondroma (osti-oh-kon-droh-mă) *n.* (*pl.* **osteochondromata**) a bone tumour composed of cartilage-forming cells. It appears as a painless mass, usually at the end of a long bone. As a small proportion of these tumours become malignant if untreated, they are excised.

osteochondrosis (osti-oh-kon-droh-sis) *n. see* osteochondritis.

osteoclasia (osteoclasis) (osti-oh-klay-ziă) *n.* **1.** (**osteoclasty**) the deliberate breaking of a malformed or malunited bone, carried out by a surgeon to correct deformity. **2.** *see* osteolysis.

osteoclasis (osti-ok-lă-sis) *n.* **1.** remodelling of bone by osteoclasts, during growth or the healing of a fracture. **2.** *see* osteoclasia.

osteoclast (oss-ti-oh-klast) *n.* **1.** a large multinucleate cell that resorbs calcified bone. **2.** a device for fracturing bone for therapeutic purposes.

osteoclastoma (osti-oh-klas-toh-mă) *n.* a rare tumour of bone, caused by proliferation of osteoclast cells.

osteocyte (oss-ti-oh-syt) *n.* a bone cell. *See also* ossification.

osteodystrophy (osti-oh-**dis**-trŏ-fi) *n.* any generalized bone disease resulting from a metabolic disorder.

osteogenesis (osti-oh-**jen**-i-sis) *n. see* ossification. *o. imperfecta* (*fragilitas ossium*) a congenital disorder in which the bones are unusually brittle and fragile.

osteogenic (osti-oh-**jen**-ik) *adj.* originating in or composed of bone tissue. *o. sarcoma see* osteosarcoma.

osteology (osti-ol-ŏji) *n.* the study of the structure and function of bones and related structures.

osteolysis (osteoclasia) (osti-ol-i-sis) *n.* dissolution of bone through disease, commonly by infection or loss of the blood supply (ischaemia) to the bone. —**osteolytic** *adj.*

osteoma (osti-oh-mă) *n.* a benign bone tumour. *cancellous o.* (*exostosis*) an outgrowth from the end of a long bone, usually rising to a point. *compact o.* (*ivory tumour*) an osteoma that is usually harmless but may rarely compress surrounding structures, as within the skull. *osteoid o.* an overgrowth of bone-forming cells, usually causing pain in the middle of a long bone.

osteomalacia (osti-oh-mă-lay-shiă) *n.* softening of the bones caused by a deficiency of vitamin D, which leads to progressive decalcification of bony tissues, often causing bone pain. The condition may become irreversible if treatment with vitamin D is not given.

osteomyelitis (osti-oh-my-ĕ-ly-tis) *n.* inflammation of bone due to infection. It can cause fracture and deformity of the bone. *acute o.* osteomyelitis occurring when bacteria enter the bone via the bloodstream; it is more common in children. There is severe pain and redness over the involved bone, accompanied by general illness and high fever. **chronic o.** osteomyelitis that may develop from partially treated acute osteomyelitis or after open fractures or surgery during which the bone is contaminated.

osteopathy (osti-**op**-ǎ-thi) *n.* a system of diagnosis and treatment based on the theory that many diseases are associated with disorders of the musculoskeletal system. Diagnosis and treatment of these disorders involves palpation, manipulation, and massage. Osteopathy provides relief for many disorders of bones and joints. —**osteopath** (ost-i-ǒ-path) *n.* —**osteopathic** (osti-ǒ-**path**-ik) *adj.*

osteopetrosis (Albers-Schönberg disease, marble-bone disease) (osti-oh-pi-**troh**-sis) *n.* a congenital abnormality in which bones become abnormally dense and brittle and tend to fracture. *See also* osteosclerosis.

osteophyte (oss-ti-ǒ-fyt) *n.* a projection of bone, usually shaped like a rose thorn, that occurs at sites of cartilage degeneration or destruction near joints and intervertebral discs.

osteoplasty (oss-ti-ǒ-plasti) *n.* plastic surgery of bones.

osteoporosis (osti-oh-por-oh-sis) *n.* loss of bony tissue, resulting in bones that are brittle and liable to fracture. Infection, injury, and synovitis can cause localized osteoporosis. Generalized osteoporosis is common in the elderly, and in women often follows the menopause. Hormone replacement therapy is preventative, and bisphosphonates can reduce or halt further bone loss. —**osteoporotic** *adj.*

osteosarcoma (osteogenic sarcoma) (osti-oh-sar-koh-mǎ) *n.* a highly malignant tumour arising from within a bone. In children the usual site for the tumour is the leg, particularly the femur. Secondary growths (metastases) are common, most frequently in the lungs (though other sites, such as the liver, may also be involved). Treatment of disease localized to the primary site is now usually by limb-sparing surgery after neoadjuvant chemotherapy, with replacement of the diseased bone by a metal prosthesis.

osteosclerosis (osti-oh-skleer-oh-sis) *n.* an abnormal increase in the density of bone, as a result of poor blood supply, chronic infection, or tumour. *See also* osteopetrosis.

An osteotome

osteotome (oss-ti-ǒ-tohm) *n.* a surgical chisel designed to cut bone.

osteotomy (osti-ot-ǒmi) *n.* a surgical operation to cut a bone into two parts, followed by realignment of the ends to allow healing. The operation may be performed to reduce pain and disability in an arthritic joint.

ostium (oss-tiǔm) *n.* (*pl.* **ostia**) (in anatomy) an opening. **o.** *abdominale* the opening of the Fallopian tube into the abdominal cavity.

-ostomy *suffix. see* -stomy.

ot- (oto-) *prefix denoting* the ear.

otalgia (oh-tal-jiă) *n.* pain in the ear.

OTC drug *n. see* over-the-counter drug.

otic (oh-tik) *adj.* relating to the ear.

otitis (oh-ty-tis) *n.* inflammation of the ear. *o. externa* inflammation of the canal between the eardrum and the external opening of the ear. *o. interna (labyrinthitis)* inflammation of the inner ear causing vertigo, vomiting, loss of balance, and deafness. *o. media* acute or chronic inflammation of the middle ear. Acute inflammation, usually due to bacterial or viral infection, causes pain and a high fever; treatment is usually with antibiotics. Chronic inflammation is associated with perforations of the eardrum; treatment involves surgical repair. *secretory o. media see* glue ear.

otoacoustic emissions (OAE) (oh-toh-ă-koo-stik) *pl. n.* tiny sounds that emerge from the inner ear either spontaneously or shortly after the ear is exposed to an external sound. An objective hearing test for infants detects otoacoustic emissions in response to a small sound.

otoconium (oh-toh-koh-niŭm) *n. see* otolith.

otolaryngology (oh-toh-la-ring-ol-ŏji) *n.* the study of diseases of the ears and larynx. **—otolaryngologist** *n.*

otolith (otoconium) (oh-toh-lith) *n.* one of the small particles of calcium carbonate associated with a macula in the saccule or utricle of the inner ear.

otology (oh-tol-ŏji) *n.* the study of diseases of the ear. **—otologist** *n.*

-otomy *suffix. see* -tomy.

otomycosis (oh-toh-my-koh-sis) *n.* a fungus infection of the ear, causing irritation and inflammation of the canal between the eardrum and the external opening of the ear.

otoplasty (pinnaplasty) (oh-toh-plasti) *n.* surgical repair or reconstruction of the ears after injury or in the correction of a congenital defect (such as bat ears).

otorhinolaryngology (oh-toh-ry-noh-la-ring-ol-ŏji) *n.* the study of ear, nose, and throat diseases (i.e. ENT disorders). **—otorhinolaryngologist** *n.*

otorrhagia (oh-toh-ray-jiă) *n.* bleeding from the ear.

otorrhoea (oh-toh-ree-ă) *n.* any discharge from the ear, commonly a purulent discharge in chronic middle ear infection (otitis media).

otosclerosis (otospongiosis) (oh-toh-skleer-oh-sis) *n.* a disorder causing deafness in adult life. An overgrowth of the bone of the inner ear leads to the stapes becoming fixed to the fenestra ovalis, so that sounds cannot be conducted to the inner ear.

otoscope (oh-toh-skohp) *n. see* auriscope.

otospongiosis (oh-toh-spunji-oh-sis) *n. see* otosclerosis.

ototoxic (oh-toh-toks-ik) *adj.* having a toxic effect on the organs of balance or hearing in the inner ear or on the vestibulocochlear nerve. Ototoxic drugs may be used in the treatment of Ménière's disease.

outbreeding (owt-breed-ing) *n.* the production of offspring by parents who are not closely related. *Compare* inbreeding.

outer ear (owt-er) *n.* the pinna and the external auditory meatus of the ear.

out-of-the-body experience *n.* a form of derealization in which there is a sensation of leaving one's body and visions of travelling through tunnels into light or of journeys on another plane of existence. It typically occurs after anaesthesia or severe illness and is often attributed to anoxia of the brain.

out-patient (owt-pay-shĕnt) *n.* a patient who receives treatment at a hospital but is not admitted to a bed in a hospital ward. Large hospitals have clinics at which out-patients can be given specialist treatment. *Compare* in-patient.

oval window (oh-văl) *n. see* fenestra (ovalis).

ovari- (ovario-) *prefix denoting* the ovary.

ovarian cancer (oh-vair-iăn) *n.* a malignant tumour of the ovary, usually a carcinoma. The incidence of the disease reaches a peak in postmenopausal women; treatment involves surgery and most cases also require combined chemotherapy and/or radiotherapy.

ovarian cyst *n.* a fluid-filled sac, one or more of which may develop in the ovary. Although most ovarian cysts are not malignant, they may reach a very large size and rotate on their stalks, thus cutting off their blood supply and causing severe abdominal pain and vomiting; in such cases the cysts require urgent surgical removal.

ovariectomy (oh-vair-i-ek-tŏmi) *n. see* oophorectomy.

ovariotomy (oh-vair-i-ot-ŏmi) *n.* literally, incision of an ovary. However, the term commonly refers to surgical removal of an ovary (oophorectomy).

ovaritis (oh-vă-ry-tis) *n. see* oophoritis.

ovary (oh-ver-i) *n.* the main female reproductive organ, which contains follicles that produce ova and steroid hormones in a regular cycle (*see* menstrual cycle). There are two ovaries, situated in the lower abdomen, one on each side of the uterus (*see* reproductive system). —**ovarian** *adj.*

overcompensation (oh-ver-kom-pen-say-shŏn) *n.* (in psychology) the situation in which a person tries to overcome a disability by making greater efforts than are required.

overt (oh-vert) *adj.* plainly to be seen or detected: applied to diseases with observable signs and symptoms.

over-the-counter drug (OTC drug) (oh-ver-thĕ-kownt-er) *n.* a drug that may be purchased directly from a pharmacist without a doctor's prescription. Current government policy is to extend the range of OTC drugs: a number have already been derestricted (e.g. ibuprofen, ranitidine) and this trend is expected to increase.

ovi (ovo-) *prefix denoting* an egg; ovum.

oviduct (oh-vi-dukt) *n. see* Fallopian tube.

ovulation (ov-yoo-lay-shŏn) *n.* the process by which an ovum is released from a mature Graafian follicle. The fluid-filled follicle distends the surface of the ovary until a thin spot breaks down and the ovum

perivitelline space
zona pellucida
ooplasm
centrosome with two centrioles
nucleus
corona radiata

A mature ovum (about X 600)

floats out and starts to travel down the Fallopian tube to the uterus.

ovum (egg cell) (oh-vŭm) n. (pl. **ova**) the mature female sex cell (see gamete).

oxalate (oks-ă-layt) n. a salt of oxalic acid. **balanced o.** a mixture of ammonium and potassium oxalates (an anticoagulant) in which blood specimens are stored before laboratory examination.

oxalic acid (oks-al-ik) n. an extremely poisonous acid found in many plants, including sorrel and the leaves of rhubarb, and in some bleaching powders. When swallowed it produces burning sensations in the mouth and throat, vomiting of blood, breathing difficulties, and circulatory collapse. Treatment is with calcium lactate or other calcium salts, lime water, or milk. Formula: $C_2H_2O_4$.

oxaluria (oks-ăl-yoor-iă) n. the presence in the urine of oxalic acid or oxalates, especially calcium oxalate.

oxazepam (oks-az-ē-pam) n. a benzodiazepine drug administered by mouth to relieve anxiety and ten-

sion and for the treatment of alcoholism.

oxidant (oks-i-dănt) n. (in biological systems) a molecule that serves as an electron acceptor. In human disease oxidants are derived from normal intracellular processes and released by inflammatory cells. They are counteracted by antioxidants, such as beta-carotene.

oxidase (oks-i-dayz) n. see oxidoreductase.

oxidation (oks-i-day-shŏn) n. a reaction in which an atom or molecule loses electrons. Many biological oxidations are effected by the removal of hydrogen atoms, which combine with an oxidizing agent. For example, glucose is oxidized during cellular respiration: $C_6H_{12}O_6 + 6O_2 \rightarrow 6CO_2 + 6H_2O$.

oxidoreductase (oks-i-doh-ri-duk-tayz) n. one of a group of enzymes that catalyse oxidation-reduction reactions. This class includes the enzymes formerly known either as dehydrogenases or as oxidases.

oximeter (oks-im-it-er) n. an instrument for measuring the proportion of oxyhaemoglobin in the blood.

oxprenolol (oks-pren-ŏ-lol) n. a drug that controls the activity of the heart (see beta blocker), administered by mouth to treat angina, high blood pressure, and abnormal heart rhythm. Trade name: **Trasicor**.

oxybutynin (oksi-bew-tin-in) n. an anticholinergic drug administered orally to reduce frequency and urgency of passing urine associated with an unstable bladder or instability of the detrusor muscle of the bladder wall.

oxycephaly (turricephaly) (oksi-sef-ăli) n. a deformity of the bones of the skull giving the head a pointed appearance. *See also* craniosynostosis. —**oxycephalic** (oksi-si-**fal**-ik) *adj.*

oxygen (oks-i-jĕn) *n.* an odourless colourless gas that makes up one-fifth of the atmosphere. Oxygen is essential to most forms of life; in humans, it is absorbed into the blood from air breathed into the lungs. Oxygen is administered therapeutically in various conditions in which the tissues are unable to obtain an adequate supply through the lungs. Symbol: O. **o. deficit** a physiological condition that exists in cells during periods of temporary oxygen shortage. **o. tent** *see* tent.

oxygenation (oksi-ji-**nay**-shŏn) *n.* the process of becoming saturated with oxygen, such as occurs in the lungs during inhalation of air.

oxygenator (oks-i-ji-nay-ter) *n.* a machine that oxygenates blood outside the body. *See also* heart-lung machine.

oxyhaemoglobin (oksi-hee-moh-**gloh**-bin) *n.* the bright-red substance formed when the pigment haemoglobin in red blood cells combines reversibly with oxygen. Oxyhaemoglobin is the form in which oxygen is transported from the lungs to the tissues. *Compare* methaemoglobin.

oxymetazoline (oksi-met-**az**-oh-leen) *n.* a sympathomimetic drug administered as a nasal spray to treat nasal congestion. Trade name: **Afrazine**.

oxyntic cells (parietal cells) (oks-**in**-tik) *pl. n.* cells of the gastric glands that secrete hydrochloric acid in the fundic region of the stomach.

oxytetracycline (oksi-tet-ră-sy-kleen) *n.* an antibiotic administered by mouth to treat infections caused by a wide variety of bacteria (*see* tetracycline). Trade name: **Terramycin**.

oxytocic (oksi-toh-sik) *n.* any agent that induces or accelerates labour by stimulating the muscles of the uterus to contract. *See also* oxytocin.

oxytocin (oksi-toh-sin) *n.* a hormone, released by the pituitary gland, that causes contraction of the uterus during labour and stimulates milk flow from the breasts by causing contraction of muscle fibres in the milk ducts. Intravenous infusions of oxytocin (Syntocinon) are used to induce uterine contractions and to control or prevent postpartum haemorrhage.

oxyuriasis (oksi-yoor-I-ă-sis) *n. see* enterobiasis.

Oxyuris (oksi-**yoor**-iss) *n. see* threadworm.

ozaena (oh-zee-nă) *n.* a disorder of the nose in which the mucous membranes inside the nose become atrophied, with the production of an offensive discharge and crusts.

ozone (oh-zohn) *n.* a poisonous gas containing three oxygen atoms per molecule. Ozone is a very powerful oxidizing agent. It is found in the atmosphere at very high altitudes (the *ozone layer*) and is responsible for absorbing a large proportion of the sun's ultraviolet radiation.

Pp

P *symbol for* phosphorus.

Pacchionian body (pak-i-oh-ni-ăn) *n. see* arachnoid. [A. Pacchioni (1665–1726), Italian anatomist]

pacemaker (payss-mayk-er) *n.* **1** a device used to produce and maintain a normal heart rate in patients who have heart block. It consists of a battery that stimulates the heart through an insulated electrode wire attached to the surface of the ventricle (*epicardial p.*) or lying in contact with the lining of the heart (*endocardial p.*). A pacemaker may be temporary, with an external battery, or it may be permanent, when the whole apparatus is surgically implanted under the skin. **2.** the part of the heart that regulates the rate at which it beats: the sinoatrial node.

pachy- *prefix denoting* **1.** thickening of a part or parts. **2.** the dura mater.

pachydactyly (pak-i-dak-tili) *n.* abnormal enlargement of the fingers and toes, occurring either as a congenital abnormality or as part of an acquired disease (such as acromegaly).

pachymeningitis (pak-i-men-in-jy-tis) *n.* inflammation of the dura mater (*see* meningitis).

pachymeninx (pak-i-mee-ninks) *n.* the dura mater, outermost of the three meninges.

pachymeter (pak-im-it-er) *n.* an instrument used to measure the thickness of the cornea. —**pachymetry** *n.*

pachysomia (pak-i-soh-miă) *n.* thickening of parts of the body, which occurs in certain diseases.

Pacinian corpuscles (pă-sin-iăn) *pl. n.* sensory receptors for touch in the skin, consisting of sensory nerve endings surrounded by capsules of membrane. They are especially sensitive to changes in pressure and therefore detect vibration particularly well. [F. Pacini (1812–83), Italian anatomist]

pack (pak) *n.* a pad of folded moistened material, such as cotton-wool, applied to the body or inserted into a cavity.

packed cell volume (PCV, haematocrit) *n.* the volume of the red cells (erythrocytes) in blood, expressed as a fraction of the total volume of the blood.

paclitaxel (pak-li-taks-ĕl) *n.* a cytotoxic anticancer drug (*see* taxane) administered by intravenous infusion to treat ovarian cancer and breast cancer that is resistant to standard therapies. Trade name: **Taxol.**

PACS *n.* picture archiving and communication system: an electronic system enabling the storage of digital images on electronic media, for later retrieval and subsequent display on high-resolution monitors. Images are moved using a hospital computer network, can be manipulated on screen, and can be viewed, simultaneously by more than one person, at local or distant sites.

pad (pad) *n.* cotton-wool, foam rubber, or other material used to protect a part of the body from friction, bruising, or other unwanted contact.

paed- (**paedo-**) *prefix denoting* children.

paediatric advanced life support (PALS) (peed-i-at-rik) *n.* a structured and algorithm-driven method of life support for use in severe medical emergencies in children.

paediatrics (peed-i-at-riks) *n.* the general medicine of childhood. Handling the sick child requires detailed knowledge of genetics, obstetrics, psychological development, management of handicaps at home and in school, and effects of social conditions on child health. *See also* child health clinic. —**paediatric** *adj.* —**paediatrician** (peed-i-ă-trish-ăn) *n.*

Paget's disease (paj-its) *n.* **1.** a chronic disease of bones, occurring in the elderly and most frequently affecting the skull, backbone, pelvis, and long bones; affected bones become thickened. There are often no symptoms, but pain, deformity, and fracture can occur. Medical name: **osteitis deformans**. **2.** a malignant condition of the nipple, resembling eczema in appearance, that is associated with underlying infiltrating cancer of the breast. [Sir J. Paget (1814–99), British surgeon]

pain (payn) *n.* an unpleasant sensation ranging from mild discomfort to agonized distress, associated with real or potential tissue damage.

Pain is a subjective response to impulses from the peripheral nerves in damaged tissue, which pass to nerves in the spinal cord, where they are subjected to a gate control. This gate modifies the subsequent passage of the impulses in accordance with descending controls from the brain. Because attention is a crucial component of pain, distraction can act as a basis for pain therapy. On the other hand, anxiety and depression focus the attention and exaggerate the pain. If the nerve pathways are damaged, the brain can increase the amplification in the pathway, maintaining the sensation as a protective mechanism.

pain clinic *n.* a clinic that specializes in techniques of long-term pain relief, such as transcutaneous electrical nerve stimulation (TENS). Pain clinics are usually directed by anaesthetists.

paint (paynt) *n.* (in pharmacy) a liquid preparation that is applied to the skin or mucous membranes. Paints usually contain antiseptics, astringents, caustics, or analgesics.

palaeo- *prefix denoting* **1.** ancient. **2.** primitive.

palate (pal-ăt) *n.* the roof of the mouth, which separates the mouth from the nasal cavity. *hard p.* the front part of the palate. It is formed by processes of the maxillae and palatine bones and is covered by mucous membrane. *soft p.* the posterior part of the palate: a movable fold of mucous membrane that tapers at the back of the mouth to form the uvula. *See also* cleft palate.

palatine bone (pal-ă-tyn) *n.* either of a pair of approximately L-shaped bones of the face that contribute to the hard palate, the nasal cavity, and the orbits.

palato- *prefix denoting* **1.** the palate. **2.** the palatine bone.

palatoplasty (pal-a-toh-plasti) *n.* plastic surgery of the roof of the mouth, usually to correct cleft palate or other congenital defects. *laser p.* laser surgery to shorten and/or stiffen the palate in the treatment of snoring.

palatoplegia (pal-ă-toh-plee-jiă) *n.* paralysis of the soft palate.

palatorrhaphy (pal-ăt-o-răfi) *n. see* staphylorrhaphy.

pali- (palin-) *prefix denoting* repetition or recurrence.

palilalia (pal-i-lay-liă) *n.* a disorder of speech in which a word spoken by the individual is rapidly and involuntarily repeated.

palindromic (pal-in-drom-ik) *adj* relapsing: describing diseases or symptoms that recur or get worse.

palliative (pal-i-ătiv) *n.* a medicine that gives temporary relief from the symptoms of a disease but does not actually cure the disease.

pallidotomy (pallidectomy) (pal-i-**dot**-ŏmi) *n.* a neurosurgical operation to destroy or modify the effects of the globus pallidus (*see* basal ganglia) for the relief of parkinsonism and other conditions in which involuntary movements are prominent. It is now performed by stereotaxy.

pallor (pal-er) *n.* abnormal paleness of the skin, due to reduced blood flow or lack of normal pigments. Pallor may indicate shock, anaemia, cancer, or other diseases.

palmar (pal-mer) *adj.* relating to the palm of the hand. *p. arches* two arterial arches (deep and superficial)

in the palm of the hand, formed by anastomosis of the ulnar and radial arteries.

palmitic acid (pal-mit-ik) *n. see* fatty acid.

palpation (pal-**pay**-shŏn) *n.* the process of examining part of the body by careful feeling with the hands and fingertips.

palpebral (pal-pi-brăl) *adj.* relating to the eyelid (*palpebra*).

palpitation (pal-pi-tay-shŏn) *n.* an awareness of the heartbeat. This is normal with fear, emotion, or exertion. It may also be a symptom of neurosis, arrhythmias, heart disease, and overactivity of the circulation.

PALS *n.* **1.** *see* paediatric advanced life support. **2.** *see* patient advocacy liaison service.

palsy (pawl-zi) *n.* paralysis. *See* Bell's palsy; cerebral palsy.

paludism (pal-yoo-dizm) *n. see* malaria.

pamidronate (pam-i-**droh**-nayt) *n. see* bisphosphonates.

pan- (pant(o)-) *prefix denoting* all; every; hence (in medicine) affecting all parts of an organ or the body; generalized.

panacea (pan-ă-**see**-ă) *n.* a medicine said to be a cure for all diseases and disorders. Unfortunately panaceas do not exist, despite the claims of many patent medicine manufacturers.

Panadol (pan-ă-dol) *n. see* paracetamol.

panarthritis (pan-arth-ry-tis) *n.* inflammation of all the structures involved in a joint. *See* arthritis.

pancarditis (pan-kar-dy-tis) *n.* an inflammatory disorder affecting the pericardium, endocardium, and heart muscle.

Pancoast syndrome (pan-kohst) *n.* pain and paralysis involving the lower branches of the brachial plexus due to infiltration by a malignant tumour of the apical region of the lung. Horner's syndrome may also be present. [H. K. Pancoast (1875–1939), US radiologist]

pancreas (pank-ri-ǎs) *n.* a compound gland, about 15 cm long, that lies behind the stomach. One end lies in the curve of the duodenum; the other end touches the spleen. It is composed of clusters (acini) of cells that secrete pancreatic juice into the duodenum via the *pancreatic duct*, which unites with the common bile duct. Interspersed among the acini are the islets of Langerhans, which secrete the hormones insulin and glucagon into the bloodstream. —**pancreatic** (pank-ri-at-ik) *adj.*

pancreatectomy (pank-ri-ǎ-tek-tŏmi) *n.* surgical removal of the pancreas, performed for tumours in the gland or because of chronic or relapsing pancreatitis. *partial p.* removal of a portion of the gland. *subtotal p.* removal of most of the gland. *total p.* (*Whipple's operation*) removal of the entire gland and part of the duodenum.

pancreatic juice *n.* the mixture of digestive enzymes secreted by the pancreas. Its production is stimulated by hormones secreted by the duodenum (*see* cholecystokinin, secretin).

pancreatic polypeptide *n.* a hormone released from the delta cells of the islets of Langerhans of the pancreas in response to protein in the small intestine. Its actions are to inhibit pancreatic bicarbonate and protein enzyme secretion and to relax the gall bladder.

pancreatin (pank-ri-ǎ-tin) *n.* an extract obtained from the pancreas, containing the pancreatic enzymes. Pancreatin is administered to treat conditions in which pancreatic secretion is deficient; for example, in pancreatitis.

pancreatitis (pank-ri-ǎ-ty-tis) *n.* inflammation of the pancreas. *acute p.* a sudden illness in which the patient experiences severe pain in the upper abdomen and back, with shock. Treatment consists of intravenous feeding and anticholinergic drugs. *chronic p.* pancreatitis that may produce symptoms similar to relapsing pancreatitis or may be painless; it leads to pancreatic failure causing malabsorption and diabetes mellitus. *relapsing p.* pancreatitis in which the symptoms of acute pancreatitis are recurrent and less severe. It may be associated with gallstones or with alcoholism.

pancreatotomy (pank-ri-ǎ-tot-ŏmi) *n.* surgical opening of the duct of the pancreas in order to inspect the duct, to join the duct to the intestine, or to inject a contrast medium.

pancreozymin (pank-ri-oh-zy-min) *n.* the name originally given to the fraction of the hormone cholecystokinin that acts on the pancreas.

pancytopenia (pan-sy-toh-pee-niǎ) *n.* a simultaneous decrease in the numbers of red cells, white cells, and platelets in the blood. It occurs in a variety of disorders, including aplastic anaemias, hypersplenism, and tumours of the bone marrow, and may occur after chemotherapy or total body irradiation.

pandemic (pan-dem-ik) *n.* an epidemic so widely spread that vast numbers of people in different countries are affected. —**pandemic** *adj.*

panic disorder (pan-ik) *n.* a condition featuring recurrent *panic attacks*: brief episodes of acute distress in which the heart beats rapidly, breathing is deep and fast, and sweating occurs. The attacks are especially common in people with agoraphobia. The condition appears to be an organic disorder with a strong psychological component.

panniculitis (Weber-Christian disease) (pă-nik-yoo-ly-tis) *n.* inflammation of the panniculus adiposus, leading to multiple tender nodules in the legs and trunk.

panniculus (pă-nik-yoo-lŭs) *n.* a membranous sheet of tissue. *p. adiposus* the fatty layer of tissue underlying the skin.

pannus (pan-ŭs) *n.* invasion of the outer layers of the cornea of the eye by tissue containing many blood vessels, which grows in from the conjunctiva.

panophthalmitis (pan-off-thal-my-tis) *n.* inflammation involving the whole of the interior of the eye.

panosteitis (pan-osti-I-tis) *n.* inflammation of all the structures of a bone.

panotitis (pan-ŏ-ty-tis) *n.* inflammation of both the middle and the inner ears.

pant- (panto-) *prefix. see* pan-.

pantothenic acid (pan-tŏ-theen-ik) *n.* a B vitamin that is a constituent of coenzyme A. It plays an important role in the transfer of acetyl groups in the body.

pantropic (pan-trop-ik) *adj.* describing a virus that can invade and affect many different tissues of the body without showing a special affinity for any one of them.

PAP *n.* primary atypical pneumonia. *See* atypical (pneumonia).

Papanicolaou test (Pap test) (pap-ă-nik-oh-lay-oo) *n.* a test to detect cancer of the cervix or lining of the uterus. *See also* cervical (smear). [G. N. Papanicolaou (1883–1962), Greek physician, anatomist, and cytologist]

papaveretum (pă-pav-er-ee-tŭm) *n. see* papaverine.

papaverine (pă-pav-er-een) *n.* an alkaloid, derived from opium, that relaxes smooth muscle. In combination with morphine and codeine (a mixture called *papaveretum*), it is administered by injection as a preanaesthetic medication and for the relief of postoperative pain.

papilla (pă-pil-ă) *n.* (*pl.* **papillae**) any small nipple-shaped protuberance. Several different kinds of papillae occur on the tongue, in association with the taste buds. *optic p. see* optic (disc). —**papillary** *adj.*

papillitis (pap-i-ly-tis) *n.* inflammation of the optic disc.

papilloedema (pap-il-ee-dee-mă) *n.* swelling of the optic disc.

papilloma (pap-i-loh-mă) *n.* a benign nipple-like growth on the surface of skin or mucous membrane. *basal-cell p. see* (seborrhoeic) keratosis. —**papillomatous** *adj.*

papillomatosis (pap-i-loh-mă-toh-sis) *n.* a condition in which many papillomas grow on an area of skin or mucous membrane.

papillotomy (pap-i-lot-ŏmi) *n.* the operation of cutting the ampulla of

Vater to widen its outlet in order to improve bile drainage and allow the passage of stones from the common bile duct. It is usually performed using a diathermy wire through a duodenoscope following ERCP.

papovavirus (pap-oh-vă-vy-rŭs) *n.* one of a group of small DNA-containing viruses producing tumours in animals and humans.

Pap test (pap) *n. see* Papanicolaou test.

papule (pap-yool) *n.* a small raised spot on the skin. —**papular** *adj.*

papulo- *prefix denoting* a papule or pimple.

papulopustular (pap-yoo-loh-pus-tew-ler) *adj.* describing a rash that contains both papules and pustules.

papulosquamous (pap-yoo-loh-skway-mŭs) *adj.* describing a rash that is both papular and scaly.

para- *prefix denoting* **1.** beside or near. **2.** resembling. **3.** abnormal.

paracentesis (pa-ră-sen-tee-sis) *n.* tapping: the process of drawing off fluid from a part of the body through a hollow needle or cannula. In ophthalmology it involves an incision into the anterior chamber of the eye.

paracetamol (acetaminophen) (pa-ră-see-tă-mol) *n.* an analgesic drug that also reduces fever. It is administered by mouth to treat mild or moderate pain, such as headache, toothache, and rheumatism. Trade names: **Calpol, Panadol, Panaleve.**

paracusis (pa-ră-kew-sis) *n.* any distortion of hearing.

paradoxical breathing (pa-ră-doks-ikăl) *n.* breathing movements in which the chest wall moves in on inspiration and out on expiration, in reverse of the normal move-ments. It may be seen in children with respiratory distress and patients with chronic airways obstruction. Crush injuries of the chest can lead to a severe degree of paradoxical breathing.

paraesthesiae (pa-ris-theez-i-ee) *pl. n.* spontaneously occurring abnormal tingling sensations, sometimes described as *pins and needles*. *Compare* dysaesthesiae.

paraffin (pa-ră-fin) *n.* one of a series of hydrocarbons derived from petroleum. *liquid p.* a mineral oil, which has been used as a laxative. *p. wax (hard p.)* a whitish mixture of solid hydrocarbons, used in medicine mainly as a base for ointments.

paraganglioma (pa-ră-gang-li-oh-mă) *n.* a benign tumour arising from paraganglion cells. Such tumours can occur around the aorta, the carotid artery (carotid body tumour), and the cervical portion of the vagus nerve (*see* glomus tumour), as well as in the abdomen and the eye.

paraganglion (pa-ră-gang-li-ŏn) *n.* one of the small oval masses of cells in the walls of the ganglia of the sympathetic nervous system, near the spinal cord. They may secrete adrenaline.

parageusia (parageusis) (pa-ră-gew-siă) *n.* abnormality of the sense of taste.

paragonimiasis (endemic haemoptysis) (pa-ră-gon-i-my-ă-sis) *n.* a tropical disease, occurring principally in the Far East, caused by the presence of the fluke *Paragonimus westermani* in the lungs. Symptoms include the coughing up of blood and dyspnoea.

parainfluenza viruses (pa-ră-in-floo-**en**-ză) *pl. n.* a group of large RNA-containing viruses that cause infections of the respiratory tract producing mild influenza-like symptoms. They are included in the paramyxovirus group (*see* myxovirus).

paraldehyde (pă-**ral**-di-hyd) *n.* an anticonvulsant drug administered by injection or enema to control seizures in status epilepticus.

paralysis (pă-**ral**-i-sis) *n.* muscle weakness that varies in its extent, its severity, and the degree of spasticity or flaccidity according to the nature of the underlying disease and its distribution in the brain, spinal cord, peripheral nerves, or muscles. *See also* diplegia, hemiplegia, paraplegia, poliomyelitis. —**paralytic** (pa-ră-**lit**-ik) *adj.*

paramedian (pa-ră-**mee**-di-ăn) *adj.* situated close to or beside the median plane.

paramedical (pa-ră-**med**-ikăl) *adj.* describing or relating to the professions closely linked to the medical profession and working in conjunction with them. Paramedical personnel in a hospital include radiographers, physiotherapists, occupational therapists, and dietitians.

paramesonephric duct (Müllerian duct) (pa-ră-mes-oh-**nef**-rik) *n.* either of a pair of ducts in the embryo that develop into the Fallopian tubes, uterus and part of the vagina.

parameter (pă-**ram**-it-er) *n.* (in medicine) a measurement of some factor, such as blood pressure, pulse rate, or haemoglobin level, that may have a bearing on the condition being investigated.

parametritis (pelvic cellulitis) (pa-ră-mi-**try**-tis) *n.* inflammation of the parametrium. The condition may be associated with puerperal infection.

parametrium (pa-ră-**mee**-triŭm) *n.* the layer of connective tissue surrounding the uterus.

paramnesia (pa-ram-**nee**-ziă) *n.* a distorted memory, such as confabulation or déjà vu.

paramyotonia congenita (pa-ră-my-ŏ-**toh**-nia kŏn-**jen**-it-ă) *n.* a rare constitutional disorder in which myotonia develops when the patient is exposed to cold. This may be due to a disorder of potassium channels.

paramyxovirus (pa-ră-**miks**-oh-vy-rŭs) *n. see* myxovirus.

paranasal sinuses (pa-ră-**nay**-zăl) *pl. n.* the air-filled spaces, lined with mucous membrane, that occur in some bones of the skull and open into the nasal cavity. They comprise the *frontal sinuses* and the *maxillary sinuses* (one pair of each), the *ethmoid sinuses* (consisting of many spaces inside the ethmoid bone), and the two *sphenoid sinuses*.

paraneoplastic syndrome (pa-ră-nee-oh-**plast**-ik) *n.* signs or symptoms that may occur in a patient with cancer but are not due directly to local effects of the cancer cells. Removal of the cancer usually leads to resolution of the problem. An example is myasthenia gravis secondary to a tumour of the thymus.

paranoia (pa-ră-**noi**-ă) *n.* a mental disorder characterized by delusions organized into a system, without hallucinations or other marked symptoms of mental illness. The same term is sometimes used more loosely for a state of mind in which the individual has a strong belief that he or she is persecuted by others.

paranoid (pa-ră-noid) *adj.* **1.** describing a mental state characterized by fixed and logically elaborated delusions. There are many causes, including paranoid schizophrenia, manic-depressive psychosis, and severe emotional stress. **2.** describing a personality distinguished by such traits as excessive sensitivity to rejection by others, suspiciousness, hostility, and self-importance.

paraparesis (pa-ră-pă-ree-sis) *n.* weakness of both legs, resulting from disease of the nervous system.

paraphasia (pa-ră-fay-ziă) *n.* a disorder of language in which unintended syllables, words, or phrases are interpolated in the patient's speech.

paraphimosis (pa-ră-fi-moh-sis) *n.* retraction and constriction of the foreskin behind the glans penis. The tight foreskin cannot be drawn back over the glans and becomes painful and swollen.

paraphrenia (pa-ră-free-niă) *n.* a mental disorder, typically seen in the elderly and deaf, that is characterized by systematic delusions and prominent hallucinations but without any other marked symptoms of mental illness. Some sufferers eventually show other symptoms of schizophrenia.

paraplegia (pa-ră-plee-jiă) *n.* paralysis of both legs, usually due to disease or injury of the spinal cord. It is often accompanied by loss of sensation below the level of the injury and disturbed bladder function. —**paraplegic** *adj.*, *n.*

parapsoriasis (pa-ră-sŏ-ry-ă-sis) *n.* a former name for the earliest phase of mycosis fungoides.

parapsychology (pa-ră-sy-kol-ŏji) *n.* the study of mental abilities that appear to defy natural law.

Paraquat (pa-ră-kwot) *n. Trademark.* the chemical compound dimethyl dipyridilium, widely used as a weed-killer. When swallowed it exerts its most serious effects upon the lungs, the tissues of which it destroys after a few days.

parasite (pa-ră-syt) *n.* any living thing that lives in or on another living organism (*see* host). Some parasites cause irritation and interfere with bodily functions; others destroy host tissues and release toxins into the body. Human parasites include fungi, bacteria, viruses, protozoa, and worms. *See also* commensal, symbiosis. —**parasitic** (pa-ră-sit-ik) *adj.*

parasiticide (pa-ră-sit-i-syd) *n.* an agent that destroys parasites (excluding bacteria and fungi). *See also* acaricide, anthelmintic, trypanocide.

parasitology (pa-ră-sit-ol-ŏji) *n.* the study and science of parasites.

parasuicide (pa-ră-soo-i-syd) *n.* a self-injuring act (such as an overdose of sleeping pills) that is not motivated by a genuine wish to die. *Compare* (attempted) suicide.

parasympathetic nervous system (pa-ră-sim-pă-thet-ik) *n.* one of the two divisions of the autonomic nervous system, having fibres that leave the central nervous system from the brain and the lower portion of the spinal cord and are distributed to blood vessels, glands, and internal organs. It is responsible for (among other effects) slowing the heart rate and constricting the pupillary muscles. The nerve endings release acetylcholine as a neurotransmitter.

parasympatholytic (pa-ră-sim-pă-thoh-lit-ik) *adj.* opposing the effects of the parasympathetic nervous system. Anticholinergic drugs have this effect.

parasympathomimetic (pa-ră-sim-pă-thoh-mi-met-ik) *adj.* having the effect of stimulating the parasympathetic nervous system. The actions of the parasympathomimetic drugs are *cholinergic* (resembling those of acetylcholine) and include stimulation of skeletal muscle, vasodilatation, depression of heart rate, increasing the tension of smooth muscle, increasing secretions (such as saliva), and constricting the pupil of the eye.

parathion (pa-ră-th'y-on) *n.* an organic phosphorus compound, used as a pesticide, that causes poisoning when inhaled, ingested, or absorbed through the skin. The symptoms are headache, sweating, salivation, lacrimation, vomiting, diarrhoea, and muscular spasms. Treatment is by administration of atropine.

parathormone (pa-ră-thor-mohn) *n. see* parathyroid hormone.

parathyroidectomy (pa-ră-th'y-roid-ek-tŏmi) *n.* surgical removal of the parathyroid glands, usually as part of the treatment of hyperparathyroidism.

parathyroid glands (pa-ră-th'y-roid) *pl. n.* two pairs of yellowish-brown endocrine glands that are situated behind, or sometimes embedded within, the thyroid gland. They are stimulated to produce

parathyroid hormone by a decrease in the amount of calcium in the blood.

parathyroid hormone (parathormone) *n.* a hormone, synthesized and released by the parathyroid glands, that controls the distribution of calcium and phosphate in the body. A deficiency of the hormone lowers blood calcium levels, causing tetany. *Compare* calcitonin.

paratyphoid fever (pa-ră-ty-foid) *n.* an infectious disease caused by the bacterium *Salmonella paratyphi* A, B, or C. Symptoms include diarrhoea, mild fever, and a pink rash on the chest. Treatment with chloramphenicol is effective. Vaccination with TAB provides temporary immunity against paratyphoid A and B.

paravertebral (pa-ră-ver-tib-răl) *adj.* close to or at the side of the backbone.

parenchyma (pă-renk-im-ă) *n.* the functional part of an organ, as opposed to the supporting tissue (*see* stroma).

parenteral (pa-rent-er-ăl) *adj.* administered by any way other than through the mouth: applied, for example, to the introduction of drugs into the body by injection. *p. feeding see* nutrition.

paresis (pă-ree-sis) *n.* muscular weakness caused by disease of the nervous system. It implies a lesser degree of weakness than paralysis, although the two words are often used interchangeably.

paries (pair-i-eez) *n.* (*pl.* **parietes**) **1.** the enveloping or surrounding part of an organ or other structure. **2.** the wall of a cavity.

parietal (pă-ry-ĕ-t'l) *adj.* of or relating to the inner walls of a body cavity, as opposed to the contents. **p. bone** either of a pair of bones forming the top and sides of the cranium. *See* skull. **p. cells** *see* oxyntic cells. **p. lobe** one of the major divisions of each cerebral hemisphere (*see* cerebrum), lying beneath the crown of the skull. It contains the sensory cortex and association areas. **p. pleura** *see* pleura.

parity (pa-riti) *n.* a term used to indicate the number of pregnancies a woman has had that have each resulted in the birth of an infant capable of survival. *See also* grand multiparity.

parkinsonism (par-kin-sŏn-izm) *n.* a clinical picture characterized by tremor, rigidity, slowness of movement, and postural instability. The patient has an expressionless face, an unmodulated voice, an increasing tendency to stoop, and a shuffling walk. Parkinsonism is a disease process affecting the basal ganglia of the brain and associated with a deficiency of the neurotransmitter dopamine. Sometimes a distinction is made between *Parkinson's disease*, a degenerative disorder associated with ageing, and parkinsonism due to other causes, notably the long-term use of antipsychotic drugs. Relief of the symptoms may be obtained with anticholinergic drugs, levodopa, dopamine-receptor agonists (e.g. bromocriptine), and apomorphine. [J. Parkinson (1755–1824), British physician]

paronychia (whitlow) (pa-roh-nik-iă) *n.* an inflamed swelling of the nail folds. *acute p.* a condition that is usually caused by infection with *Staphylococcus aureus. chronic p.* paronychia that occurs mainly in those who habitually engage in wet work; it is associated with secondary infection with *Candida albicans.*

parosmia (pa-roz-miă) *n.* any disorder of the sense of smell.

parotid gland (pă-rot-id) *n.* one of a pair of salivary glands situated in front of each ear.

parotitis (pa-rŏ-ty-tis) *n.* inflammation of the parotid salivary glands. *See* mumps (infectious parotitis).

parous (pa-rŭs) *adj.* having given birth to one or more children.

paroxetine (pă-roks-ĕ-teen) *n.* an antidepressant drug that acts by prolonging the action of the neurotransmitter serotonin (5-hydroxytryptamine) in the brain (*see* SSRI). It is taken by mouth. Trade name: **Seroxat**.

paroxysm (pa-rŏk-sizm) *n.* **1.** a sudden violent attack, especially a spasm or convulsion. **2.** the abrupt worsening of symptoms or recurrence of disease. —**paroxysmal** (pa-rŏk-siz-măl) *adj.*

paroxysmal dyspnoea *n.* attacks of breathlessness occurring at night due to left ventricular heart failure.

paroxysmal tachycardia *n.* abnormally increased heart rate due to impulses generated anywhere in the heart outside the natural pacemaker (sinoatrial node), for example in the atrial muscle (*paroxysmal atrial tachycardia, PAT*).

parrot disease (pa-rŏt) *n. see* psittacosis.

pars (parz) *n.* a specific part of an

organ or other structure, such as any of parts of the pituitary gland.

Parse's nursing theory (parz-iz) *n.* a theory that views patients as taking an active and continuous role in their development, being free to select the means of achieving a particular way of living. Nurse and patient should work together to derive the meaning of a particular situation for the patient to enable the planning of health-care intervention. [R. Parse (20th century), nurse theorist]

parthenogenesis (par-thin-oh-jen-i-sis) *n.* reproduction in which an organism develops from an unfertilized ovum. It is common in plants and occurs in some lower animals (e.g. aphids).

partially sighted register (par-shă-li) *n.* (in Britain) a list of persons who have poor sight but are not technically blind. In general their sight is adequate to permit the performance of tasks for which some vision is essential. *Compare* blind register.

partogram (par-toh-gram) *n.* a graphic record of the course of labour.

parturition (par-tewr-ish-ŏn) *n.* childbirth. *See* labour. —**parturient** (par-tewr-i-ĕnt) *adj.*

parvi- *prefix denoting* small size.

pascal (pas-kăl) *n.* the SI unit of pressure, equal to 1 newton per square metre. Symbol: Pa.

Paschen bodies (pah-skĕn) *pl. n.* particles that occur in the cells of skin rashes in patients with cowpox or smallpox; they are thought to be the virus particles. [E. Paschen (1860–1936), German pathologist]

passive movement (pas-iv) *n.*

movement not brought about by a patient's own efforts. Passive movements are induced by manipulation of the joints by a physiotherapist. *Compare* active movement.

Pasteurella (pas-cher-el-ă) *n.* a genus of small rodlike Gram-negative bacteria that are parasites of animals and humans. *P. multocida* a species that usually infects animals but may be transmitted to humans through bites or scratches.

pasteurization (pas-cher-I-zay-shŏn) *n.* the treatment of milk by heating it to 65°C for 30 minutes, or to 72°C for 15 minutes, followed by rapid cooling, to kill such bacteria as those of tuberculosis and typhoid.

pastille (pas-t'l) *n.* a medicinal preparation containing gelatine and glycerine that is dissolved in the mouth so that the medication is applied to the mouth or throat.

PAT *n. see* paroxysmal (atrial) tachycardia.

Patau syndrome (pat-ow) *n.* a chromosome disorder in which there are three no. 13 chromosomes (instead of the usual two), causing abnormal brain development, severe mental retardation, and defects in the heart, kidney, and scalp. Affected individuals rarely survive. [K. Patau (20th century), US geneticist]

patch test (pach) *n.* a test to discover which allergen is responsible for contact dermatitis in a patient. Very low concentrations of different allergens are applied under a patch on the back: a positive test will show an eczematous reaction.

patella (pă-tel-ă) *n.* the lens-shaped bone that forms the kneecap. It is situated in front of the knee in the tendon of the quadriceps muscle of the thigh. *See also* sesamoid bone. —**patellar** (pă-tel-er) *adj.*

patellar reflex *n.* the knee jerk, in which stretching the muscle at the front of the thigh by tapping its tendon below the kneecap causes a reflex contraction of the muscle, so that the leg kicks.

patellectomy (pat-ĕ-lek-tŏmi) *n.* surgical excision of the patella.

patent (pay-tĕnt) *adj.* open; unblocked. *p. ductus arteriosus see* ductus arteriosus.

path- (patho-) *prefix denoting* disease.

pathogen (pa-thŏ-jen) *n.* a microorganism, such as a bacterium, that parasitizes an animal (or plant) or a human and produces a disease.

pathogenesis (pa-thŏ-jen-i-sis) *n.* the origin and development of a disease. —**pathogenetic** (pa-thoh-ji-net-ik) *adj.*

pathogenic (pa-thŏ-jen-ik) *adj.* capable of causing disease. The term is applied to a parasitic microorganism (especially a bacterium) in relation to its host. —**pathogenicity** *n.*

pathognomonic (pa-thŏg-noh-mon-ik) *adj.* describing a symptom or sign that is characteristic of or unique to a particular disease.

pathological (pa-thŏ-loj-ikăl) *adj.* relating to or arising from disease. *p. fracture see* fracture.

pathology (pă-thol-ŏji) *n.* the study of disease processes with the aim of understanding their nature and causes. *clinical p.* the application of the knowledge of disease processes to the treatment of patients. —**pathologist** *n.*

-pathy *suffix denoting* **1.** disease. **2.** therapy.

patient advocacy liaison service (PALS) (pay-shĕnt ad-vŏ-kă-si lee-ay-zŏn) *n.* an advocacy service for patients in acute trusts and Primary Care Trusts that presents patients' concerns and complaints to the trust. It has taken on some of the services provided by the Community Health Council.

patient allocation (al-ŏ-kay-shŏn) *n.* a method of organizing nursing care in which a nurse is allocated to care holistically for all the needs of a patient on a daily basis. *Compare* task allocation.

patient-controlled analgesia (PCA) *n.* a form of pain control, used especially postoperatively, in which the patient holds a device with a button that, when pressed, administers a preset dose of an analgesic (usually morphine) into the patient's bloodstream.

Paul-Bunnell test (pawl-bŭ-nel) *n.* a haemagglutination test used in the diagnosis of glandular fever. [J. R. Paul (1893–1971) and W. W. Bunnell (1902–66), US physicians]

Paul's tube (pawlz) *n.* a glass tube with a projecting rim, used to drain the bowel after it has been brought to the surface of the abdomen and opened. [F. T. Paul (1851–1941), British surgeon]

PBC *n. see* (primary biliary) cirrhosis.

PBM *n.* peak bone mass.

p.c. (**post cibum**) Latin: after food, used as a direction in prescriptions.

PCA *n. see* patient-controlled analgesia.

PCG *n. see* Primary Care Group.

PCP *n.* Pneumocystis carinii pneumonia. *See* Pneumocystis.

PCT *n.* *see* Primary Care Trust.

PCV *n.* *see* packed cell volume.

PCWP *n.* *see* pulmonary (capillary wedge pressure).

PDA *n.* *see* (patent) ductus arteriosus.

PDP *n.* *see* personal development plan.

PE *n.* pulmonary embolus. *See* (pulmonary) embolism.

peak expiratory flow rate (PEFR) (peek eks-**pir**-ă-ter-i floh rayt) *n.* the rate at which a person can expel air from the lungs: a reliable measure of lung reserves in tests of vital capacity.

Pearson bed (peer-sŏn) *n.* a special type of hospital bed for nursing patients with fractures.

peau d'orange (poh daw-**rahnj**) *n.* a dimpled appearance of the skin over a breast tumour, resembling the surface of an orange. The skin is thickened and the openings of hair follicles and sweat glands are enlarged.

PECT *n.* positron emission computed tomography (*see* positron emission tomography).

pecten (pek-tin) *n.* **1.** the middle section of the anal canal. **2.** a sharp ridge on the upper branch of the pubis (part of the hip bone). —**pectineal** (pek-**tin**-iăl) *adj.*

pectoral (pek-ter-ăl) *adj.* relating to the chest or breast. **p. girdle** *see* shoulder girdle. **p. muscles** the chest muscles: the pectoralis major, which draws the arm forward across the chest, and the pectoralis minor, which depresses the shoulder.

pectoriloquy (pek-ter-il-ŏ-kwi) *n.*

abnormal transm— tient's voice soun— chest wall so that th— heard through a ste—

pectus (pek-tŭs) *n.* breast. **p. carinatum** chest. **p. excavatum** see

pedicle (ped-ikŭl) *n.* **1.** neck of tissue connectin— mours to the normal t— which they have develop— plastic surgery) a narro— tube of skin by means of piece of skin used for graf— mains attached to its origin— **3.** (in anatomy) any slender— like process.

pediculicide (pi-dik-yoo-li-sy— an agent that kills lice; example— clude benzyl benzoate, carbaryl, — permethrin.

pediculosis (pi-dik-yoo-loh-sis) — an infestation with lice whic— causes intense itching. **p. capitis** in— festation with *head lice*, which is quite common in schoolchildren and does not indicate poor hygiene; it may be treated with malathion, carbaryl, or permethrin lotions or by use of a nit comb. **p. corporis** infestation with *body lice*, which affects vagrants, tramps, etc. *Pubic lice (Phthirus pubis*, the crab louse) are commonly sexually transmitted and respond to the same treatment as head lice.

Pediculus (pi-**dik**-yoo-lŭs) *n.* a widely distributed genus of lice. *P. humanus capitis* the head louse. *P. humanus corporis* the body louse, which in some parts of the world transmits relapsing fever and typhus. *See also* pediculosis.

peduncle (pi-**dunk**-ŭl) *n.* a narrow

cess or stalklike structure, serving as a connection or support.

EP *n. see* positive end expiratory pressure.

FR *n. see* peak expiratory flow ate.

EG *n. see* (percutaneous endoscopic) gastrostomy.

el-Ebstein fever (pel-eb-styn) *n.* a recurrent fever characteristic of patients with lymphoma or Hodgkin's disease. [P. K. Pel (1852–1919), Dutch physician; W. Ebstein (1836–1912), German physician]

pellagra (pel-ag-ră) *n.* a nutritional disease due to a deficiency of nicotinic acid (a B vitamin). It is common in maize-eating communities. The symptoms of pellagra are scaly dermatitis on exposed surfaces, diarrhoea, and depression.

pellet (pel-it) *n.* a small pill, especially one used as an implant.

pellicle (pel-ikŭl) *n.* a thin layer of skin, membrane, or any other substance.

pelvic-floor exercises (pel-vik) *pl. n. see* Kegel exercises.

pelvic girdle (hip girdle) *n.* the bony structure to which the bones of the lower limbs are attached. It consists of the right and left hip bones.

pelvic inflammatory disease (PID) *n.* an acute or chronic condition in which the uterus, Fallopian tubes, and ovaries are inflamed and infected. The infection spreads from an adjacent infected organ (such as the appendix), ascends from the vagina (as in the case of chlamydial infection), or may be blood-borne (such as tuberculosis). The main feature is lower abdominal pain that may be severe; blocking of the Fallopian tubes is a common result;

this can lead to ectopic pregnancy or infertility. In the chronic state, when pelvic adhesions have developed, surgical removal of the diseased tissue may be necessary.

pelvimetry (pel-**vim**-itri) *n.* the measurement of the four internal diameters of the pelvis, using an instrument called a *pelvimeter*. Pelvimetry helps in determining whether it will be possible for a fetus to be delivered in the normal way.

pelvis (pel-vis) *n.* (*pl.* **pelves**) **1.** the bony structure formed by the hip bones, sacrum, and coccyx (see illustration). The hip bones are fused at the back to the sacrum to form a rigid structure that protects the organs of the lower abdomen and provides attachment for the bones and muscles of the lower limbs. **2.** the cavity within the bony pelvis. **3.** any structure shaped like a basin.

The male pelvis (ventral view)

renal p. the expanded part of the ureter in the kidney. —**pelvic** *adj.*

pemphigoid (bullous pemphigoid) (pem-fig-oid) *n.* a chronic itchy blistering disorder of the elderly. The blisters most commonly occur on the limbs and persist for several days, unlike those of pemphigus. Pemphigoid is an autoimmune disease and responds to treatment with corticosteroids or immunosuppressant drugs. *ocular p.* a potentially blinding disease in which there is blistering and scarring of the conjunctiva and adhesions to the eyelid.

pemphigus (pemphigus vulgaris) (pem-fig-ŭs) *n.* a rare but serious autoimmune skin disease marked by successive outbreaks of blisters. The blisters are superficial and do not remain intact for long; the mouth and other mucous membranes, as well as the skin, are usually affected. A number of milder variants of the disease exist.

Pendred's syndrome (pen-drinds) *n.* goitre associated with congenital deafness due to deficiency of peroxidase, an enzyme that is essential for the utilization of iodine. [V. Pendred (1869–1946), British physician]

-penia *suffix denoting* lack or deficiency.

penicillamine (pen-i-sil-ă-meen) *n.* a drug that binds metals and therefore aids their excretion (*see* chelating agent). It is administered by mouth to treat Wilson's disease, metal poisoning, and severe rheumatoid arthritis. Trade names: **Distamine, Pendramine.**

penicillin (pen-i-sil-in) *n.* any one of a number of antibiotics derived

from *Penicillium* moulds and used to treat infections caused by a wide variety of bacteria. Some patients are allergic to penicillin and develop such reactions as skin rashes, swelling of the throat, and fever. *p. G* (or *benzylpenicillin*) a form of penicillin usually administered by injection but taken orally to treat dental abscesses. *p. V* (or *phenoxymethylpenicillin*) an orally administered form of penicillin. *semisynthetic p.* one of a number of antibiotics derived from the penicillins, such as amoxicillin, ampicillin, and flucloxacillin.

penicillinase (pen-i-sil-in-ayz) *n.* an enzyme, produced by some bacteria, that is capable of antagonizing the antibacterial action of penicillin. Purified penicillinase may be used to treat reactions to penicillin.

Penicillium (pen-i-sil-iŭm) *n.* a genus of mouldlike fungi that commonly grow on decaying fruit, bread, or cheese. Some species are pathogenic to humans, causing diseases of the skin and respiratory tract. *P. rubrum* the major natural source of the antibiotic penicillin.

penile prosthesis (pee-nyl) *n. see* prosthesis.

penis (pee-nis) *n.* the male organ that carries the urethra, through which urine and semen are discharged (see illustration). Most of the organ is composed of erectile tissue (corpus cavernosum and corpus spongiosum), which becomes filled with blood under conditions of sexual excitement so that the penis is erected. *See also* glans, prepuce. —**penile** *adj.*

pent- (penta-) *prefix denoting* five.

pentamidine (pen-tam-i-deen) *n.* a

- corpus cavernosum
- corpus spongiosum
- urethra
- glans penis
- prepuce
- opening of urethra

The penis (median section)

drug effective against protozoans and used in the treatment of *Pneumocystis carinii* pneumonia in AIDS patients and leishmaniasis. It is administered by injection or from an inhaler. Trade name: **Pentacarinat**.

pentazocine (pen-**taz**-oh-seen) *n.* a potent opioid analgesic drug administered by mouth, injection, or in suppositories to relieve moderate or severe pain. Trade name: **Fortral**.

pentose (**pen**-tohz) *n.* a simple sugar with five carbon atoms, such as for example, ribose or xylose.

pentostatin (pen-tŏ-**stat**-in) *n.* a cytotoxic drug that is used in treating hairy cell leukaemia. It is administered by intravenous injection. Trade name: **Nipent**.

pentosuria (pen-tohs-**yoor**-iǎ) *n.* an inborn defect of sugar metabolism causing abnormal excretion of pentose in the urine.

Peplau's model (**pep**-lowz) *n.* a model for nursing based on interpersonal relations. It emphasizes that the therapeutic nurse–patient relationship is an integral part of nursing practice and that the nurse's role evolves as a result of it. *See also* nursing models. [H. Peplau (1909–), US nurse theorist]

peppermint (**pep**-er-mint) *n.* an oil extracted from a species of mint (*Mentha piperita*), used as a carminative and flavouring agent.

pepsin (**pep**-sin) *n.* an enzyme in the stomach that begins the digestion of proteins by splitting them into peptones (*see* peptidase). It is produced by the action of hydrochloric acid on *pepsinogen*, which is secreted by the gastric glands.

pepsinogen (pep-**sin**-ŏ-jěn) *n. see* pepsin.

peptic (**pep**-tik) *adj.* **1.** relating to pepsin. **2.** relating to digestion. **p. ulcer** a breach in the lining (mucosa) of the digestive tract produced by digestion of the mucosa by pepsin and acid. This may occur when pepsin and acid are present in abnormally high concentrations. *See* duodenal ulcer, gastric (ulcer), oesophageal ulcer.

peptidase (**pep**-tid-ayz) *n.* one of a group of digestive enzymes that split proteins in the stomach and intestine into their constituent amino acids.

peptide (**pep**-tyd) *n.* a molecule consisting of two or more amino acids linked by bonds between the amino group and the carboxyl group. *See also* polypeptide.

peptone (**pep**-tohn) *n.* a large protein fragment produced by the action of enzymes on proteins in the first stages of protein digestion.

peptonuria (pep-tohn-**yoor**-iǎ) *n.*

peri-arrest period

the presence in the urine of peptones.

perception (per-**sep**-shŏn) n. (in psychology) the process by which information about the world, received by the senses, is analysed and made meaningful.

percussion (per-**kush**-ŏn) n. the technique of examining part of the body by tapping it with the fingers or an instrument (plessor) and sensing the resultant vibrations. It is used to detect the presence of fluid or abnormal solidification or enlargement in different organs.

percutaneous (per-kew-**tay**-niŭs) adj. through the skin: often applied to the route of administration of drugs in ointments, etc., which are absorbed through the skin. *p. endoscopic gastrostomy see* gastrostomy. *p. epididymal sperm aspiration see* PESA. *p. nephrolithotomy see* nephrolithotomy. *p. transhepatic cholangiopancreatography see* cholangiopancreatography.

perforation (per-fer-ay-shŏn) n. the creation of a hole in an organ, tissue, or tube. This may occur in the course of a disease, such as duodenal ulcer, colonic diverticulitis, or stomach cancer. Treatment is usually by surgical repair of the perforation, but conservative treatment with antibiotics may result in spontaneous healing. Perforation may also be caused accidentally by instruments (for example a curette may perforate the uterus) or by injury (for example to the eardrum).

performance indicators (PIs) (per-**for**-mănss) *pl.* n. statistical information, based on quantitative measures of the resources and activities of the NHS, produced by

health authorities and sent to the Department of Health. This enables comparisons of performance of one section with that achieved by another to be analysed and published.

perfusion (per-few-zhŏn) n. **1.** the passage of fluid through a tissue, especially the passage of blood through the lung tissue to pick up oxygen in the alveoli and release carbon dioxide. **2.** the deliberate introduction of fluid into a tissue, usually by injection into the blood vessels supplying the tissue.

perfusion scan n. a technique for demonstrating an abnormal blood supply to an organ by injecting a radioactive tracer or contrast medium. Areas not being perfused show up as holes on gamma-camera images. *See also* ventilation-perfusion scanning.

pergolide (per-gŏ-lyd) n. a drug that is used in the treatment of parkinsonism. It is administered by mouth. Trade name: **Celance**.

peri- *prefix denoting* near, around, or enclosing.

periadenitis (pe-ri-ad-in-I-tis) n. inflammation of tissues surrounding a gland.

perianal haematoma (external haemorrhoid) (pe-ri-ay-nāl) n. a small painful swelling beside the anus, occurring after a bout of straining to pass faeces or coughing. Perianal haematomas are caused by the rupture of a small vein in the anus.

peri-arrest period (pe-ri-ă-**rest**) n. the recognized period, either just before or just after a full cardiac arrest, when the patient's condition is very unstable and care must be taken to prevent progression or regression into a full cardiac arrest.

periarteritis nodosa (pe-ri-ar-ter-I-tis) *n. see* polyarteritis nodosa.

periarthritis (pe-ri-arth-**ry**-tis) *n.* inflammation of tissues around a joint capsule, including tendons and bursae. *chronic p.* a common cause of pain and stiffness of the shoulder; it usually responds to local steroid injections or physiotherapy.

peribulbar (pe-ri-**bul**-ber) *adj.* (in ophthalmology) denoting the area around the eye.

pericard- (**pericardio-**) *prefix denoting* the pericardium.

pericardiectomy (**pericardectomy**) (pe-ri-kar-di-**ek**-tŏmi) *n.* surgical removal of the pericardium. It is used in the treatment of chronic constrictive pericarditis and chronic pericardial effusion (*see* pericarditis).

pericardiocentesis (pe-ri-kar-di-oh-sen-**tee**-sis) *n.* removal of excess fluid from within the pericardium by means of needle aspiration.

pericardiorrhaphy (pe-ri-kar-di-o-**ráfi**) *n.* the repair of wounds in the pericardium, such as those due to injury or surgery.

pericardiostomy (pe-ri-kar-di-ost-ŏmi) *n.* an operation in which the pericardium is opened and the fluid within drained via a tube. It is sometimes used in the treatment of septic pericarditis.

pericardiotomy (**pericardotomy**) (pe-ri-kar-di-ot-ŏmi) *n.* surgical opening or puncture of the pericardium. It is required to gain access to the heart in heart surgery and to remove excess fluid from within the pericardium.

pericarditis (pe-ri-kar-**dy**-tis) *n.*

acute or chronic inflammation of the pericardium. Pericarditis may be seen alone or as part of pancarditis. It has numerous causes, including virus infections, uraemia, and cancer. *acute p.* pericarditis characterized by fever, chest pain, and a pericardial friction rub. Fluid may accumulate within the pericardial sac (*pericardial effusion*). *chronic constrictive p.* chronic thickening of the pericardium, which interferes with activity of the heart and has many features in common with heart failure.

pericardium (pe-ri-**kar**-diŭm) *n.* the membrane surrounding the heart. *fibrous p.* the outer portion of the pericardium, which completely encloses the heart and is attached to the large blood vessels emerging from the heart. *serous p.* the internal portion of the pericardium: a closed sac of serous membrane containing a very small amount of fluid, which prevents friction between the two surfaces as the heart beats. —**pericardial** *adj.*

pericardotomy (pe-ri-kar-**dot**-ŏmi) *n. see* pericardiotomy.

perichondritis (pe-ri-kon-**dry**-tis) *n.* inflammation of cartilage and surrounding soft tissues, usually due to chronic infection. A common site is the external ear.

perichondrium (pe-ri-**kon**-driŭm) *n.* the dense layer of fibrous connective tissue that covers the surface of cartilage.

pericranium (pe-ri-**kray**-niŭm) *n.* the periosteum of the skull.

pericystitis (pe-ri-sis-**ty**-tis) *n.* inflammation in the tissues around the bladder, causing pain in the pelvis, fever, and symptoms of cystitis. It usually results from infection in the Fallopian tubes or uterus.

perifolliculitis (pe-ri-fŏ-lik-yoo-ly-tis) *n.* inflammation around the hair follicles.

perihepatitis (pe-ri-hep-ă-ty-tis) *n.* inflammation of the membrane covering the liver. It is usually associated with abnormalities of the liver or chronic peritonitis.

perilymph (pe-ri-limf) *n.* the fluid between the bony and membranous labyrinths of the ear.

porimonopauco (po ri mon ŏ pawz) *n.* the period of time around the menopause in which marked changes in the menstrual cycle occur, usually accompanied by hot flushes, and in which no 12 consecutive months of amenorrhoea have yet occurred.

perimeter (per-im-it-er) *n.* an instrument for mapping the absolute extent of the visual field and detecting any gaps or defects. —**perimetry** *n.*

perimetritis (pe-ri-mi-try-tis) *n.* inflammation of the membrane on the outer surface of the uterus. The condition may be associated with parametritis.

perimetrium (pe-ri-mee-triŭm) *n.* the peritoneum of the uterus.

perimysium (pe-ri-mis-iŭm) *n.* the fibrous sheath that surrounds each bundle of muscle fibres.

perinatal (pe-ri-nay-t'l) *adj.* relating to the period starting a few weeks before birth and including the birth and a few weeks after birth. *p. mortality rate* the number of stillbirths and first-week or neonatal deaths per 1000 live births.

perindopril (pĕ-rin-dŏ-pril) *n. see* ACE inhibitor.

perineal (pe-ri-nee-ăl) *adj.* relating to the perineum. *p. descent* abnormal bulging down of the perineum due to weakness of the pelvis floor muscles. *p. pouch see* ileal pouch. *p. tear* any injury to the perineum, which may be sustained during childbirth. It may involve only the perineal muscles (second-degree tear), the external and internal anal sphincters (third-degree tear), or the anal sphincters and rectal mucosa (fourth-degree tear).

perineoplasty (pe-ri-nee-oh-plasti) *n.* an operation designed to enlarge the vaginal opening by incising the hymen and part of the perineum (*Fenton's operation*).

perineorrhaphy (pe-ri-ni-o-răfi) *n.* the surgical repair of a damaged perineum. The damage is usually the result of a tear in the perineum sustained during childbirth.

perinephric (pe-ri-nef-rik) *adj.* around the kidney. *p. abscess* a collection of pus around the kidney, usually secondary to pyonephrosis.

perinephritis (pe-ri-ni-fry-tis) *n.* inflammation of the tissues around the kidney, usually due to spread of infection from the kidney itself. The patient has pain in the loins, fever, and fits of shivering.

perineum (pe-ri-nee-ŭm) *n.* the region of the body between the anus and the urethral opening, including both skin and underlying muscle.

perineurium (pe-ri-newr-iŭm) *n.* the sheath of connective tissue that surrounds individual bundles of nerve fibres in a large nerve.

periocular (pe-ri-ok-yoo-ler) *adj.* adjacent to the eyeball.

periodic fever (peer-i-od-ik) *n. see* malaria.

periodontal (pe-ri-ŏ-don-t'l) *adj.* denoting or relating to the tissues surrounding the teeth. **p. disease** disease of the tissues that support and attach the teeth – the gums, periodontal membrane, and alveolar bone: the most common cause of tooth loss in older people. **p. membrane (p. ligament)** the ligament around a tooth, by which it is attached to the bone.

periodontium (pe-ri-ŏ-don-tiŭm) *n.* the tissues, collectively, surrounding the teeth: the gums (gingiva), periodontal membrane, and alveolar bone.

periodontology (pe-ri-ŏ-don-tol-ŏji) *n.* the branch of dentistry concerned with the tissues that support and attach the teeth and the prevention and treatment of periodontal disease.

periorbital (pe-ri-or-bit-ăl) *adj.* **1.** around the eye socket (orbit). **2.** relating to the periosteum within the orbit.

periosteotome (pe-ri-ost-i-ŏ-tohm) *n.* an instrument used for cutting the periosteum and separating it from the underlying bone.

periosteum (pe-ri-ost-iŭm) *n.* a layer of dense connective tissue that covers the surface of a bone and provides attachment for muscles, tendons, and ligaments. The outer layer of the periosteum contains a large number of blood vessels; the inner layer contains osteoblasts and fewer blood vessels. —**periosteal** *adj.*

periostitis (pe-ri-ost-I-tis) *n.* inflammation of the periosteum. **acute p.** periostitis that results from direct injury to the bone and is associated with a haematoma, which may later become infected. **chronic p.** periostitis that is often due to an inflammatory disease, such as tuberculosis or syphilis, or to a chronic ulcer overlying the bone involved.

peripheral nervous system (per-if-er-ăl) *n.* all parts of the nervous system lying outside the central nervous system. It includes the cranial nerves and spinal nerves and their branches and the autonomic nervous system.

peripheral neuropathy *n. see* neuropathy.

peripheral vascular disease (PVD) *n.* any disease of the blood vessels outside the heart, especially in the extremities, most commonly due to atherosclerosis. Examples are intermittent claudication and Raynaud's disease.

periphlebitis (pe-ri-fli-by-tis) *n.* inflammation of the tissues around a vein: seen as an extension of phlebitis.

periproctitis (pe-ri-prok-ty-tis) *n.* inflammation of the tissues around the rectum and anus.

perisalpingitis (pe-ri-sal-pin-jy-tis) *n.* inflammation of the peritoneal membrane on the outer surface of a Fallopian tube.

perisplenitis (pe-ri-spli-ny-tis) *n.* inflammation of the external coverings of the spleen.

peristalsis (pe-ri-stal-sis) *n.* a wavelike movement that progresses along some of the hollow muscular tubes of the body, such as the intestines. It occurs involuntarily, induced by distension of the walls of the tube. Alternate contraction and relaxation of the circular and longi-

— liver
— kidney
— pancreas
— stomach
— duodenum
— transverse colon
— peritoneal cavity
— mesentery
— jejunum
— ileum
— bladder
— pubic symphysis
— rectum

Sagittal section of the abdomen to show arrangement of the peritoneum

tudinal muscles tends to push the contents of the tube forward. —**peristaltic** *adj.*

peritendinitis (pe-ri-ten-di-ny-tis) *n. see* tenosynovitis.

peritomy (per-it-ŏmi) *n.* an eye operation in which an incision of the conjunctiva is made in a complete circle around the cornea.

peritoneoscope (pe-ri-tŏn-ee-ŏ-skohp) *n. see* laparoscope.

peritoneum (pe-ri-tŏn-ee-ŭm) *n.* the serous membrane of the abdominal cavity (see illustration). *parietal p.* the part of the peritoneum that lines the walls of the abdomen. *visceral p.* the part of the peritoneum that covers the abdominal organs. *See also* mesentery, omentum. —**peritoneal** *adj.*

peritonitis (pe-ri-tŏn-I-tis) *n.* in-

flammation of the peritoneum. *primary p.* peritonitis caused by bacteria spread via the bloodstream. Symptoms are diffuse abdominal pain and swelling, with fever and weight loss. *secondary p.* peritonitis due to perforation or rupture of an abdominal organ, such as the vermiform appendix, allowing access of bacteria and irritant digestive juices to the peritoneum. This produces sudden severe abdominal pain and shock. Treatment is usually by surgical repair of the perforation.

peritonsillar abscess (pe-ri-ton-sil-er) *n. see* quinsy.

peritrichous (pe-ri-try-kŭs) *adj.* describing bacteria in which the flagella cover the entire cell surface.

perityphlitis (pe-ri-tif-ly-tis) *n.* Ar-

chaic. inflammation of the tissues around the caecum.

periureteritis (pe-ri-yoor-i-ter-I-tis) *n.* inflammation of the tissues around a ureter. This is usually associated with inflammation of the ureter itself (*see* ureteritis) often behind an obstruction caused by a stone or stricture.

PERLA pupils equal, react to light and accommodation: used in hospital notes.

perle (perl) *n.* a soft capsule containing medicine.

perleche (per-lesh) *n.* dryness and cracking of the corners of the mouth, sometimes with infection. Perleche may be caused by persistent lip licking or by a vitamin-deficient diet.

permeability (per-mi-ă-bil-iti) *n.* the ability of membranes to allow soluble substances to pass through them. *See also* semipermeable membrane. —**permeable** (per-mi-ăbŭl) *adj.*

permethrin (per-meeth-rin) *n.* a synthetic derivative of the naturally occurring insecticide pyrethrin that is applied externally to treat head lice, pubic lice, and scabies. Trade name: **Lyclear**.

pernicious (per-nish-ŭs) *adj.* describing diseases that are highly dangerous or likely to result in death if untreated. *p. anaemia* a form of anaemia resulting from deficiency of vitamin B_{12}, due either to failure to produce intrinsic factor or to dietary deficiency of the vitamin. It is characterized by defective production of red blood cells and the presence of megaloblasts in the bone marrow.

pernio (per-ni-oh) *n.* the medical name for a chilblain (*see* chilblains).

perniosis (per-ni-oh-sis) *n. see* chilblains.

pero- *prefix denoting* deformity; defect.

peromelia (pe-roh-mee-liă) *n.* congenital deformity of one or more limbs.

peroneal (pe-rŏ-nee-ăl) *adj.* relating to or supplying the outer (fibular) side of the leg.

peroneus (pe-rŏ-nee-ŭs) *n.* one of the muscles of the leg that arises from the fibula and helps to turn the foot outwards.

peroral (per-or-ăl) *adj.* through the mouth.

perphenazine (per-fen-ă-zeen) *n.* a phenothiazine antipsychotic drug administered by mouth or injection to treat schizophrenia and mania, to relieve anxiety, tension, and agitation, and to prevent nausea and vomiting. Trade name: **Fentazin**.

perseveration (per-sev-er-ay-shŏn) *n.* **1.** excessive persistence at a task that prevents the individual from turning his attention to new situations. It is a symptom of organic disease of the brain and sometimes of obsessional neurosis. **2.** the phenomenon in which an image continues to be perceived briefly in the absence of the object. This is a potentially serious neurological disorder.

persistent vegetative state (PVS) (per-sist-ĕnt) *n.* the condition of living like a vegetable, without consciousness or the ability to initiate voluntary action, as a result of brain damage. People in the vegetative state may sometimes give the appearance of being awake and conscious, with open eyes. They may make random movements of the limbs or head and may pick or rub with the fingers, but there is no response to any form of communication and no reason to suppose that there is any awareness of the environment. *Compare* locked-in syndrome.

personal development plan (PDP) (per-son-ăl) *n.* an individualized plan developed by nurses and other health-care professionals to further their commitment to continuing professional development.

personality (per-sŏn-al-iti) *n.* (in psychology) an enduring disposition to act and feel in particular ways that differentiate one individual from another.

personality disorder *n.* a deeply ingrained maladaptive pattern of behaviour, which persists through many years and causes suffering, either to the patient or to other people (or to both). *See* antisocial personality disorder, hysterical, paranoid, schizoid personality.

perspiration (per-sper-ay-shŏn) *n.* sweat or the process of sweating. *insensible p.* sweat that evaporates immediately from the skin and is therefore not visible. *sensible p.* sweat that is visible on the skin in the form of drops.

Perthes' disease (per-tiz) *n. see* Legg-Calvé-Perthes disease.

pertussis (per-tus-iss) *n. see* whooping cough.

pes (payz) *n.* (in anatomy) the foot or a part resembling a foot. *p. clavus see* claw-foot. *p. planus see* flat-foot.

PESA (percutaneous epididymal sperm aspiration) *n.* a method of removing spermatozoa directly from the epididymis, a new technique used in assisted conception. The sperm are then used to fertilize egg cells in vitro.

pessary (pess-er-i) *n.* **1.** a plastic device, often ring-shaped, that fits into the vagina and keeps the uterus in position: used to treat prolapse. **2.** **(vaginal suppository)** a plug or cylinder of soft material containing a drug that is fitted into the vagina for the treatment of such disorders as vaginitis.

pesticide (pest-i-syd) *n.* a chemical agent, such as parathion, used to kill insects or other organisms harmful to crops and other cultivated plants.

PET *n. see* positron emission tomography.

petechiae (pi-tee-ki-ee) *pl. n.* small round flat dark-red spots caused by bleeding into the skin or beneath the mucous membrane.

pethidine (peth-i-deen) *n.* a potent opioid analgesic drug with mild sedative action, administered by mouth or injection to relieve moderate or severe pain.

petit mal (pe-tee mal) *n. see* epilepsy.

Petri dish (pe-tri) *n.* a flat shallow circular glass or plastic dish with a pillbox-like lid, used to hold solid agar or gelatin media for culturing bacteria. [J. R. Petri (1852–1921), German bacteriologist]

petrissage (pay-tri-sahzh) *n.* kneading: a form of massage in which the skin is lifted up, pressed down and squeezed, and pinched and rolled.

petrositis (pet-roh-sy-tis) *n.* inflammation of the petrous part of the temporal bone, usually due to an extension of mastoiditis.

petrous bone (pet-rŭs) *n. see* temporal (bone).

Peutz-Jeghers syndrome (puuts-**yeg**-erz) *n.* a hereditary disorder in which the presence of multiple polyps in the lining of the small intestine (intestinal polyposis) is associated with pigmented areas (similar to freckles) around the lips, on the inside of the mouth, and on the palms and soles. [J. L. A. Peutz (1886–1957), Dutch physician; H. J. Jeghers (1904–), US physician]

-pexy *suffix denoting* surgical fixation.

Peyer's patches (py-erz) *pl. n.* oval masses of lymphoid tissue on the mucous membrane lining the small intestine. [J. C. Peyer (1653–1712), Swiss anatomist]

Peyronie's disease (pay-roh-neez) *n.* a dense fibrous plaque in the penis. The penis curves or angulates at this point on erection and pain often results. [F. de la Peyronie (1678–1747), French surgeon]

PGD *n. see* preimplantation genetic diagnosis.

pH *n.* a measure of the concentration of hydrogen ions in a solution, and therefore of its acidity or alkalinity. A pH of 7 indicates a neutral solution, a pH below 7 indicates acidity, and a pH in excess of 7 indicates alkalinity.

phaco- (phako-) *prefix denoting* the lens of the eye.

phacoemulsification (phako-emulsification) (fakŏ-i-mul-si-fi-kay-shŏn) *n.* a widely used method of cataract extraction in which a high-frequency ultrasound probe is used to break up a cataract so that it can be removed through a very small incision.

phaeochromocytoma (fi-oh-kroh-moh-sy-toh-mă) *n.* a small vascular tumour of the medulla of the adrenal gland. Many of these tumours function by their uncontrolled and irregular secretion of the hormones adrenaline and noradrenaline. They cause attacks of raised blood pressure, increased heart rate, palpitations, and headache.

phag- (phago-) *prefix denoting* **1.** eating. **2.** phagocytes.

phage (fayj) *n. see* bacteriophage.

-phagia *suffix denoting* a condition involving eating.

phagocyte (fag-ŏ-syt) *n.* a cell that is able to engulf and digest bacteria, protozoa, cells and cell debris, and other small particles. Phagocytes include many white blood cells and macrophages, which play a major role in the body's defence mechanism. —**phagocytic** *adj.*

phagocytosis (fag-ŏ-sy-**toh**-sis) *n.* the engulfment and digestion of bacteria and other foreign particles by a phagocyte. *Compare* pinocytosis.

phakic (fay-kik) *adj.* denoting the state in which the natural crystalline lens of the eye is still in place, as contrasted with aphakic (*see* aphakia).

phako- *prefix. see* phaco-.

phalanges (fă-**lan**-jeez) *n.* (*sing.* **phalanx**) the bones of the fingers and toes (digits). The first digit (thumb/big toe) has two phalanges. Each of the remaining digits has three phalanges. —**phalangeal** *adj.*

phalangitis (fal-ăn-jy-tis) *n.* inflammation of a finger or toe, caused by infection of the soft tissues, bone, or joints or by rheumatic diseases. *See also* dactylitis.

phalanx (fal-anks) *n. see* phalanges.

phalloplasty (fal-oh-plasti) *n.* surgical reconstruction or repair of the penis, performed to correct a congenital deformity or following injury to the penis.

phallus (fal-ŭs) *n.* the embryonic penis, before the urethral duct has reached its final state of development.

phantom limb (fan-tŏm) *n.* the sensation that an arm or leg, or part of an arm or leg, is still attached to the body after it has been amputated. Pain or other sensations may seem to come from the amputated part.

phantom pregnancy *n. see* pseudocyesis.

phantom tumour *n.* a swelling, in the abdomen or elsewhere, caused by local muscular contraction or the accumulation of gases, that mimics a swelling caused by a tumour. The condition is usually associated with emotional disorder.

pharmaceutical (farm-ă-sewt-ikăl) *adj.* relating to pharmacy.

pharmacist (farm-ă-sist) *n.* a person who is qualified by examination and registered and authorized to dispense medicines.

pharmaco- *prefix denoting* drugs.

pharmacodynamics (farm-ă-koh-dy-nam-iks) *n.* the interaction of drugs with cells. It includes such factors as the binding of drugs to cells, their uptake, and intracellular metabolism.

pharmacokinetics (farm-ă-koh-ki-net-iks) *n.* the study of how drugs are handled within the body, in-

cluding their absorption, distribution, metabolism, and excretion.

pharmacology (farm-ă-kol-ŏji) *n.* the science of the properties of drugs and their effects on the body. —**pharmacological** *adj.* —**pharmacologist** *n.*

pharmacopoeia (farm-ă-kŏ-pee-ă) *n.* a book containing a list of the drugs used in medicine, with details of their formulae, methods of preparation, dosages, standards of purity, etc.

pharmacy (farm-ăsi) *n.* **1.** the preparation and dispensing of drugs. **2.** premises registered to dispense medicines and sell poisons.

pharyng- (pharyngo-) *prefix denoting* the pharynx.

pharyngeal (fa-rin-jee-ăl) *adj.* of or relating to the pharynx. *p. pouch* (*branchial pouch, visceral pouch*) any of the paired segmented pouches in the side of the throat of the early embryo. They give rise to the tympanic cavity, the parathyroid glands, the thymus, and probably the thyroid gland. *p. reflex see* gag reflex.

pharyngectomy (fa-rin-jek-tŏmi) *n.* surgical removal of part of the pharynx.

pharyngitis (fa-rin-jy-tis) *n.* inflammation of the pharynx. It produces sore throat and may be associated with tonsillitis.

pharyngocele (fă-ring-oh-seel) *n.* a pouch or cyst opening off the pharynx (*see* branchial cyst).

pharyngolaryngeal (fă-ring-oh-la-rin-jee-ăl) *adj.* relating to both the pharynx and the larynx.

pharyngoscope (fă-ring-ŏ-skohp) *n.* an endoscope for the examination of the pharynx.

pharyngotympanic tube (få-ring-oh-tim-**pan**-ik) *n. see* Eustachian tube.

pharynx (fa-rinks) *n.* a muscular tube, lined with mucous membrane, that extends from the beginning of the oesophagus (gullet) up to the base of the skull. It communicates with the posterior nares, Eustachian tube, mouth, larynx, and oesophagus. The pharynx acts as a passageway for food, as an air passage from the nasal cavity and mouth to the larynx, and as a resonating chamber for the sounds produced in the larynx. *See* hypopharynx, nasopharynx, oropharynx.

PHC *n.* primary health care. *See* primary care.

phenazocine (fin-az-oh-seen) *n.* an opioid analgesic drug administered by mouth for rapid relief of moderate or severe pain. Trade name: **Narphen**.

phenelzine (fen-ĕl-zeen) *n.* a drug administered by mouth to relieve depression and anxiety (*see* MAO inhibitor). Trade name: **Nardil**.

phenindione (fen-in-di-ohn) *n.* an anticoagulant drug administered by mouth to prevent or treat thrombosis in the blood vessels of the heart and limbs. Trade name: **Dindevan**.

pheniodol (fin-I-ŏ-dol) *n.* an iodine-containing compound that is used as a contrast medium during X-ray examination of the gall bladder (*see* cholecystography).

phenobarbital (phenobarbitone) (fee-noh-**bar**-bit-al) *n.* a barbiturate drug administered by mouth or injection as an anticonvulsant in the treatment of epilepsy. Phenobarbital is no longer commonly prescribed.

phenol (carbolic acid) (fee-nol) *n.* a strong disinfectant used for cleansing wounds, treating inflammations of the mouth, throat, and ear, and as a preservative in injections. It is administered as solution, ointments, and lotions and is highly toxic if taken by mouth.

phenomenology (fin-om-in-ol-ŏji) *n.* the study of occurrences forming part of human experiences. Concerned with describing the facts of the immediate situation, rather than speculating about causes, it helps nurses and patients to understand the phenomena in question and may lead to an improved understanding of oneself and others.

phenothiazines (fee-noh-**th'y**-ă-zeenz) *pl. n.* a group of chemically related compounds with various pharmacological actions. Some (e.g. chlorpromazine) are antipsychotic drugs; others (e.g. piperazine) are anthelmintics.

phenotype (fee-noh-typ) *n.* the observable characteristics of an individual, which result from interaction between his genotype and the environment.

phenoxybenzamine (fin-oks-i-ben-ză-meen) *n.* a drug that dilates blood vessels (*see* alpha blocker). It is administered by mouth or injection to reduce high blood pressure in patients with phaeochromocytoma. Trade name: **Dibenyline**.

phenoxymethylpenicillin (fin-oks-i-meth-il-pen-i-sil-in) *n. see* penicillin.

phentolamine (fen-**tol**-ă-meen) *n.* a drug that dilates blood vessels (*see* alpha blocker) and is administered by mouth or injection to reduce high blood pressure in patients with phaeochromocytoma. Trade name: **Rogitine**.

phenylalanine (fee-nyl-al-ă-neen) *n.* an essential amino acid that is readily converted to tyrosine. Blockade of this metabolic pathway gives rise to phenylketonuria.

phenylbutazone (fee-nyl-bew-tă-zohn) *n.* an analgesic drug that reduces fever and inflammation (*see* NSAID) and is administered by mouth or injection to relieve pain in refractory ankylosing spondylitis. Trade name: **Butacote**.

phenylephrine (fee-nyl-ef-reen) *n.* a drug that constricts blood vessels (*see* sympathomimetic). It is given by injection to increase blood pressure, in a nasal spray to relieve nasal congestion, and in eye drops to dilate the pupils. Trade names: **Fenox**, **Minims Phenylephrine**.

phenylketonuria (PKU) (fee-nyl-kee-tŏn-yoor iă) *n.* an inherited defect of protein metabolism (*see* inborn error of metabolism) causing an excess of the amino acid phenylalanine in the blood, which damages the nervous system and leads to severe mental retardation. The gene responsible for phenylketonuria is recessive, so that a child is affected only if both parents are carriers of the defective gene.

phenytoin (fen-i-toh-in) *n.* an anticonvulsant drug administered by mouth or injection to control major and focal epileptic seizures. Trade name: **Epanutin**.

phial (fy-ăl) *n.* a small glass bottle for storing medicines or poisons.

Philadelphia chromosome (fil-ă-del-fiă) *n.* an abnormal chromosome (number 22) found in the blood cells of patients with chronic myeloid leukaemia.

-philia *suffix denoting* morbid craving or attraction.

phimosis (fy-moh-sis) *n.* narrowing of the opening of the foreskin, which cannot therefore be drawn back over the underlying glans penis.

phleb- (phlebo-) *prefix denoting* a vein or veins.

phlebectomy (fli-bek-tŏmi) *n.* the surgical removal of a vein (or part of a vein), sometimes performed for the treatment of varicose veins in the legs (*varicectomy*).

phlebitis (fli-by-tis) *n.* inflammation of the wall of a vein, which is most commonly seen in the legs as a complication of varicose veins. A segment of vein becomes painful and tender and the surrounding skin feels hot and appears red. Thrombosis commonly develops (*see* thrombophlebitis). Treatment consists of elastic support and administration of drugs, such as phenylbutazone.

phlebography (fli-bog-răfi) *n. see* venography.

phlebolith (flee-boh-lith) *n.* a stonelike structure that results from deposition of calcium in a venous blood clot.

phlebothrombosis (flee-boh-throm-boh-sis) *n.* obstruction of a vein by a blood clot, without preceding inflammation of its wall. It is most common within the deep veins of the calf of the leg (*deep vein thrombosis, DVT*). The affected leg may become swollen and tender and the clot may become detached and give rise to pulmonary embolism. Prolonged immobility, heart failure, pregnancy, injury, and surgery predispose to thrombosis by encouraging sluggish blood flow. Anticoagulant drugs (such as heparin and warfarin) are used in prevention and treatment.

phlebotomy (venesection) (fli-**bot**-ŏmi) *n.* the surgical opening or puncture of a vein in order to remove blood (in the treatment of polycythaemia) or to infuse fluids, blood, or drugs in the treatment of many conditions.

phlegm (flem) *n.* a nonmedical term for sputum.

phlegmasia (fleg-**may**-ziă) *n.* inflammation. *p. alba dolens see* white leg.

phlycten (flik-tĕn) *n.* a small pinkish-yellow nodule surrounded by a zone of dilated blood vessels that occurs in the conjunctiva or in the cornea. Phlyctens are thought to be due to a type of allergy to certain bacteria.

phobia (foh-biă) *n.* a pathologically strong fear of a particular event or thing. Avoiding the feared situation may severely restrict one's life and cause much suffering. Treatment is with behaviour therapy, especially desensitization and flooding. Psychotherapy and drug therapy are also useful.

-phobia *suffix denoting* morbid fear or dread.

phocomelia (foh-koh-**mee**-liă) *n.* congenital absence of the upper arm and/or upper leg, the hands or feet or both being attached to the trunk by a short stump.

pholcodine (fol-kŏ-deen) *n.* a drug that suppresses coughs and reduces irritation in the respiratory system (*see* antitussive). It is administered

by mouth in cough mixtures. Trade names: **Famel, Galenphol.**

phon- (phono-) *prefix denoting* sound or voice.

phonation (foh-**nay**-shŏn) *n.* the production of vocal sounds, particularly speech.

phoniatrics (foh-ni-at-riks) *n.* the study of the voice and its disorders.

phonocardiogram (foh-noh-**kar**-di-ŏ-gram) *n. see* electrocardiophonography. —**phonocardiography** (foh-noh-kar-di-og-răfi) *n.*

phonophobia (foh-noh-foh-biă) *n.* excessive sensitivity to certain specific sounds. *See* hyperacusis, misophonia.

phonosurgery (foh-noh-**serj**-er-i) *n.* surgery performed on the larynx externally or endoscopically to improve or modify the quality of the voice.

-phoria *suffix denoting* (in ophthalmology) an abnormal deviation of the eyes or turning of the visual axis.

phosgene (fos-jeen) *n.* a poisonous gas developed during World War I. It is a choking agent, acting on the lungs to produce oedema, with consequent respiratory and cardiac failure.

phosphagen (fos-fă-jĕn) *n.* creatine phosphate (*see* creatine).

phosphataemia (fos-fă-tee-miă) *n.* the presence of phosphates in the blood. Sodium, calcium, potassium, and magnesium phosphates are normal constituents.

phosphatase (fos-fă-tayz) *n.* one of a group of enzymes capable of catalysing the hydrolysis of phosphoric acid esters. Phosphatases are important in the absorption and metabolism of carbohydrates, nucleotides, and phospholipids and are essential in the calcification of bone. *acid p.* a phosphatase present in kidney, semen, serum, and the prostate gland. *alkaline p.* a phosphatase that occurs in teeth, developing bone, plasma, kidney, and intestine.

phosphate (fos-fayt) *n.* any salt or ester of phosphoric acid.

phosphatidylcholine (fos-fat-i-dil-koh-leen) *n. see* lecithin.

phosphaturia (phosphuria) (fos-fat-*yoor*-iă) *n.* the presence of an abnormally high concentration of phosphates in the urine, making it cloudy. The condition may be associated with the formation of calculi in the kidneys or bladder.

phosphocreatine (fos-foh-kree-ă-teen) *n.* creatine phosphate (*see* creatine).

phospholipid (fos-foh-**lip**-id) *n.* a lipid containing a phosphate group as part of the molecule. Phospholipids are constituents of all tissues and organs, especially the brain. They are involved in many of the body's metabolic processes. Examples are cephalins, lecithins, and plasmalogens.

phosphonecrosis (fos-foh-nek-roh-sis) *n.* the destruction of tissues caused by excessive amounts of phosphorus in the system. The tissues likely to suffer are the liver, kidneys, muscles, bones, and the cardiovascular system.

phosphorus (fos-fer-us) *n.* a nonmetallic element that is toxic in its pure state. Phosphorus compounds are major constituents in the tissues of both plants and animals. In humans, phosphorus is mostly concentrated in bone. Symbol: P.

phot- (photo-) *prefix denoting* light.

photalgia (foh-tal-jiă) *n.* pain in the eye caused by very bright light.

photoablation (foh-toh-ăb-lay-shŏn) *n.* the use of light or lasers to destroy tissue.

photochemotherapy (foh-toh-kee-moh-th'e-ră-pi) *n. see* photodynamic therapy, PUVA.

photocoagulation (foh-toh-koh-ag-yoo-lay-shŏn) *n.* **1.** the destruction of tissue by heat released from the absorption of light shone on it. In eye disorders the technique is used to destroy diseased retinal tissue and to produce scarring between the retina and choroid, thus binding them together, in cases of retinal detachment. **2.** a method of arresting bleeding by causing coagulation, usually using an infrared light source.

photodermatosis (foh-toh-der-mă-**toh**-sis) *n.* any of various diseases caused by exposure to light of varying wavelength (*see* photosensitivity). The face and neck are most commonly affected. A common photodermatosis is *polymorphic light eruption*, which appears with the first sunshine of spring and abates by late summer. The photodermatoses include certain porphyrias.

photodynamic therapy (PDT, photoradiation therapy, phototherapy, photochemotherapy) (foh-toh-dy-**nam**-ik th'e-ră-pi) *n.* a treatment for some types of superficial cancers. A photosensitizing agent is injected into the bloodstream and remains in cancer cells for a longer time than in normal cells. Exposure to laser radiation produces an active form of oxygen that destroys the treated cancer cells. The laser radiation can be directed through a fibreoptic bronchoscope into the airways, through a gastroscope into the oesophagus, or through a cystoscope into the bladder.

photomicrograph (foh-toh-my-krŏ-grahf) *n. see* micrograph.

photophobia (foh-toh-**foh**-biă) *n.* an abnormal intolerance of light, in which exposure to light produces intense discomfort of the eyes with tight contraction of the eyelids. Photophobia may be associated with migraine, measles, German measles, or meningitis.

photophthalmia (foh-tof-**thal**-miă) *n.* inflammation of the eye due to exposure to light. It is usually caused by the damaging effect of ultraviolet light on the cornea, for example in snow blindness.

photoradiation (foh-toh-ray-di-ay-shŏn) *n. see* photodynamic therapy.

photorefractive keratectomy (PRK) (foh-toh-ri-frak-tiv) *n. see* keratectomy.

photoretinitis (foh-toh-ret-in-I-tis) *n.* damage to the retina of the eye caused by looking at the sun without adequate protection for the eyes. The central part of the visual field may be permanently lost (*sun blindness*).

photosensitivity (foh-toh-sen-si-tiv-iti) *n.* abnormal reaction of the skin to sunlight, which characterizes certain skin diseases (*see* photodermatosis). Drugs, such as tetracyclines, phenothiazines, and NSAIDs, can also cause photosensitivity. —**photosensitive** *adj.*

phototherapeutic keratec-

tomy (foh-toh-th'e-ră-**pew**-tik) *n. see* keratectomy.

phototherapy (foh-toh-**th'e**-ră-pi) *n.* the treatment of disorders by exposing the patient to light. Phototherapy using fluorescent light is used to treat jaundice in the newborn, as the blue range of the light decomposes bilirubin. *See also* photodynamic therapy.

phototoxicity (foh-toh-toks-**iss**-iti) *n.* damage caused by prolonged exposure to light. *retinal p.* damage to the retina of the eye as a result of prolonged exposure to light.

photuria (foht-**yoor**-iă) *n.* the excretion of phosphorescent urine, due to the presence of certain compounds containing phosphorus.

phren- (phreno-) *prefix denoting* **1.** the mind or brain. **2.** the diaphragm. **3.** the phrenic nerve.

-phrenia *suffix denoting* a condition of the mind.

phrenic (fren-ik) *adj.* **1.** relating to the mind. **2.** relating to the diaphragm. *p. avulsion* the surgical removal of a section of the phrenic nerve, which paralyses the diaphragm: formerly used as a means of resting a lung infected with tuberculosis. *p. crush* surgical crushing of a portion of the phrenic nerve, paralysing part of the diaphragm, which is then pushed upwards and presses on the lung, partially collapsing it: formerly used in the treatment of tuberculosis. *p. nerve* the nerve that supplies the muscles of the diaphragm. On each side it arises in the neck and passes downwards between the lungs and the heart.

Phthirus (thi-rŭs) *n.* a widely distributed genus of lice. *P. pubis* the crab (or pubic) louse, a common parasite of humans that lives permanently attached to the body hair, particularly that of the pubic or perianal regions. *See also* pediculosis.

phthisis (th'y-sis) *n.* **1.** any disease resulting in wasting of tissues. *p. bulbi* a shrunken eyeball that has lost its function due to disease or damage. **2.** a former name for pulmonary tuberculosis.

phycomycosis (fy-koh-my-**koh**-sis) *n.* a disease caused by parasitic fungi of the genera *Rhizopus*, *Absidia*, and *Mucor*. The fungi grow within the blood vessels of the lungs and nervous tissue, causing blood clots that cut off the blood supply (*see* infarction). Treatment with the antibiotic amphotericin B has proved effective.

physi- (physio-) *prefix denoting* **1.** physiology. **2.** physical.

physical (fiz-ikăl) *adj.* (in medicine) relating to the body rather than to the mind. *p. sign* a sign that a doctor can detect when examining a patient, such as abnormal dilation of the pupils or the absence of a knee-jerk reflex.

physical medicine *n.* the medical specialty that is concerned with the diagnosis and management of rheumatic diseases and the rehabilitation of patients with physical disabilities. *See also* rheumatology.

physician (fiz-**ish**-ăn) *n.* a registered medical practitioner who specializes in the diagnosis and treatment of disease by other than surgical means. *See also* Doctor.

physiological saline (fiz-i-ŏ-**loj**-ikăl) *n.* a 0.9% solution of sodium chloride in water, used for maintaining living cells

physiological solution *n.* one of a group of solutions, including Ringer's solution, used to maintain tissues in a viable state. These solutions contain specific concentrations of substances that are vital for normal tissue function.

physiology (fiz-i-**ol**-ŏji) *n.* the science of the functioning of living organisms and of their component parts. —**physiological** *adj.* —**physiologist** *n.*

physiotherapy (fiz-i-oh-**th'e**-ră-pi) *n.* the branch of treatment that employs physical methods to promote healing, including the use of light, heat, electric current, ultrasound, massage, manipulation, hydrotherapy, and remedial exercise.

physo- *prefix denoting* air or gas.

phyt- (phyto-) *prefix denoting* plants; of plant origin.

phytomenadione (fy-toh-men-ă-dy-ohn) *n.* a form of vitamin K that is used as an antidote to overdosage with anticoagulant drugs. It promotes the production of prothrombin, essential for the normal coagulation of blood. Trade name: **Konakion**.

phytotherapy (fy-toh-**th'e**-ră-pi) *n.* medical treatment based exclusively on plant extracts and products. Plants have provided a wide range of important drugs, but any drugs derived directly from plants should be extracted, purified, assayed, and tested before being used as medication.

pia (pia mater) (pee-ă) *n.* the innermost of the three meninges surrounding the brain and spinal cord. It contains numerous finely branching blood vessels that supply the nerve tissue within.

pian (pi-ahn) *n. see* yaws.

pica (py-kă) *n.* the indiscriminate eating of non-nutritious or harmful substances, such as grass, stones, or clothing. It is common in early childhood but may also be found in mentally handicapped and psychotic patients.

PICC *n.* peripherally inserted central catheter. *See* central venous catheter.

Pick's disease (piks) *n.* **1.** a cause of dementia. The damage is mainly in the frontal and temporal lobes of the brain. [A. Pick (1851–1924), Czech psychiatrist] **2.** a syndrome in constrictive pericarditis, in which there is hepatic enlargement, ascites, and pleural effusion. [F. Pick (1867–1926), Czech physician]

picornavirus (pi-kor-nă-vy-rŭs) *n.* one of a group of small RNA-containing viruses. The group includes Coxsackie viruses, polioviruses, and rhinoviruses.

picric acid (trinitrophenol) (pik-rik) *n.* a yellow crystalline solid used as a dye and as a tissue fixative.

PICU *n.* paediatric intensive care unit: *see* intensive care.

PID *n.* **1.** *see* pelvic inflammatory disease. **2.** *see* prolapsed intervertebral disc.

Pierre Robin syndrome (p'yair roh-ban) *n.* a congenital disease in which affected infants have a very small lower jawbone (mandible) and a cleft palate. They are susceptible to feeding and respiratory problems. [Pierre Robin (1867–1950), French dentist]

piezoelectric (peets-oh-i-lek-trik) *adj.* denoting or relating to an electrically generated pulse or polarity that is caused by pressure.

pigeon chest (pij-ŏn) *n.* forward protrusion of the breastbone resulting in deformity of the chest. The condition is painless and harmless. Medical name: **pectus carinatum.**

pigeon toes *n.* an abnormal posture in which the toes are turned inwards. It is often associated with knock-knee.

pigment (pig-mĕnt) *n.* a substance giving colour. Physiologically important pigments include the blood pigments (especially haemoglobin), the bile pigments, and retinal pigment (*see* rhodopsin).

pigmentation (pig-mĕn-tay-shŏn) *n.* coloration produced in the body by the deposition of one pigment, especially in excessive amounts. Pigmentation may be produced by natural pigments, such as melanin, or by foreign material, such as lead or arsenic in chronic poisoning.

PIH *n.* pregnancy-induced hypertension. *See* pre-eclampsia.

piles (pylz) *pl. n. see* haemorrhoids.

pill (pil) *n.* **1.** a small ball of variable size, shape, and colour, sometimes coated with sugar, that contains one or more medicinal substances in solid form. It is taken by mouth. **2. the Pill** *see* oral contraceptive.

pillar (pil-er) *n.* (in anatomy) an elongated apparently supportive structure.

pilo- *prefix denoting* hair.

pilocarpine (py-loh-kar-peen) *n.* a parasympathomimetic drug used as a miotic to counteract the effects of phenylephrine and to reduce the pressure inside the eye in glaucoma. It is administered as eye drops. Trade name: **Minims Pilocarpine.**

pilomotor nerves (py-loh-**moh**-ter) *pl. n.* sympathetic nerves that supply muscle fibres in the skin, around the roots of hairs. Activity of the sympathetic nervous system causes the muscles to contract, resulting in goose flesh.

pilonidal sinus (py-loh-**ny**-d'l) *n.* a short tract leading from an opening in the skin in the cleft at the top of the buttocks and containing hairs. The sinus may be recurrently infected, leading to pain and the discharge of pus.

pilosebaceous (py-loh-si-bay-ŏhŭs) *adj.* relating to the hair follicles and their associated sebaceous glands.

pilosis (py-loh-sis) *n.* the abnormal growth of hair.

pilus (py-lŭs) *n.* a hair.

pimel- (pimelo-) *prefix denoting* fat; fatty.

pimozide (pim-oh-zyd) *n.* an antipsychotic drug administered by mouth to relieve hallucinations and delusions occurring in schizophrenia. Trade name: **Orap**.

pimple (pim-pŭl) *n.* a small inflamed swelling on the skin that contains pus. It may be the result of bacterial infection of a skin pore that has become obstructed with fatty secretions from the sebaceous glands. *See also* acne.

PIN *n. see* prostatic intraepithelial neoplasia.

pineal gland (pineal body) (pin-i-ăl) *n.* a pea-sized mass of nerve tissue attached by a stalk to the posterior wall of the third ventricle of the brain. It functions as a gland, secreting the hormone melatonin. Anatomical name: **epiphysis**.

pinguecula (ping-wek-yoo-lă) *n.* a degenerative change in the conjunctiva of the eye, seen most commonly in the elderly. Thickened yellow triangles develop on the conjunctiva at the inner and outer margins of the cornea.

pink disease *n.* a severe illness of children of the teething age, marked by pink cold clammy hands and feet, heavy sweating, raised blood pressure, rapid pulse, and photophobia. Affected infants are very prone to secondary infection, which may be fatal. The condition may be an allergic reaction to mercury; it has virtually disappeared since all mercury-containing paediatric preparations have been banned. Medical names: **acrodynia, erythroedema, erythromelalgia**.

pink eye *n. see* conjunctivitis.

pinna (auricle) (pin-ă) *n.* the flap of skin and cartilage that projects from the head at the exterior opening of the external auditory meatus of the ear.

pinnaplasty (pin-ă-plasti) *n. see* otoplasty.

pinocytosis (pee-noh-sy-toh-sis) *n.* the intake of small droplets of fluid by a cell by cytoplasmic engulfment. *Compare* phagocytosis.

pins and needles (pinz) *pl. n. see* paraesthesiae.

pinta (pin-tă) *n.* a skin disease, prevalent in tropical America, that seems to affect only the dark-skinned races. It is caused by the spirochaete *Treponema carateum*. Symptoms include thickening and eventual loss of pigment of the skin, particularly on the hands, wrists, feet, and ankles.

pinworm (pin-werm) *n. see* threadworm.

piperazine (pi-pe-ră-zeen) n. a drug that is administered by mouth to treat infestations by roundworms and threadworms. Trade name: **Pripsen**.

piriform fossae (pi-ri-form) pl. n. two pear-shaped depressions that lie on either side of the opening to the larynx.

piroxicam (py-roks-i-kam) n. a nonsteroidal anti-inflammatory drug (see NSAID) administered by mouth, injection, or topically to relieve pain and stiffness in osteoarthritis, rheumatoid arthritis, gout, and ankylosing spondylitis. Trade name: **Feldene**.

PIs pl. n. see performance indicators.

pisiform bone (py-si-form) n. the smallest bone of the wrist (see carpus): a pea-shaped bone that articulates with the triquetral bone and, indirectly by cartilage, with the ulna.

pit (pit) n. (in anatomy) a hollow or depression.

pithiatism (pith-I-ă-tizm) n. the treatment of certain disorders by persuading the patient that all is well.

pitting (pit-ing) n. the formation of depressed scars, as occurs on the skin following acne. **p. oedema** oedema in which fingertip pressure leaves temporary indentations in the skin.

pituitary apoplexy (pit-yoo-it-eri) n. acute intrapituitary haemorrhage, usually into an existing tumour, presenting as severe headache and collapse. It is a medical emergency.

pituitary gland (hypophysis) n. the master endocrine gland: a pea-sized body attached to the hypothal-amus at the base of the skull. The anterior lobe of the gland (*adenohypophysis*) secretes thyroid-stimulating hormone, ACTH, gonadotrophins (LH and FSH), growth hormone, prolactin, lipotrophin, and melanocyte-stimulating hormone. The posterior lobe (*neurohypophysis*) secretes vasopressin and oxytocin.

pityriasis (pit-i-ry-ă-sis) n. (originally) any of a group of skin diseases typified by the development of fine branlike scales. **p. alba** a common condition in children in which pale scaly patches occur on the face. **p. capitis** see dandruff. **p. rosea** a common skin rash, believed to be viral in origin, that starts with a single patch on the trunk and is followed by an eruption of oval pink scaly macules. The rash clears completely in about eight weeks. **p. versicolor** a common chronic infection of the skin caused by the fungus *Pityrosporum orbiculare*, a normal inhabitant of the scalp that in susceptible people changes to a pathogenic form on the trunk.

Pityrosporum (pit-i-ros-pŏ-rŭm) n. a genus of yeasts producing superficial infections of the skin. *P. orbiculare* a normal inhabitant of the scalp that can become pathogenic in susceptible individuals (see pityriasis).

pivmecillinam (piv-mes-il-in-am) n. a penicillin-type antibiotic used to treat urinary-tract and other infections. It is administered by mouth. Trade name: **Selexid**.

pivot joint (piv-ŏt) n. see trochoid joint.

pixel (piks-ĕl) n. short for 'picture element', the smallest individual component of an electronically produced image. *See* digital (image).

pizotifen (piz-ot-i-fen) *n.* an antihistamine drug used to prevent severe migraine attacks. Administered by mouth, it acts by inhibiting the effects of serotonin. Trade name: **Sanomigran**.

PKU *n. see* phenylketonuria.

placebo (plă-see-boh) *n.* a medicine that is ineffective but may help to relieve a condition because the patient has faith in its powers. New drugs are tested against placebos in clinical trials.

placenta (plă-sent-ă) *n.* an organ within the uterus by means of which the embryo is attached to the wall of the uterus. Its primary function is to provide the embryo with nourishment, eliminate its wastes, and exchange respiratory gases. It also functions as a gland, secreting chorionic gonadotrophin, progesterone, and oestrogens. *See also* afterbirth. **p. praevia** a placenta situated wholly or partially in the lower and noncontractile part of the uterus. When this becomes elongated and stretched during the last few weeks of pregnancy, and the cervix becomes stretched either before or during labour, placental separation and haemorrhage will occur. If the placenta is situated entirely before the presenting part of the fetus, delivery must be by Caesarean section. —**placental** *adj.*

placentography (plas-en-tog-răfi) *n.* radiography of the pregnant uterus in order to determine the position of the placenta. This method is now superseded by the use of ultrasound.

plagiocephaly (play-ji-oh-sef-ăli)

n. any distortion or lack of symmetry in the shape of the head, usually due to irregularity in the closure of the sutures between the bones of the skull.

plague (playg) *n.* **1.** any epidemic disease with a high death rate. **2.** an acute epidemic disease of rats and other wild rodents caused by the bacterium *Yersinia pestis*, which is transmitted to humans by rat fleas. **bubonic p.** the most common form of the disease, characterized by acute painful swellings of the lymph nodes (*see* bubo). In favourable cases the buboes burst and then heal; in other cases bleeding under the skin can lead to ulcers, which may prove fatal. *pneumonic p.* a serious form of plague in which the lungs are affected. *septicaemic p.* a serious form of plague in which bacteria enter the bloodstream.

plane (playn) *n.* a level or smooth surface, especially any of the hypothetical flat surfaces used to divide the body (*see* coronal, sagittal).

planning (plan-ing) *n.* the stage of the nursing process in which an individual *care plan* is produced, stating the patient's problem(s), the objective, the goal or expected outcome, the nursing intervention, and the time or date by which the objective is expected to be achieved or by which the problem should be reviewed.

plantar (plan-ter) *adj.* relating to the sole of the foot (*planta*). **p. arch** the arch in the sole of the foot formed by anastomosing branches of the plantar arteries. **p. fasciitis** (*policeman's heel*) inflammation of the point of attachment of the fascia in the sole of the foot to the calcaneus, causing pain and tenderness of the heel. *p. reflex* a reflex obtained by drawing a bluntly pointed object along the outer border of the sole of the foot. The normal (flexor) response is a bunching and downward movement of the toes. *Compare* Babinski reflex. *p. wart see* wart.

plaque (plak) *n.* **1.** a layer composed of bacteria in an organic matrix that forms on the surface of a tooth, principally at its neck. It may cause caries or periodontal disease. **2.** a raised patch on the skin formed by enlarging or coalescing papules. **3.** a deposit, consisting of a fatty core covered with a fibrous cap, that develops on the inner wall of an atheromatous artery. **4.** any flattened patch or localized area of abnormality on a body surface.

-plasia *suffix denoting* formation; development.

plasm- (plasmo-) *prefix denoting* **1.** blood plasma. **2.** protoplasm or cytoplasm.

plasma (blood plasma) (plaz-mǎ) *n.* the straw-coloured fluid in which the blood cells are suspended. It consists of a solution of various inorganic salts of sodium, potassium, calcium, etc., with a high concentration of protein and a variety of trace substances.

plasma cells *pl. n.* antibody-producing cells found in blood-forming tissue and also in the epithelium of the lungs and gut. They develop in the bone marrow, lymph nodes, and spleen when antigens stimulate B-lymphocytes to produce the precursor cells that give rise to them.

plasmacytoma (plaz-mǎ-sy-toh-mǎ) *n.* a malignant tumour of

plasma cells, usually occurring as a single tumour in bone marrow or more rarely soft tissue (*extramedullary p.*) and often known as a 'solitary myeloma'. However, it may be multiple, in which case it is classifed as a multiple myeloma.

plasmapheresis (plaz-mǎ-fer-ee-sis) *n.* a method of removing a quantity of plasma from the blood. Blood is withdrawn from the patient and allowed to settle. The plasma is then drawn off and the blood cells transfused back into the patient.

plasmin (fibrinolysin) (plaz-min) *n.* an enzyme that digests the protein fibrin. Its function is the dissolution of blood clots (*see* fibrinolysis).

plasminogen (plaz-min-ŏ-jĕn) *n.* a substance normally present in the blood plasma that may be activated to form plasmin. *See* fibrinolysis. *p. activator* any enzyme that converts plasminogen to plasmin, of which there are two types: tissue-type plasminogen activator and urokinase-like plasminogen activator.

Plasmodium (plaz-moh-diŭm) *n.* a genus of protozoans that live as parasites within the red blood cells and liver cells of humans. Four species cause malaria in humans: *P. vivax, P. ovale, P. falciparum,* and *P. malariae.*

plaster (plah-ster) *n.* adhesive tape used in shaped pieces or as a bandage to keep a dressing in place.

plaster of Paris (POP) *n.* a preparation of gypsum (calcium sulphate) that sets hard when water is added. It is used in dentistry and orthopaedics for preparing plaster casts.

plastic lymph (plast-ik) *n.* a transparent yellowish liquid produced in a wound or other site of inflammation, in which connective tissue cells and blood vessels develop during healing.

plastic surgery *n.* a branch of surgery dealing with the reconstruction of parts of the body deformed or damaged by burns, major accidents, or cancer. It also includes the correction of congenital defects, such as cleft lip, and the replacement of parts of the body that have been lost. *aesthetic p. s. (cosmetic surgery)* plastic surgery performed simply to improve appearance.

plastron (plas-tron) *n.* the breastbone (sternum) together with the costal cartilages attached to it.

-plasty *suffix denoting* plastic surgery.

platelet (thrombocyte) (playt-lit) *n.* a disc-shaped cell structure, 1–2 μm in diameter, present in the blood. Platelets have several functions, all relating to the arrest of bleeding (*see* blood coagulation). *See also* thrombopoiesis.

platy- *prefix denoting* broad or flat.

platyhelminth (plat-i-hel-minth) *n.* see flatworm.

platysma (plă-tiz-mă) *n.* a broad thin sheet of muscle that extends from below the collar bone to the angle of the jaw. It depresses the jaw.

play (play) *n.* any spontaneous or organized activity that provides enjoyment, entertainment, amusement, or diversion. Play in childhood is essential to enable holistic development.

pledget (plej-it) *n.* a small wad of dressing material, such as lint, used either to cover a wound or sore or as a plug. Mounted on an instrument,

it is used during operations to wipe away blood and other fluids.

-plegia *suffix denoting* paralysis.

pleio- (pleo-) *prefix denoting* **1.** multiple. **2.** excessive.

pleocytosis (plee-oh-sy-toh-sis) *n.* the presence of an abnormally large number of lymphocytes in the cerebrospinal fluid.

pleomorphism (plee-oh-mor-fizm) *n.* the condition in which an individual assumes a number of different forms during its life cycle. The malarial parasite (*Plasmodium*) displays pleomorphism.

pleoptics (plee-op-tiks) *n.* special techniques practised by orthoptists for developing normal function of the macula, in people whose macular function has previously been disturbed because of strabismus (squint).

plessor (plexor) (ples-er) *n.* a small hammer used to investigate nervous reflexes and in the technique of percussion.

plethora (pleth-er-ă) *n.* any excess of any bodily fluid, especially blood (*see* hyperaemia). —**plethoric** (pleth-o-rik) *adj.*

plethysmography (pleth-iz-mog-răfi) *n.* the process of recording the changes in the volume of a limb caused by alterations in blood pressure. The limb is inserted into a fluid-filled watertight casing (*oncometer*) and the pressure variations in the fluid are recorded.

pleur- (pleuro-) *prefix denoting* **1.** the pleura. **2.** the side of the body.

pleura (ploor-ă) *n.* the covering of the lungs (*visceral p.*) and of the inner surface of the chest wall (*parietal p.*), consisting of a closed sac of serous membrane. Fluid secreted by the membrane lubricates the opposing surfaces so that they can slide painlessly over each other during breathing. —**pleural** *adj.*

parietal pleura —

visceral pleura —

pleural cavity —

chest wall —

diaphragm

The pleura

pleural cavity (ploor-ăl) *n.* the space between the visceral and parietal pleura, which is normally very small as the pleural membranes are in close contact.

pleurectomy (ploor-ek-tŏmi) *n.* surgical removal of part of the pleura, which is sometimes done to prevent further recurrences of spontaneous pneumothorax or to remove diseased areas of pleura.

pleurisy (ploor-i-si) *n.* inflammation of the pleura, often due to pneumonia in the underlying lung. The pleural surfaces become slightly sticky, so that there is pain on deep breathing. Pleurisy is always associated with some other disease in the lung, chest wall, diaphragm, or abdomen.

pleurocele (ploor-oh-seel) *n.* herniation of the pleura.

pleurocentesis (thoracentesis, thoracocentesis) (ploor-oh-sen-tee-sis) *n.* the insertion of a hollow needle into the pleural cavity

through the chest wall in order to withdraw fluid, blood, pus, or air.

pleurodesis (ploor-oh-dee-sis) *n.* a treatment for pneumothorax in which adhesions between the parietal and visceral pleura are induced by injecting a substance (e.g. silver nitrate) into the pleural cavity.

pleurodynia (ploor-oh-din-iă) *n.* severe paroxysmal pain arising from the muscles between the ribs. It is often thought to be of rheumatic origin.

pleurolysis (pneumolysis) (ploor-ol-i-sis) *n.* surgical stripping of the parietal pleura from the chest wall to allow the lung to collapse. The procedure was formerly used to help tuberculosis to heal.

pleuropneumonia (ploor-oh-new-moh-niă) *n.* inflammation involving both the lung and pleura. *See* pleurisy, pneumonia.

pleuropneumonia-like organisms (PPLO) *pl. n. see* mycoplasma.

plexor (pleks-er) *n. see* plessor.

plexus (pleks-ŭs) *n.* a network of nerves or blood vessels. *See* brachial plexus.

PLF *n.* (serum) *p*lacental *f*ementin: a storage protein, levels of which are used for monitoring placental function from conception until delivery.

plica (plik-ă) *n.* a fold of tissue. —**plicate** *adj.*

plication (pli-kay-shŏn) *n.* a surgical technique in which the size of a hollow organ is reduced by taking tucks or folds in the walls.

ploidy (ployd-i) *n.* the condition of having multiple the normal number of chromosomes for the species. An increase in ploidy in the cells of a malignant tumour usually indicates greater aggressiveness and ability to invade.

plombage (plom-bah*zh*) *n.* a surgical technique used to correct retinal detachment. A small piece of silicone plastic is sewn on the outside of the eyeball to produce an indentation over the retinal hole or tear to allow the retina to reattach.

plumbism (plum-bizm) *n.* lead poisoning. *See* lead.

Plummer's disease (plum-erz) *n.* a hyperfunctioning, usually benign, adenoma of the thyroid gland, which can be palpated and appears as a 'hot nodule' on radioactive thyroid scanning. [H. S. Plummer (1874–1937), US physician]

Plummer–Vinson syndrome (vin-sŏn) *n.* a disorder characterized by difficulty in swallowing associated with severe iron deficiency anaemia. [H. S. Plummer and P. P. Vinson (1890–1959), US physicians]

pluri- *prefix denoting* more than one; several.

PMB *n.* postmenopausal bleeding.

PMS *n. see* premenstrual syndrome.

pneo- *prefix denoting* breathing; respiration.

pneum- **(pneumo-)** *prefix denoting* **1.** the presence of air or gas. **2.** the lung(s). **3.** respiration.

pneumat- **(pneumato-)** *prefix denoting* **1.** the presence of air or gas. **2.** respiration.

pneumatocele (new-mat-oh-seel) *n.* herniation of lung tissue.

pneumatosis (new-mă-**toh**-sis) *n.* the occurrence of gas cysts in abnormal sites in the body. *p. cystoides intestinalis* the occurrence of multiple gas cysts in the walls of the lower intestines.

pneumaturia (new-măt-**yoor**-iă) *n.*

the presence in the urine of bubbles of air or other gas, due to the formation of gas by bacteria infecting the urinary tract or to a fistula between the urinary tract and bowel.

pneumocephalus **(pneumocele)** (new-moh-sef-ă-lŭs) *n.* the presence of air within the skull, usually resulting from a fracture passing through one of the air sinuses.

pneumococcus (new-moh-**kok**-ŭs) *n.* (*pl.* **pneumococci**) the bacterium *Streptococcus pneumoniae*, which is associated with pneumonia and pneumococcal meningitis. —**pneumococcal** *adj.*

pneumoconiosis (new-moh-koh-ni-**oh**-sis) *n.* a group of lung diseases caused by inhaling dust. In practice industrial exposure to coal dust (*see* coal-worker's pneumoconiosis), silica (*see* silicosis), and asbestos (*see* asbestosis) produces most of the cases of pneumoconiosis.

Pneumocystis (new-moh-**sis**-tis) *n.* a genus of protozoans. *P. carinii* the cause of pneumonia in immunosuppressed patients, usually following intensive chemotherapy or in patients with AIDS. *See also* opportunist.

pneumocyte (new-moh-syt) *n.* a type of cell that lines the walls separating the air sacs (*see* alveolus) in the lungs.

pneumoencephalography (new-moh-en-sef-ă-**log**-răfi) *n.* a technique used in the X-ray diagnosis of disease within the skull. Air is introduced into the ventricles of the brain to displace the cerebrospinal fluid, thus acting as a contrast medium. X-ray photographs show the size and disposition of the ventricles and the subarachnoid spaces.

The technique has largely been superseded by CT and MRI scanning.

pneumogastric (new-moh-**gas**-trik) *adj.* relating to the lungs and stomach. *p. nerve* the vagus nerve.

pneumograph (new-moh-grahf) *n.* an instrument used to record the movements made during respiration.

pneumolysis (new-mol-i-sis) *n. see* pleurolysis.

pneumomycosis (new-moh-my-koh-sis) *n.* any infection of the lungs caused by fungi, such as aspergillosis.

pneumon- (pneumono-) *prefix* denoting the lung(s).

pneumonectomy (new-mŏ-**nek**-tŏmi) *n.* surgical removal of a lung, usually for cancer.

pneumonia (new-moh-niǎ) *n.* inflammation of the lung caused by bacteria, in which the alveoli become filled with inflammatory cells and the lung becomes solid (*see* consolidation). The symptoms include fever, malaise, cough, and chest pain, and there are shadows on the chest X-ray. Treatment with antibiotics is usually effective. *bronchopneumonia* pneumonia that starts in the small bronchi and spreads into the alveoli. *hypostatic p.* pneumonia that develops in dependant parts of the lung in people who are otherwise ill, chilled, or immobilized. *lobar p.* pneumonia that affects whole lobes of either or both lungs. *See also* atypical (pneumonia), viral pneumonia. *Compare* pneumonitis.

pneumonitis (new-mŏ-ny-tis) *n.* inflammation of the lung that is confined to the walls of the alveoli and often caused by viruses or unknown

agents. It may be acute and transient or chronic, leading to increasing respiratory disability. It does not respond to antibiotics but corticosteroids may be helpful. *Compare* pneumonia.

pneumoperitoneum (new-moh-pe-ri-tŏn-ee-ŭm) *n.* air or gas in the peritoneal or abdominal cavity, usually due to a perforation of the stomach or bowel. It may be induced for diagnostic purposes (*see* laparoscopy).

pneumoradiography (new-moh-ray-di-og-răfi) *n.* X-ray examination of part of the body using a gas, such as air or carbon dioxide, as a contrast medium. The technique is now little used apart from double contrast examinations of the bowel.

pneumoretinopexy (new-moh-ret-in-oh-peks-i) *n.* a surgical technique in which an inert gas bubble is injected into the eye to press and seal breaks in the retina. When the retina is flat, a laser beam or cryoretinopexy is applied to cause scarring and permanently seal the tear.

pneumothorax (new-moh-**thor**-aks) *n.* air in the pleural cavity, which results from breach of the lung surface or chest wall and causes the lung to collapse. *artificial p.* the deliberate injection of air into the pleural cavity to collapse the lung: a former treatment for pulmonary tuberculosis. *spontaneous p.* pneumothorax that occurs without any apparent cause, in otherwise healthy people. *tension p.* pneumothorax in which a breach in the lung surface acts as a valve, admitting air into the pleural cavity when the patient breathes in but preventing its escape when breathing out.

traumatic p. pneumothorax that results from injuries to the chest.

pneumotonometer (new-moh-toh-**nom**-it-er) *n.* an instrument that blows a puff of air at the cornea to cause flattening and hence measure intraocular pressure. It is commonly used by optometrists in tests for glaucoma.

-pnoea *suffix denoting* a condition of breathing.

POAG *n.* primary open-angle glaucoma. *See* glaucoma.

pock (pok) *n.* a small pus-filled eruption on the skin characteristic of chickenpox and smallpox rashes. *See also* pustule.

pocket resuscitation mask (pok-it) *n.* a compressible and easily carried mask, which can be expanded and fitted over the mouth and nose of a nonbreathing patient in order to perform mouth-to-mouth resuscitation through a small valve without contact between the mouth of the rescuer and that of the patient.

pod- *prefix denoting* the foot.

podagra (pŏ-**dag**-ră) *n.* gout of the foot, especially the big toe.

podalic version (pŏ-**dal**-ik) *n.* altering the position of a fetus in the uterus so that its feet will emerge first at birth. *See also* version.

podopompholyx (poh-doh-**pom**-foh-liks) *n. see* pompholyx.

-poiesis *suffix denoting* formation; production.

poikilo- *prefix denoting* variation; irregularity.

poikilocyte (**poi**-kil-oh-syt) *n.* an abnormally shaped erythrocyte. *See also* poikilocytosis.

poikilocytosis (poi-kil-oh-sy-toh-sis) *n.* the presence of poikilocytes

in the blood. Poikilocytosis is particularly marked in myelofibrosis but can occur to some extent in almost any blood disease.

poikilothermic (poi-kil-oh-**therm**-ik) *adj.* cold-blooded: being unable to regulate the body temperature, which fluctuates according to that of the surroundings. *Compare* homoiothermic. —**poikilothermy** *n.*

poison (poi-zŏn) *n.* any substance that irritates, damages, or impairs the activity of the body's tissues. The term is usually reserved for substances, such as arsenic, cyanide, and strychnine, that are harmful in relatively small amounts.

polar body (poh-ler) *n.* one of the small cells produced by division of an oocyte that does not develop into a functional egg cell. *See* oogenesis.

pole (pohl) *n.* (in anatomy) the extremity of the axis of the body, an organ, or a cell.

poli- (polio-) *prefix denoting* the grey matter of the nervous system.

policeman's heel (pŏ-lees-**mănz**) *n. see* plantar (fasciitis).

polioencephalitis (poh-li-oh-en-sef-ă-ly-tis) *n.* a virus infection of the brain, causing particular damage to the grey matter of the cerebral hemispheres and the brainstem. The term is now usually restricted to infections of the brain by the poliomyelitis virus.

polioencephalomyelitis (poh-li-oh-en-sef-ă-loh-my-ĕ-ly-tis) *n.* any virus infection of the central nervous system affecting the grey matter of the brain and spinal cord. Rabies is the outstanding example.

poliomyelitis (infantile paralysis, polio) (poh-li-oh-my-ĕ-ly-tis) *n.* an infectious virus disease affecting the central nervous system. Immunization, using the Sabin vaccine or the Salk vaccine, is highly effective. *abortive p.* poliomyelitis in which only the throat and intestines are infected and the symptoms are those of a stomach upset or influenza. *bulbar p.* paralytic poliomyelitis in which the muscles of the respiratory system are affected. *nonparalytic p.* a form of the disease in which the symptoms of abortive poliomyelitis are accompanied by muscle stiffness. *paralytic p.* a less common form of polio in which the symptoms of the milder forms of the disease are followed by weakness and eventual paralysis of the muscles. *See also* post-polio syndrome.

poliovirus (poh-li-oh-vy-rŭs) *n.* one of a small group of RNA-containing viruses causing poliomyelitis. They are included within the picornavirus group.

Politzer's bag (pol-it-zerz) *n.* a flexible rubber bag for inflating the middle ear through the Eustachian tube. [A. Politzer (1835–1920), Austrian otologist]

pollex (pol-eks) *n.* (*pl.* **pollices**) the thumb.

pollinosis (poli-noh-sis) *n.* a more precise term than hay fever for an allergy due to the pollen of grasses, trees, or shrubs.

poly- *prefix denoting* **1.** many; multiple. **2.** excessive. **3.** generalized; affecting many parts.

polyarteritis nodosa (periarteritis nodosa) (poli-ar-ter-I-tis noh-doh-să) *n.* a disease of unknown cause in which there is patchy inflammation of the walls of the arteries. It is one of the connective-tissue diseases. Common manifestations include arthritis, skin rashes, asthma, hypertension, and kidney failure.

polyarthritis (poli-arth-ry-tis) *n.* disease involving several joints, either together or in sequence, causing pain, stiffness, swelling, tenderness, and loss of function. Rheumatoid arthritis is the most common cause.

polycystic disease of the kidneys (poli-sis-tik) *n.* an inherited disorder in which the substance of both kidneys is largely replaced by numerous cysts. Symptoms, including haematuria, urinary tract infection, and hypertension, are associated with chronic kidney failure.

polycystic ovary syndrome (POS) *n.* a hormonal disorder characterized by incomplete development of Graafian follicles in the ovary due to inadequate secretion of luteinizing hormone; the follicles fail to ovulate and remain as multiple cysts distending the ovary. *See also* Stein-Leventhal syndrome.

polycythaemia (poli-sy-theem-iă) *n.* an increase in the packed cell volume (haematocrit) in the blood. This may be due either to a decrease in the total volume of the plasma (*relative p.*) or to an increase in the total volume of the red cells (*absolute p.*). The latter may occur as a primary disease or as a secondary condition in association with various respiratory or circulatory disorders and with certain tumours. *p. vera* (*p. rubra vera, erythraemia, Vaquez-Osler disease*) a disease in which absolute polycythaemia is often accompanied by an increase in the numbers of white blood cells and platelets. Symptoms include headache, thromboses, cyanosis, plethora, and itching.

polydactylism (poli-**dak**-til-izm) *n.* see hyperdactylism.

polydipsia (poli-**dip**-siă) *n.* abnormally intense thirst: a symptom of diabetes mellitus and diabetes insipidus.

polymer (**pol**-im-er) *n.* a substance formed by the linkage of a large number of smaller molecules known as *monomers.* An example of a monomer is glucose, whose molecules link together to form glycogen, a polymer.

polymorph (polymorphonuclear leucocyte) (**pol**-i-morf) *n.* a type of white blood cell with a lobed nucleus and granular cytoplasm. *See* basophil, eosinophil, neutrophil.

polymorphic light eruption (poli-**mor**-fik) *n.* see photodermatosis.

polymyalgia rheumatica (poli-my-**al**-jiă roo-**mat**-ikă) *n.* a rheumatic disease causing aching and progressive stiffness of the muscles of the shoulders and hips after inactivity. It is typically associated with loss of appetite, fatigue, night sweats, and a raised ESR. The condition is most common in the elderly and is often associated with temporal arteritis. The symptoms respond rapidly and effectively to corticosteroid treatment.

polymyositis (poli-my-oh-**sy**-tis) *n.* a generalized disease of the muscles that may be acute or chronic. It particularly affects the muscles of the shoulder and hip girdles, which are weak and tender to the touch. Relief of the symptoms is obtained with

corticosteroid drugs. *See also* dermatomyositis.

polymyxin B (poli-**miks**-in) *n.* an antibiotic used to treat severe infections caused by Gram-negative bacteria. Formulated with other drugs, it is administered as a solution or ointment for ear and eye infections.

polyneuritis (poli-newr-**I**-tis) *n.* see (peripheral) neuropathy.

polyneuropathy (poli-newr-**op**-ă-thi) *n.* see (peripheral) neuropathy.

polyopia (poli oh **pi**ă) *n.* the sensation of multiple images of one object. It is sometimes experienced by people with early cataract. *See also* diplopia.

polyp (polypus) (**pol**-ip) *n.* a growth, usually benign, protruding from a mucous membrane. Polyps are commonly found in the nose and sinuses, giving rise to obstruction, chronic infection, and discharge. Other sites include the ear, the stomach, and the colon, where they may eventually become malignant. Polyps are usually removed surgically (see polypectomy). *juvenile p.* a polyp that occurs in the intestine (usually colon or rectum) of infants or young people; sometimes they are multiple (*see* polyposis). Most juvenile polyps are benign. *See also* Peutz-Jeghers syndrome.

polypectomy (poli-**pek**-tŏmi) *n.* the surgical removal of a polyp. The technique used depends upon the site and size of the polyp, but it is often done by cutting across the base using a wire loop (snare) through which is passed a coagulating diathermy current.

polypeptide (poli-**pep**-tyd) *n.* a molecule consisting of three or more amino acids linked together by peptide bonds. Protein molecules are polypeptides.

polyphagia (poli-fay-jiă) *n.* gluttonous excessive eating.

polypharmacy (poli-farm-ă-si) *n.* treatment of a patient with more than one type of medicine.

polyploid (pol-i-ploid) *adj.* describing cells, tissues, or individuals in which there are three or more complete sets of chromosomes. *Compare* diploid, haploid. —**polyploidy** *n.*

polypoid (pol-i-poid) *adj.* having the appearance of a polyp.

polyposis (poli-poh-sis) *n.* a condition in which numerous polyps form in an organ or tissue. *familial adenomatous p.* (*p. coli*) a hereditary disease in which multiple adenomas develop in the gastrointestinal tract, usually the colon or rectum, at an early age. As these polyps invariably become malignant, patients are usually advised to undergo total removal of the affected bowel. *See also* Peutz-Jeghers syndrome. *Compare* pseudopolyposis.

polypus (pol-i-pŭs) *n. see* polyp.

polyradiculitis (**polyradiculopathy**) (poli-ră-dik-yoo-ly-tis) *n.* any disorder of the peripheral nerves (*see* neuropathy) in which the brunt of the disease falls on the nerve roots where they emerge from the spinal cord.

polysaccharide (poli-sak-eryd) *n.* a carbohydrate formed from many monosaccharides joined together in long linear or branched chains. Examples are glycogen and cellulose.

polyserositis (poli-seer-oh-sy-tis) *n.* inflammation of the membranes that line the chest, abdomen, and joints, with accumulation of fluid in the cavities.

polysomnograph (poli-som-noh-graf) *n.* a record of measurements of various bodily parameters during sleep. It is used in the diagnosis of sleep disorders, such as obstructive sleep apnoea.

polyspermia (poli-sper-miă) *n.* **1.** excessive formation of semen. **2.** *see* polyspermy.

polyspermy (**polyspermia**) (poli-sper-mi) *n.* fertilization of a single ovum by more than one spermatozoon: the development is abnormal and the embryo dies.

polyuria (poli-yoor-iă) *n.* the production of large volumes of dilute urine. The phenomenon may be due simply to excessive liquid intake or to disease, particularly diabetes mellitus, diabetes insipidus, and kidney disorders.

POM *n. see* prescription only medicine.

pompholyx (pom-foh-liks) *n.* eczema of the palms (*cheiropompholyx*) and soles (*podopompholyx*). Because the horny layer of the skin in these parts is so thick the vesicles typical of eczema cannot rupture. There is intense itching until the skin eventually peels. Pompholyx is commonest in early adulthood.

pons (ponz) *n.* any portion of tissue that joins two parts of an organ. *p. Varolii* the part of the brainstem that links the medulla oblongata and the thalamus. It contains numerous nerve tracts between the cerebral cortex and the spinal cord. [C. Varolius (1543–75), Italian anatomist] —**pontine** (pon-teen) *adj.*

POP *n. see* plaster of Paris.

popliteus (pop-lit-iŭs) *n.* a flat triangular muscle at the back of the knee joint, between the femur and tibia, that helps to flex the knee. —**popliteal** *adj.*

pore (por) *n.* a small opening. *sweat p.* the opening of a sweat gland on the surface of the skin.

porencephaly (por-en-sef-ăli) *n.* an abnormal communication between the lateral ventricle and the surface of the brain. This is usually a consequence of brain injury or cerebrovascular disease.

porphin (por-fin) *n.* a complex nitrogen-containing ring structure and parent compound of the porphyrins.

porphyria (por-fi-riă) *n.* one of a group of rare inborn errors of metabolism in which there are deficiencies in the enzymes involved in the biosynthesis of haem. The accumulation of the enzyme's substrate gives rise to the features of the disorder, which include the excretion of porphyrins and their derivatives in the urine, which may change colour on standing. *acute intermittent p.* a hereditary hepatic porphyria marked by recurrent attacks of acute abdominal pain, constipation, and psychotic behaviour. *erythropoietic p.* any porphyria in which the defect is primarily in the bone marrow. *hepatic p.* any porphyria in which the defect is primarily in the liver. *p. cutanea tarda* a hereditary or acquired hepatic porphyria in which light-exposed areas of the skin become blistered and fragile (*see* photodermatosis).

porphyrin (por-fi-rin) *n.* one of a number of pigments derived from porphin, which are widely distributed in living things. All porphyrins form chelates with iron, magnesium, zinc, nickel, copper, and cobalt. These chelates are constituents of haemoglobin, myohaemoglobin, the cytochromes, and chlorophyll. *See also* protoporphyrin IX.

porphyrinuria (por-fi-rin-yoor-iă) *n.* the presence in the urine of porphyrins, sometimes causing discoloration. *See* porphyria.

porta (por-tă) *n.* the aperture in an organ through which its associated vessels pass. Such an opening occurs in the liver (*p. hepatis*). —**portal** *adj.*

portacaval anastomosis (portacaval shunt) (por-tă-kay-văl) *n.* **1.** a surgical technique in which the hepatic portal vein is joined to the inferior vena cava, thus bypassing the liver. It is used in the treatment of portal hypertension. **2.** any of the natural communications between the branches of the hepatic portal vein in the liver and the inferior vena cava.

portal hypertension (por-t'l) *n.* a state in which the pressure within the hepatic portal vein is increased, causing enlargement of the spleen and ascites. The commonest cause is cirrhosis. Treatment is by diuretic drugs, by surgery (*see* portacaval anastomosis), or by implanting a stent within the liver to join portal tract veins to a hepatic vein tributary.

portal system *n.* a vein or group of veins that terminates at both ends in a capillary bed. *hepatic p. s.* the best known portal system, consisting of the portal vein and its tributaries.

portal vein *n.* a vein that conveys blood from the stomach, intestines, spleen, and pancreas to the liver.

port-wine stain (port-wyn) *n. see* naevus.

POS *n. see* polycystic ovary syndrome.

position (pŏ-zish-ŏn) *n.* a posture or attitude assumed by a patient in order to facilitate nursing, diagnostic, or surgical procedures (see illustration).

genupectoral position

lithotomy position

Trendelenburg's position

semi-prone position

Types of position

positive end expiratory pressure (PEEP) (poz-it-iv) *n.* a technique used with the mechanical ventilation of patients with respiratory failure. The pressure at the end of expiration is kept sufficiently high to maintain the partial inflation of the lungs to prevent alveolar collapse.

positive pressure ventilation (PPV) *n.* the forcible passage of air into the lungs to stimulate breathing movements. *See also* respirator.

positron (poz-i-tron) *n.* an electrically charged particle, released in some radioactive decays, that has the same mass as an electron but opposite charge. It has a very short lifetime as it quickly reacts with an electron to produce gamma rays.

positron emission tomography (PET, positron emission computed tomography, PECT) *n.* a cross-sectional imaging technique of nuclear medicine that enables evaluation of the metabolic activity of tissues of the brain, chest, and abdomen by measuring their uptake of injected radioisotopes (e.g. fluorodeoxyglucose, using fluorine-18, to examine glucose metabolism). As the radioisotope is metabolized, it emits positrons, which are annihilated with the production of gamma rays; these are detected by the PET scanner and used to construct images.

posology (pŏ-sol-ŏji) *n.* the science of the dosage of medicines.

posseting (poss-it-ing) *n.* the regurgitation of a small amount of milk, usually with some wind, by a baby after feeding.

Possum (poss-ŭm) *n.* a device that enables severely paralysed patients to use typewriters, telephones, and other machines. Modern Possums are operated by micro-switches that require only the slightest movement in any limb. The name derives from *Patient-Operated Selector Mechanism* (POSM).

post- *prefix denoting* **1.** following; after. **2.** (in anatomy) behind.

postcibal (pohst-sy-băl) *adj.* occurring after eating.

postcoital (pohst-koh-i-t'l) *adj.* occurring after sexual intercourse. **p. contraception** prevention of pregnancy after intercourse has taken place. This can be achieved by two spaced oral doses of an oestrogen combined with a progestogen, or of a progesterone only, taken within 72 hours of unprotected intercourse; or the insertion of an IUCD. *p. test* a test used in the investigation of infertility. A specimen of cervical mucus, taken 6–24 hours after coitus in the postovulatory phase of the menstrual cycle, is examined under a microscope for the presence of motile spermatozoa.

postconcussional syndrome (pohst-kŏn-**kush**-ŏn-ăl) *n.* persistent headaches, giddiness, and lack of concentration that may follow a head injury.

postepileptic (pohst-epi-**lep**-tik) *adj.* occurring after an epileptic fit.

posterior (poss-teer-i-er) *adj.* situated at or near the back of the body or an organ. *p. chamber* the rear section of the eye, behind the lens, which is filled with vitreous humour.

postero- *prefix denoting* posterior.

postganglionic (pohst-gang-li-on-ik) *adj.* describing a neurone in a nerve pathway that starts at a ganglion and ends at the muscle or gland that it supplies. *Compare* preganglionic.

postgastrectomy syndrome (pohst-gas-**trek**-tŏmi) *n. see* dumping syndrome.

posthitis (poss-th'y-tis) *n.* inflammation of the foreskin. This usually occurs in association with balanitis (*see* balanoposthitis).

posthumous birth (poss-tew-mŭs) *n.* **1.** delivery of a child by Caesarean section after the mother's death. **2.** birth of a child after the father's death.

postmature (pohst-mă-tewr) *adj.* describing a baby born after 42 weeks of gestation (calculated from the first day of the last menstrual period). —**postmaturity** *n.*

postmenopause (pohst-men-ŏ-pawz) *n.* the period of a woman's life after the menopause.

postmicturition dribble (pohst-mik-tewr-ish-ŏn drib-ĕl) *n.* a lower urinary tract symptom in which a dribble occurs after voiding has been completed, often after leaving the toilet. It is quite common in men but is not caused by benign prostatic hyperplasia. *Compare* terminal dribble.

post mortem (pohst mor-tĕm) Latin: after death. *See* autopsy.

postnasal space (pohst-nay-zăl) *n. see* nasopharynx.

postnatal (pohst-nay-t'l) *adj.* following childbirth. *p. depression* sadness affecting a woman after childbirth. It ranges from a fleeting misery (so-called *baby blues*) that affects about half of all women after the birth of their first baby, to a pathological condition: *see* puerperal (depression).

postoperative (pohst-**op**-er-ă-tiv) *adj.* following operation: referring to the condition of a patient or to the treatment given at this time.

postpartum (pohst-**par**-tŭm) *adj.* relating to the period of a few days immediately after birth.

post-polio syndrome (pohst-**poh**-li-oh) *n.* insidious numbness in muscles, together with fatigue and pain, that develops 15–20 years after an attack of poliomyelitis. It may be caused by loss of nerve cells that have been under greater strain than normal; there is no evidence of reactivation of the poliovirus.

postprandial (pohst-**pran**-di-ăl) *adj.* occurring after eating.

Post-Registration Education and Practice Project (pohst-rej-i-stray-shŏn) *n.* see PREPP.

post-traumatic stress disorder (PTSD) (pohst-traw-**mat**-ik) *n.* an anxiety disorder caused by the major personal stress of a serious or frightening event, such as exposure to warfare or a disaster involving many casualties. The sufferer experiences the persistent recurrence of images or memories of the event, together with nightmares, insomnia, a sense of isolation, guilt, irritability, and loss of concentration.

postviral fatigue syndrome (pohst-vy-răl) *n.* see CFS/ME.

potassium (pŏ-**tas**-iŭm) *n.* a mineral element and an important constituent of the human body. It is the main base ion of intracellular fluid. High concentrations occur particularly in kidney failure and may lead to arrhythmia and finally to cardiac arrest. Low values result from fluid loss, e.g. due to vomiting or diarrhoea, and this may lead to general muscle paralysis. Symbol: K.

potassium-channel activator *n.* a drug that enhances the movement of potassium ions through the protein channels in cell membranes, reducing the sensitivity of smooth muscle cells in the walls of arteries to the normal stimuli to contract. The result is widening of the arteries. Potassium-channel activators, such as *nicorandil* (Icorel), are used for improving the blood supply to the heart muscle in angina pectoris.

potassium chloride *n.* a salt of potassium administered by mouth or injection to prevent and treat potassium deficiency, especially during treatment with certain diuretics. Trade name: **Slow-K**.

potassium hydroxyquinoline (hy-droks-i-**kwin**-ŏ-leen) *n.* a salt of potassium that has antifungal, antibacterial, and deodorant activities.

potassium permanganate (per-**mang**-ă-nayt) *n.* a salt of potassium used for disinfecting and cleansing wounds and as a general skin antiseptic. It irritates mucous membranes and is poisonous if taken into the body.

Potter syndrome (**pot**-er) *n.* a congenital condition characterized by absence of kidneys, resulting in decreased amniotic fluid (*see* oligohydramnios) and compression of the fetus. Affected babies have poorly developed lungs, a characteristic wrinkled and flattened facial appearance, and leg deformities and do not usually survive. [E. L. Potter (20th century), US pathologist]

Pott's disease (pots) *n.* tuberculosis of the backbone. Untreated, it can lead to a hunchback deformity. [P. Pott (1714–88), British surgeon]

Pott's fracture (pot) n. see fracture.

pouch (powch) n. **1.** (in anatomy) a small sac-like structure, especially occurring as an outgrowth of a larger structure. *p. of Douglas* a pouch of peritoneum occupying the space between the rectum and uterus. [J. Douglas (1675–1742), British anatomist] **2.** (in surgery) a sac created from a loop of intestine and used to replace a section of rectum that has been surgically removed, for example in ulcerative colitis. *See also* ileal pouch.

poultice (fomentation) (pohl-tis) n. a preparation of hot moist material applied to any part of the body to increase local circulation, alleviate pain, or soften the skin.

Poupart's ligament (poo-parz) n. see inguinal (ligament). [F. Poupart (1661–1708), French anatomist]

powder (pow-der) n. (in pharmacy) a medicinal preparation consisting of a mixture of two or more drugs in the form of fine particles.

pox (poks) n. **1.** an infectious disease causing a skin rash. **2.** a rash of pimples that become pus-filled, as in chickenpox and smallpox.

poxvirus (poks-vy-rŭs) n. one of a group of large DNA-containing viruses including those that cause smallpox (variola) and cowpox (vaccinia).

PPLO pl. n. see mycoplasma.

PPS n. plasma protein solution.

PPV n. see positive pressure ventilation.

PR per rectum.

practice nurse (prak-tis) n. a trained nurse caring for the patients of one or more general practitioners in the consulting room and on domiciliary consultations. In Britain practice nurses are usually employed by GPs but may also be employed by community trusts as district nurses.

Prader orchidometer (prah-der) n. see orchidometer.

Prader-Willi syndrome (prah-der vil-i) n. a congenital condition in which obesity is associated with mental retardation and small genitalia; diabetes mellitus frequently develops in affected individuals. [A. Prader and H. Willi (20th century), Swiss paediatricians]

pravastatin (prǎ-vas-tǎ-tin) n. a drug taken by mouth to reduce abnormally high levels of cholesterol in the blood (see statin). Trade name: **Lipostat**.

praziquantel (praz-i-kwon-tel) n. an anthelmintic drug used to eliminate tapeworms and schistosomes. It is administered by mouth. Trade name: **Cysticide**.

prazosin (praz-oh-sin) n. a drug used in the treatment of high blood pressure (hypertension) by reducing peripheral vascular resistance (see alpha blocker). It is administered by mouth. Trade name: **Hypovase**.

pre- prefix denoting **1.** before; preceding. **2.** (in anatomy) in front of; anterior to.

precancerous (pree-kan-ser-ŭs) adj. describing a nonmalignant condition that is known to become malignant if left untreated.

precipitin (pri-sip-it-in) n. any antibody that combines with its antigen to form a complex that is seen as a precipitate. The precipitin reaction is a useful means of confirming the identity of an unknown antigen or establishing that a serum contains antibodies to a known disease. *See also* agglutination.

precocious puberty (pri-koh-shŭs) *n.* the development in girls of breasts or pubic hair before the age of six or menstruation before the age of eight, and in boys the development of pubic hair or other adult sexual features below the age of nine. In girls 90% of cases have no underlying abnormalities, but in boys approximately half have a serious underlying cause, of which malignant testicular or adrenal tumours are the most common.

precocity (pri-kos-iti) *n.* an acceleration of normal development. The intellectually precocious child has a high IQ and may become isolated from his contemporaries or frustrated at school. —**precocious** *adj.*

precordium (pree-kor-diŭm) *n.* the region of the thorax immediately over the heart. —**precordial** *adj.*

precursor (pri-ker-ser) *n.* a substance from which another, usually more biologically active, substance is formed. For example, trypsinogen is the precursor of the enzyme trypsin.

predigestion (pree-dy-jes-chŏn) *n.* the partial digestion of foods by artificial means before they are taken into the body.

predisposition (pree-dis-pŏ-zish-ŏn) *n.* a tendency to be affected by a particular disease or kind of disease. *See also* diathesis.

prednisolone (pred-nis-ŏ-lohn) *n.* a synthetic corticosteroid used to treat rheumatic diseases, inflammatory and allergic conditions, and some cancers. It is administered by mouth, injected into joints, or applied in creams, lotions, ointments, or drops. Trade names: **Deltacortril, Deltastab, Precortisyl, Prednesol, Predsol.**

pre-eclampsia (pregnancy-induced hypertension, PIH) (pree-i-klamp-siă) *n.* high blood pressure (greater than 140/90 mmHg) developing during pregnancy in a woman whose blood pressure was previously normal. It is often accompanied by excessive fluid retention and less often by the the presence of protein in the urine. *See also* eclampsia.

prefrontal leucotomy (pree-frun-t'l) *n. see* leucotomy.

prefrontal lobe *n.* the region of the brain at the very front of each cerebral hemisphere. The functions of the lobe are concerned with emotions, memory, learning, and social behaviour.

preganglionic (pree-gang-li-on-ik) *adj.* describing fibres in a nerve pathway that end in a ganglion, where they form synapses with postganglionic fibres.

pre-gangrene (pree-gang-reen) *n.* the penultimate stage of vascular insufficiency before gangrene sets in; the term is usually applied to ischaemia of the lower limb.

pregnancy (preg-năn-si) *n.* the period during which a woman carries a developing fetus, normally in the uterus (*compare* ectopic pregnancy). Pregnancy lasts for approximately 266 days, from conception until the baby is born, or 280 days from the first day of the last menstrual period (*see* Naegele rule). *See also* pseudocyesis (phantom pregnancy).

p. test any of several methods used to demonstrate whether or not a woman is pregnant. Most pregnancy tests are based on the detection, by immunological methods, of a hormone, human chorionic gonadotrophin, in the urine or in the serum. —**pregnant** *adj.*

pregnancy-induced hypertension (PIH) *n. see* pre-eclampsia.

pregnanediol (preg-nayn-dy-ol) *n.* a steroid that is formed during the metabolism of the female sex hormone progesterone. It occurs in the urine during pregnancy and certain phases of the menstrual cycle.

pregnenolone (preg-neen-ŏ-lohn) *n.* a steroid synthesized in the adrenal glands, ovaries, and testes. Pregnenolone is an important intermediate product in steroid hormone synthesis.

preimplantation genetic diagnosis (PGD) (pree-im-plahn-tay-shŏn) *n.* prenatal genetic diagnosis extended to the earliest stages of embryonic development, before implantation occurs.

premature beat (prem-ă-tewr) *n. see* ectopic beat.

premature birth *n. see* preterm birth.

premedication (pree-med-i-kay-shŏn) *n.* drugs administered to a patient before an operation. Premedication usually comprises injection of a sedative (e.g. a benzodiazepine) together with a drug, such as hyoscine, to dry up the secretions of the lungs (which might otherwise be inhaled during anaesthesia).

premenstrual syndrome (PMS) (pree-**men**-stroo-ăl) *n.* a group of symptoms experienced in varying degrees by women of reproductive age in the week before menstruation. These include altered mental stability, fatigue, bloating, breast tenderness, and headaches. Treatments include stress management, salt restriction and low-dose diuretics to relieve fluid retention, simple analgesia for aches and pains, and the contraceptive pill because suppression of ovulation often relieves the symptoms.

premolar (pree-moh-ler) *n.* either of the two teeth on each side of each jaw behind the canines and in front of the molars in the adult dentition.

prenatal diagnosis (antenatal diagnosis) (pree-nay-t'l) *n.* diagnostic procedures carried out on pregnant women in order to discover genetic or other abnormalities in the developing fetus. Ultrasound scanning (*see* ultrasonography) remains the cornerstone of prenatal diagnosis. Other tests include estimation of the level of alpha-fetoprotein in the mother's serum and the amniotic fluid; chromosome and enzyme analysis of fetal cells obtained by amniocentesis or, at an earlier stage of pregnancy, by chorionic villus sampling; and examination of fetal blood obtained by fetoscopy or cordocentesis. *See also* preimplantation genetic diagnosis.

preoperative (pree-op-er-ă-tiv) *adj.* before operation: referring to the condition of a patient or to treatment, such as sedation, given at this time.

prepatellar bursitis (pree-pă-tel-er) *n. see* housemaid's knee.

PREPP *n.* (in the UK) Post-Registration Education and Practice Project: a project, launched by the UKCC, that aims to establish standards of practice and principles of education beyond registration to provide for competent and cost-effective nursing, midwifery, and health visiting.

prepubertal (pree-pew-ber-t'l) *adj.* relating to or occurring in the period before puberty.

prepuce (foreskin) (pree-pewss) *n.* the fold of skin that grows over the glans penis. On its inner surface modified sebaceous glands (*preputial glands*) secrete a lubricating fluid over the glans. —**preputial** (pree-pew-shăl) *adj.*

presby- (presbyo-) *prefix denoting* old age.

presbyacusis (prezbi-ă-kew-sis) *n.* the progressive sensorineural deafness that occurs with age.

presbyopia (prezbi-oh-piă) *n.* difficulty in reading at the usual distance and in performing other close work, due to the decline with age in the ability of the eye to focus on close objects.

prescribed disease (pri-skrybd) *n.* one of a number of illnesses (currently 48) arising as a result of employment requiring close contact with a hazardous substance or circumstance. Examples include decompression sickness in divers and infections such as anthrax in those handling wool.

prescription (pri-skrip-shŏn) *n.* a written direction from a registered medical practitioner to a pharmacist for preparing and dispensing a drug.

prescription only medicine (POM) *n.* a legal category of drugs that can only be dispensed with a prescription.

presenility (pree-sin-il-iti) *n.* pre-mature ageing of the mind and body, so that a person shows the reduction in mental and physical abilities normally found only in old age. *See also* dementia, progeria. —**presenile** (pree-see-nyl) *adj.*

present (pri-zent) *vb.* **1.** (of a patient) to come forward for examination and treatment because of experiencing specific symptoms (*presenting symptoms*). **2.** (in obstetrics) *see* presentation.

presentation (prez-ĕn-tay-shŏn) *n.* the part of the fetus that is closest to the birth canal and can be felt on inserting the finger into the vagina. Normally the head presents (*cephalic p.*). However, the buttocks may present (*see* breech presentation), or, if the fetus lies transversely across the uterus, the shoulder or arm may present.

pressor (pres-er) *n.* an agent that raises blood pressure. *See* vasoconstrictor.

pressure area (presh-er) *n.* any of the areas of the body where a bone is close to the skin surface, so that pressure on that area (e.g. by lying in bed) deprives the overlying tissues of their blood supply (*see* bedsore).

pressure index (PI) (in-deks) *n.* the ratio of the pressure in the posterior tibial artery to that in the brachial artery, which reflects the degree of arterial obstruction in the artery of the lower limb.

pressure point *n.* a point at which an artery lies over a bone on which it may be compressed by finger pressure, to arrest haemorrhage beyond.

pressure sore *n. see* bedsore.

pressure support ventilation (PSV) *n.* the form of mechanical ventilation used to assist patients with respiratory failure who are able to provide some breathing. It is adjusted to supplement the patient's inadequate efforts.

presystole (pree-**sis**-tŏ-li) *n.* the period in the cardiac cycle just preceding systole.

preterm birth (premature birth) (pree-term) *n.* birth of a baby before 37 weeks (259 days) of gestation (calculated from the first day of the mother's last menstrual period); a birth at less than 23 weeks is at present incompatible with life. Conditions affecting preterm babies may include respiratory distress syndrome, feeding difficulties, inability to maintain normal body temperature, apnoea, infection, necrotizing enterocolitis, and brain haemorrhages. Supportive treatment is provided in an incubator in a neonatal unit.

preventive medicine (pri-**ven**-tiv) *n.* the branch of medicine whose main aim is the prevention of disease.

priapism (pry-ă-pizm) *n.* a persistent and usually painful erection of the penis that requires urgent decompression; if painless, treatment is less urgent. The condition may result from the administration of alprostadil or a similar drug or it may occur in patients with sickle-cell disease or those on haemodialysis.

prickle cells (prik-ŭl) *pl. n.* cells with cytoplasmic processes that form intercellular bridges. The germinative layer of the epidermis is sometimes called the *prickle cell layer*.

prickly heat (prik-li) *n.* an itchy rash of small raised red spots. It oc-

curs usually on the face, neck, back, chest, and thighs in hot moist weather. The only treatment is removal of the patient to a cool (air-conditioned) place. Medical name: **miliaria**.

prilocaine (pril-oh-kayn) *n.* a local anaesthetic used particularly in ear, nose, and throat surgery and in dentistry. It is applied in a solution to mucous membranes or injected. Trade name: **Citanest**.

primaquine (pry-mă-kween) *n.* a drug used to treat malaria. It is administered by mouth, usually in combination with other antimalarial drugs, such as chloroquine.

primary care (pry-**mer**-i) *n.* comprehensive health care for individuals and families in the community provided through an integrated network of services covering the treatment of common illness and injuries, maternal and child health problems, the care and rehabilitation of people with long- and short-term handicaps and disabilities, and health education. In the UK the delivery of primary care is based on general practitioner services. It works best where there is a multidisciplinary team approach to care. *Compare* secondary care, tertiary care.

Primary Care Group (PCG) *n.* one of a number of groups of local health-care and social-care professionals, patients, and Health Authority representatives who take devolved responsibility for the health-care needs of their local community. The PCGs aim to improve the health of, and address health inequalities in, their communities; develop primary care and community services across the local area; and advise on, or commission directly, a range of hospital services for patients. By 2004 all PCGs are expected to become Primary Care Trusts and the role of Health Authorities will become increasingly diminished.

Primary Care Trust (PCT) *n.* one of a group of free-standing statutory bodies within the National Health Service, accountable to their local Health Authority. PCTs have the same overall functions as Primary Care Groups but are able to commission local care and are responsible for the provision of community services, such as social work, health visiting, etc.

primary nursing *n.* a method of organizing nursing care in which one nurse (the *primary nurse*) is responsible for assessing the patient, planning appropriate care, and evaluating the progress of that patient throughout his or her stay in hospital and on discharge.

primary teeth *pl. n. see* dentition.

prime (prym) *vb.* (in chemotherapy) to administer small doses of a cytotoxic drug to a patient prior to high-dose chemotherapy and/or radiotherapy. This causes proliferation of the primitive bone marrow cells and aids subsequent regeneration of the bone marrow.

prime mover *n. see* agonist.

primidone (pry-mid-ohn) *n.* an anticonvulsant drug administered by mouth to treat major epilepsy. Trade name: **Mysoline**.

primigravida (pry-mi-grav-id-ă) *n.* a woman experiencing her first pregnancy.

primipara (pry-**mip**-er-ă) *n.* a

woman who has given birth to one infant capable of survival.

primordial (pry-**mor**-di-ăl) *adj.* (in embryology) describing cells or tissues that are formed in the early stages of embryonic development.

P–R interval *n.* the interval on an electrocardiogram between the onset of atrial activity and ventricular activity.

prion (pree-on) *n.* a constituent protein of brain cells that, in an abnormal form, accumulates in and destroys brain tissue. This form is very stable and is resistant and is thought to interact with normal prion protein in such a way as to convert it to abnormal prion. Prions are now widely accepted as being the causal agents of Creutzfeldt-Jakob disease and other spongiform encephalopathies.

PRK *n. see* (photorefractive) keratectomy.

p.r.n. (pro re nata) Latin: as required, used as a direction in prescriptions.

pro- *prefix denoting* **1.** before; preceding. **2.** a precursor. **3.** in front of.

probang (proh-bang) *n.* a long flexible rod with a small sponge, ball, or tuft at the end, used to remove obstructions from the larynx or oesophagus.

probe (prohb) *n.* a thin rod of pliable metal with a blunt swollen end. The instrument is used for exploring cavities, wounds, fistulae, or sinus channels. *See also* heater-probe.

probenecid (proh-ben-ĕ-sid) *n.* a drug that reduces the level of uric acid in the blood (*see* uricosuric drug), administered by mouth in the treatment of gout. Trade name: **Benemid**.

problem-solving approach (prob-lĕm-sol-ving) n. a method of planning work involving assessment, problem identification, planning, implementation, and evaluation. See nursing process.

procainamide (proh-kayn-ă-myd) n. a drug that slows down the activity of the heart and is administered by mouth or injection to control abnormal heart rhythm. Trade name: **Pronestyl**.

procaine (procaine hydrochloride) (proh-kayn) n. a local anaesthetic administered by injection for spinal anaesthesia. It was formerly used in dentistry. Trade name: **Novutex**.

procarbazine (proh-kar-bă-zeen) n. a drug that inhibits growth of cancer cells by preventing cell division and is administered by mouth to treat such cancers as Hodgkin's disease.

process (proh-ses) n. (in anatomy) a thin prominence or protuberance.

prochlorperazine (proh-klor-per-ă-zeen) n. a phenothiazine antipsychotic drug used to treat schizophrenia and other mental disorders, migraine, vertigo, nausea, and vomiting. It is administered by mouth, injection, or in suppositories. Trade name: **Stemetil**.

procidentia (pros-i-den-shiă) n. the complete prolapse of an organ, especially the uterus, which protrudes from the vaginal opening.

proct- (procto-) prefix denoting the anus and/or rectum.

proctalgia (proctodynia) (prok-tal-jiă) n. pain in the rectum or anus. p. fugax severe pain that sud-

denly affects the rectum and may last for minutes or hours. There is no structural disease and the pain is probably due to muscle spasm.

proctatresia (prok-tă-tree-ziă) n. see imperforate (anus).

proctectasia (prok-tek-tay-ziă) n. enlargement or widening of the rectum, usually due to long-standing constipation.

proctectomy (prok-tek-tŏmi) n. surgical removal of the rectum. It is usually performed for cancer of the rectum and may require the construction of a permanent opening in the colon (see colostomy).

proctitis (prok-ty-tis) n. inflammation of the rectum. Symptoms are tenesmus, diarrhoea, and often bleeding. Proctitis is always present in ulcerative colitis and sometimes in Crohn's disease, but may occur independently (idiopathic p.).

proctocele (rectocele) (prok-toh-seel) n. bulging or pouching of the rectum, usually a forward protrusion of the rectum into the posterior wall of the vagina in association with prolapse of the uterus.

proctoclysis (prok-tok-li-sis) n. an infusion of fluid into the rectum: formerly used to replace fluid but rarely employed now.

proctocolectomy (prok-toh-kŏ-lek-tŏmi) n. a surgical operation in which the rectum and colon are removed. Removal of the whole rectum and colon (panproctocolectomy) requires either a permanent opening of the ileum (see ileostomy) or the construction of an ileal pouch.

proctocolitis (prok-toh-kŏ-ly-tis) n. inflammation of the rectum and colon, usually due to ulcerative colitis. See also proctitis.

proctodynia (prok-toh-**din**-iă) *n.* see proctalgia.

proctogram (prok-tŏ-gram) *n.* an X-ray photograph of the rectum taken after the introduction into it of a contrast medium. *defecating p.* a proctogram that demonstrates problems of abnormal defecation.

proctology (prok-tol-ŏji) *n.* the study of disorders of the rectum and anus.

proctorrhaphy (prokt-o-răfi) *n.* a surgical operation to stitch tears of the rectum or anus.

proctoscope (prok-tŏ-skohp) *n.* an illuminated instrument through which the lower part of the rectum and the anus may be inspected. —**proctoscopy** *n.*

proctosigmoiditis (prok-toh-sig-moid-I-tis) *n.* inflammation of the rectum and the sigmoid colon. *See also* proctocolitis.

proctotomy (prok-tot-ŏmi) *n.* incision into the rectum or anus to relieve stricture of these canals or to open an imperforate anus.

procyclidine (proh-sy-kli-deen) *n.* an anticholinergic drug administered by mouth to reduce muscle tremor and rigidity in parkinsonism. Trade names: **Arpicolin**, **Kemadrin**.

prodromal (proh-droh-măl) *adj.* relating to the period of time between the appearance of the first symptoms of an infectious disease and the development of a rash or fever. *p. rash* a rash that precedes the full rash of an infectious disease.

prodrome (proh-drohm) *n.* a symptom indicating the onset of a disease.

proenzyme (zymogen) (proh-en-zym) *n.* the inactive form in which certain enzymes (e.g. digestive enzymes) are originally produced and secreted.

proflavine (proh-**flay**-vin) *n.* a dye used as an antiseptic in the form of skin applications and eye drops.

profunda (proh-**fun**-dă) *adj.* describing blood vessels that are deeply embedded in the tissues they supply.

profundaplasty (proh-**fun**-dă-plasti) *n.* surgical enlargement of the junction of the femoral artery and its deep branch, a common operation to relieve narrowing by atherosclerosis at this point.

progeria (proh-jeer-iă) *n.* a very rare condition in which all the signs of old age appear and progress in a child, so that 'senility' is reached before puberty.

progesterone (proh-jest-er-ohn) *n.* a steroid hormone secreted by the corpus luteum of the ovary, the placenta, and also (in small amounts) by the adrenal cortex and testes. It is responsible for preparing the endometrium of the uterus for pregnancy.

progestogen (proh-jest-oh-jĕn) *n.* one of a group of naturally occurring or synthetic steroid hormones, including progesterone, that maintain the normal course of pregnancy. Progestogens are used to treat premenstrual tension, amenorrhoea, and abnormal bleeding from the uterus. Because they prevent ovulation, progestogens are a major constituent of oral contraceptives and other forms of hormonal contraception.

proglottis (proh-glot-iss) *n.* (*pl.* **proglottids** or **proglottides**) one of the segments of a tapeworm. Mature segments, situated at the posterior end of the worm, each consist mainly of a branched uterus packed with eggs.

prognathism (prog-nă-thizm) *n.* the state of one jaw being markedly larger than the other and therefore in front of it. —**prognathic** (prog-nath-ik) *adj.*

prognosis (prog-noh-sis) *n.* an assessment of the future course and outcome of a patient's disease.

progressive (prŏ-gres-iv) *adj.* (of a disease) increasing in severity or extent; expected to get worse.

progressive supranuclear palsy *n.* a progressive neurological disorder resulting from degeneration of the motor neurones, basal ganglia, and brainstem. Starting in late middle age, it is characterized by a staring facial expression due to impaired ability to move the eyes up and down, progressing to difficulties in swallowing, speech, balance, and movement and general spasticity.

proguanil (proh-gwan-il) *n.* a drug that kills malaria parasites and is administered by mouth in the prevention and treatment of malaria. Trade name: **Paludrine**.

proinsulin (proh-ins-yoo-lin) *n.* a substance produced in the pancreas from which the hormone insulin is derived.

Project 2000 (proj-ekt) *n.* a scheme for nurse education introduced by the UKCC in 1989. Student nurses gain a diploma in higher education as well as their registered nurse qualification.

projection (prŏ-jek-shŏn) *n.* (in psychology) the attribution of one's own qualities to other people. This is one of the defence mechanisms; people who cannot tolerate their own feelings may cope by imagining that other people have those feelings.

prolactin (lactogenic hormone, luteotrophic hormone, luteotrophin) (proh-lak-tin) *n.* a hormone, synthesized and stored in the anterior pituitary gland, that stimulates milk production after childbirth and also stimulates production of progesterone by the corpus luteum in the ovary.

prolactinoma (proh-lak-tin-oh-mă) *n.* a benign tumour (an adenoma) of the pituitary gland that secretes excessive amounts of prolactin. Symptoms include a loss of sexual drive, amenorrhoea or impotence, and sometimes production of milk from the nipples of both men and women. If the tumour is large enough it may compress and damage adjacent structures.

prolapse (proh-laps) *n.* downward displacement of an organ or tissue from its normal position. *p. of the rectum* descent of the rectum to lie outside the anus. *p. of the uterus* descent of the cervix, or the whole of the uterus, into the vagina. The cervix may be visible at the vaginal opening or the uterus may be completely outside the vagina. It is often caused by stretching and tearing of the supporting tissues during childbirth.

prolapsed intervertebral disc (PID) *n.* a 'slipped disc': protrusion of the pulpy inner material of an intervertebral disc through the fibrous outer coat, causing pressure on adjoining nerve roots, ligaments, etc. Treatment is by rest, traction,

proliferate (prŏ-lif-er-ayt) *vb.* to grow rapidly by cell division: applied particularly to malignant tumours. —**proliferation** *n.*

proline (proh-leen) *n.* an amino acid found in many proteins.

promazine (proh-mă-zeen) *n.* a phenothiazine antipsychotic drug administered by mouth or injection to relieve agitation, confusion, and restlessness.

promethazine (proh-meth-ă-zeen) *n.* a powerful antihistamine drug administered by mouth or injection to treat allergic conditions and insomnia. It is also used as an antiemetic. Trade name: **Phenergan**.

promontory (prom-ŏn-ter-i) *n.* (in anatomy) a projecting part of an organ or other structure.

pronation (proh-nay-shŏn) *n.* the act of turning the hand so that the palm faces downwards. In this position the radius and ulna are crossed. *Compare* supination.

pronator (proh-nay-ter) *n.* any muscle that causes pronation of the forearm and hand.

prone (prohn) *adj.* **1.** lying with the face downwards. **2.** (of the forearm) in the position in which the palm of the hand faces downwards. *Compare* supine.

propantheline (proh-panth-ĕ-leen) *n.* an anticholinergic drug that decreases activity of smooth muscle (*see* antispasmodic) and is administered by mouth to treat disorders of the digestive system and enuresis (bed wetting). Trade name: **Pro-Banthine**.

properdin (proh-per-din) *n.* a group of substances in blood plasma that, in combination with complement and magnesium ions, is capable of destroying certain bacteria and viruses.

prophase (proh-fayz) *n.* the first stage of mitosis and of each division of meiosis, in which the chromosomes become visible under the microscope.

prophylactic (pro-fil-ak-tik) *n.* an agent that prevents the development of a condition or disease.

prophylaxis (pro-fil-aks-iss) *n.* any means taken to prevent disease, such as immunization. —**prophylactic** *adj.*

propranolol (proh-pran-ŏ-lol) *n.* a drug (*see* beta blocker) administered by mouth or injection to treat abnormal heart rhythm, angina, and high blood pressure and to relieve anxiety. Trade name: **Inderal**.

proprietary name (prŏ-pry-ĕt-er-i) *n.* (in pharmacy) the trade name of a drug: the name assigned to it by the firm that manufactured it.

proprioceptor (proh-pri-ŏ-sep-ter) *n.* a specialized sensory nerve ending (*see* receptor) that monitors internal changes in the body brought about by movement and muscular activity. Proprioceptors in muscles and tendons assist in coordinating muscular activity.

proptosis (prop-toh-sis) *n.* forward displacement of an organ, especially the eye (*see* exophthalmos).

propylthiouracil (proh-pil-th'y-oh-yoor-ă-sil) *n.* a drug that reduces thyroid activity and is administered by mouth to treat thyrotoxicosis and to prepare patients for surgical removal of the thyroid gland.

Proscar (pros-kar) *n. see* finasteride.

prosop- (prosopo-) *prefix denoting* the face.

prostaglandin (pros-tă-**gland**-in) *n.* one of a group of hormone-like substances present in a wide variety of tissues and body fluids. Prostaglandins have many actions; for example, they cause contraction of smooth muscle (including that of the uterus) and dilatation of blood vessels, they are mediators in the process of inflammation, and they are involved in the production of mucus in the stomach. Synthetic prostaglandins are used to induce labour or produce abortion, to treat peptic ulcers, and in the treatment of newborn babies with congenital heart disease.

prostate cancer (pros-tayt) *n.* a malignant tumour (carcinoma) of the prostate gland, a common form of cancer in elderly men. In most men it progresses slowly over many years and gives symptoms similar to those of benign enlargement of the prostate (*see* prostate gland).

prostatectomy (pros-tă-tek-tŏmi) *n.* surgical removal of some or all of the prostate gland. The operation is necessary to relieve retention of urine due to enlargement of the prostate or to reduce lower urinary tract symptoms thought to be due to benign prostatic hyperplasia. It can be performed through the bladder (*transvesical p.*), through the surrounding capsule of the prostate (*retropubic p.*), or through the urethra (*transurethral p.*). **radical** (or *total*) *p.* removal of the prostate with its capsule and the seminal vesicles, performed for the treatment of prostate cancer confined to the gland. *See also* resection.

prostate gland *n.* a male accessory sex gland that opens into the urethra just below the bladder and vas deferens. During ejaculation it secretes an alkaline fluid that forms part of the semen. The prostate may become enlarged in elderly men (*benign prostatic hyperplasia, BPH*). This may result in obstruction of the neck of the bladder and is treated by surgery (*see* prostatectomy, resection) or by means of drugs.

The prostate gland and associated structures (median view)

prostate specific antigen (PSA) *n.* an enzyme produced by the glandular epithelium of the prostate. Increased quantities are secreted when the gland enlarges and levels of PSA in the blood are significantly elevated in cancer of the prostate.

prostatic intraepithelial neoplasia (PIN) (pros-tat-ik) *n.* abnormal cells in the prostate that are not cancer, but are associated with cancer within the prostate. Typically, PIN will be found in prostate biopsies taken because levels of prostate specific antigen are elevated.

prostatitis (pros-tă-ty-tis) *n.* inflammation of the prostate gland. This may be due to bacterial infection and can be either acute or chronic.

prostatocystitis (pros-tă-toh-sis-ty-tis) *n.* inflammation of the prostate gland associated with inflammation of the urinary bladder.

prostatorrhoea (pros-tă-tŏ-ree-ă) *n.* an abnormal discharge of thin watery fluid from the prostate gland. This occurs in some patients with acute prostatitis.

prosthesis (pros-th'ee-sis) *n. (pl.* **prostheses**) any artificial device that is attached to the body as a substitute for a missing or nonfunctional part. Prostheses include artificial limbs, hearing aids and cochlear implants, dentures, and implanted pacemakers. *See also* implant. *penile p.* a malleable, semirigid, or inflatable rod inserted into the corpora cavernosa of the penis to produce rigidity sufficient for vaginal penetration in men with impotence. —**prosthetic** (pros-thet-ik) *adj.*

prosthodontics (prosthetic dentistry) (pros-thoh-don-tiks) *n.* the branch of dentistry concerned with the provision of dentures, bridges, and implant-retained prostheses.

prostration (pros-tray-shŏn) *n.* extreme exhaustion.

protamine (proh-tă-meen) *n.* one of a group of simple proteins that can be conjugated with nucleic acids to form nucleoproteins. *p. zinc insulin* a combination of protamine, insulin, and zinc that is absorbed much more slowly than ordinary insulin and thus reduces the frequency of injections.

protanopia (proh-tă-noh-piă) *n. see* Daltonism.

protease (proh-ti-ayz) *n.* any enzyme that catalyses the splitting of a protein.

protease inhibitor *n.* one of a class of antiviral drugs used in the treatment of HIV infection and AIDS. They inhibit the action of protease produced by HIV, required by viral growth and replication. Protease inhibitors include *indinavir* (Crixivan), *lopinavir* (Kaletra), and *nelfinavir* (Norvir).

protein (proh-teen) *n.* one of a group of organic compounds made up of one or more chains of amino acids. Proteins are essential constituents of the body; they form the structural material of muscles, tissues, organs, etc., and are equally important as regulators of function, as enzymes and hormones. Proteins are synthesized in the body from their constituent amino acids, which are obtained from the digestion of protein in the diet.

proteinuria (proh-tin-yoor-iă) *n. see* albuminuria.

proteolysis (proh-ti-ol-i-sis) *n.* the process whereby protein molecules are broken down by proteolytic enzymes into their constituent amino acids, which are then absorbed into the bloodstream. —**proteolytic** (proh-ti-ŏ-lit-ik) *adj.*

proteolytic enzyme *n.* a digestive enzyme that causes the breakdown of protein.

proteose (proh-ti-ohz) *n.* a product

of the hydrolytic decomposition of protein.

Proteus (proh-ti-ŭs) *n.* a genus of rodlike Gram-negative flagellate highly motile bacteria common in the intestines and in decaying organic material. *P. vulgaris* a species that can cause urinary tract infections.

prothrombin (PT) (proh-**throm**-bin) *n.* a substance, present in blood plasma, that is the inactive precursor from which the enzyme thrombin is derived during the process of blood coagulation. *See also* coagulation factors. **p. time** *(PT)* the time taken for blood clotting to occur in a sample of blood to which calcium and thromboplastin have been added; a prolonged PT indicates a deficiency of coagulation factors. Measurement of PT is used to control anticoagulant therapy (e.g. with warfarin).

proto- *prefix denoting* **1.** first. **2.** primitive; early. **3.** a precursor.

proton-pump inhibitor (proh-ton-pump) *n.* a drug that reduces gastric acid secretion by blocking an enzyme (the *proton pump*) within the oxyntic (parietal) cells of the gastric glands. Proton-pump inhibitors include omeprazole and lansoprazole; they are used for treating gastric and duodenal ulcers, reflux oesophagitis, and the hypersecretion caused by gastrinomas.

protopathic (proh-tŏ-**path**-ik) *adj.* describing the ability to perceive only strong stimuli of pain, heat, etc. *Compare* epicritic.

protoplasm (proh-tŏ-plazm) *n.* the material of which living cells are made, which includes the cytoplasm and nucleus. —**protoplasmic** *adj.*

protoporphyrin IX (proh-toh-**por**-fi-rin) *n.* the most common type of porphyrin found in nature. It is a constituent of haemoglobin, myohaemoglobin, and the commoner chlorophylls.

protozoa (proh-tŏ-**zoh**-ă) *pl. n.* a group of microscopic single-celled organisms. Most protozoa are free-living but some, such as *Plasmodium* and *Leishmania*, are important disease-causing parasites of humans. *See also* amoeba. —**protozoan** *adj., n.*

protuberance (prŏ-**tew**-ber-ăns) *n.* (in anatomy) a rounded projecting part.

proud flesh (prowd) *n.* a large amount of soft granulation tissue that may develop during the healing of a wound of large surface area.

provitamin (proh-**vit**-ă-min) *n.* a substance that is not itself a vitamin but can be converted to a vitamin in the body. An example is β-carotene, which can be converted into vitamin A.

proximal (proks-i-măl) *adj.* (in anatomy) situated close to the origin or point of attachment or close to the median line of the body. *Compare* distal.

Prozac (proh-zak) *n. see* fluoxetine.

prune belly syndrome (Eagle-Barrett syndrome) (proon) *n.* a hereditary condition, occurring exclusively in males, characterized by a deficiency of abdominal muscles, complex malformation of the urinary tract, and bilateral undescended testes. The lungs may be underdeveloped. The name derives from the typically wrinkled appearance of the skin over the abdomen.

prurigo (proor-**I**-goh) *n.* an intensely

itchy eruption. *Besnier's p.* chronic lichenified atopic eczema. *nodular p.* a condition of unknown cause, usually found in atopic individuals (*see* atopy), in which severely itching nodules mostly occur on the distal limbs. *p. of pregnancy* prurigo occurring in the middle trimester of pregnancy, affecting mainly the abdomen and the extensor surfaces of the limbs. It may recur in later pregnancies.

pruritus (proor-I-tŭs) *n.* itching; the predominant symptom of atopic eczema, lichen planus, and many other skin diseases. It also occurs in the elderly and may be a manifestation of psychological illness. Perineal itching is common: itching of the vulva in women (*p. vulvae*) may be accompanied by itching of the anal region (*p. ani*), although the latter is more common in men. Causes of perineal itching include poor hygiene, candidosis, threadworms, and itchy skin diseases (such as eczema).

prussic acid (prus-ik) *n. see* hydrocyanic acid.

PSA *n. see* prostate specific antigen.

psammoma (sam-oh-mă) *n.* a tumour containing gritty sandlike particles (*p. bodies*). It is typical of cancer of the ovary but may also be found in the meninges.

pseud- (pseudo-) *prefix denoting* superficial resemblance to; false.

pseudarthrosis (nearthrosis) (s'yood-arth-**roh**-sis) *n.* a 'false' joint, formed around a displaced bone end after dislocation or between the bone ends of a fracture that fails to unite.

pseudoangina (s'yoo-doh-an-jy-nă) *n.* pain in the centre of the chest in the absence of heart disease. It is associated with anxiety and may be part of the effort syndrome.

pseudocholinesterase (s'yoo-doh-koh-lin-**est**-er-ayz) *n.* an enzyme found in the blood and other tissues that breaks down acetylcholine, but much more slowly than cholinesterase.

pseudocoxalgia (s'yoo-doh-koks-al-jiă) *n. see* Legg-Calvé-Perthes disease.

pseudocrisis (s'yoo-doh-**kry**-sis) *n.* a false crisis: a sudden but temporary fall of temperature in a patient with fever.

pseudocyesis (phantom pregnancy) (s'yoo-doh-sy-**ee**-sis) *n.* a condition in which a nonpregnant woman exhibits symptoms of pregnancy, e.g. enlarged abdomen, morning sickness, and absence of menstruation. The condition usually has an emotional basis.

pseudocyst (s'yoo-doh-sist) *n.* a fluid-filled space without a proper wall or lining, within an organ. *pancreatic p.* a pseudocyst, filled with pancreatic juice, that may develop in cases of chronic pancreatitis or as a complication of acute pancreatitis. It may cause episodes of abdominal pain accompanied by a rise in the level of enzymes in the blood. Treatment is by surgical drainage, usually by marsupialization.

pseudodementia (s'yoo-doh-di-men-shă) *n.* **1.** a condition in which symptoms of dementia, including memory disorders, are caused by depression rather than organic brain disease. It is most commonly seen in elderly depressed individuals. **2.** *see* Ganser state.

pseudohermaphroditism (s'yoo-doh-her-**maf**-rō-dyt-izm) *n.* a congenital abnormality in which the external genitalia of a male or a female resemble those of the opposite sex.

pseudohypertrophy (s'yoo-doh-hy-per-trō-fi) *n.* increase in the size of an organ or structure caused by excessive growth of cells that have a packing or supporting role. The result is usually a decline in the efficiency of the organ. —**pseudohypertrophic** (s'yoo-doh-hy-per-trof-ik) *adj.*

pseudohypoparathyroidism (s'yoo-doh-hy-poh-pa-**rā-th'y**-roid-izm) *n.* a syndrome of mental retardation, restricted growth, and bony abnormalities due to a genetic defect that causes lack of response to parathyroid hormone. *See also* Albright's hereditary osteodystrophy.

pseudologia fantastica (s'yoo-doh-**loh** jiā fan-**tas**-tik ā) *n.* the telling of elaborate and fictitious stories as if they were true. It is sometimes a feature of chronic mental illness and of personality disorders, particularly psychopathy.

pseudomembranous colitis (s'yoo-doh-**mem**-brān-ŭs) *n. see* colitis.

Pseudomonas (s'yoo-doh-**moh**-năs) *n.* a genus of rodlike motile pigmented Gram-negative bacteria. Most live in soil and decomposing organic matter. *P. aeruginosa* a species that occurs in pus from wounds; it is associated with urinary tract infections. *P. pseudomallei* the causative agent of melioidosis.

pseudomyxoma (s'yoo-doh-miks-**oh**-mă) *n.* a mucoid tumour of the peritoneum, often seen in association with myxomas of the ovary.

pseudo-obstruction (s'yoo-doh-ŏb-**struk**-shŏn) *n.* obstruction of the alimentary canal without mechanical narrowing of the bowel. It is usually associated with abnormality of the nerve supply to the muscles of the bowel. *See also* ileus, Hirschsprung's disease.

pseudoplegia (s'yoo-doh-**plee**-jiā) *n.* paralysis of the limbs not associated with organic abnormalities. It may be a symptom of conversion disorder.

pseudopodium (s'yoo-doh-**poh**-diŭm) *n.* (*pl.* **pseudopodia**) a temporary and constantly changing extension of the body of an amoeba or an amoeboid cell. Pseudopodia engulf bacteria and other particles as food and are responsible for the movements of the cell.

pseudopolyposis (s'yoo doh-pol-i-**poh**-sis) *n.* a condition in which the bowel lining (mucosa) is covered by elevated or protuberant plaques (*pseudopolyps*) that are not true polyps but abnormal growth of inflamed mucosa. It is usually found in chronic ulcerative colitis.

pseudoxanthoma elasticum (s'yoo-doh-zanth-**oh**-mă i-lass-tik-ŭm) *n.* a hereditary disease in which elastic fibres (*see* elastic tissue) become calcified. The skin becomes lax and yellowish nodules develop in affected areas; this is accompanied by degenerative changes in the blood vessels.

psilosis (sy-loh-sis) *n. see* sprue.

psittacosis (parrot disease, ornithosis) (sit-ă-koh-sis) *n.* an endemic infection of birds, especially parrots, budgerigars, canaries, finches, pigeons, and poultry, caused by the bacterium

Chlamydia psittaci. The infection is transmitted to humans by inhalation from handling the birds or by contact with feathers, faeces, or cage dust, but person-to-person transmission also occurs. The symptoms include fever, dry cough, severe muscle pain, and headache; occasionally a severe generalized systemic illness results. The condition responds to tetracycline or erythromycin.

psoas (psoas major) (soh-ăs) *n.* a muscle in the groin that acts jointly with the iliacus muscle to flex the hip joint. A smaller muscle (*p. minor*) has the same action but is often absent.

psoralen (sor-ah-lĕn) *n. see* PUVA.

psoriasis (sŏ-ry-ă-sis) *n.* a chronic skin disease in which scaly pink patches form on the elbows, knees, scalp, and other parts of the body. Psoriasis is one of the commonest skin diseases in Britain, but its cause is not known. It sometimes occurs in association with arthritis (*psoriatic arthritis*). Occasionally the disease may be very severe, affecting much of the skin and causing considerable disability in the patient. —**psoriatic** (sor-i-at-ik) *adj.*

PSV *n. see* pressure support ventilation.

psych- (psycho-) *prefix denoting* **1.** the mind; psyche. **2.** psychology.

psyche (sy-ki) *n.* the mind or the soul; the mental (as opposed to the physical) functioning of the individual.

psychedelic (sy-ki-del-ik) *adj.* describing drugs, such as cannabis and LSD, that can induce changes in the level of consciousness of the mind.

psychiatrist (si-ky-ă-trist) *n.* a medically qualified physician who specializes in the study and treatment of mental disorders.

psychiatry (si-ky-ă-tri) *n.* the study of mental disorders and their diagnosis, management, and prevention. —**psychiatric** (sy-ki-at-rik) *adj.*

psychic (sy-kik) *adj.* **1.** of or relating to the psyche. **2.** relating to parapsychological phenomena.

psychoanalysis (sy-koh-ă-**nal**-i-sis) *n.* a school of psychology and a method of treating mental disorders based upon the teachings of Sigmund Freud (1856–1939). Psychoanalysis employs the technique of free association in the course of intensive psychotherapy in order to bring repressed fears and conflicts to the conscious mind, where they can be dealt with (*see* repression). —**psychoanalyst** (sy-koh-**an**-ă-list) *n.* —**psychoanalytic** (sy-koh-an-ă-lit-ik) *adj.*

psychodrama (sy-koh-drah-mă) *n.* a form of group psychotherapy in which individuals acquire insight into themselves by acting out situations from their past with other group members. *See* group therapy.

psychodynamics (sy-koh-dy-nam-iks) *n.* the study of the mind in action. —**psychodynamic** *adj.*

psychogenic (sy-koh-jen-ik) *adj.* having an origin in the mind rather than in the body. The term is applied particularly to symptoms and illnesses.

psychogeriatrics (sy-koh-je-ri-at-riks) *n.* the branch of psychiatry that deals with the mental disorders of old people. —**psychogeriatric** *adj.*

psychologist (sy-kol-ŏ-jist) *n.* a

person who is engaged in the scientific study of the mind. *clinical p.* a psychologist trained in aspects of the assessment and treatment of the ill and handicapped. He or she usually works in a hospital. *educational p.* a psychologist trained in aspects of the cognitive and emotional development of children. He or she usually works in close association with schools.

psychology (sy-kol-ŏji) *n.* the science concerned with the study of behaviour and its related mental processes. The different schools of psychology include behaviourism, cognitive psychology, psychoanalysis, and gestaltism. —**psychological** (sy-kŏ-loj-ikăl) *adj.*

psychometrics (sy-koh-met-riks) *n.* the measurement of individual differences in psychological functions (such as intelligence and personality) by means of standardized tests. —**psychometric** *adj.*

psychomotor (sy-koh-moh-ter) *adj.* relating to muscular and mental activity. The term is applied to disorders in which muscular activities are affected by cerebral disturbance.

psychoneuroimmunology (sy-koh-newr-oh-im-yoo-nol-ŏji) *n.* the study of the effects of the mind on the functioning of the immune system, especially in relation to the influence of the mind on susceptibility to disease and the progression of a disease.

psychoneurosis (sy-koh-newr-oh-sis) *n.* a neurosis that is manifest in psychological rather than organic symptoms.

psychopath (sy-koh-path) *n.* a person who behaves in an antisocial

way and shows little or no guilt for antisocial acts and little capacity for forming emotional relationships with others. *See also* antisocial personality disorder. —**psychopathic** *adj.* —**psychopathy** (sy-kop-ă-thi) *n.*

psychopathology (sy-koh-pă-thol-ŏji) *n.* **1.** the study of mental disorders, with the aim of explaining and describing aberrant behaviour. *Compare* psychiatry. **2.** the symptoms, collectively, of a mental disorder. —**psychopathological** *adj.*

psychopharmacology (sy-koh-farm-ă-kol-ŏji) *n.* the study of the effects of drugs on mental processes and behaviour, particularly psychotropic drugs.

psychophysiology (sy-koh-fiz-i-ol-ŏji) *n.* the branch of psychology that records physiological measurements, such as heart rate and size of the pupil, and relates them to psychological events. —**psychophysiological** *adj.*

psychosexual development (sy-koh-seks-yoo-ăl) *n.* the process by which an individual becomes more mature in his sexual feelings and behaviour. Gender identity, sex-role behaviour, and choice of sexual partner are the three major areas of development.

psychosis (sy-koh-sis) *n.* one of a group of mental disorders that feature loss of contact with reality. The psychoses include schizophrenia, major disorders of affect (*see* manic-depressive psychosis), major paranoid states, and organic mental disorders. Psychotic disorders may feature delusions, hallucinations, severe thought disturbances, abnormal alteration of mood, poverty of thought, and grossly abnormal behaviour. Many cases of psychotic illness respond well to antipsychotic drugs. —**psychotic** (sy-kot-ik) *adj.*

psychosomatic (sy-koh-sŏ-**mat**-ik) *adj.* relating to or involving both the mind and body: usually applied to illnesses, such as asthma and peptic ulcer, that are caused by the interaction of mental and physical factors.

psychosurgery (sy-koh-**ser**-jer-i) *n.* surgery on the brain to relieve psychological symptoms, such as severe chronic anxiety, depression, and untreatable pain. —**psychosurgical** *adj.*

psychotherapy (sy-koh-**th'e-răpi**) *n.* psychological (as opposed to physical) methods for treating mental disorders and psychological problems. There are many different approaches to psychotherapy, including psychoanalysis, client-centred therapy, group therapy, and family therapy. *See also* behaviour therapy, counselling. —**psychotherapeutic** (sy-koh-th'e-ră-**pew**-tik) *adj.* —**psychotherapist** *n.*

psychoticism (sy-kot-i-sizm) *n.* a dimension of personality derived from psychometric tests, which appears to indicate a degree of emotional coldness and some cognitive impairment.

psychotropic (sy-koh-**trop**-ik) *adj.* describing drugs that affect mood. Antidepressants, sedatives, stimulants, and antipsychotics are psychotropic.

PT *n. see* prothrombin.

PTC *n. see* (percutaneous transhepatic) cholangiopancreatography.

pterion (teer-i-ŏn) *n.* the point on the side of the skull at which the sutures between the parietal, temporal, and sphenoid bones meet.

pteroylglutamic acid (te-roh-il-gloo-**tam**-ik) *n. see* folic acid.

pterygium (tĕ-**rij**-iŭm) *n.* a triangular overgrowth of the cornea, usually the inner side, by thickened and degenerative conjunctiva.

pterygo- *prefix denoting* the pterygoid process.

pterygoid process (te-ri-goid) *n.* either of two large processes of the sphenoid bone.

ptomaine (toh-mayn) *n.* any of various substances, such as putrescine, cadaverine, and neurine, produced in decaying foodstuffs and responsible for the unpleasant taste and smell of such foods. Ptomaines themselves are harmless, but they are often associated with toxic bacteria.

ptosis (blepharoptosis) (toh-sis) *n.* drooping of the upper eyelid. This may be due to a disorder of the oculomotor nerve, a disease of the eye muscles, or myasthenia gravis; it may also occur as part of Horner's syndrome or as an isolated congenital feature. It is also associated with the pain of a cluster headache.

-ptosis *suffix denoting* a lowered position of an organ or part; prolapse.

PTSD *n. see* post-traumatic stress disorder.

PTTK *n.* partial thromboplastin time with kaolin, also known as activated partial thromboplastin time (*APTT*): a method for estimating the degree of anticoagulation induced by heparin therapy for venous thrombosis.

ptyal- (ptyalo-) *prefix denoting* saliva.

ptyalin (ty-ă-lin) *n.* an enzyme (an amylase) found in saliva.

ptyalism (sialorrhoea) (ty-ă-lizm) *n.* the excessive production of saliva: a symptom of certain nervous disorders, poisoning, or infection (rabies). *Compare* dry mouth.

ptyalith (ty-ă-lith) *n.* a stone (calculus) in a salivary gland or duct.

ptyalography (ty-ă-log-răfi) *n.* see sialography.

puberty (pew-ber-ti) *n.* the time at which the onset of sexual maturity occurs and the reproductive organs become functional (*see* gonadarche). It is manifested in both sexes by the appearance of secondary sexual characteristics and in girls by the start of menstruation. *See also* precocious puberty. **—pubertal** *adj.*

pubes (pew-beez) *n.* **1.** the body surface that overlies the pubis, at the front of the pelvis. **2.** *see* pubis. **—pubic** *adj.*

pubiotomy (pew-bi-ot-ŏmi) *n.* an operation to divide the pubic bone near the symphysis, now only rarely performed during childbirth to increase the size of an abnormally small pelvis or to facilitate access to the base of the bladder and the urethra during complex urological procedures.

pubis (pew-bis) *n.* (*pl.* **pubes**) a bone forming the lower and anterior part of each side of the hip bone (*see also* pelvis). The two pubes meet at the front of the pelvis at the *pubic symphysis*. *See also* pubes.

public health medicine (pub-lik) *n.* the branch of medicine concerned with assessing needs and trends in health and disease of populations as distinct from individuals. Formerly known as *community*

or *social medicine*, it includes epidemiology, health promotion, health service planning and evaluation, communicable disease control, and environmental hazards.

public health nurse *n.* see health visitor.

public health physician *n.* (in Britain) a doctor of consultant status with special postgraduate training in public health medicine, formerly known as a *community physician*.

pudendal (pew-den-d'l) *adj.* relating to the pudendum. *p. block* anaesthesia of the pudendum and surrounding areas by injecting a local anaesthetic into the nerves that supply them. It is performed to relieve the pain of the expulsive stage of labour. *See also* nerve block. *p. nerve* the nerve that supplies the lowest muscles of the pelvic floor and the anal sphincter. It is often damaged in childbirth, causing incontinence.

pudendum (pew-den-dŭm) *n.* (*pl.* **pudenda**) the external genital organs, especially those of the female (*see* vulva).

puerperal (pew-er-per-ăl) *adj.* relating to childbirth or the period that immediately follows it. *p. depression* a state of pathological sadness that sometimes affects a woman soon after the birth of her baby. In some cases it becomes serious enough to require admission to hospital, where careful supervision and treatment are essential as there is a risk that the woman may kill herself or her baby. *p. infection* infection of the female genital tract arising as a complication of childbirth. *p. pyrexia* a temperature of 38°C occurring on any two days within 14 days of childbirth or miscarriage.

puerperium (pew-er-**peer**-iŭm) *n.* the period of up to about six weeks after childbirth, during which the uterus returns to its normal size.

Pulex (**pew**-leks) *n.* a genus of widely distributed fleas. *P. irritans* the human flea: a common parasite whose bite may give rise to intense irritation and bacterial infection.

pulmo- (pulmon(o)-) *prefix denoting* the lung(s).

pulmonary (**pul**-mŏn-er-i) *adj.* relating to, associated with, or affecting the lungs. *p. artery* the artery that conveys deoxygenated blood from the heart to the lungs for oxygenation. *p. capillary wedge pressure (PCWP)* pressure of blood in the left atrium of the heart, which indicates the adequacy of the pulmonary circulation. It is measured using a catheter wedged in the most distal segment of the pulmonary artery. *p. circulation see* circulation. *p. embolism see* embolism. *p. hypertension* raised blood pressure within the blood vessels supplying the lungs. Pulmonary hypertension may complicate pulmonary embolism, septal defects, heart failure, diseases of the mitral valve, and chronic lung diseases. *p. stenosis* congenital narrowing of the outlet of the right ventricle of the heart. Severe pulmonary stenosis may produce angina pectoris, faintness, and heart failure. The defect is corrected by surgery. *p. surfactant see* surfactant. *p. tuberculosis see* tuberculosis. *p. valve see* semilunar valve. *p. vein* a vein carrying oxygenated blood from the lung to the left atrium.

pulp (pulp) *n.* **1.** a soft mass of tissue (for example, of the spleen). **2.** the mass of connective tissue containing blood vessels and nerve fibres at the centre of a tooth (*p. cavity*). **3.** the fleshy cushion on the flexor surface of the fingertip.

pulsatile (**puls**-ă-tyl) *adj.* characterized by regular rhythmical beating.

pulsation (pul-**say**-shŏn) *n.* a rhythmical throbbing or beating, as of the heart or arteries.

pulse (puls) *n.* a series of pressure waves within an artery caused by contractions of the left ventricle and corresponding with the heart rate. It is easily detected over certain superficial arteries (*p. points* – see illustration). The average adult pulse rate at rest is 60–80 per minute, but exercise, injury, illness, and emotion may produce much faster rates.

pulseless disease (**puls**-lis) *n. see* Takayasu's disease.

pulseless electrical activity (electromechanical dissociation) *n.* the appearance of normal-looking complexes on the electrocardiogram that are, however, associated with a state of cardiac arrest. It is usually caused by large pulmonary emboli, cardiac tamponade, tension pneumothorax, severe disturbance of body salt levels, severe haemorrhage, or hypothermia causing severe lack of oxygen to the heart muscle.

pulsus alternans (**pul**-sus awl-**ter**-nanz) *n.* a pulse in which there is a regular alternation of strong and weak beats without changes in the length of the cycle.

pulsus paradoxus (pa-ră-**doks**-ŭs) *n.* a large fall in systolic blood pressure and pulse volume when the patient breathes in. It is seen in constrictive pericarditis, pericardial effusion, and asthma.

pulvis (pul-vis) *n.* (in pharmaceutics) a powder.

punch-drunk syndrome *n.* a group of symptoms consisting of progressive dementia, tremor of the hands, and epilepsy. It is a consequence of repeated blows to the head that have been severe enough to cause concussion.

punctate (punk-tayt) *adj.* spotted or dotted.

punctum (punk-tŭm) *n.* (*pl.* **puncta**) (in anatomy) a point or small area. *puncta lacrimalia* the two openings of the tear ducts in the inner corners of the upper and lower eyelids. *See* lacrimal (apparatus).

puncture (punk-cher) **1.** *n.* a wound made accidentally or deliberately by a sharp object or instrument. *needle p.* a puncture using a hollow needle to withdraw a sample of tissue (especially from the liver, bone marrow, or breast) for examination for diagnostic purposes. *See also* lumbar (puncture). **2.** *vb.* to pierce a tissue with a sharp instrument.

PUO *n.* pyrexia of unknown origin. *See* fever.

pupil (pew-pil) *n.* the circular opening in the centre of the iris, through which light passes into the lens of the eye. —**pupillary** (pew-pil-er-i) *adj.*

pupillary reflex (light reflex) *n.* the reflex change in the size of the pupil according to the amount of light entering the eye.

pupilloplasty (pew-pil-oh-plasti) *n.* a surgical procedure to alter the shape or function of the pupil. It is usually performed to repair a pupil damaged after trauma.

purgation (per-gay-shŏn) *n.* the use of drugs to stimulate intestinal activity and clear the bowels. *See* laxative.

purgative (per-gă-tiv) *n. see* laxative.

The pulse points

purine (pewr-reen) *n.* a nitrogenous compound with a two-ring molecular structure. Examples of purines are adenine and guanine, which occur in nucleic acids, and uric acid.

Purkinje cells (per-kin-ji) *pl. n.* nerve cells found in great numbers in the cortex of the cerebellum. [J. E. Purkinje (1787–1869), Bohemian physiologist]

Purkinje fibres *pl. n. see* atrioventricular bundle.

purpura (per-pew-ră) *n.* a skin rash resulting from bleeding into the skin from blood capillaries; the rash is made up of individual purple spots (*see* petechiae). Purpura may be due either to defects in the blood capillaries (*nonthrombocytopenic p.*) or to a deficiency of blood platelets (*thrombocytopenic p.*). **idiopathic thrombocytopenic p.** an autoimmune disease in which the platelets are destroyed, leading to spontaneous bruising. A mild acute form affects children; a more serious chronic form typically affects adults. *See also* thrombocytopenia, Henoch-Schönlein purpura.

purulent (pewr-uu-lĕnt) *adj.* forming, consisting of, or containing pus.

pus (pus) *n.* a thick yellowish or greenish liquid formed at the site of an established infection. Pus contains dead white blood cells, both living and dead bacteria, and fragments of dead tissue. *See also* mucopus, seropus.

push-bang technique (puush-bang) *n.* a technique for removing a stone from the ureter. It consists of 'pushing' the stone back into the renal pelvis, where it can be destroyed by lithotripsy ('bang').

pustule (pus-tewl) *n.* a small blister on the skin that contains pus.

putamen (pew-tay-men) *n.* a part of the lenticular nucleus (*see* basal ganglia).

putrefaction (pew-tri-fak-shŏn) *n.* the process whereby proteins are decomposed by bacteria. This is accompanied by the formation of amines (such as putrescine and cadaverine) having a strong and very unpleasant smell.

PUVA (photochemotherapy) *n.* psoralen + ultraviolet A: the combination of *psoralen*, a light-sensitive drug, and exposure to long-wave (315–400 nm) ultraviolet light (UVA). It is principally used for treating psoriasis.

PV per vagina.

PVD *n. see* peripheral vascular disease.

PVS *n. see* persistent vegetative state.

py- (pyo-) *prefix denoting* pus; a purulent condition.

pyaemia (py-ee-miă) *n.* blood poisoning by pus-forming bacteria released from an abscess. Widespread formation of abscesses may develop, with fatal results. *Compare* sapraemia, septicaemia, toxaemia.

pyarthrosis (py-arth-roh-sis) *n.* an infected joint filled with pus. Drainage, combined with antibiotic treatment, is necessary.

pyel- (pyelo-) *prefix denoting* the pelvis of the kidney.

pyelitis (py-ĕ-ly-tis) *n.* inflammation of the pelvis of the kidney, usually caused by a bacterial infection. The patient experiences pain in the loins, shivering, and a high temperature. Treatment is by the administration of a suitable antibiotic, together with analgesics and a high fluid intake.

pyelocystitis (py-ĕ-loh-sis-ty-tis) n. inflammation of the renal pelvis and urinary bladder (see pyelitis, cystitis).

pyelogram (py-ĕ-loh-gram) n. an X-ray picture obtained by pyelography.

pyelography (urography) (py-ĕ-log-răfi) n. X-ray examination of the pelvis of the kidney using radio-paque contrast material. *retrograde p.* pyelography in which fine catheters are passed up the ureter to the kidneys at cystoscopy and contrast material is injected directly into the renal pelvis. *See also* urography.

pyelolithotomy (py-ĕ-loh-lith-ot-ŏmi) n. surgical removal of a stone from the kidney through an incision made in the pelvis of the kidney.

pyelonephritis (py-ĕ-loh-ni-fry-tis) n. bacterial infection of the kidney substance. *acute p.* pyelonephritis in which the patient has pain in the loins, a high temperature, and shivering fits. Treatment is by the administration of an appropriate antibiotic. *chronic p.* pyelonephritis in which the kidneys become small and scarred and kidney failure ensues. Vesicoureteric reflux in childhood is one of the causes.

pyeloplasty (py-ĕ-loh-plasti) n. an operation to relieve obstruction at the junction of the pelvis of the kidney and the ureter. *See* hydronephrosis, Dietl's crisis.

pyelotomy (py-ĕ-lot-ŏmi) n. surgical incision into the pelvis of the kidney. This operation is usually undertaken to remove a stone (see pyelolithotomy).

pyg- (pygo-) *prefix denoting* the buttocks.

pykno- *prefix denoting* thickness or density.

pyknolepsy (pik-noh-lep-si) n. *Obsolete.* a very high frequency of absence attacks (see epilepsy).

pyl- (pyle-) *prefix denoting* the portal vein.

pylephlebitis (portal pyaemia) (py-li-fli-by-tis) n. septic inflammation and thrombosis of the hepatic portal vein, resulting from the spread of infection within the abdomen. The condition causes fever, liver abscesses, and ascites. Treatment is by antibiotic drugs and surgical drainage of abscesses.

pylethrombosis (py-li-throm-boh-sis) n. obstruction of the portal vein by a blood clot (see thrombosis), resulting from such conditions as pylephlebitis and cirrhosis of the liver. Portal hypertension is a frequent result.

pylor- (pyloro-) *prefix denoting* the pylorus.

pylorectomy (py-lor-ek-tŏmi) n. a surgical operation in which the muscular outlet of the stomach (pylorus) is removed. *See* antrectomy, pyloroplasty.

pyloric stenosis (py-lor-ik) n. narrowing of the pylorus. This causes delay in passage of the stomach contents to the duodenum, which leads to repeated vomiting. Pyloric stenosis in adults is caused by a peptic ulcer close to the pylorus or by a cancerous growth invading it. *congenital hypertrophic p. s.* pyloric stenosis that occurs in babies about 3–5 weeks old (particularly boys) in which the thickened pyloric muscle can be felt as a nodule. Treatment is by pyloromyotomy.

pyloromyotomy (Ramstedt's operation) (py-lor-oh-my-ot-ŏmi) *n.* a surgical operation in which the muscle around the pylorus is divided down to the lining (mucosa) in order to relieve congenital pyloric stenosis.

pyloroplasty (py-lor-oh-plasti) *n.* a surgical operation in which the pylorus is widened by a form of reconstruction. It is done to allow the contents of the stomach to pass more easily into the duodenum.

pylorospasm (py-lor-oh-spazm) *n.* closure of the pylorus due to muscle spasm, leading to delay in the passage of stomach contents to the duodenum and vomiting. It is usually associated with duodenal or pyloric ulcers.

pylorus (py-lor-ŭs) *n.* the lower end of the stomach, which leads to the duodenum. It terminates at a ring of muscle (*pyloric sphincter*), which contracts to close the opening by which the stomach communicates with the duodenum. —**pyloric** *adj.*

pyo- *prefix. see py-.*

pyocele (py-oh-seel) *n.* a swelling caused by an accumulation of pus in a part of the body.

pyocolpos (py-oh-kol-pos) *n.* the presence of pus in the vagina.

pyocyanin (py-oh-sy-ă-nin) *n.* an antibiotic substance produced by the bacterium *Pseudomonas aeruginosa*. It is used in medicine principally to attack Gram-positive bacteria.

pyoderma gangrenosum (py-oh-der-mă gang-ri-noh-sŭm) *n.* an acute destructive ulcerating process of the skin, especially the legs. It

may be associated with ulcerative colitis or Crohn's disease or with rheumatoid arthritis or other forms of arthritis affecting many joints.

pyogenic (py-oh-jen-ik) *adj.* causing the formation of pus. **p. granuloma** a common rapidly growing nodule on the surface of the skin. Resembling a redcurrant or (if large) a raspberry, it is composed of small blood vessels and therefore bleeds readily after the slightest injury.

pyometra (py-oh-mee-tră) *n.* the presence of pus in the uterus.

pyomyositis (py-oh-my-oh-sy-tis) *n.* bacterial or fungal infection of a muscle resulting in painful inflammation.

pyonephrosis (py-oh-ni-froh-sis) *n.* obstruction and infection of the kidney resulting in pus formation. A kidney stone is the usual cause of the obstruction, and the kidney becomes distended by pus and destroyed by the inflammation. Treatment is urgent nephrectomy under antibiotic cover.

pyopericarditis (py-oh-pe-ri-kardy-tis) *n.* inflammation of the pericardium, with the formation of pus.

pyopneumothorax (py-oh-new-moh-thor-aks) *n.* pus and gas or air in the pleural cavity. The condition can arise if air is introduced during attempts to drain the pus from an empyema, or if a hydropneumothorax becomes infected.

pyorrhoea (py-ŏ-ree-ă) *n.* a former name for periodontal disease.

pyosalpinx (py-oh-sal-pinks) *n.* the accumulation of pus in a Fallopian tube.

pyosis (py-oh-sis) *n.* the formation and discharge of pus.

pyothorax (py-oh-thor-aks) *n. see* empyema.

pyr- (pyro-) *prefix denoting* **1.** fire. **2.** a burning sensation. **3.** fever.

pyramid (pi-ră-mid) *n.* **1.** one of the conical masses that make up the medulla of the kidney. **2.** one of the elongated bulging areas on the anterior surface of the medulla oblongata in the brain. —**pyramidal** (pi-ram-i-d'l) *adj.*

pyramidal cell *n.* a type of neurone found in the cerebral cortex, with a pyramid-shaped cell body.

pyramidal system *n.* a collection of nerve fibres in the central nervous system that extend from the motor cortex in the brain to the spinal cord and are responsible for initiating movement. They form a pyramid in the medulla oblongata.

pyrazinamide (py-ră-zin-ă-myd) *n.* a drug administered by mouth, usually in combination with other drugs, to treat tuberculosis. Trade name: **Zinamide**.

pyret- (pyreto-) *prefix denoting* fever.

pyrexia (py-reks-iă) *n. see* fever.

pyridostigmine (pi-ri-doh-stig-meen) *n.* a drug that inhibits the enzyme cholinesterase and is used to treat myasthenia gravis. It has a more prolonged action and is less toxic than neostigmine.

pyridoxal phosphate (pi-ri-doks-ăl) *n.* a derivative of vitamin B_6 that is an important coenzyme in certain reactions of amino-acid metabolism. *See* transamination.

pyridoxine (vitamin B_6) (pi-ri-doks-een) *n. see* vitamin B.

pyrimethamine (pi-ri-meth-ă-meen) *n.* a drug administered by mouth for the prevention and treatment of malaria, either alone or in combination with dapsone; it is also used in the treatment of toxoplasmosis. Trade name: **Daraprim**.

pyrimidine (pi-rim-i-deen) *n.* a nitrogen-containing compound with a ring molecular structure. The commonest pyrimidines are cytosine, thymine, and uracil, which form the nucleotides of nucleic acids.

pyrogen (py-roh-jen) *n.* any substance or agent producing fever. —**pyrogenic** *adj.*

pyromania (py-roh-may-niă) *n.* an excessively strong impulse to set things on fire. —**pyromaniac** *adj., n.*

pyrosis (py-roh-sis) *n.* another name (chiefly US) for heartburn.

pyruvic acid (pyruvate) (py-roo-vik) *n.* a compound, derived from carbohydrates, that may be oxidized in the Krebs cycle to yield carbon dioxide and energy in the form of ATP.

pyuria (py-yoor-iă) *n.* the presence of pus in the urine, making it cloudy. This is a sign of bacterial infection in the urinary tract.

Qq

QALYs *pl. n. see* quality-adjusted life years.

q.d.s. (quater die sumendus) Latin: four times a day, used as a direction in prescriptions.

Q fever *n.* an acute infectious disease of many animals, including cattle, sheep, goats, deer, and dogs, that is caused by a rickettsia, *Coxiella burnetii*. It is transmitted to humans primarily through inhalation of infected particles or consumption of contaminated unpasteurized milk, but also via ticks acting as vectors. A severe influenza-like illness develops, sometimes with pneumonia, after an incubation period of up to three weeks. Treatment with tetracyclines or chloramphenicol is effective. *See also* typhus.

QRS complex *n.* the element of an electrocardiogram that precedes the S–T segment and indicates ventricular contraction.

Q–T interval *n.* the interval on an electrocardiogram that contains the deflections produced by ventricular contraction.

quadratus (kwod-**ray**-tŭs) *n.* any of various four-sided muscles. *q. femoris* a flat muscle at the head of the femur, responsible for lateral rotation of the thigh.

quadri- *prefix denoting* four.

quadriceps (**kwod**-ri-seps) *n.* one of the great extensor muscles of the legs. It is situated in the thigh and is subdivided into four distinct portions: the *rectus femoris*, *vastus lateralis*, *vastus medialis*, and *vastus intermedius*.

quadriplegia (tetraplegia) (kwod-ri-**plee**-jiǎ) *n.* paralysis affecting all four limbs. —**quadriplegic** *adj.*, *n.*

quality-adjusted life years (QALYs) (**kwol**-iti-ǎ-just-id) *pl. n.* a quantitative measure, in terms of years of good-quality life, of the value of a medical procedure or service to a group of patients with similar medical conditions.

quality assurance (ǎ-shor-ǎns) *n.* a programme used in health-care services as a means of measuring the satisfaction of consumers for services given by all professional disciplines. *See* nursing audit, performance indicators. *q. a. tool* a model used by nurses to measure the quality of nursing care. It involves observation of patients, listening to reports, reviewing the care plans, and then scoring to a predetermined schedule (such as *Qualpacs* or *Monitor*).

quality circle *n.* a strategy utilized to develop and maintain nursing standards. It relies heavily on enthusiastic representatives from all disciplines participating in the process of standard development, in order to foster a personal commitment to a quality service.

Qualpacs (**kwol**-paks) *n. see* quality assurance (tool).

quantitative digital radiography (kwon-ti-tă-tiv dij-i-t'l) *n.* a method of detecting osteoporosis. A narrow X-ray beam is directed at the area of interest (usually the spine and hip), which enables a measurement to be made of its calcium content (density).

quarantine (kwo-răn-teen) *n.* the period for which a person (or animal) is kept in isolation to prevent the spread of a contagious disease. Different diseases have different quarantine periods.

quartan fever (kwor-t'n) *n.* a type of malaria, caused by *Plasmodium malariae*, in which there is a three-day interval between fever attacks.

Queckenstedt test (kwek-ĕn-stet) *n.* a part of the routine lumbar puncture procedure. It is used to determine whether or not the flow of cerebrospinal fluid is blocked in the spinal cord. [H. H. G. Queckenstedt (1876–1918), German physician]

quickening (kwik-ĕn-ing) *n.* the first movement of a fetus in the uterus that is felt by the mother, usually after about 16 weeks of pregnancy.

quiescent (kwi-es-ĕnt) *adj.* describing a disease that is in an inactive or undetectable phase.

quinidine (kwin-i-deen) *n.* a drug that slows down the activity of the heart and is administered by mouth to control abnormal and increased heart rhythm. Trade name: **Kinidin Durules**.

quinine (kwin-een) *n.* a drug used to prevent and treat malaria, now largely replaced by more effective less toxic drugs except in cases of malaria due to *Plasmodium falciparum*. Small doses of quinine are used to treat muscular cramps. It is administered by mouth or injection; large doses can cause severe poisoning (*see* cinchonism).

quinism (kwin-izm) *n.* the symptoms of overdosage or too prolonged treatment with quinine. *See* cinchonism.

quinolone (kwin-ŏ-lohn) *n.* one of a group of chemically related synthetic antibiotics that includes ciprofloxacin, nalidixic acid, and ofloxacin. These drugs are often useful for treating infections with organisms that have become resistant to other antibiotics. They are administered by mouth.

quinsy (kwin-zi) *n.* pus in the space between the tonsil and the wall of the pharynx. The patient has severe pain with difficulty in opening the mouth (trismus) and swallowing. Treatment is with antibiotics; surgical incision of the abscess may be necessary. Medical name: **peritonsillar abscess**.

quotidian fever (kwoh-tid-iăn) *n.* a severe type of malaria, caused by *Plasmodium falciparum*, in which the interval between fever attacks varies from a few hours to two days.

quotient (kwoh-shĕnt) *n. see* intelligence quotient, respiratory quotient.

Q wave *n.* the downward deflection on an electrocardiogram that indicates the beginning of ventricular contraction.

Rr

rabbit fever (rab-it) *n. see* tularaemia.

rabies (hydrophobia) (ray-beez) *n.* an acute virus disease of the central nervous system that may be transmitted to humans by a bite from an infected dog. Symptoms include malaise, fever, difficulty in breathing, salivation, and painful muscle spasms of the throat induced by swallowing. In the later stages of the disease the mere sight of water induces convulsions and paralysis; death occurs within 4–5 days. Injections of rabies vaccine and antiserum may prevent the disease from developing in a person bitten by an infected animal. —**rabid** (rab-id) *adj.*

racemose (ras-i-mohs) *adj.* resembling a bunch of grapes. The term is applied particularly to a compound gland the secretory part of which consists of a number of small sacs.

rachi- (rachio-) *prefix denoting* the spine.

rachis (ray-kis) *n. see* backbone.

rachischisis (ray-kis-ki-sis) *n. see* spina bifida.

rachitic (ră-kit-ik) *adj.* afflicted with rickets.

rad (rad) *n.* a former unit of absorbed dose of ionizing radiation. It has been replaced by the gray.

radial (ray-di-ăl) *adj.* relating to or associated with the radius. *r. artery* a branch of the brachial artery, beginning at the elbow and passing down the forearm, around the wrist, and into the palm of the hand. *r. nerve* an important mixed sensory and motor nerve of the arm, forming the largest branch of the brachial plexus. *r. reflex* flexion of the forearm (and sometimes also of the fingers) that occurs when the lower end of the radius is tapped.

radiation (ray-di-ay-shŏn) *n.* energy in the form of waves or particles, such as gamma rays, X-rays, ultraviolet rays, visible light, and infrared rays (radiant heat). *r. sickness* an acute illness caused by extreme exposure to rays emitted by radioactive substances, e.g. X-rays or gamma rays. Very high doses cause death within hours. Lower doses cause immediate symptoms of nausea, vomiting, and diarrhoea followed by damage to the bone marrow, loss of hair, and bloody diarrhoea; these can occur after radiotherapy.

radical treatment (rad-ikăl) *n.* vigorous treatment that aims at the complete cure of a disease rather than the mere relief of symptoms. *Compare* conservative treatment.

radicle (rad-ikŭl) *n.* (in anatomy) **1.** a small root. **2.** the initial fibre of a nerve or the origin of a vein. —**radicular** (ră-dik-yoo-ler) *adj.*

radiculitis (ră-dik-yoo-ly-tis) *n.* inflammation of the root of a nerve. *See* polyradiculitis.

radio- *prefix denoting* **1.** radiation. **2.** radioactive substances.

radioactivity (ray-di-oh-ak-**tiv**-iti) *n.* disintegration of the nuclei of certain elements, with the emission of energy in the form of alpha, beta, or gamma rays. Naturally occurring radioactive elements include radium and uranium. *See also* radioisotope. —**radioactive** *adj.*

radioallergosorbent test (RAST) (ray-di-oh-al-er-joh-**sor**-bĕnt) *n.* a blood test that identifies allergen-specific immunoglobulin E (IgE).

radioautography (ray-di-oh-aw-tog-răfi) *n. see* autoradiography.

radiobiology (ray-di-oh-by-**ol**-ŏji) *n.* the study of the effects of radiation on living tissues. —**radiobiologist** *n.*

radiodermatitis (ray-di-oh-dermă-ty-tis) *n.* inflammation of the skin after exposure to ionizing radiation. The skin becomes dry, hairless, and atrophied, losing its colouring.

radiographer (ray-di-og-ră-fer) *n.* a person who is trained in the technique either of taking X-ray pictures or other images of parts of the body (*diagnostic r.*) or of treatment by radiotherapy (*therapeutic r.*).

radiography (ray-di-og-răfi) *n.* diagnostic radiology: traditionally, the technique of examining the body by directing X-rays through it to produce images (*radiographs*) on photographic film or a fluoroscope. It now also includes the production of images by computerized tomography and nuclear medicine. Radiography is used to produce images of disease in all parts of the body, to be interpreted by radiologists for

physicians and surgeons. *computerized r.* radiography in which photographic film is replaced by a charged plate, from which charge is knocked off by exposure to X-rays. The resultant image is read by a laser beam, then stored digitally or printed out. *digital r.* (*DR*) radiography in which X-ray images are acquired in digital format, allowing the storage of images on hard disk and their subsequent retrieval and interpretation using TV monitors.

radioimmunoassay (ray-di-ohim-yoo-noh-**ass**-ay) *n.* the technique of using radioactive antibodies as tracers to estimate the levels of natural substances, especially hormones, in the blood, which act as antigens. The amount of radioactivity trapped is a measure of the amount of the antigen present.

radioimmunolocalization (ray-di-oh-im-yoo-noh-loh-kăl-I-zay-shŏn) *n.* a method of identifying the site of a tumour (e.g. colorectal cancer) that relies on its uptake of radioactive isotopes attached to an appropriate anticancer immune cell.

radioisotope (ray-di-oh-**I**-sŏ-tohp) *n.* an isotope of an element that emits alpha, beta, or gamma radiation during its decay into another element. Artificial radioisotopes, such as iodine-131 and cobalt-60, are produced by bombarding elements with beams of neutrons. They are widely used in medicine as tracers and as sources of radiation for the different techniques of radiotherapy.

radiologist (ray-di-**ol**-ŏ-jist) *n.* a doctor specialized in the interpretation of X-rays and other scanning techniques for the diagnosis of disease. *interventional r.* a specialist in the use of imaging to guide interventional radiology techniques.

radiology (ray-di-**ol**-ōji) *n.* the branch of medicine involving the study of radiographs or other imaging technologies (such as ultrasound and magnetic resonance imaging) to diagnose or treat disease. *diagnostic r. see* radiography. *interventional r.* the performance of therapeutic or diagnostic procedures under the control of an appropriate imaging technique, such as X-ray fluoroscopy, ultrasound, computerized tomography, or magnetic resonance imaging. *therapeutic r. see* radiotherapy.

radiolucent (ray-di-oh-**loo**-sĕnt) *adj.* having the property of being transparent to X-rays. Gases are relatively radiolucent to X-rays and can be used as a negative contrast medium in X-ray examinations.

radionuclide (ray-di-oh-**new**-klyd) *n.* a substance containing a radioactive atomic nucleus, which can be used as a tracer for diagnosis in nuclear medicine.

radiopaque (ray-di-oh-oh-**payk**) *adj.* having the property of absorbing, and therefore being opaque to, X-rays. Radiopaque materials, such as those containing iodine or barium, are used as contrast media in radiography.

radio pill (ray-di-oh) *n.* a capsule containing a miniature radio transmitter that can be swallowed by a patient. During its passage through the digestive tract a radio pill transmits information about internal conditions (acidity, etc.).

radiosensitive (ray-di-oh-sen-**sit**-iv) *adj.* describing certain forms of

cancer cell that are particularly susceptible to radiation and are likely to be dealt with successfully by radiotherapy.

radiosensitizer (ray-di-oh-**sen**-sit-I-zer) *n.* a substance that increases the sensitivity of cells to radiation. The presence of oxygen and other compounds with a high affinity for electrons will increase radiosensitivity, as will chemotherapy drugs, such as fluorouracil, used concurrently with radiotherapy.

radiotherapist (ray-di-oh-**th**'e-ră-pist) *n.* a doctor who specializes in treatment with radiotherapy.

radiotherapy (ray-di-oh-**th**'e-răpi) *n.* therapeutic radiology: the treatment of disease with penetrating radiation, such as X-rays, beta rays, or gamma rays. Beams of radiation may be directed at a diseased part from a distance (*see* teletherapy), or radioactive material, in the form of needles, wires, or pellets, may be implanted in the body. *See also* brachytherapy.

radium (ray-diŭm) *n.* a radioactive metallic element that emits its alpha and gamma rays during its decay into other elements. The gamma radiation was formerly employed in radiotherapy for the treatment of cancer. Symbol: Ra.

radius (ray-di-ŭs) *n.* the outer and shorter bone of the forearm (*compare* ulna). It partially revolves about the ulna, permitting pronation and supination of the hand. —**radial** *adj.*

radix (ray-diks) *n. see* root.

radon (ray-don) *n.* a radioactive gaseous element that is produced during the decay of radium. It emits alpha and gamma radiation. Symbol: Rn. *r. seeds* sealed capsules containing radon, used in radiotherapy for the treatment of cancer but now largely replaced by newer agents and techniques.

RAI *n.* see Relatives Assessment Interview.

RAISSE *n.* Relatives Assessment Interview for Schizophrenia in a secure environment (see Relatives Assessment Interview).

rale (rahl) *n.* see crepitation.

raloxifene (ral-oks-i-feen) *n.* a drug used to prevent osteoporosis that develops after the menopause. It mimics the protective action of oestrogen in the bones by acting selectively on oestrogen receptors; unlike hormone replacement therapy, it does not relieve menopausal symptoms. It is administered by mouth. Trade name: **Evista**.

ramipril (ram-i-pril) *n.* see ACE inhibitor.

Ramstedt's operation (rahm-stets) *n.* see pyloromyotomy. [W. C. Ramstedt (1867–1963), German surgeon]

ramus (ray-mus) *n.* (*pl.* **rami**) **1.** a branch, especially of a nerve fibre or blood vessel. **2.** a thin process projecting from a bone.

range of movement (ROM) (raynj) *n.* an observational measure of joint flexibility.

ranitidine (ra-nit-i-deen) *n.* an H₂-receptor antagonist (see antihistamine) used in the treatment of gastric and duodenal ulcers and reflux oesophagitis. It may be administered by mouth, intravenously, or intramuscularly. Trade name: **Zantac**.

ranula (ran yoo-lă) *n.* a cyst found under the tongue, formed when the

duct leading from a salivary or mucous gland is obstructed and distended.

raphe (ray-fi) *n.* a line, ridge, seam, or crease in a tissue or organ; for example, the furrow that passes down the centre of the dorsal surface of the tongue.

rarefaction (rair-i-fak-shŏn) *n.* thinning of bony tissue sufficient to cause decreased density of bone to X-rays, as in osteoporosis.

rash (rash) *n.* a temporary eruption on the skin, usually typified by reddening, which may be accompanied by itching. A rash may be a local skin reaction or the outward sign of a disorder affecting the body.

Rasmussen's encephalitis (ras-muus-ĕnz) *n.* a focal encephalitis, found most commonly in children, that results in continual focal seizures (see epilepsy). The underlying cause is unknown but it may be due to a viral infection. [G. L. Rasmussen (1904–), US anatomist]

raspatory (rah-spă-ter-i) *n.* a file-like surgical instrument used for scraping the surface of bone.

A rib raspatory

raspberry tumour (rahz-be-ri) *n.* an adenoma of the umbilicus.

RAST *n.* see radioallergosorbent test.

rat-bite fever (sodokosis) (rat-byt) *n.* a disease, contracted from the bite of a rat, due to infection by either the bacterium *Spirillum* *minus*, which causes ulceration of the skin and recurrent fever, or by the fungus *Streptobacillus moniliformis*, which causes inflammation of the skin, muscular pains, and vomiting. Both infections respond well to penicillin.

rationalization (rash-ŏn-ă-ly-zay-shŏn) *n*. (in psychiatry) the explanation of events or behaviour in terms that avoid giving the true reasons.

Raynaud's disease (ray-nohz) *n*. a condition of unknown cause in which the arteries of the fingers are unduly reactive and enter spasm when the hands are cold. This produces attacks of pallor, numbness, and discomfort in the fingers. Gangrene or ulceration of the fingertips may result. Warm gloves and peripheral vasodilators may relieve the condition. *R. phenomenon* a similar condition resulting from atherosclerosis, ingestion of ergot derivatives, or use of vibrating tools. [M. Raynaud (1834–81), French physician]

RBC *n*. red blood cell (*see* erythrocyte).

RCC *n*. red cell concentrate.

RDA *n*. recommended daily allowance (of a nutrient).

reaction (ri-ak-shŏn) *n*. **1.** the response to a stimulus. **2.** the interaction of two or more substances that results in chemical changes in them. **3.** the effect produced by an allergen (*see* allergy).

reactive (ri-ak-tiv) *adj*. describing mental illnesses that are precipitated by events in the psychological environment. *r. hypoglycaemia see* hypoglycaemia.

reagent (ree-ay-jĕnt) *n*. a compound that reacts with another, especially one used to detect the presence of the other compound.

reagin (ree-ă-jin) *n*. a type of antibody, formed against an allergen, that remains fixed in various tissues. Subsequent contact with the allergen causes damage to the tissue and the release of histamine and serotonin, which are responsible for the allergic reaction (*see* anaphylaxis).

real-time imaging (reel-tym) *n*. the rapid acquisition and manipulation of ultrasound information from a scanning probe by electronic circuits to enable images to be produced on TV screens almost instantaneously. Using similar techniques, the instantaneous display of other imaging modalities, such as CT scanning and magnetic resonance imaging, can now be achieved.

reboxetine (reb-oks-i-teen) *n*. an antidepressant drug that acts by inhibiting reabsorption of the neurotransmitter noradrenaline, thus prolonging its action in the brain. It is administered by mouth. Trade name: **Edronax**.

recall (ri-kawl) **1.** *n*. the process of eliciting a representation (especially an image) of a past experience. **2.** *vb*. to elicit such a representation.

receptaculum (ree-sep-tak-yoo-lŭm) *n*. the dilated portion of a tubular anatomical part. *r.* (or *cisterna*) *chyli* the dilated end of the thoracic duct, into which lymph vessels from the lower limbs and intestines drain.

receptor (ri-sep-ter) *n*. **1.** a cell or group of cells specialized to detect changes in the environment and trigger impulses in the sensory nervous system. All sensory nerve endings act as receptors. *See* exteroceptor, interoceptor, proprioceptor. **2.** a specialized area of cell membrane that can bind with a specific hormone (e.g. *oestrogen r.*), neurotransmitter (e.g. *adrenergic r.*), drug, or other chemical, thereby initiating a change within the cell.

recess (ri-ses) *n.* (in anatomy) a hollow chamber or a depression in an organ or other part.

recessive (ri-ses-iv) *adj.* describing a gene (or its corresponding characteristic) whose effect is shown in the individual only when its allele is the same, i.e. when two such alleles are present (the *double recessive* condition). *Compare* dominant. *See also* autosomal. —**recessive** *n.*

recipient (ri-sip-iĕnt) *n.* a person who receives something from a donor, such as a blood transfusion or a kidney transplant.

recombinant DNA (ri-kom-bin-ănt) *n.* DNA that contains genes from different sources that have been combined by the techniques of genetic engineering. Genetic engineering is therefore also known as *recombinant DNA technology.*

recovery position (ri-kuv-eri) *n.* a first-aid position into which an unconscious but breathing patient can be laid to afford maximum protection to the airway. It involves lying the patient on his or her side, with the uppermost leg bent at the knee and hip and the lower arm behind the back to prevent rolling into a position in which the patient could smother or choke.

recrudescence (ree-kroo-des-ĕns) *n.* a fresh outbreak of a disorder in a patient after a period during which its signs and symptoms had died down.

rect- (recto-) *prefix denoting* the rectum.

rectocele (rek-toh-seel) *n. see* proctocele.

rectopexy (rek-toh-peks-i) *n.* the surgical fixation of a prolapsed rectum.

rectosigmoid (rek-toh-**sig**-moid) *n.* the region of the large intestine around the junction of the sigmoid colon and the rectum.

rectovesical (rek-toh-ves-ikăl) *adj.* relating to the rectum and the urinary bladder.

rectum (rek-tŭm) *n.* the terminal part of the large intestine, which runs from the sigmoid colon to the anal canal. Faeces are stored in the rectum before defecation. —**rectal** (rek-t'l) *adj.*

rectus (rek-tŭs) *n.* any of several straight muscles. *r. abdominis* a long flat muscle that extends bilaterally along the entire length of the front of the abdomen. *r. femoris see* quadriceps. *r. muscles of the orbit* some of the extrinsic eye muscles.

recumbent (ri-kum-bĕnt) *adj.* lying down. —**recumbency** *n.*

recurrent (ri-ku-rĕnt) *adj.* (in anatomy) describing a structure, such as a nerve or blood vessel, that turns back on its course, forming a loop.

red blood cell (RBC) *n. see* erythrocyte.

Reductil (ri-duk-til) *n. see* sibutramine.

reduction (ri-duk-shŏn) *n.* (in surgery) the restoration of a displaced part of the body, such as a hernia or a dislocated joint, to its normal position by manipulation or operation.

reduction division *n.* the first division of meiosis, in which the chromosome number is halved.

referred pain (synalgia) (ri-ferd) *n.* pain felt in a part of the body other than where it might be expected. An abscess beneath the diaphragm, for example, may cause a referred pain in the shoulder area. The confusion arises because sensory nerves from different parts of the body share common pathways when they reach the spinal cord.

reflection (ri-flek-shŏn) *n.* the careful consideration of personal actions, including the ability to review, analyse, and evaluate situations during or after events. It is an essential part of the learning process that will result in new methods of approaching and understanding nursing practice.

reflex (ree-fleks) *n.* an automatic or involuntary response to a stimulus, which is brought about by relatively simple nervous circuits without consciousness being necessarily involved. *See* conditioned reflex, Moro reflex, patellar reflex, plantar (reflex), pupillary reflex, rooting reflex. *r.* **arc** the nervous circuit involved in a reflex, being at its simplest a sensory nerve with a receptor, linked at a synapse in the brain or spinal cord with a motor nerve, which supplies a muscle or gland. See illustration.

reflexology (ree-fleks-ol-ŏji) *n.* a complementary therapy based on the theory that reflex points on the feet correspond with all body parts.

Firm pressure is applied to the relevant reflex points using the thumb or fingers. Reflexology is said to be able to help with specific illnesses and may also restore the body's natural balance and harmony.

reflux (ree-fluks) *n.* a backflow of liquid, against its normal direction of movement. *See* gastro-oesophageal reflux, (reflux) oesophagitis, vesicoureteric reflux.

refraction (ri-frak-shŏn) *n.* the change in direction of light rays when they pass obliquely from one transparent medium to another, of a different density. Refraction occurs as light enters the eye and passes through the cornea, lens, etc., to come to a focus on the retina. **error of r.** (**refractive error**) an abnormality of the eye, such as astigmatism or long- or short-sightedness, in which a blurred image forms on the

A reflex arc

retina due to abnormal focusing. —**refractive** (ri-frak-tiv) *adj.*

refractive surgery *n.* any surgical procedure that has as its primary objective the correction of any refractive error. It includes such procedures as lens extraction, LASIK, LASEK, photorefractive keratectomy, and thermokeratoplasty.

refractometer (ree-frak **tom**-it-er) *n. see* optometer.

refractory (ri-**frakt**-er-i) *adj.* unresponsive: applied to a condition that fails to respond satisfactorily to a given treatment.

refractory period *n.* (in neurology) the time of recovery needed for a nerve cell that has just transmitted a nerve impulse or for a muscle fibre that has just contracted. During the refractory period a normal stimulus will not bring about excitation of the cell.

regeneration (ri-jen-er-ay-shŏn) *n.* the natural regrowth of a tissue or other part lost through injury.

regimen (rej-i-men) *n.* (in therapeutics) a prescribed systematic form of treatment, such as a diet or a course of drugs, for curing disease or improving health.

regional ileitis (ree-jŏn-ăl) *n. see* Crohn's disease.

registered nurse (rej-is-terd) *n. see* nurse.

registrar (specialist registrar) (rej-i-strar) *n.* (in a hospital) a registered doctor who undergoes a training programme in a chosen specialty in order to obtain a Certificate of Completion of Specialist Training and be eligible to apply for a consultant post. The post of specialist registrar replaced those of *registrar* and *senior registrar*.

regression (ri-**gresh**-ŏn) *n.* **1.** (in psychiatry) reversion to a more immature level of functioning. **2.** the stage of a disease during which the signs and symptoms disappear and the patient recovers.

regurgitation (ri-ger-ji-**tay**-shŏn) *n.* **1.** the bringing up of undigested material from the stomach to the mouth (*see* vomiting). **2.** the flowing back of a liquid in a direction opposite to the normal one.

rehabilitation (ree-ă-bil-i-**tay**-shŏn) *n.* **1.** (in physical medicine) the treatment of an ill, injured, or disabled patient with the aim of restoring normal health and function. **2.** any means for restoring the independence of a patient after disease or injury.

reiki (ray-ki) *n.* a complementary therapy based on an ancient healing system rediscovered in the 20th century by a Buddhist monk. It involves the therapist putting his or her hands on or very close to the patient to boost the patient's natural invisible energy fields. It is often used as an adjunct to other therapies and is said to be helpful for many conditions.

Reiter's syndrome (ry-terz) *n.* a condition, usually affecting young men, characterized by urethritis, conjunctivitis, and polyarthritis. No causative agent has been positively identified, although a virus may be implicated. [H. Reiter (1881–1969), German physician]

rejection (ri-jek-shŏn) *n.* (in transplantation) the destruction by immune mechanisms of a tissue grafted from another individual. Antibodies, complement, clotting factors, and platelets are involved in the failure of the graft to survive. Allograft rejection is a vigorous response that can be modified by drugs (such as ciclosporin and corticosteroids) and antibodies against T-cells; xenograft rejection is an acute response that is at present beyond therapeutic control.

relapse (ri-laps) *n.* a return of disease symptoms after recovery had apparently been achieved or the worsening of an apparently recovering patient's condition.

relapsing fever (ri-laps-ing) *n.* an infectious disease caused by bacteria of the genus *Borrelia*, which is transmitted by ticks or lice and results in recurrent fever. The first episode of fever is accompanied by severe headache and aching muscles and joints. Subsequent attacks are milder and occur at intervals of 3–10 days.

relative density (rel-ă-tiv) *n.* the ratio of the density of a substance at a specified temperature to the density of a reference substance (for liquids, this is water at 4°C). It was formerly known as *specific gravity*.

Relatives Assessment Interview (RAI) *n.* an assessment tool designed to identify the perceptions and coping skills of relatives of patients with mental health problems. The *Relatives Assessment Interview for Schizophrenia in a secure environment* (*RAISSE*) is a form of the RAI adapted to examine the effects of a secure environment on the course of schizophrenia.

relaxant (ri-laks-ănt) *n.* an agent that reduces tension and strain, particularly in muscles (*see* muscle relaxant).

relaxation (ree-laks-ay-shŏn) *n.* (in

physiology) the diminution of tension in a muscle, which occurs when it ceases to contract. *r. therapy* treatment by teaching a patient to decrease his anxiety by reducing the tone in his muscles.

relaxin (ri-laks-in) *n.* a hormone, secreted by the placenta in the terminal stages of pregnancy, that causes the cervix of the uterus to dilate and prepares the uterus for the action of oxytocin during labour.

Relenza (ri-lenz-ă) *n. see* zanamivir.

rem (rem) *n.* a former unit dose of ionizing radiation; it was replaced by the sievert.

REM *n.* rapid eye movement: the stage of sleep during which the muscles of the eyeballs are in constant motion behind the eyelids. REM usually coincides with dreaming.

remission (ri-mish-ŏn) *n.* **1.** a lessening in the severity of symptoms or their temporary disappearance during the course of an illness. **2.** a reduction in the size of a cancer and the symptoms it is causing.

remittent fever (ri-mit-ĕnt) *n. see* fever.

renal (ree-năl) *adj.* relating to or affecting the kidneys. *r. artery* either of two large arteries arising from the abdominal aorta and supplying the kidneys. *r. cell carcinoma see* hypernephroma. *r. function tests* tests for assessing the function of the kidneys, which include measurements of the specific gravity of urine, creatinine clearance time, and blood urea levels, as well as intravenous urography and renal angiography. *r. tubule* (*uriniferous tubule*) the fine tubular part of a nephron, through which water and certain dissolved substances are re-absorbed back into the blood.

reni- (reno-) *prefix denoting* the kidney.

renin (ree-nin) *n.* an enzyme released into the blood by the kidney in response to stress. It produces angiotensin, which causes constriction of blood vessels and thus an increase in blood pressure. Excessive production of renin results in renal hypertension.

rennin (ren-in) *n.* an enzyme produced in the stomach that coagulates milk. It converts caseinogen (milk protein) into insoluble casein in the presence of calcium ions. This ensures that the milk remains in the stomach, exposed to protein-digesting enzymes, for as long as possible.

renography (isotope renography) (ri-nog-răfi) *n.* the radiological study of the kidneys by a gamma camera following the intravenous injection of a radioactive tracer, which is concentrated and excreted by the kidneys. A graph of the radioactivity in each kidney gives information on its function and rate of drainage.

reovirus (ree-oh-vy-rŭs) *n.* one of a group of small RNA-containing viruses that infect both respiratory and intestinal tracts without producing specific or serious diseases (and were therefore termed respiratory enteric orphan viruses). *Compare* echovirus.

repetitive strain injury (RSI) (ri-pet-it-iv) *n.* pain with associated loss of function in a limb resulting from its repeated movement or sustained static loading. Tenosynovitis and tendovaginitis of the wrist associated with typing or operating a word processor is the injury most frequently encountered.

replantation (ree-plahn-tay-shŏn) *n.* **1.** a developing specialty for the reattachment of severed limbs (or parts of limbs) and other body parts (e.g. the nose). It employs techniques of microsurgery to rejoin nerves and vessels. **2. (reimplantation)** (in dentistry) the reinsertion of a tooth into its socket after its accidental or deliberate removal. —**replant** *vb.*

replication (rep-li-kay-shŏn) *n.* the process by which DNA makes copies of itself when the cell divides. The two strands of the DNA molecule unwind and each strand directs the synthesis of a new strand complementary to itself.

repolarization (ri-poh-ler-I-zay-shŏn) *n.* the process in which the membrane of a nerve cell returns to its normal electrically charged state after a nerve impulse has passed.

repositor (ri-poz-it-er) *n.* an instrument used to return a displaced part of the body to its normal position.

repression (ri-presh-ŏn) *n.* (in psychoanalysis) the process of excluding an unacceptable wish or an idea from conscious mental life. The repressed material may give rise to symptoms.

reproductive system (ree-prŏ-duk-tiv) *n.* the combination of organs and tissues associated with the process of reproduction. In males it includes the testes, vasa deferentia, prostate gland, seminal vesicles, urethra, and penis; in females it includes the ovaries, Fallopian tubes, uterus, vagina, and vulva. *See* illustrations.

Male reproductive system

Female reproductive system

research ethics committee (ri-serch) n. (in Britain) a group of lay people, medical practitioners, and other experts set up to monitor research investigations that involve the use of human subjects.

resection (ri-sek-shŏn) n. surgical removal of a portion of any part of the body. *submucous r.* removal of part of the cartilage septum of the nose that has become deviated, usually by injury. *transurethral r. of the prostate* (*TUR* or *TURP*) an operation performed when the prostate gland becomes enlarged. It involves removal of portions of the gland through the urethra using an instrument called a *resectoscope*.

resectoscope (ri-sek-tŏ-skohp) n. *see* (transurethral) resection.

reserve volume (ri-zerv) n. the extra volume of air that an individual could inhale (*inspiratory r. v.*, *IRV*) or exhale (*expiratory r. v.*, *ERV*) if not breathing to the limit of his or her capacity.

residual urine (ri-zid-yoo-ăl) n.

urine remaining in the bladder after micturition.

residual volume (RV) n. the volume of air that remains in the lungs after the individual has breathed out as much as he or she can. This volume is increased in emphysema.

resistance (ri-zist-ăns) n. **1.** the degree of immunity that the body possesses. **2.** the degree to which a disease or disease-causing organism remains unaffected by antibiotics or other drugs.

resolution (rez-ŏ-loo-shŏn) n. **1.** the stage during which inflammation gradually disappears. **2.** the degree to which individual details can be distinguished by the eye, as through a microscope.

resonance (rez-ŏn-ăns) n. the sound produced by percussion of a part of the body during a physical examination. *See also* vocal resonance.

resorption (ri-sorp-shŏn) n. loss of substance through physiological or pathological means.

respiration (res-per-**ay**-shŏn) *n.* the process of gaseous exchange between an organism and its environment. **external** *r.* breathing: the stage of respiration in which oxygen is taken up by the capillaries of the lung alveoli and carbon dioxide is released from the blood. **internal** *r.* the stage of respiration in which oxygen is released to the tissues and carbon dioxide absorbed by the blood. *See also* lung. —**respiratory** (rĕs-**pir**-ă-ter-i) *adj.*

respirator (res-per-**ayt**-er) *n.* **1.** a device used to maintain the breathing movements of paralysed patients. *cuirass r.* a type of respirator in which the patient is enclosed, except for the head and limbs, in an airtight container in which the air pressure is decreased and increased mechanically. This draws air into and out of the lungs, through the normal air passages. *Drinker r.* (*iron lung*) a respirator that works on a similar principle to the cuirass respirator but also encloses the limbs. *positive-pressure r.* a respirator that blows air into the patient's lungs via a tube passed either through the mouth into the trachea or through a tracheostomy. **2.** a face mask for administering oxygen or other gas or for filtering harmful fumes, dust, etc. *See also* artificial respiration.

respiratory distress syndrome (hyaline membrane disease) *n.* the condition of a newborn infant in which the lungs are imperfectly expanded. Breathing is rapid, laboured, and shallow. The condition is most common and serious among preterm infants. It is treated by careful nursing, intravenous fluids, and oxygen, with or without

positive pressure by a respirator. Surfactant administered at birth has produced encouraging results.

respiratory quotient (RQ) *n.* the ratio of the volume of carbon dioxide transferred from the blood into the alveoli to the volume of oxygen absorbed into the alveoli. The RQ is usually about 0.8.

respiratory syncytial virus (RSV) *n.* a paramyxovirus (*see* myxovirus) that causes infections of the nose and throat. It is a major cause of bronchiolitis and pneumonia in young children.

respiratory system *n.* the combination of organs and tissues associated with breathing. It includes the nasal cavity, pharynx, larynx, trachea, bronchi, and lungs.

response (ri-**spons**) *n.* the way in which the body or part of the body reacts to a stimulus.

responsibility (ri-spons-i-**bil**-iti) *n.* (in nursing) the state of being answerable for one's performance according to the terms of reference of the Code of Professional Conduct (see Appendix 12). It involves demonstrating commitment and trustworthiness during the performance of care through devolved authority. Nurses (whether registered or not) are responsible for their actions at all times.

restenosis (ree-sti-**noh**-sis) *n.* recurrent stenosis, usually in a blood vessel after such procedures as angioplasty or insertion of a stent.

restless legs syndrome (Ekbom's syndrome) (rest-lis) *n.* a condition in which a sense of uneasiness, restlessness, and itching, often accompanied by twitching and pain, is felt in the calves of the legs when sitting or lying down, especially in bed at night. The cause is unknown: it may be inadequate circulation, peripheral neuropathy, deficiency of iron, vitamin B_{12}, or folic acid, or a reaction to antipsychotic or antidepressant drugs.

rest pain (rest) *n.* pain, usually experienced in the feet, that indicates an extreme degree of ischaemia.

resuscitation (ri-sus-i-**tay**-shŏn) *n.* the process of reviving someone who appears to be dead; for example by cardiac massage or artificial respiration. *r. mannikin* a life-size model of a person for practising all aspects of basic and advanced life support.

retardation (ree-tar-**day**-shŏn) *n.* the slowing down of a process. *psychomotor r.* a marked slowing down of activity and speech. It is a symptom of severe depression. *See also* mental retardation.

retching (**rech**-ing) *n.* repeated unavailing attempts to vomit.

rete (**ree**-ti) *n.* a network of blood vessels, nerve fibres, or other strands of interlacing tissue in the structure of an organ.

retention (ri-**ten**-shŏn) *n.* inability to pass urine, which is retained in the bladder. The condition may be acute and painful or chronic and painless. The commonest cause of spontaneous *acute urinary r. (AUR)* is enlargement of the prostate gland in men.

retention cyst *n.* a cyst that arises when the outlet of the duct of a gland is blocked.

retention defect *n.* (in psychology) a memory defect in which items that have been registered in

the memory are lost from storage. It is a feature of dementia.

reticular (ri-**tik**-yoo-ler) *adj.* (of tissues) resembling a network; branching. *r. fibres* branching fibres of connective tissue that form a delicate supportive meshwork around blood vessels, muscle fibres, glands, nerves, etc. *r. formation* a network of nerve pathways and nuclei throughout the brainstem, connecting motor and sensory nerves to and from the spinal cord, the cerebellum and the cerebrum, and the cranial nerves.

reticulocyte (ri-**tik**-yoo-loh-syt) *n.* an immature red blood cell (erythrocyte). Reticulocytes normally comprise about 1% of the total red cells.

reticulocytosis (ri-tik-yoo-loh-sy-toh-sis) *n.* an increase in the proportion of reticulocytes in the bloodstream: a sign of increased output of new red cells from the bone marrow.

reticuloendothelial system (RES) (ri-tik-yoo-loh-en-doh-**theel**-iăl) *n.* a community of phagocytes that is spread throughout the body. The RES is concerned with defence against microbial infection and with the removal of worn-out blood cells from the bloodstream. *See also* spleen.

reticulosis (ri-tik-yoo-**loh**-sis) *n.* abnormal overgrowth, usually malignant, of any of the cells of the lymphatic glands or the immune system. *See* Burkitt's lymphoma, Hodgkin's disease, lymphoma, mycosis fungoides.

reticulum (ri-**tik**-yoo-lŭm) *n.* a network of tubules or blood vessels. *See* endoplasmic reticulum.

retin- (retino-) *prefix denoting* the retina.

retina (ret-in-ă) *n.* the light-sensitive layer that lines the interior of the eye. The inner part of the retina, next to the cavity of the eyeball, contains rods and cones (light-sensitive cells) and their associated nerve fibres. The outer part (*retinal pigment epithelium*, *RPE*) is pigmented to prevent the passage of light. —**retinal** (ret-in-ăl) *adj.*

retinaculum (ret-in-ak-yoo-lŭm) *n.* (*pl.* **retinacula**) a thickened band of tissue that serves to hold various tissues in place.

retinal (retinene) (ret-in-al) *n.* the aldehyde of retinol (vitamin A). *See also* rhodopsin.

retinal artery occlusion *n.* blockage of an artery supplying blood to the retina, usually as a result of thrombosis or embolism. *branch r. a. o.* blockage of one of the branches of the central retinal artery, which results in visual field loss in the area of the retina supplied by the occluded vessel. *central r. a. o.* blockage of the central retinal artery, which enters the eye at the optic disc, usually resulting in sudden painless loss of vision.

retinal detachment (detached retina) *n.* separation of the inner nervous layer of the retina from the outer pigmented layer (retinal pigment epithelium), causing loss of vision in the affected part of the retina. The condition can be treated surgically by creating patches of scar tissue between the retina and the choroid (*see* cryosurgery, photocoagulation); this, combined with plombage, allows reattachment of the retina.

retinal vein occlusion *n.* blockage of a vein carrying blood from the retina. *branch r. v. o.* blockage of one of the small branches of the central retinal vein, resulting in painless reduction of vision in the affected area. *central r. v. o.* blockage of the central retinal vein, which leaves the eye at the optic disc, usually resulting in sudden painless reduction of vision.

retinene (ret-in-een) *n. see* retinal.

retinitis (ret-i-ny-tis) *n.* inflammation of the retina. *r. pigmentosa* a noninflammatory hereditary condition that is characterized by progressive degeneration of the retina due to malfunctioning of the retinal pigment epithelium. Night blindness and limited peripheral vision starting in childhood may progress to complete loss of vision.

retinoblastoma (ret-in-oh-blas-toh-mă) *n.* a rare malignant tumour of the retina, occurring in infants.

retinoid (ret-in-oid) *n.* one of a group of drugs derived from vitamin A that act on the skin to cause drying and peeling and a reduction in oil (sebum) production. Retinoids include isotretinoin and tretinoin; they are used in the treatment of severe acne, psoriasis, ichthyosis, and other skin disorders. Possible side-effects, which may be serious, include severe fetal abnormalities (if taken by pregnant women), toxic effects on babies (if taken by breast-feeding mothers), and liver and kidney damage.

retinol (ret-in-ol) *n. see* vitamin A.

retinopathy (ret-in-op-ă-thi) *n.* any of various disorders of the retina resulting in impairment or loss of vision. *AIDS r.* retinopathy that occurs as a complication of AIDS. *diabetic r.* retinopathy resulting from diabetes, in which haemorrhaging or exudation may occur, either from damaged vessels into the retina or from new abnormal vessels into the vitreous humour (*see* neovascularization).

retinopexy (ret-in-oh-peks-i) *n.* any surgical procedure used to repair a retinal detachment. *See* pneumoretinopexy, cryoretinopexy.

retinoschisis (ret-in-osk-i-sis) *n.* splitting of the layers of the retina with accumulation of fluid between the layers. This usually progresses very slowly compared to other types of retinal detachment.

retinoscope (ret-in-oh-skohp) *n.* an instrument used to determine the power of spectacle lenses required to correct errors of refraction of the eye. —**retinoscopy** (ret-in-os-kŏ-pi) *n.*

retinotomy (ret-in-ot-ŏmi) *n.* a surgical incision into the retina.

retraction (ri-trak-shŏn) *n.* **1.** (in obstetrics) the quality of uterine muscle fibres of remaining shortened after contracting during labour. This results in a gradual progression of the fetus downward through the pelvis. *r. ring* a depression in the uterine wall marking the junction between the actively contracting muscle fibres of the upper segment and the muscle fibres of the lower segment of the uterus. This depression is not always visible and is normal. *Compare* Bandl's ring. **2.** (in dentistry) the drawing back of one or more teeth into a better position by an orthodontic appliance.

retractor (ri-trak-ter) *n.* a surgical instrument used to expose the oper-

wound retractor

abdominal retractor

Retractors

ation site by drawing aside the cut edges of skin, muscle, or other tissues. See illustration.

retro- *prefix denoting* at the back or behind.

retrobulbar neuritis (optic neuritis) (ret-roh-**bulb**-er) *n.* inflammation of the optic nerve behind the eye, causing increasingly blurred vision. Retrobulbar neuritis is one of the symptoms of multiple sclerosis but it can also occur as an isolated lesion.

retroflexion (ret-roh-flek-shŏn) *n.* the bending backward of an organ or part of an organ, especially the abnormal bending backwards of the upper part of the uterus.

retrograde (ret-roh-grayd) *adj.* going backwards, or moving in the opposite direction to the normal. *See also* (retrograde) amnesia, (retrograde) pyelography.

retrogression (ret-roh-**gresh**-ŏn) *n.* return to a less complex state or condition; regression.

retrolental fibroplasia (ret-roh-len-t'l) *n.* the abnormal proliferation of fibrous tissue immediately behind the lens of the eye, leading to blindness. It is most commonly seen in newborn preterm infants, in whom it is associated with high concentrations of inhaled oxygen.

retro-ocular (ret-roh-**ok**-yoo-ler) *adj.* behind the eye.

retroperitoneal fibrosis (RPF) (ret-roh-pe-ri-tŏn-**ee**-ăl) *n.* a condition in which a dense plaque of fibrous tissue develops behind the peritoneum adjacent to the abdominal aorta. The ureters become encased and hence obstructed, causing acute anuria and renal failure. The obstruction can be relieved by nephrostomy or the insertion of double J stents. In the acute phase steroid administration may help, but in established RPF ureterolysis is required.

retroperitoneal space *n.* the region between the posterior parietal peritoneum and the front of the lumbar vertebrae. This space contains important structures, including the kidneys, adrenal glands, pancreas, lumbar spinal nerve roots, sympathetic ganglia and nerves, and the abdominal aorta and its major branches.

retropharyngeal (ret-roh-fǎ-rin-ji-ǎl) *adj.* behind the pharynx. **r. abscess** a collection of pus in the tissues behind the pharynx, resulting in difficulty in swallowing, pain, and fever.

retropubic (ret-roh-**pew**-bik) *adj.* behind the pubis. **r. prostatectomy** *see* prostatectomy.

retropulsion (ret-roh-**pul**-shŏn) *n.* a compulsive tendency to walk backwards. It is a symptom of parkinsonism.

retrospection (ret-roh-**spek**-shŏn) *n.* (in psychology) the systematic reviewing of past experiences.

retroversion (ret-roh-**ver**-shŏn) *n.*

an abnormal position of the uterus in which it is tilted backwards, with the base lying in the pouch of Douglas, against the rectum, instead of on the bladder.

retrovirus (ret-roh-vy-rŭs) *n.* an RNA-containing virus that can convert its genetic material into DNA, which enables it to become integrated into the DNA of its host's cells. Retroviruses include HIV and viruses implicated in the development of some cancers.

Rett's syndrome (rets) *n.* a disorder affecting young girls, in which stereotyped movements and social withdrawal appear during early childhood. Intellectual development is often impaired and special educational help is needed. [A. Rett (20th century), Austrian paediatrician]

revascularization (ri-vas-kew-ler-I-zay-shŏn) *n.* **1.** the regrowth of blood vessels following disease or injury so that normal blood supply to an organ, tissue, or part is restored. **2.** the surgical operation of re-establishing the blood supply to a tissue or organ by means of a blood-vessel graft. **coronary r.** re-establishing blood flow through the coronary arteries, usually by means of a coronary artery bypass graft.

Reye's syndrome (rayz) *n.* a rare disorder occurring in childhood. It is characterized by the symptoms of encephalitis combined with evidence of liver failure. Treatment is aimed at controlling cerebral oedema and correcting metabolic abnormalities, but there is a significant mortality and there may be residual brain damage. The cause is not known, but aspirin has been implicated and this drug should not be used in children below the age of 15 unless specifically indicated. [R. D. K. Reye (1912–77), Australian histopathologist]

RF *n. see* rheumatic fever.

RGN *n.* registered general nurse: *see* nurse.

rhabdomyosarcoma (rab-doh-my-oh-sar-koh-mǎ) *n.* a rare malignant tumour, usually of childhood, originating in, or showing the characteristics of, striated muscle.

rhagades (rag-ǎ-deez) *pl. n.* cracks or long thin scars in the skin, particularly around the mouth. The fissures around the mouth and nose of babies with congenital syphilis eventually heal to form rhagades.

rhegmatogenous (reg-mǎ-toj-i-nǔs) *adj.* resulting from a break or tear. *r. retinal detachment* retinal detachment as a consequence of a tear in the retina.

rheo- *prefix denoting* **1.** a flow of liquid. **2.** an electric current.

rhesus factor (Rh factor) (ree-sǔs) *n.* a group of antigens that may or may not be present on the surface of the red blood cells; it forms the basis of the rhesus blood group system. Most people have the rhesus factor, i.e. they are *Rh-positive*. People who lack the factor are termed *Rh-negative*. Incompatibility between Rh-positive and Rh-negative blood is an important cause of blood transfusion reactions and of haemolytic disease of the newborn. *See also* blood group.

rheumatic fever (RF, acute rheumatism) (roo-mat-ik) *n.* a disease affecting mainly children and young adults that arises as a delayed complication of infection of the upper respiratory tract with haemolytic streptococci. The main features are fever, arthritis, Sydenham's chorea, and inflammation of the heart muscle, its valves, and the membrane surrounding the heart. The infection is treated with antibiotics (e.g. penicillin) and bed rest. *chronic rheumatic heart disease* a complication of rheumatic fever, in which there is scarring and chronic inflammation of the heart and its valves leading to heart failure, murmurs, and damage to the valves.

rheumatism (room-ǎ-tizm) *n.* any disorder in which aches and pains affect the muscles and joints. *See* rheumatoid arthritis, rheumatic fever, osteoarthritis, gout.

rheumatoid arthritis (room-ǎ-toid) *n.* a form of arthritis that is a disease of the synovial lining of joints. It involves the joints of the fingers, wrists, feet, and ankles, with later involvement of the hips, knees, shoulders, and neck. Diagnosis is supported by a blood test and by X-rays revealing typical changes around the affected joints. Treatment relies upon a variety of drugs, including anti-inflammatory analgesics, steroids, immunosuppressants, and gold salts, and some diseased joints can be replaced by prosthetic surgery (*see* arthroplasty).

rheumatology (room-ǎ-tol-ǒji) *n.* the medical specialty concerned with the diagnosis and management of disease involving joints, tendons, muscles, ligaments, and associated structures. *See also* physical medicine. —**rheumatologist** *n.*

Rh factor *n. see* rhesus factor.

rhin- (rhino-) *prefix denoting* the nose.

rhinitis (ry-**ny**-tis) *n.* inflammation of the mucous membrane of the nose. *acute r. see* (common) cold. *allergic r. see* hay fever. *atrophic r.* rhinitis in which the mucous membrane becomes thinned and fragile. *perennial r.* (*vasomotor r.*) rhinitis in which there is overgrowth of, and increased secretion by, the membrane.

rhinology (ry-**nol**-ŏji) *n.* the branch of medicine concerned with disorders of the nose and nasal passages.

rhinomycosis (ry-noh-my-**koh**-sis) *n.* fungal infection of the lining of the nose.

rhinophyma (ry-noh-**fy**-mă) *n.* a bulbous craggy swelling of the nose, usually in men. It is a complication of rosacea and in no way related to alcohol intake.

rhinoplasty (**ry**-noh-plasti) *n.* surgery to alter the shape of the nose.

rhinorrhoea (ry-nŏ-**ree**-ă) *n.* a persistent watery mucous discharge from the nose, as in the common cold.

rhinoscopy (ry-**nosk**-ŏ-pi) *n.* examination of the interior of the nose using a speculum or endoscope.

rhinosinusitis (ry-noh-sy-nŭs-**I**-tis) *n.* inflammation of the lining of the nose and paranasal sinuses, caused by allergies, infection, immune deficiencies, mucociliary transport abnormalities, trauma, drugs, or tumours. *See* rhinitis, sinusitis.

rhinosporidiosis (ry-noh-sper-id-i-**oh**-sis) *n.* a fungal infection of the mucous membranes of the nose, larynx, eyes, and genitals that is characterized by the formation of polyps.

rhinovirus (**ry**-noh-vy-rŭs) *n.* any one of a group of RNA-containing

viruses that cause respiratory infections resembling the common cold. They are included in the picornavirus group.

rhiz- (rhizo-) *prefix denoting* a root.

rhizotomy (ry-**zot**-ŏmi) *n.* a surgical procedure in which selected nerve roots are cut at the point where they emerge from the spinal cord. The posterior (sensory) nerve roots are cut for the relief of intractable pain; the anterior (motor) nerve roots are sometimes cut for the relief of severe muscle spasm or dystonia.

rhodopsin (visual purple) (roh-**dop**-sin) *n.* a pigment in the retina of the eye consisting of retinal and a protein. The presence of rhodopsin is essential for vision in dim light. *See* rod.

rhombencephalon (rom-ben-**sef**-ă-lon) *n. see* hindbrain.

rhomboid (**rom**-boid) *n.* either of two muscles situated in the upper part of the back, between the backbone and shoulder blade. They help to move the shoulder blade backwards and upwards.

rhonchus (**ronk**-ŭs) *n.* (*pl.* **rhonchi**) an abnormal musical noise produced by air passing through narrowed bronchi. It is heard through a stethoscope, usually when the patient breathes out.

rhythm method (**rith**-ĕm) *n.* a contraceptive method in which sexual intercourse is restricted to the days at the beginning and end of the menstrual cycle when conception is least likely to occur (*safe period*). The method depends for its reliability on the woman having uniform regular periods and its failure rate is higher than with mechanical methods.

rib (rib) *n.* a curved strip of bone forming part of the skeleton of the thorax. There are 12 pairs of ribs. The head of each rib articulates with one of the 12 thoracic vertebrae of the backbone; the other end is attached to a costal cartilage. **false r.** any of the three pairs of ribs below the true ribs. Each is connected by its cartilage to the rib above it. **floating r.** any of the last two pairs of ribs, which end freely in the muscles of the body wall. **true r.** any of the first seven pairs of ribs, which are connected directly to the sternum by their costal cartilages. Anatomical name: **costa**.

ribavirin (ry-bă-vy-rin) *n.* an antiviral drug effective against a range of DNA and RNA viruses, including the herpes group, respiratory syncytial virus, hepatitis C virus, and those causing several strains of influenza and Lassa fever. It is administered by a small-particle aerosol inhaler or by mouth. Trade names: **Rebetol, Virazole**.

riboflavin (vitamin B₂) (ry-boh-flay-vin) *n. see* vitamin B.

ribonuclease (ry-boh-new-kli-ayz) *n.* an enzyme, located in the lysosomes of cells, that splits RNA at specific places in the molecule.

ribonucleic acid (ry-boh-new-klee-ik) *n. see* RNA.

ribose (ry-bohz) *n.* a pentose sugar that is a component of RNA and several coenzymes. Ribose is also involved in intracellular metabolism.

ribosome (ry-bŏ-sohm) *n.* a particle, consisting of RNA and protein, that occurs in cells and is the site of protein synthesis in the cell (*see* translation). —**ribosomal** *adj.*

ricewater stools (rys-waw-ter) *pl. n. see* cholera.

ricin (ry-sin) *n.* a highly toxic albumin obtained from castor-oil seeds (*Ricinus communis*) that inhibits protein synthesis and becomes attached to the surface of cells, resulting in gastroenteritis, hepatic congestion and jaundice, and cardiovascular collapse. *See also* immunotoxin.

rickets (rik-its) *n.* a disease of childhood in which the bones do not harden due to a deficiency of vitamin D. *See also* osteomalacia. **renal r.** a type of rickets that is due to impaired kidney function causing bone-forming minerals to be excreted in the urine, which results in softening of the bones.

rickettsiae (ri-ket-si-ee) *pl. n.* (*sing.* **rickettsia**) a group of very small nonmotile spherical or rod-like parasitic bacteria that cannot reproduce outside the bodies of their hosts. They cause such illnesses as rickettsial pox, Rocky Mountain spotted fever, and typhus. Rickettsiae infect arthropods (ticks, mites, etc.), through whom they can be transmitted to humans. —**rickettsial** (ri-ket-si-ăl) *adj.*

rickettsial pox *n.* a disease of mice caused by the microorganism *Rickettsia akari* and transmitted to humans by mites: it produces chills, fever, muscular pain, and a rash similar to that of chickenpox. *See also* typhus.

ridge (rij) *n.* **1.** (in anatomy) a crest or a long narrow protuberance, e.g. on a bone. **2.** (in dental anatomy) *see* alveolus.

Riedel's struma (reed-ĕlz) *n.* a rare fibrosing destructive disorder of the thyroid gland that may spread to adjacent tissues and obstruct the airway. It is sometimes associated with fibrosis in other parts of the body, such as the bile duct or retroperitoneal fibrosis. [B. M. C. L. Riedel (1846–1916), German surgeon]

rifampicin (rif-am-pi-sin) n. an antibiotic administered by mouth to treat various infections, particularly tuberculosis. Trade names: **Rifadin, Rimactane**.

rigidity (ri-jid-iti) n. (in neurology) resistance to the passive movement of a limb that persists throughout its range. It is a symptom of parkinsonism. *Compare* spasticity.

rigor (ry-ger) n. an abrupt attack of shivering and a sensation of coldness, accompanied by a rapid rise in body temperature. This often marks the onset of a fever and may be followed by a feeling of heat, with copious sweating. *r. mortis* the stiffening of a body that occurs within some eight hours of death, due to chemical changes in muscle tissue. It starts to disappear after about 24 hours.

riluzole (ril-yoo-zohl) n. a drug used to prolong the lives of patients with amyotrophic lateral sclerosis. It is administered by mouth. Trade name: **Rilutek**.

rima (ry-mă) n. (in anatomy) a cleft. *r. glottidis* the space between the vocal folds.

ring (ring) n. (in anatomy) *see* annulus.

ring block n. a circumferential ring of local anaesthetic solution used to block the nerves of a digit for purposes of minor surgery (*see* nerve block). Precautions are necessary to

avoid vascular damage leading to gangrene.

Ringer's solution (Ringer's mixture) (ring-erz) n. a clear colourless physiological solution of sodium chloride, potassium chloride, and calcium chloride prepared with recently boiled pure water. [S. Ringer (1835–1910), British physiologist]

ringworm (ring-werm) n. *see* tinea.

Rinne's test (rin-iz) n. a test to determine whether deafness is conductive or sensorineural. A vibrating tuning fork is held first in the air, close to the ear, and then with its base placed on the mastoid process. If the sound conducted by air is heard louder than the sound conducted by bone the test is positive and the deafness sensorineural; a negative result indicates conductive deafness. [H. A. Rinne (1819–68), German otologist]

RIP n. raised intracranial pressure. *See* intracranial (pressure).

risk factor (risk) n. an attribute, such as a habit (e.g. cigarette smoking) or exposure to some environmental hazard, that leads the individual concerned to have a greater likelihood of developing an illness. The relationship is one of probability and as such can be distinguished from a causal agent.

risperidone (ris-pe-ri-dohn) n. an atypical antipsychotic drug used in the treatment of schizophrenia and other psychoses in patients unresponsive to conventional antipsychotics. Side-effects are fewer and less severe than those of conventional antipsychotics. Trade name: **Risperdal**.

risus sardonicus (ry-sŭs sar-don-ik-ŭs) *n.* an abnormal grinning expression resulting from involuntary prolonged contraction of facial muscles, as seen in tetanus.

Ritter's disease (rit-erz) *n. see* staphylococcal scalded skin syndrome. [G. Ritter von Rittershain (1820–83), German physician]

rituximab (rit-uks-i-mab) *n.* a monoclonal antibody administered by intravenous infusion to treat some types of non-Hodgkin's lymphoma that have not responded to standard chemotherapy. Trade name: **Mabthera**.

rivastigmine (ry-vă-stig-meen) *n.* see acetylcholinesterase inhibitor.

river blindness *n. see* onchocerciasis.

RMN *n.* registered mental nurse: see nurse.

RN *n.* registered nurse: see nurse.

RNA (ribonucleic acid) *n.* a nucleic acid, occurring in the nucleus and cytoplasm of cells, that is concerned with synthesis of proteins (*see* messenger RNA, ribosome, transfer RNA, translation). In some viruses RNA is the genetic material.

RNMH *n.* registered nurse for the mentally handicapped: see nurse.

Rocky Mountain spotted fever (spotted fever, tick fever) *n.* a disease of rodents and other small mammals in the USA caused by the microorganism *Rickettsia rickettsii* and transmitted to humans by ticks. Symptoms include fever, muscle pains, and a profuse reddish rash like that of measles. Treatment with tetracycline or chloramphenicol is effective. *See also* typhus.

rod (rod) *n.* one of the two types of light-sensitive cells in the retina of the eye (*compare* cone). Rods are

necessary for seeing in dim light. They contain the pigment rhodopsin, which is bleached in the light and regenerated in the dark. When all the pigment is bleached (i.e. in bright light) the rods no longer function. *See also* dark adaptation, light adaptation.

rodent ulcer (roh-děnt) *n. see* basal cell carcinoma.

roentgen (ront-gĕn) *n.* a unit of exposure dose of X- or gamma-radiation.

rofecoxib (rof-i-koks-ib) *n.* an anti-inflammatory drug (*see* COX-2 inhibitor) that is taken by mouth in the treatment of osteoarthritis. Trade name: **Vioxx**.

role playing (rohl-play-ing) *n.* acting out another person's expected behaviour, usually in a contrived situation, in order to understand that person better. It is used in family psychotherapy, in teaching social skills to patients, and also in the training of psychiatric (and other) staff.

ROM *n. see* range of movement.

Romanowsky stains (roh-mă-nof-ski) *pl. n.* a group of stains used for microscopical examination of blood cells, consisting of variable mixtures of thiazine dyes with eosin. [D. L. Romanowsky (1861–1921), Russian physician]

Romberg's sign (rom-bergz) *n.* a finding on examination suggesting a sensory disorder affecting those nerves that transmit information to the brain about the position of the limbs and joints and the tension in the muscles. The patient is unable to maintain an upright posture with the eyes closed. [M. Romberg (1795–1873), German neurologist]

rongeur (rawn-*zher*) *n.* powerful biting forceps for cutting tissue, particularly bone.

root (root) *n.* **1.** (in neurology) a bundle of nerve fibres at its emergence from the spinal cord. **2.** (in dentistry) the part of a tooth that is not covered by enamel and is normally attached to the alveolar bone by periodontal fibres. *r. canal treatment* the procedure of removing the remnants of the pulp of a tooth, cleaning and shaping the canal inside the tooth, and filling the root canal. **3.** the origin of any structure, i.e. the point at which it diverges from another structure. Anatomical name: **radix**.

root end resection *n. see* apicectomy.

rooting reflex (root-ing) *n.* a primitive reflex present in newborn babies: if the cheek is stroked near the mouth, the infant will turn its head to the same side to suckle.

Roper, Logan, and Tierney model (roh-per loh-găn teer-ni) *n.* a model for nursing that emphasizes the importance of the patient's ability to perform activities of daily living. Individuals are seen as being engaged in various activities of living throughout their lifespan; during their lives they will fluctuate between total independence and total dependence, according to age, circumstance, and health status. Nursing should provide assistance with these activities when needed. *See also* nursing models. [N. Roper, W. Logan, and A. Tierney (20th century), British nurse theorists]

ropinirole (roh-pin-i-rohl) *n.* a dopamine receptor agonist used to treat Parkinson's disease, either alone or in conjunction with levodopa. It is administered by mouth. Trade name: **Requip**.

Rorschach test (ror-shahk) *n.* a test to measure aspects of personality, consisting of ten inkblots in colour and black and white. The responses to the different inkblots are used to derive hypotheses about the subject. [H. Rorschach (1884–1922), Swiss psychiatrist]

rosacea (roh-zay-shiă) *n.* a chronic inflammatory disease of the face in which the skin becomes abnormally flushed. The disease occurs in both sexes and at all ages but is most common in women in their thirties.

roseola (roseola infantum, exanthem subitum) (roh-zee-ŏ-lă) *n.* a condition of young children in which a fever lasting for three or four days is followed by a rose-coloured rash that fades after two days. It is caused by human herpesvirus 6.

rostrum (ros-trŭm) *n.* (*pl.* **rostra**) (in anatomy) a beaklike projection, such as that on the sphenoid bone. —**rostral** *adj.*

rotator (roh-tay-ter) *n.* a muscle that brings about rotation of a part.

rotavirus (roh-tă-vy-rus) *n.* any member of a genus of viruses that occur in birds and mammals and cause diarrhoea (often severe) in children. The viruses are excreted in the faeces of infected individuals and are usually transmitted in food prepared with unwashed hands.

Rothera's test (roth-er-ăz) *n.* a method of testing urine for the presence of acetone or acetoacetic acid – a sign of diabetes mellitus. [A. C. H. Rothera (1880–1915), Australian biochemist]

Roth spot (roht) *n.* a pale area surrounded by haemorrhage sometimes seen in the retina of those who have bacterial endocarditis, septicaemia, or leukaemia. [M. Roth (1839–1915), Swiss physician]

roughage (ruf-ij) *n. see* dietary fibre.

rouleau (roo-loh) *n.* (*pl.* **rouleaux**) a cylindrical structure in the blood formed from several red blood cells piled one upon the other and adhering by their rims.

round ligaments (rownd) *pl. n.* the fibromuscular bands that pass from the uterus along the broad ligaments to terminate in the labia majora.

round window *n. see* fenestra (rotunda).

roundworm (rownd-werm) *n. see* nematode.

Rovsing's sign (rov-singz) *n.* pain in the right iliac fossa induced by pressure on the left iliac fossa: a sign of acute appendicitis. [N. T. Rovsing 1868–1927), Danish surgeon]

Roy's model (roiz) *n.* a model for nursing based on the assumption that individuals are constantly adapting to changes in their environment. Adaptive responses to environmental stimuli are by means of innate or acquired mechanisms and work within the modes of physiological function, the concept of 'self', role function, and interdependence. Nursing should aim to promote and support these adaptive responses. *See also* nursing models. [C. Roy (1939–   ), US nurse theorist]

RPE *n.* retinal pigment epithelium. *See* retina.

-rrhagia (-rrhage) *suffix denoting* excessive or abnormal flow or discharge from an organ or part.

-rrhaphy *suffix denoting* surgical sewing; suturing.

-rrhexis *suffix denoting* splitting or rupture of a part.

-rrhoea *suffix denoting* a flow or discharge from an organ or part.

RSCN *n.* registered sick children's nurse: *see* nurse.

RSI *n. see* repetitive strain injury.

RSV *n. see* respiratory syncytial virus.

RTA *n.* road-traffic accident.

rubefacient (roo-bi-fay-shĕnt) *n.* an agent that causes reddening and warming of the skin. Rubefacients are often used as counterirritants for the relief of muscular pain.

rubella (roo-bel-ă) *n. see* German measles.

rubeola (roo-bee-ŏ-lă) *n. see* measles.

rubidium-81 (roo-bid-iŭm) *n.* an artificial radioactive isotope, with a half-life of about four hours, that decays into krypton-81m, emitting radiations. It is used in ventilation-perfusion scanning.

rubor (roo-ber) *n.* redness: one of the four classical signs of inflammation in a tissue. *See also* calor, dolor, tumor.

ruga (roo-gă) *n.* (*pl.* **rugae**) a fold or crease, especially one of the folds of mucous membrane that line the stomach.

rule of nines (rool nynz) *n.* a method for quickly assessing the area of the body covered by burns in order to assist calculation of the amount of intravenous fluid to be given. The body is divided into areas of skin comprising approximately 9% each of the total body surface. These are as follows: each arm = 9%, the head = 9%, each leg = 18%, the back of the torso = 18%, the front of the torso = 18%, with the external genitalia making up the final 1%.

rumination (roo-mi-nay-shŏn) *n.* (in psychiatry) an obsessional type of thinking in which the same thoughts or themes are experienced repetitively. The thoughts are irrational and resisted by the patient.

rupture (rup-cher) **1.** *n. see* hernia. **2.** *n.* the bursting apart or open of an organ or tissue; for example, the splitting of the membranes enclosing an infant during childbirth. **3.** *vb.* (of tissues, etc.) to burst apart or open.

Russell-Silver syndrome (rus-ĕl sil-ver) *n.* a congenital condition characterized by short stature, a triangular face with a small mandible (lower jaw), and asymmetry of the body. [A. Russell (20th century), British pathologist; H. K. Silver (1918–), US paediatrician]

Russell traction *n.* a form of traction used to align a fractured femur. The lower leg is supported in a sling just below the knee and pulling forces are exerted upwards and longitudinally by means of pulleys and weights. [R. H. Russell (1860–1933), Australian surgeon]

RV *n. see* residual volume.

RVF *n.* right ventricular failure. *See* heart failure.

Ryle's tube (rylz) *n.* a thin flexible tube of rubber or plastic, which is inserted into the stomach through the mouth or nose of a patient and is used for withdrawing fluid from the stomach or for giving a test meal. [J. A. Ryle (1889–1950), British physician]

Ss

SA *n. see* (sinus) arrhythmia.

Sabin vaccine (say-bin) *n.* an oral vaccine against poliomyelitis. [A. B. Sabin 1906–93), US bacteriologist]

sac (sak) *n.* a pouch or baglike structure. Sacs can enclose natural cavities in the body, e.g. in the lungs (*see* alveolus), or they can be pathological, as in a hernia.

saccades (sa-kah-deez) *pl. n.* voluntary rapid movements of the eyes, usually when changing the point of fixation on an object (e.g. when reading).

sacchar- (saccharo-) *prefix denoting* sugar.

saccharide (sak-eryd) *n.* a carbohydrate. *See also* disaccharide, monosaccharide, polysaccharide.

saccharine (sak-er-een) *n.* a sweetening agent. Saccharine is 400 times as sweet as sugar and has no energy content. It is very useful as a sweetener in diabetic and low-calorie foods.

Saccharomyces (sak-er-oh-my-seez) *n. see* yeast.

sacculated (sak-yoo-layt-id) *adj.* pursed out with small pouches or sacs.

saccule (sacculus) (sak-yool) *n.* the smaller of the two membranous sacs within the vestibule of the ear. It contains a macula, which responds to gravity and relays information to the brain about the position of the head.

sacralization (say-krä-ly-zay-shŏn) *n.* abnormal fusion of the fifth lumbar vertebra with the sacrum.

sacral nerves (say-krăl) *pl. n.* the five pairs of spinal nerves that emerge from the spinal column in the sacrum. The nerves carry sensory and motor fibres from the upper and lower leg and from the anal and genital regions.

sacral vertebrae *pl. n. see* sacrum.

sacro- *prefix denoting* the sacrum.

sacrococcygeal (say-kroh-kok-sij-iăl) *adj.* relating to or between the sacrum and the coccyx.

sacroiliac (say-kroh-il-i-ak) *adj.* relating to the sacrum and the ilium.

sacroiliitis (say-kroh-il-i-I-tis) *n.* inflammation of the sacroiliac joint. Involvement of both joints is a common feature of ankylosing spondylitis and associated rheumatic diseases. The resultant low back pain and stiffness may be alleviated by rest and use of anti-inflammatory analgesics.

sacrum (say-krŭm) *n.* (*pl. sacra*) a curved triangular element of the backbone consisting of five fused vertebrae (*sacral vertebrae*). It articulates with the last lumbar vertebra above, the coccyx below, and the hip bones laterally. *See also* vertebra. —**sacral** *adj.*

SAD (seasonal affective disorder) (sad) *n.* a disorder in which the mood of the affected person changes according to the season of the year. Typically, with the onset of winter, there is depression, general slowing of mind and body, excessive sleeping, and overeating. These symptoms resolve with the coming of spring and are also relieved by phototherapy. There is evidence that mood is related to light, which suppresses the release of the hormone melatonin from the pineal gland, but the mechanism by which light acts as an antidepressant is unclear.

saddle-nose (sa-d'l-nohz) *n.* flattening of the bridge of the nose, such as may occur in congenital syphilis.

sadism (say-dizm) *n.* sexual excitement in response to inflicting pain upon other people. *See also* masochism, sexual deviation. —**sadist** *n.* —**sadistic** (să-dis-tik) *adj.*

safe period (sayf) *n. see* rhythm method.

sagittal (saj-it'l) *adj.* describing the dorsoventral plane that extends down the long axis of the body, dividing it into right and left halves. *s. suture* the immovable joint between the two parietal bones of the skull.

SAH *n. see* subarachnoid haemorrhage.

salaam attacks (să-lahm) *pl. n. see* infantile (spasms).

salbutamol (sal-bew-tă-mol) *n.* a drug that stimulates beta-adrenergic receptors (*see* sympathomimetic). It is administered by mouth, injection, or inhalation as a bronchodilator to relieve asthma, chronic bronchitis, and emphysema. Trade names: **Aerolin, Airomir, Asmasal, Ventolin.**

salicylate (să-lis-i-layt) *n.* a salt of salicylic acid. *See* methyl salicylate.

salicylic acid (sal-i-sil-ik) *n.* a drug that causes the skin to peel and de-

stroys bacteria and fungi. It is applied to the skin to treat ulcers, dandruff, eczema, psoriasis, warts, and corns.

salicylism (sal-i-sil-izm) *n.* poisoning due to an overdose of aspirin or other salicylate-containing compounds. The main symptoms are headache, dizziness, tinnitus, disturbances of vision, and vomiting.

saline (normal saline) (say-lyn) *n.* a solution containing 0.9% sodium chloride. Saline may be used clinically as a diluent for drugs administered by injection and as a plasma substitute.

saliva (să-ly-vă) *n.* the alkaline liquid secreted by the salivary glands and the mucous membrane of the mouth. Its principal constituents are water and mucus, which keep the mouth moist and lubricate food, and enzymes (e.g. amylase) that begin the digestion of starch. *See also* dry mouth. —**salivary** (să-ly-ver-i) *adj.*

salivary gland *n.* a gland that produces saliva. There are three pairs of salivary glands: the parotid

parotid gland

parotid duct (Stensen's duct)

tongue

sublingual gland

submandibular gland

Salivary glands

glands, sublingual glands, and submandibular glands (see illustration).

salivary stone *n. see* sialolith.

salivation (sal-i-vay-shŏn) *n.* the secretion of saliva by the salivary glands of the mouth, increased in response to the chewing action of the jaws or to the thought, taste, smell, or sight of food. *See also* ptyalism.

Salk vaccine (sawlk) *n.* a vaccine against poliomyelitis. It is administered by injection. [J. E. Salk (1914–95), US bacteriologist]

salmeterol (sal-mee-ter-ol) *n.* a sympathomimetic drug used as a bronchodilator to treat severe asthma. It is administered by metered-dose aerosol inhaler. Trade name: **Serevent.**

Salmonella (sal-mŏ-nel-ă) *n.* a genus of Gram-negative motile rod-like bacteria that inhabit the intestines of animals and humans. Certain species cause such diseases as food poisoning, gastroenteritis, and septicaemia. *S. paratyphi* a species that causes paratyphoid fever. *S. typhi* a species that causes typhoid fever.

salmonellosis (sal-mŏ-nel-oh-sis) *n.* an infestation of the digestive system by bacteria of the genus *Salmonella. See also* food poisoning.

salping- (salpingo-) *prefix denoting* **1.** the Fallopian tube. **2.** the auditory canal (meatus).

salpingectomy (sal-pin-jek-tŏmi) *n.* the surgical removal of a Fallopian tube. The operation involving both tubes is a permanent and completely effective method of sterilization.

salpingitis (sal-pin-jy-tis) *n.* in-

flammation of a tube, most commonly of one or both of the Fallopian tubes caused by bacterial infection spreading from the vagina or uterus or carried in the blood. *acute s.* salpingitis in which there is sharp pain in the lower abdomen. The infection may spread to the peritoneum (*see* peritonitis); in severe cases the tubes may become blocked with scar tissue.

salpingography (sal-ping-og-răfi) *n.* radiography of one or both Fallopian tubes after a radiopaque substance has been introduced into them via an injection into the uterus. *standardized selective s.* salpingography combined with tubal catheterization, which enables occluded tubes to be restored to patency.

salpingolysis (sal-ping-ol-i-sis) *n.* a surgical operation carried out to restore patency to blocked Fallopian tubes; it involves the division and removal of adhesions around the ovarian ends of the tubes.

salpingo-oophorectomy (sal-ping-oh-oh-ŏ-fŏ-rek-tŏmi) *n.* surgical removal of a Fallopian tube and the ovary associated with it.

salpingo-oophoritis (sal-ping-oh-oh-ŏ-fŏ-ry-tis) *n.* inflammation of a Fallopian tube and an ovary.

salpingostomy (sal-ping-ost-ŏmi) *n.* the surgical creation of an artificial opening in a blocked Fallopian tube in order to restore its patency.

salpinx (sal-pinks) *n.* (in anatomy) a tube, especially a Fallopian tube or the external auditory meatus.

salt (sawlt) *n.* (in chemistry) a compound formed when the hydrogen in an acid is replaced by a metal. An acid and a base react together to form a salt and water. *common s. see* sodium chloride. *s. depletion* excessive loss of sodium chloride from the body. This may result from sweating, persistent vomiting or diarrhoea, or loss of fluid in wounds. The main symptoms are muscular weakness and cramps.

salvage procedure (sal-vij) *n.* surgical measures to palliate the worst effects of a tumour but with no aim to effect a cure.

sanatorium (san-ă-tor-iŭm) *n.* **1.** a hospital or institution for the rehabilitation and convalescence of patients of any kind. **2.** an institution for patients who have suffered from pulmonary tuberculosis.

sandfly fever (sand-fly) *n.* a viral influenza-like disease transmitted to humans by the bite of the sandfly *Phlebotomus papatasii* Sandfly fever occurs principally in countries surrounding the Persian Gulf and the tropical Mediterranean.

sandwich therapy (sand-wich) *n.* a combination of treatments in which one type of therapy (e.g. a surgical operation) is 'sandwiched' between exposures to another treatment (e.g. pre- and postoperative radiotherapy). *See also* combined therapy.

sangui- (**sanguino-**) *prefix denoting* blood.

sanguineous (sang-win-iŭs) *adj.* **1.** containing, stained, or covered with blood. **2.** (of tissues) containing more than the normal quantity of blood.

sanies (say-ni-eez) *n.* a foul-smelling watery discharge from a wound or ulcer, containing serum, blood, and pus.

SANS *n. see* Schedule for Assessment of Negative Symptoms.

saphena (să-fee-nă) *n. see* saphenous vein.

saphena varix *n.* an abnormal dilatation of the terminal section of the long saphenous vein in the groin.

saphenous nerve (să-fee-nŭs) *n.* a large branch of the femoral nerve that supplies the skin from the knee to below the ankle with sensory nerves.

saphenous vein (saphena) *n.* either of two superficial veins of the leg, draining blood from the foot. *long s. v.* the longest vein in the body, running from the foot to the groin. *short s. v.* the vein that runs up the back of the calf.

saponity (să-pon-i-fy) *vb.* (in chemistry) to hydrolyse an ester with a hydroxide, especially a fat with a hydroxide to form a soap. —**saponification** *n.*

sapr- (**sapro-**) *prefix denoting* **1.** putrefaction. **2.** decaying matter.

sapraemia (sap-ree-miă) *n.* blood poisoning by toxins of saprophytic bacteria. *Compare* pyaemia, septicaemia, toxaemia.

saprophyte (sap-roh-fyt) *n.* any free-living organism that lives and feeds on the dead and putrefying tissues of animals or plants. *Compare* parasite. —**saprophytic** (sap-roh-fit-ik) *adj.*

sarc- (**sarco-**) *prefix denoting* **1.** flesh or fleshy tissue. **2.** muscle.

sarcoid (sar-koid) **1.** *adj.* fleshy. **2.** *n.* a fleshy tumour.

sarcoidosis (Boeck's disease) (sar-koid-oh-sis) *n.* a chronic disorder of unknown cause in which the lymph nodes in many parts of the body are enlarged and granulomas develop in the lungs, liver, and spleen. The skin, nervous system, eyes, and salivary glands are also commonly affected, and the condition has features similar to tuberculosis.

sarcolemma (sar-koh-**lem**-ă) n. the cell membrane that encloses a muscle cell (muscle fibre).

sarcoma (sar-koh-mă) n. any cancer of connective tissue. These tumours may occur in any part of the body; they arise in fibrous tissue, muscle, fat, bone, cartilage, synovium, blood and lymphatic vessels, and various other tissues. *See also* chondrosarcoma, fibrosarcoma, leiomyosarcoma, liposarcoma, lymphangiosarcoma, osteosarcoma, rhabdomyosarcoma. —**sarcomatous** *adj.*

sarcomatosis (sar-koh-mă-toh-sis) n. sarcoma that has spread widely throughout the body, most commonly through the bloodstream.

sarcoplasm (myoplasm) (sar-koh-plazm) n. the cytoplasm of muscle cells.

Sarcoptes (sar-kop-teez) n. a genus of small oval mites. *S. scabiei* the scabies mite. The female tunnels into the skin, where it lays its eggs. The presence of the mites causes severe irritation, which eventually leads to scabies.

sartorius (sar-tor-iŭs) n. a narrow ribbon-like muscle at the front of the thigh. The longest muscle in the body, the sartorius flexes the leg on the thigh and the thigh on the abdomen.

SAS n. sleep apnoea syndrome (*see* (obstructive) sleep apnoea).

saucerization (saw-ser-I-zay-shŏn) n. **1.** an operation in which tissue is cut away from a wound to form a saucer-like depression. It is carried out to facilitate healing of injuries or disorders in which bone is infected. **2.** the concave appearance of the upper surface of a vertebra that has been fractured by compression.

Sayre's jacket (say-erz) n. a plaster of Paris cast used to support the backbone when the vertebrae have been severely damaged by disease, such as tuberculosis. [L. A. Sayre (1820–1900), US surgeon]

SBE n. *see* subacute bacterial endocarditis.

SBS n. *see* short bowel syndrome.

scab (skab) n. a hard crust of dried blood, serum, or pus that develops over a sore, cut, or scratch.

scabicide (skay-bi-syd) n. a drug that kills the mites causing scabies.

scabies (skay-beez) n. a skin infection caused by the mite *Sarcoptes scabiei*. Scabies is typified by severe itching, red papules, and often secondary infection. The mites pass from person to person by close contact. Commonly infected areas are the penis, nipples, and the finger webs. Treatment is by application of a scabicide, usually permethrin or malathion, to all areas of the body from the neck down; benzyl benzoate may be used but is more irritant.

scala (skay-lă) n. one of the spiral canals of the cochlea.

scald (skawld) n. a burn produced by a hot liquid or vapour, such as boiling water or steam.

scale (skayl) **1.** n. any of the flakes of dead epidermal cells shed from the skin. **2.** *vb.* to scrape deposits of calculus from the teeth (*see* scaler).

scalenus (skay-leen-ŭs) *n.* one of four paired muscles of the neck (*s. anterior, medius, minimus,* and *posterior*). They are responsible for raising the first and second ribs in inspiration and for bending the neck forward and to either side.

scalenus syndrome (thoracic outlet syndrome) *n.* the group of symptoms caused by compression of the subclavian artery and the lower roots of the brachial plexus against the outlet of the upper thoracic vertebrae. Loss of sensation and wasting may be found in the affected arm, which may also be painful.

scaler (skayl-er) *n.* an instrument for removing calculus from the teeth. It may be a hand instrument or one energized by rapid ultrasonic vibrations.

scalp (skalp) *n.* the skin that covers the cranium and is itself covered with hair.

scalpel (skal-pĕl) *n.* a small pointed surgical knife with a straight handle and usually detachable disposable blades of various shapes.

scan (skan) **1.** *n.* examination of the body or a part of the body using ultrasonography, computerized tomography (CT), magnetic resonance imaging (MRI), or scintigraphy. **2.** *n.* the image obtained from such an examination. **3.** *vb.* to examine the body using any of these techniques.

scanning speech (skan-ing) *n.* a disorder of articulation in which the syllables are inappropriately separated and equally stressed. It is caused by cerebellar disease.

scaphocephaly (skaf-oh-sef-ăli) *n.*

an abnormally long and narrow skull due to premature closure of the sagittal suture. —**scaphocephalic** (skaf-oh-si-fal-ik) *adj.*

scaphoid bone (skay-foid) *n.* a boat-shaped bone of the wrist (*see* carpus). It articulates with the trapezium and trapezoid bones in front, with the radius behind, and with the capitate and lunate medially. It is commonly injured by falls; for example, a *scaphoid fracture* is usually caused by a fall onto the outstretched hand.

scapul- (scapulo-) *prefix denoting* the scapula.

scapula (skap-yoo-lă) *n.* (*pl.* **scapulas** or **scapulae**) the shoulder blade: a triangular bone, a pair of which form the back part of the shoulder girdle. —**scapular** *adj.*

scar *n.* a permanent mark left after wound healing. *hypertrophic s.* an abnormal raised scar that tends to settle after a year or so, as distinct from a keloid, which is not only permanent but tends to extend beyond the original wound.

scarification (ska-rifi-kay-shŏn) *n.* the process of making a series of shallow cuts or scratches in the skin to allow a substance, such as a droplet of smallpox vaccine, to penetrate the body.

scarlatina (skar-lă-tee-nă) *n. see* scarlet fever.

scarlet fever (skar-lit) *n.* a highly contagious disease caused by toxin-producing bacteria of the genus *Streptococcus.* The symptoms include fever, tonsillitis, and a widespread scarlet rash; the tongue is also affected, becoming bright red. Treatment with antibiotics reduces the risk of secondary complications, such as ear and kidney inflammation. Medical name: **scarlatina**. *Compare* German measles.

Scarpa's triangle (skar-pǎz) *n. see* femoral (triangle). [A. Scarpa (1747–1832), Italian anatomist and surgeon]

scat- (scato-) *prefix denoting* faeces.

SCBU *n. see* special care baby unit.

SCC *n. see* squamous cell carcinoma.

Schedule for Assessment of Negative Symptoms (SANS) (shed-yool) *n.* an assessment tool designed to identify 20 negative symptoms of schizophrenia (apathy, social withdrawal, lack of spontaneity, etc.), which are numerically graded on a scale from 0 to 5.

Scheuermann's disease (shoi-er-manz) *n.* a form of osteochondritis affecting the vertebrae. It develops in adolescents and causes spinal pain and outward curvature of the spine (kyphosis). [H. W. Scheuermann (1877–1960), Danish surgeon]

Schick test (shik) *n.* a test to determine whether a person is susceptible to diphtheria. A small quantity of diphtheria toxin is injected under the skin; a patch of reddening and swelling shows that the person has no immunity. [B. Schick (1877–1967), US paediatrician]

Schilling test (shil-ing) *n.* a test used to assess a patient's capacity to absorb vitamin B_{12} from the bowel. Radioactive vitamin B_{12} is given by mouth and urine collected. A patient with pernicious anaemia will excrete less than 5% of the original dose over a period of 24 hours. [R. F. Schilling (1919–), US physician]

schindylesis (skin-di-lee-sis) *n.* a form of synarthrosis (immovable joint) in which a crest of one bone fits into a groove of another.

-schisis *suffix denoting* a cleft or split.

schisto- *prefix denoting* a fissure; split.

Schistosoma (Bilharzia) (shist-ŏ-soh-mǎ) *n.* a genus of blood flukes, three species of which are important parasites of humans causing the tropical disease schistosomiasis.

schistosomiasis (bilharziasis) (shist-ŏ-soh-**my**-ǎ-sis) *n.* a tropical disease caused by blood flukes of the genus *Schistosoma*. The disease is contracted when larvae penetrate the skin of anyone bathing in infected water. Adult flukes eventually settle in the blood vessels of the intestine (*S. mansoni* and *S. japonicum*) or bladder (*S. haematobium*); the release of their spiked eggs causes anaemia, inflammation, and the formation of scar tissue. Additional symptoms include diarrhoea, dysentery, cirrhosis of the liver, haematuria, and cystitis. The disease is treated with praziquantel.

schiz- (schizo-) *prefix denoting* a split or division.

schizoid personality (skits-oid) *n.* a personality characterized by solitariness, emotional coldness to others, inability to experience pleasure, lack of response to praise and criticism, withdrawal into a fantasy world, excessive introspection, and eccentricity of behaviour. *See* personality disorder.

schizophrenia (skits-ŏ-freen-iǎ) *n.* a severe mental disorder (or group of disorders) characterized by a disintegration of the process of thinking, of contact with reality, and of emotional responsiveness. The patient suffers from hallucinations and delusions and feels that his thoughts, sensations, and actions are controlled by, or shared with, others. Treatment is with phenothiazines and other antipsychotic drugs and with vigorous psychological and social management and rehabilitation. *catatonic s.* schizophrenia in which there are marked motor disturbances; this form is now rare. *hebephrenic s. see* hebephrenia. *paranoid s.* schizophrenia characterized by prominent delusions. *simple s.* schizophrenia in which increasing social withdrawal and personal ineffectiveness are the major changes. —**schizophrenic** (skits-ŏ-fren-ik) *adj.*

Schizophrenia Nursing Assessment Protocol (SNAP) *n.* a tool used by mental health nurses to assess major issues for patients with mental health problems and their families.

Schlatter's disease (shlat-erz) *n. see* Osgood-Schlatter disease.

Schlemm's canal (shlemz) *n.* a channel in the eye, at the junction of the cornea and the sclera, through which the aqueous humour drains. [F. Schlemm (1795–1858), German anatomist]

Schmidt's syndrome (sh'mitz) *n.* the autoimmune destruction of the thyroid, the adrenals, and the beta cells of the islets of Langerhans, causing type 1 diabetes mellitus. It is often associated with failure of the ovaries (causing an early menopause), parathyroids, and the parietal cells of the gastric glands (causing pernicious anaemia). [M.

B. Schmidt (1863– 1949), German physician]

Schönlein-Henoch purpura *n. see* Henoch-Schönlein purpura.

school health service (skool) *n.* (in Britain) a service concerned with the early detection of physical and emotional abnormalities in schoolchildren and their subsequent treatment and surveillance.

school nurse *n.* a registered nurse who has undertaken a course in the health care of school-age children. A member of the school health service, a school nurse is responsible for monitoring growth and development, conducting routine examinations, and treating minor ailments.

Schwann cells (shwon) *pl. n.* the cells that lay down the myelin sheath around the axon of a medullated nerve fibre. [T. Schwann (1810–82), German anatomist and physiologist]

Schwannoma (shwon-oh-mǎ) *n. see* neurofibroma.

Schwartze's operation (shvarts-ĕz) *n.* an operation to open and drain the air cells in the mastoid in severe cases of mastoiditis. [H. H. R. Schwartze (1837–1910), German otologist]

sciatica (sy-at-ik-ǎ) *n.* pain felt down the back and outer side of the thigh, leg, and foot. It is usually caused by degeneration of an intervertebral disc, which protrudes laterally to compress a spinal nerve root. The onset may be sudden, brought on by an awkward lifting or twisting movement.

sciatic nerve (sy-at-ik) *n.* the major nerve of the leg and the nerve with the largest diameter. It runs down behind the thigh from the lower end of the spine.

SCID *n. see* severe combined immune deficiency.

scintigram (sin-ti-gram) *n.* a diagram showing the distribution of radioactive tracer in a part of the body, produced by recording the flashes of light given off by a scintillator as it is struck by radiation of different intensities. This technique is called *scintigraphy*. By scanning the body, section by section, a 'map' of the radioactivity in various regions is built up, aiding the diagnosis of cancer or other disorders. Such a record is known as a *scinti-scan*.

scintillator (sin-ti-lay-ter) *n.* a substance that produces a fluorescent flash when struck by high-energy radiation, such as beta or gamma rays. A scintillator forms the basis of a gamma camera. *See also* scintigram.

scintiscan (sin-ti-skan) *n. see* scintigram.

scirrhous (si-rŭs) *adj.* describing carcinomas that are stony hard to the touch. Such a carcinoma is known as a *scirrhus*.

scissor leg (siz-er) *n.* a disability in which one leg becomes permanently crossed over the other as a result of spasticity of its adductor muscles or deformity of the hip. The condition occurs in children with brain damage and in adults after strokes.

scissura (scissure) (si-zhor-ă) *n.* a cleft or splitting, such as the splitting open of tissues when a hernia forms.

scler- (sclero-) *prefix denoting* **1.**

hardening or thickening. **2.** the sclera. **3.** sclerosis.

sclera (sclerotic coat) (skleer-ă) *n.* the white fibrous outer layer of the eyeball. At the front of the eye it becomes the cornea. *See* eye. —**scleral** *adj.*

scleritis (skleer-I-tis) *n.* inflammation of the sclera.

scleroderma (skleer-oh-**der**-mă) *n.* thickening of the skin, either localized (*see* morphoea) or generalized, resulting in waxy ivory-coloured areas. Scleroderma may be an autoimmune disease. Systemic sclerosis is a related multisystem disorder.

scleromalacia (skleer-oh-mă-**lay**-shiă) *n.* thinning of the sclera (white of the eye) as a result of inflammation.

sclerosis (skleer-**oh**-sis) *n.* hardening of tissue, usually due to scarring (fibrosis) after inflammation or to ageing. It can affect the lateral columns of the spinal cord and the medulla of the brain (*amyotrophic lateral s.* (*ALS*) or *Lou Gehrig's disease*), causing progressive muscular paralysis (*see* motor neurone disease). *See also* arteriosclerosis, atherosclerosis, multiple sclerosis, systemic (sclerosis), tuberous (sclerosis).

sclerotherapy (skleer-oh-**th'e**-ră-pi) *n.* treatment of varicose veins by the injection of an irritant solution. This causes thrombophlebitis, which encourages obliteration of the varicose vein by thrombosis and subsequent scarring. Sclerotherapy is also used for treating haemorrhoids and oesophageal varices.

sclerotic (skleer-ot-ik) **1.** (**sclerotic coat**) *n. see* sclera. **2.** *adj.* affected with sclerosis.

sclerotome (skleer-ŏ-tohm) *n.* a surgical knife used in the operation of sclerotomy.

sclerotomy (skleer-ot-ŏmi) *n.* an operation in which an incision is made in the sclera.

scolex (skoh-leks) *n.* (*pl.* **scolices**) the head of a tapeworm. Suckers and/or hooks on the scolex enable the worm to attach itself to the wall of its host's gut.

scoliosis (skoh-li-oh-sis) *n.* lateral (sideways) deviation of the backbone, caused by congenital or acquired abnormalities of the vertebrae, muscles, and nerves. *See also* kyphosis, kyphoscoliosis.

-scope *suffix denoting* an instrument for observing or examination.

scopolamine (skŏ-pol-ă-meen) *n.* *see* hyoscine.

scorbutic (skor-bew-tik) *adj.* affected with scurvy.

scoring system (skor-ing) *n.* any of various methods in which the application of an agreed numerical scale is used as a means of estimating the degree of a clinical situation, e.g. the severity of an injury, the degree of patient recovery, or the extent of malignancy. *See* Glasgow scoring system, Gleason grade, injury scoring system.

scoto- *prefix denoting* darkness.

scotoma (skoh-toh-mă) *n.* (*pl.* **scotomata**) a small area of abnormally less sensitive or absent vision in the visual field, surrounded by normal sight.

scotometer (skoh-tom-it-er) *n.* an instrument used for mapping defects in the visual field. *See also* perimeter.

scotopic (skoh-top-ik) *adj.* relating to or describing conditions of poor illumination. *s. vision* vision in dim light in which the rods of the retina are involved (*see* dark adaptation).

screening test (skreen-ing) *n.* a test carried out on a large number of apparently healthy people to separate those who probably have a specified disease from those who do not. Examples are the Guthrie test, cervical smears, and Forrest screening. *See also* genetic screening.

scrofula (skrof-yoo-lă) *n.* tuberculosis of lymph nodes, usually those in the neck, causing the formation of abscesses. Treatment with antituberculous drugs is effective. The disease, which is now rare, most commonly affects young children. —**scrofulous** *adj.*

scrofuloderma (skrof-yoo-loh-der-mă) *n.* tuberculosis of the skin in which the skin breaks down over suppurating tuberculous glands, with the formation of irregular-shaped ulcers with blue-tinged edges. Treatment is with antituberculous drugs.

scrototomy (skroh-tot-ŏmi) *n.* an operation in which the scrotum is surgically explored, usually undertaken to investigate patients with probable obstructive azoospermia.

scrotum (skroh-tŭm) *n.* the paired sac that holds the testes and epididymides outside the abdominal cavity. Its function is to allow the production and storage of spermatozoa to occur at a lower temperature than that of the abdomen. —**scrotal** *adj.*

scrub typhus (tsutsugamushi disease) (skrub) *n.* a disease, widely distributed in SE Asia, caused by the parasitic microorganism *Rickettsia tsutsugamushi* and transmitted to humans through the bite of mites. Symptoms include headache, chills, high temperature, a red rash, a cough, and delirium. A small ulcer forms at the site of the bite. Scrub typhus is treated with tetracycline antibiotics. *See also* rickettsiae, typhus.

scrum-pox (skrum-poks) *n.* a form of herpes simplex found in rugby players and wrestlers. It is caused by abrasive contact.

scurvy (sker-vi) *n.* a disease that is caused by a deficiency of vitamin C, which in humans cannot be synthesized and must be obtained from fresh fruit and vegetables. The first sign of scurvy is swollen bleeding gums, and a rash of tiny bleeding spots around the hair follicles is characteristic; this may be followed by subcutaneous bleeding. Vitamin C is used both in treatment and to prevent scurvy occurring in those at risk.

scybalum (sib-ă-lŭm) *n.* a lump or mass of hard faeces.

SDH *n. see* (subdural) haematoma.

seasickness (see-sik-nis) *n. see* motion sickness.

seasonal affective disorder (see-zŏ-năl) *n. see* SAD.

seat-belt syndrome (seet-belt) *n.* thoracic injuries that arise from violent contact with a restraining seat belt in motor vehicle accidents occurring at high speeds.

sebaceous cyst (si-bay-shŭs) *n.* **1. (epidermoid cyst, wen)** a pale or flesh-coloured dome-shaped cyst that commonly occurs in adults, especially on the face, neck, or trunk. It is firm, with a central dot, and contains keratin. It is usually removed surgically. **2.** a cyst of the se-

baceous glands occurring in multiple form in a rare inherited condition, *steatocystoma multiplex*.

sebaceous gland *n.* any of the simple or branched glands in the skin that secrete an oily substance, sebum. They open into hair follicles and their secretion is produced by the disintegration of their cells.

seborrhoea (seb-ŏ-ree-ă) *n.* excessive secretion of sebum by the sebaceous glands. The glands are enlarged, especially on the nose and central face. The condition predisposes to acne and is common at puberty. Seborrhoea is sometimes associated with a kind of eczema (seborrhoeic eczema). —**seborrhoeic** *adj.*

sebum (see-bŭm) *n.* the oily substance secreted by the sebaceous glands. Sebum provides a thin film of fat over the skin, which slows the evaporation of water; it also has an antibacterial effect.

secondary care (sek-ŏnd-er-i) *n.* health care provided by medical specialists or hospital staff members for a patient whose primary care was provided by the general practitioner who first diagnosed or treated the patient. Secondary care cannot be accessed directly by patients. For example, a general practitioner who accepts a patient with an unusual skin condition may refer the patient to a dermatologist, who then becomes the source of secondary care. *Compare* tertiary care.

secondary prevention *n.* the avoidance or alleviation of the serious consequences of disease by early detection.

secondary sexual characteristics *pl. n.* the physical characteristics that develop after puberty. In boys they include the growth of facial and pubic hair and the breaking of the voice. In girls they include the growth of pubic hair and the development of the breasts.

second-level nurse (sek-ŏnd levĕl) *n.* a person who, having completed a nursing course, provides nursing care under the direction of a first-level nurse. A second-level nurse participates in the assessment and implementation of nursing care and works in a team with other nurses, medical and paramedical staff, and social workers. *See* enrolled nurse.

second messenger *n.* an organic molecule that acts within a cell to initiate the response to a signal carried by a chemical messenger (e.g. a hormone) that does not itself enter the cell. Examples of second messengers are inositol triphosphate and cyclic AMP.

secretin (si-kree-tin) *n.* a hormone secreted from the duodenum when acidified food leaves the stomach. Secretin stimulates the secretion of relatively enzyme-free alkaline juice by the pancreas and of bile by the liver.

secretion (si-kree-shŏn) *n.* **1.** the process by which a gland isolates constituents of the blood or tissue fluid and chemically alters them to produce a substance that it discharges for use by the body or excretes. **2.** the substance that is produced by a gland.

section (sek-shŏn) **1.** *n.* (in surgery) the act of cutting (the cut or division made is also called a section). **2.** *n.* (in imaging) a three-dimensional reconstruction of a body scan obtained by computerized tomography or magnetic resonance imaging. **3.** *n.* (in microscopy) a thin slice of the specimen to be examined under a microscope. **4.** *vb.* to issue an order for compulsory admission to a psychiatric hospital under the appropriate section of the Mental Health Act.

Section 47 *n.* a section of the National Assistance Act 1948 that enables a local authority to arrange for the compulsory removal to a place of care of a person who is unwilling to go voluntarily from his or her own home. It can be applied to individuals who are suffering from a grave chronic disease, or are physically incapacitated, or are living in insanitary conditions because of old age or infirmity.

security object (si-kewr-iti objĭkt) *n.* a particular item that brings comfort and a sense of security to a young child, often for a number of years. Security objects are usually associated in some way with bed and sleep. There is no reason to suppose that they are in any way undesirable, at any age.

sedation (si-day-shŏn) *n.* the production of a restful state of mind, particularly by the use of drugs (*see* sedative).

sedative (sed-ă-tiv) *n.* a drug that has a calming effect, relieving anxiety and tension. *See also* anxiolytic.

sedimentation rate (sed-i-mentay-shŏn) *n.* the rate at which solid particles sink in a liquid under the influence of gravity. *See also* ESR (erythrocyte sedimentation rate).

segment (seg-mĕnt) *n.* (in anatomy) a portion of a tissue or an organ (e.g. the uterus or the eye), usually distinguishable from other portions by lines of demarcation.

Seidlitz powder (sed-lits) *n.* a mixture of sodium bicarbonate, sodium potassium tartrate, and tartaric acid, taken as a laxative when dissolved in water.

selective serotonin reuptake inhibitor (si-lek-tiv) *n. see* SSRI.

selegiline (sel-ej-i-leen) *n.* a selective MAO inhibitor used in the treatment of parkinsonism. It is administered by mouth. Trade names: **Eldepryl, Zelapar**.

selenium (si-lee-niŭm) *n.* a trace element that has important antioxidant properties. It is also known to be an essential component of the enzyme that catalyses the production of triiodothyronine (T_3) from thyroxine (T_4) in the thyroid gland. Symbol: Se.

selenium sulphide (sul-fyd) *n.* a selenium compound with antifungal properties, used to treat dandruff and scalp infections. It is administered in a shampoo. Trade names: **Lenium, Selsun**.

self-actualization (self-ak-tew-ă-ly-zay-shŏn) *n.* the tendency to realize and fulfil one's maximum potential. *See* Maslow's hierarchy of human needs.

self-care (self-kair) *n.* the practice of activities that are necessary to sustain life and health, normally initiated and carried out by the individual for him- or herself.

self-catheterization (self-kath-it-er-I-zay-shŏn) *n. see* intermittent self-catheterization.

self-inflating bag (self-in-flayt-ing) *n.* a device for delivering emergency artificial ventilation by means of a tight-fitting face mask, a laryngeal mask, or an endotracheal tube. It consists of a stiff plastic bag, which is squeezed to deliver its gas contents into the patient's airway; when the pressure is released, it is reinflated from the atmosphere or an attached oxygen supply.

sella turcica (sel-ă ter-sik-ă) *n.* a depression in the body of the sphenoid bone that encloses the pituitary gland.

semeiology (see-mi-ol-ŏji) *n. see* symptomatology.

semen (seminal fluid) (see-men) *n.* the fluid ejaculated from the penis at sexual climax. Each ejaculate may contain 300–500 million sperms suspended in a fluid secreted by the prostate gland and seminal vesicles with a small contribution from Cowper's glands. —**seminal** (sem-in-ăl) *adj.*

semi- *prefix denoting* half.

semicircular canals (sem-i-ser-kew-ler) *pl. n.* three tubes that form part of the membranous labyrinth of the ear. They are concerned with balance and each canal registers movement in a different plane.

semilunar cartilage (sem-i-loo-ner) *n.* one of a pair of crescent-shaped cartilages in the knee joint situated between the femur and tibia.

semilunar valve *n.* either of the two valves in the heart situated at the origin of the aorta (*aortic valve*) and the pulmonary artery (*pulmonary valve*). Each consists of three flaps (cusps), which maintain the flow of blood in one direction.

seminal analysis *n.* analysis of a specimen of semen, which should be obtained after five days of abstinence from coitus, in order to assess male fertility. It includes determinations of the concentration and motility of the sperm and detection of the presence of abnormal forms of sperm. *See also* sperm count.

seminal vesicle *n.* either of a pair of male accessory sex glands that open into the vas deferens. The seminal vesicles secrete most of the liquid component of semen.

seminiferous tubule (sem-in-if-er-ŭs) *n.* any of the long convoluted tubules that make up the bulk of the testis.

seminoma (sem-in-oh-mă) *n.* a malignant tumour of the testis, appearing as a swelling, often painless, in the scrotum. The best treatment for localized disease is orchidectomy. A similar tumour occurs in the ovary (*see* dysgerminoma).

semipermeable membrane (sem-i-per-mi-ăbŭl) *n.* a membrane that allows the passage of some molecules but not others. Semipermeable membranes are used clinically in haemodialysis.

semiprone (sem-i-prohn) *adj.* describing the position of a patient lying face downwards, but with one or both knees flexed to one side. *Compare* prone, supine.

senescence (si-nes-ĕns) *n.* the condition of ageing, which is often marked by a decrease in physical and mental abilities. —**senescent** *adj.*

Sengstaken tube (sengz-tay-kĕn) *n.* a tube containing a triple lumen and inflatable balloons that is passed down the oesophagus to the stomach to compress bleeding oesophageal varicose veins. [R. W. Sengstaken (1923–), US neurosurgeon]

senile dementia (see-nyl) *n.* loss of the intellectual faculties, often associated with behavioural deterioration, beginning for the first time in old age. *See also* dementia.

senility (sin-il-iti) *n.* the state of physical and mental deterioration that is associated with the ageing process. —**senile** *adj.*

senna (sen-ă) *n.* the dried fruits of certain shrubs of the genus *Cassia*, administered by mouth as a stimulant laxative to relieve constipation. Trade name: **Senokot**.

sensation (sen-say-shŏn) *n.* a feeling: the result of messages from the body's sensory receptors registering in the brain as information about the environment.

sense (sens) *n.* one of the faculties by which the qualities of the external environment are appreciated – sight, hearing, smell, taste, or touch. **s. organ** a collection of specialized cells (receptors), connected to the nervous system, that is capable of responding to a particular stimulus from either outside or inside the body.

sensibility (sen-si-bil-iti) *n.* the ability to be affected by, and respond to, changes in the surroundings. Sensibility is a characteristic of cells of the nervous system.

sensible (sen-sibŭl) *adj.* **1.** perceptible to the senses. **2.** capable of sensibility.

sensitive (sen-sit-iv) *adj.* possessing the ability to respond to a stimulus.

sensitivity (sen-sit-iv-iti) *n.* the degree to which a disease-causing organism responds to treatment by antibiotics or other drugs.

sensitization (sen-si-ty-zay-shŏn)

n. **1.** alteration of the responsiveness of the body to the presence of foreign substances. In the development of an allergy, an individual becomes sensitized to a particular allergen. The phenomena of sensitization are due to the production of antibodies. **2.** (in behaviour therapy) a form of aversion therapy in which anxiety-producing stimuli are associated with the unwanted behaviour.

sensory (sen-ser-i) *adj.* relating to the input division of the nervous system, which carries information from receptors throughout the body towards the brain and spinal cord. *s. cortex* the region of the cerebral cortex responsible for receiving incoming information relayed by sensory nerve pathways from all parts of the body. *s. deprivation* a condition resulting from partial or complete absence of sensory stimuli, leading to confusion and disorientation. *s. nerve see* nerve.

sentinel lymph node (sent-i-nêl) *n.* the first lymph node to show evidence of metastasis of a malignant tumour (e.g. breast cancer) via the lymphatic system. Absence of cancer cells in the sentinel node indicates that more distal lymph nodes will also be free of metastasis.

sepsis (sep-sis) *n.* the putrefactive destruction of tissues by disease-causing bacteria or their toxins.

sept- (septi-) *prefix denoting* **1.** seven. **2. (septo-)** a septum, especially the nasal septum. **3.** sepsis.

septal defect (sep-t'l) *n.* a hole in the partition (septum) between the left and right halves of the heart. This congenital condition is due to an abnormality of heart development in the fetus. It may be found between the two atria (*atrial s. d.*, *ASD*) or between the ventricles (*ventricular s. d.*, *VSD*). A septal defect permits abnormal circulation of blood from the left side of the heart to the right, which results in excessive blood flow through the lungs. Pulmonary hypertension develops and heart failure may occur. Large defects are closed surgically but small defects do not require treatment.

septic (sep-tik) *adj.* relating to or affected with sepsis. *s. arthritis* infection in a joint, which becomes swollen, hot, and tender; movement is painful and very restricted. The infecting organism enters the joint via the bloodstream or through a penetrating injury.

septicaemia (septi-seem-iă) *n.* widespread destruction of tissues due to absorption of disease-causing bacteria or their toxins from the bloodstream. *meningococcal s. see* meningitis. *Compare* pyaemia, sapraemia, toxaemia.

Septrin (sep-trin) *n. see* co-trimoxazole.

septum (sep-tŭm) *n.* (*pl.* **septa**) a partition or dividing wall within an anatomical structure. —**septal** *adj.* —**septate** (sep-tayt) *adj.*

sequela (si-kwee-lă) *n.* (*pl.* **sequelae**) any disorder or pathological condition that results from a preceding disease or accident.

sequestration (see-kwes-tray-shŏn) *n.* **1.** the formation of a sequestrum and its separation from the surrounding tissue. **2.** a separated part of an organ occurring as a developmental anomaly.

sequestrectomy (see-kwes-trek-

tōmi) *n.* surgical removal of a sequestrum.

sequestrum (si-kwes-trŭm) *n.* (*pl.* **sequestra**) a portion of dead bone formed in an infected bone in chronic osteomyelitis. It can cause irritation and the formation of pus, which may discharge through a sinus, and is usually surgically removed.

ser- (sero-) *prefix denoting* **1.** serum. **2.** serous membrane.

serine (se-reen) *n.* see amino acid.

serooonvert (seer-oh-kŏn-vert) *vb.* to produce specific antibodies in response to the presence of an antigen (e.g. a vaccine or a virus). In AIDS patients seroconversion is accompanied by a sore throat, swollen lymph nodes, fever, and aches and pains. —**seroconversion** *n.*

serology (si-rol-ŏji) *n.* the study of blood serum and its constituents, particularly their contribution to the protection of the body against disease. —**serological** *adj.*

seropus (seer-oh-pus) *n.* a mixture of serum and pus, which forms, for example, in infected blisters.

serosa (si-roh-să) *n.* see serous membrane.

serositis (seer-oh-sy-tis) *n.* inflammation of a serous membrane. See polyserositis.

serotherapy (seer-oh-th'e-ră-pi) *n.* the use of serum containing known antibodies (see antiserum) to treat a patient with an infection or to confer temporary passive immunity upon a person at special risk.

serotonin (5-hydroxytryptamine, 5HT) (se-rŏ-toh-nin) *n.* a compound widely distributed in the tissues, particularly in the blood platelets, intestinal wall, and central nervous system. It is thought to play a role in inflammation similar to that of histamine and it is involved in the genesis of a migrainous headache. Serotonin also acts as a neurotransmitter, and its levels in the brain are believed to have an important effect on mood. See also 5HT₁ agonist, SSRI.

serotype (seer-oh-typ) *n.* a category into which material is placed based on its serological activity, particularly in terms of the antigens it contains or the antibodies that may be produced against it.

serous (seer-ŭs) *adj.* **1.** relating to or containing serum. **2.** resembling serum or producing a fluid resembling serum.

serous membrane (serosa) *n.* a smooth transparent membrane lining certain large cavities of the body, such as the abdomen (see peritoneum) and chest (see pleura). The *parietal* portion of the membrane lines the walls of the cavity, and the *visceral* portion covers the organs concerned. The two form a closed sac, the inner surface of which is moistened by a thin fluid derived from blood serum, allowing frictionless movement of organs within their cavities. *Compare* mucous membrane.

serpiginous (ser-pij-in-ŭs) *adj.* describing a creeping or extending skin lesion, especially one with a wavy edge.

serrated (ser-ayt-id) *adj.* having a saw-toothed edge. —**serration** *n.*

sertraline (ser-tră-leen) *n.* an antidepressant drug that acts by prolonging the action of the neurotransmitter serotonin (5-hydroxytryptamine) in the brain (*see* SSRI). It is taken by mouth. Trade name: **Lustral**.

serum (blood serum) (seer-ŭm) *n.* the fluid that separates from clotted blood or blood plasma that is allowed to stand. Serum is essentially similar in composition to plasma but lacks fibrinogen and other substances that are used in the coagulation process. *s. sickness* a reaction that sometimes occurs 7–12 days after injection of a quantity of foreign antigen. Large immune complexes are deposited in the arteries, kidneys, and joints, causing vasculitis, nephritis, and arthritis.

sesamoid bone (ses-ă-moid) *n.* an oval nodule of bone that lies within a tendon and slides over another bony surface. The patella (kneecap) is a sesamoid bone.

sessile (se-syl) *adj.* (of a tumour) attached directly by its base without a stalk.

severe combined immune deficiency (SCID) (sĕ-veer kŏm-bynd) *n.* a rare disorder that usually manifests itself within the first three months of life by severe bacterial, fungal, and viral infection and failure to thrive. It is due to reduced numbers of T- and B-lymphocytes.

Sever's disease (see-verz) *n.* apophysitis caused by pulling at the point of insertion of the Achilles tendon into the calcaneus (heel bone), causing heel pain. [J. W. Sever (20th century), US orthopaedic surgeon]

sexarche (seks-ar-ki) *n.* the age when a person first engages in sexual intercourse.

sex chromatin (seks) *n.* chromatin found only in female cells and believed to represent a single X

chromosome in a nondividing cell. It can be used to discover the sex of a baby before birth by examination of cells obtained by amniocentesis or chorionic villus sampling.

sex chromosome *n.* a chromosome involved in the determination of the sex of the individual. Women have two X chromosomes; men have one X chromosome and one Y chromosome. *Compare* autosome.

sex hormone *n.* any steroid hormone, produced mainly by the ovaries or testes, that is responsible for controlling sexual development and reproductive function. Oestrogens and progesterone are the female sex hormones; androgens are the male sex hormones.

sex-linked (seks-linkt) *adj.* describing genes (or the characteristics controlled by them) that are carried on the sex chromosomes. The genes for certain disorders, e.g. haemophilia, are carried on the X chromosome; these genes are disorders and described as *X-linked*.

sexology (seks-ol-ŏji) *n.* the study of sexual matters, including anatomy, physiology, behaviour, and techniques.

sexual deviation (seks-yoo-ăl) *n.* any sexual behaviour regarded as abnormal by society. The deviation may relate to the sexual object (as in fetishism) or the activity engaged in (for example, sadism and exhibitionism).

sexual intercourse (in-ter-kors) *n. see* coitus.

sexually transmitted disease (STD) *n.* any disease transmitted by sexual intercourse, formerly known as *venereal disease*. STDs include AIDS, syphilis, gonorrhoea, genital herpes, *Chlamydia* infection, and soft sore. The medical specialty concerned with STDs is *genitourinary medicine*.

SFD *adj.* small for dates: *see* intrauterine (growth retardation).

SFS *n. see* Social Functioning Scale.

SGA *adj.* small for gestational age.

SGOT *n.* serum glutamic oxaloacetic transaminase. *See* aspartate aminotransferase.

SGPT *n.* serum glutamic pyruvic transaminase. *See* alanine aminotransferase.

sheath (sheeth) *n.* (in anatomy) the layer of connective tissue that envelops structures such as nerves, arteries, tendons, and muscles.

Sheehan's syndrome (shee-ănz) *n.* subnormal activity of the pituitary gland, causing amenorrhoea and infertility, resulting from a reduction in its blood supply, due to a major haemorrhage in pregnancy. [H. L. Sheehan (20th century), British pathologist]

Shigella (shig-el-ă) *n.* a genus of nonmotile rodlike Gram-negative bacteria normally present in the intestinal tract. Some species are pathogenic. *S. dysenteriae* a species associated with bacillary dysentery.

shigellosis (shig-el-oh-sis) *n.* an infestation of the digestive system by bacteria of the genus *Shigella*, causing bacillary dysentery.

shin bone (shin) *n. see* tibia.

shingles (shing-ŭlz) *n. see* herpes (zoster).

Shirodkar's operation (shi-rod-karz) *n.* an operation in which the neck (cervix) of the uterus is closed by means of a purse-string suture in order to prevent miscarriage. [N. V.

Shirodkar (1900–71), Indian obstetrician]

shock (shok) *n.* the condition associated with circulatory collapse, when the arterial blood pressure is too low to maintain an adequate supply of blood to the tissues. The patient has a cold sweaty pallid skin, a weak rapid pulse, irregular breathing, dry mouth, dilated pupils, and a reduced flow of urine. Shock may be due to a decrease in the volume of blood, as occurs after haemorrhage, dehydration, burns, etc., or it may be caused by reduced activity of the heart, as in coronary thrombosis. It may also be due to widespread dilation of the veins so that there is insufficient blood to fill them. This may be caused by the presence of bacteria in the bloodstream (*bacteraemic* or *toxic s.*); a severe allergic reaction (*anaphylactic s.*: *see* anaphylaxis); drug overdosage, e.g. overdosage of insulin produces hypoglycaemia (*insulin s.*); or emotional shock (*neurogenic s.*). *See also* spinal shock.

short bowel syndrome (SBS) (short) *n.* a malabsorption disorder in children due to congenital abnormalities, ischaemia, or vascular injury.

short circuit (ser-kit) *n. see* anastomosis.

short-sightedness (short-syt-id-nis) *n. see* myopia.

short Synacthen test (sin-ak-thĕn) *n.* a test used to assess the ability of the adrenal cortex to produce cortisol. Serum cortisol is measured before and then 30 minutes after an intramuscular injection of 250 µg tetracosactide (Synacthen), an analogue of ACTH.

shoulder (shohl-der) *n.* the ball-and-socket joint (*see* enarthrosis) between the glenoid cavity of the scapula and the upper end (head) of the humerus. The joint is surrounded by a capsule closely associated with many tendons.

shoulder girdle (pectoral girdle) *n.* the bony structure to which the bones of the upper limbs are attached. It consists of the right and left scapulas and clavicles.

show (shoh) *n. Informal.* a discharge of blood-stained mucus from the vagina that occurs at the start of labour.

shunt (shunt) *n.* a passage connecting two anatomical channels and diverting blood or other fluid (e.g. cerebrospinal fluid) from one to the other. It may occur as a congenital abnormality (as in septal defects of the heart) or be surgically created. *See also* anastomosis.

SIADH *n. see* syndrome of inappropriate secretion of antidiuretic hormone.

sial- (sialo-) *prefix denoting* **1.** saliva. **2.** a salivary gland.

sialadenitis (sy-ăl-ad-i-ny-tis) *n.* inflammation of a salivary gland.

sialagogue (sy-al-ŏ-gog) *n.* a drug that promotes the secretion of saliva. Parasympathomimetic drugs have this action.

sialography (ptyalography) (sy-ă-log-răfi) *n.* X-ray examination of the salivary glands, after introducing, via a cannula, a quantity of radiopaque material into the ducts of the parotid and submandibular glands in the mouth.

sialolith (sy-al-oh-lith) *n.* a stone (calculus) in a salivary gland or duct. The flow of saliva is ob-

structed, causing swelling and intense pain.

sialorrhoea (sy-ă-lŏ-ree-ă) *n. see* ptyalism.

Siamese twins (conjoined twins) (sy-ă-meez) *pl. n.* identical twins that are physically joined together at birth. The condition ranges from twins joined only by the umbilical blood vessels to those in whom conjoined heads or trunk are inseparable.

sib (sib) *n. see* sibling.

SIB *n.* self-injurious behaviour. *See* (attempted) suicide, parasuicide.

sibilant (sib-i-lănt) *adj.* whistling or hissing. The term is applied to certain high-pitched abnormal sounds heard through a stethoscope.

sibling (sib) (sib-ling) *n.* one of a number of children of the same parents, i.e. a brother or sister.

sibutramine (sy-boo-tră-meen) *n.* a drug that acts on the central nervous system to suppress the appetite: it inhibits the reuptake of noradrenaline and serotonin. Sibutramine is administered by mouth in the treatment of obesity, mainly for those with a body mass index of 30 or over who have failed to respond to standard weight-reduction measures. Trade name: **Reductil**.

sickle-cell disease (drepanocytosis) (sik-ŭl-sel) *n.* a hereditary blood disease that mainly affects people of African ancestry. It occurs when the sickle-cell gene has been inherited from both parents and is characterized by the production of an abnormal type of haemoglobin, which precipitates in the red blood cells when the blood is deprived

silicosis

of oxygen. The affected cells are distorted into the characteristic sickle shape and are rapidly removed from the circulation, leading to anaemia.

sickle-cell trait *n.* the carrier condition of sickle-cell disease, in which the defective gene is inherited from only one parent. It generally causes no symptoms.

side-effect (syd-i-fekt) *n.* an unwanted effect produced by a drug in addition to its desired therapeutic effects. Side-effects may be harmful (adverse drug reactions).

sidero- *prefix denoting* iron.

sideropenia (sid-er-oh-pee-niă) *n.* iron deficiency. This may result from dietary inadequacy; increased requirement of iron by the body, as in pregnancy or childhood; or increased loss of iron from the body, usually due to chronic bleeding.

siderosis (sid-er-oh-sis) *n.* the deposition of iron oxide dust in the lungs, occurring in silver finishers, arc welders, and haematite miners. Pulmonary fibrosis may develop if fibrogenic dusts such as silica are also inhaled.

SIDS *n.* sudden infant death syndrome: *see* cot death.

sievert (see-vŭt) *n.* the SI unit of dose equivalent, being the dose equivalent when the absorbed dose of ionizing radiation multiplied by the stipulated dimensionless factors is 1 J kg⁻¹. The sievert has replaced the rem. Symbol: Sv.

sigmoid- *prefix denoting* the sigmoid colon.

sigmoid colon (sigmoid flexure) (sig-moid) *n.* the S-shaped terminal part of the descending colon, which leads to the rectum.

sigmoidectomy (sig-moid-ek-tŏmi) *n.* removal of the sigmoid colon by surgery. It is performed for tumours, severe diverticular disease, or sigmoid volvulus.

sigmoidoscope (sig-moid-ŏ-skohp) *n.* an instrument inserted through the anus in order to inspect the interior of the rectum and sigmoid colon.

sigmoidoscopy (sig-moid-osk-ŏpi) *n.* examination of the rectum and sigmoid colon with a sigmoidoscope. It is used in the investigation of diarrhoea or rectal bleeding, particularly to detect colitis or cancer of the rectum.

sigmoidostomy (sig-moid-ost-ŏmi) *n.* an operation in which the sigmoid colon is brought through the abdominal wall and opened. *See* colostomy.

sign (syn) *n.* an indication of a particular disorder that is observed by a physician but is not apparent to the patient. *Compare* symptom.

sildenafil (sil-den-ă-fil) *n.* a drug administered orally for the treatment of erectile impotence. During sexual stimulation, it causes smooth muscle relaxation and increased blood flow to the corpus cavernosum of the penis, which results in erection. Trade name: **Viagra**.

silicone (sil-i-kohn) *n.* any of a group of synthetic organic compounds of silicon that are water-repellant and are used in medicine in prostheses and as lubricants and adhesives.

silicosis (sil-i-koh-sis) *n.* a lung disease – a form of pneumoconiosis – produced by inhaling silica dust particles. It affects workers in hard-rock mining and tunnelling, quarrying, stone dressing, and boiler scaling. Silica stimulates fibrosis of lung tissue, which produces progressive breathlessness and considerably increased susceptibility to tuberculosis.

silver nitrate (sil-ver ny-trayt) *n.* a salt of silver with caustic, astringent, and disinfectant properties. It is applied in solutions or creams to destroy warts and to treat skin injuries, including burns. Formula: $AgNO_3$.

simethicone (activated dimeticone) (si-meth-i-kohn) *n.* a silicone-based material with antifoaming properties, used in the treatment of infantile colic and often incorporated into antacid remedies. Trade names: **Dentinox, Infacol**.

Simmonds disease (sim-önz) *n.* loss of sexual function, loss of weight, and other features of hypopituitarism caused by trauma or tumours or occurring in women after childbirth complicated by bleeding (postpartum haemorrhage). [M. Simmonds (1855–1925), German physician]

Sims's position (simz-iz) *n.* the left-sided knees-up position commonly assumed by patients undergoing examinations of the anus and rectum or vagina. [J. M. Sims (1813–83), US gynaecologist]

SIMV *n. see* (synchronized) intermittent mandatory ventilation.

simvastatin (sim-vas-tă-tin) *n.* a drug administered by mouth to reduce abnormally high levels of cholesterol in the blood (*see* statin). Trade name: **Zocor**.

sinew (sin-yoo) *n.* a tendon.

singer's nodule (sing-erz) *n.* a pearly white nodule that may develop on the vocal folds of people who use their voice excessively or in those with poor vocal technique.

singultus (sing-gul-tŭs) *n. see* hiccup.

sinistr- (sinistro-) *prefix denoting* left or the left side.

sino- (sinu-) *prefix denoting* **1.** a sinus. **2.** the sinus venosus.

sinoatrial node (SA node) (sy-noh-ay-tri-ăl) *n.* the pacemaker of the heart: a microscopic area of specialized cardiac muscle located in the upper wall of the right atrium near the entry of the vena cava. Fibres of the SA node contract at around 70 times per minute. Following each contraction, the impulse spreads along connecting fibres to the atrioventricular node. Impulses arriving at the SA node accelerate or decrease the heart rate.

sinogram (sy-noh-gram) *n.* an X-ray photograph of a sinus that has been injected with a radiopaque substance. —**sinography** (sy-nog-răfi) *n.*

sinus (sy-nŭs) *n.* **1.** an air cavity within a bone, especially any of the cavities within the bones of the face or skull (*see* paranasal sinuses). **2.** any wide channel containing blood, usually venous blood. *s. arrhythmia see* arrhythmia. *s. venosus* a chamber in the embryonic heart that becomes part of the right atrium after birth. **3.** a pocket or bulge in a tubular organ, especially a blood vessel. **4. (sinus tract)** an infected tract leading from a focus of infection to the surface of the skin or a hollow organ. *See* pilonidal sinus.

sinusitis (sy-nŭs-I-tis) *n.* inflammation of one or more of the

The skeleton

skull

mandible

cervical vertebrae

clavicle

scapula

ribs

sternum

humerus

thoracic vertebrae

lumbar vertebrae

ilium

ulna

sacrum

radius

metacarpals

carpals

phalanges

coccyx

femur

patella

tibia

fibula

tarsals

phalanges

metatarsals

paranasal sinuses. It is often associated with rhinitis and may be acute or chronic. Symptoms may include pain, purulent discharge from the nose, nasal obstruction, and disturbances of the sense of smell. Persistent cases require treatment with antibiotics, decongestants, or steroid nose drops; surgery, such as sinus washouts or antrostomy, is occasionally required.

sinusoid (sy-new-soid) *n.* a small blood vessel found in certain organs, such as the adrenal gland and liver.

siphonage (sy-fŏn-ij) *n.* the transfer of liquid from one container to another by means of a bent tube. The procedure is used in gastric lavage.

Sipple's syndrome (sip-ĕlz) *n. see* MENS. [J. H. Sipple (1930–), US physician]

sitz bath (sits) *n.* a fairly shallow hip bath. Sitz baths of cold and hot water, rapidly alternated, were formerly used for the treatment of a variety of sexual disorders.

SI units (Système International d'Unités) *pl. n.* the internationally agreed system of units, based on the metre-kilogram-second system, now in use for all scientific purposes. See Appendix 11.

Sjögren's syndrome (sher-grenz) *n.* an autoimmune condition affecting the salivary and lacrimal glands, resulting in a dry mouth and dryness of the eyes. In the systemic form of the disease other glands may be affected, causing dryness of the airways, vagina, or skin. The syndrome may occur secondarily to other conditions, such as rheumatoid arthritis. [H. S. C. Sjögren (20th century), Swedish ophthalmologist]

skatole (methyl indole) (skat-ohl) *n.* a derivative of the amino acid tryptophan, excreted in the urine and faeces.

skeletal muscle (skel-i-t'l) *n. see* striated muscle.

skeleton (skel-i-tŏn) *n.* the rigid framework of connected bones that gives form to the body, protects and supports its soft organs and tissues, and provides attachments for muscles and a system of levers essential for locomotion. *appendicular s.* the bones of the limbs. *axial s.* the bones of the head and trunk. See illustration. —**skeletal** *adj.*

skia- *prefix denoting* shadow.

skier's thumb (gamekeeper's thumb) (skee-erz) *n.* rupture and consequent instability of the ulnar collateral ligament on the inside of the thumb between the metacarpal and proximal (first) phalanx, caused by forced abduction of the thumb.

skill mix (skil miks) *n.* the various skill levels of health-service staff required either within a particular discipline or for the total staff within a health authority.

skin (skin) *n.* the outer covering of the body, consisting of an outer layer, the epidermis, and an inner layer, the dermis (see illustration). The epidermis protects the body from injury and from invasion by parasites. It also helps to prevent the body from becoming dehydrated. The combination of erectile hairs, sweat glands, and blood capillaries in the skin form part of the temperature-regulating mechanism of the body. The skin also acts as an organ of excretion (by the secretion of sweat) and as a sense organ (it contains receptors that are sensitive to heat, cold, touch, and pain). Anatomical name: **cutis**. **s. graft** a portion of healthy skin cut from one area of the body and used to cover a part that has lost its skin, usually as a result of injury, burns, or operation. *See also* split-skin graft.

ski-stick injury (skee-stik) *n.* a penetrating injury by a ski stick.

skull (skul) *n.* the skeleton of the head and face, which is made up of 22 bones. It can be divided into the cranium, which encloses the brain, and the face, including the lower jaw (mandible). (See illustration.) All the bones of the skull except the mandible are connected to each other by immovable joints (*see* suture). The skull contains cavities for the eyes and nose and a large opening at its base (foramen magnum) through which the spinal cord passes.

Section through the skin

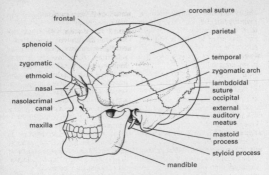

frontal
coronal suture
sphenoid
parietal
zygomatic
temporal
ethmoid
zygomatic arch
nasal
lambdoidal suture
nasolacrimal canal
occipital
maxilla
external auditory meatus
mastoid process
styloid process
mandible

Side view of the skull

SLE *n.* systemic lupus erythematosus: *see* lupus (erythematosus).

sleep (sleep) *n.* a state of natural unconsciousness, during which the brain's activity is not apparent (apart from the continued maintenance of basic bodily functions, such as breathing) but can be detected by means of an electroencephalogram (EEG). *See also* REM.

sleep apnoea *n.* cessation of breathing during sleep. *central s. a.* sleep apnoea in which there is no evidence of any voluntary efforts to breathe. *obstructive s. a. (syndrome) (OSA(S), s. a. syndrome, SAS)* sleep apnoea in which airflow from the nose and mouth is restricted, resulting in more than five episodes of apnoea per hour of sleep associated with significant daytime sleepiness; snoring is a feature, but not

universal. In children it is usually caused by enlarged tonsils; adult patients are often obese. Complications of prolonged OSA include heart failure and hypertension.

sleeping sickness (African trypanosomiasis) (sleep-ing) *n.* a disease of tropical Africa caused by the presence in the blood of the parasitic protozoans *Trypanosoma gambiense* or *T. rhodesiense*, which are transmitted through the bite of tsetse flies. Initial symptoms include fever, headache, and chills, followed later by enlargement of the lymph nodes, anaemia, and pains in the limbs and joints. The parasites eventually invade the minute blood vessels supplying the central nervous system, causing drowsiness and lethargy.

sleep paralysis *n.* a terrifying inability to move or speak while remaining fully alert. It occurs in up to 60% of patients with narcolepsy and may occur in other conditions, such as severe anxiety.

sleep-walking (sleep-wawk-ing) *n. see* somnambulism.

sling (sling) *n.* a bandage arranged to support and rest an injured limb so that healing is not hindered by activity. The most common sling is a triangular bandage tied behind the neck to support the weight of a broken arm.

slipped disc (slipt) *n. see* prolapsed intervertebral disc.

slit lamp (slit) *n.* a device for providing a narrow beam of light, used in conjunction with a special microscope. It can be used to examine minutely the structures within the eye, one layer at a time.

slough (sluf) *n.* dead tissue, such as skin, that separates from healthy tissue after inflammation or infection.

slow virus (sloh) *n.* one of a group of infective disease agents now more commonly known as prions.

SMA *n. see* spinal muscular atrophy.

small bowel (smawl) *n.* the small intestine (*see* intestine). *s.-b.* **enema** (*enteroclysis*) a technique for examining the jejunum and ileum in which barium sulphate is injected through a tube passing through the mouth into the small bowel and then a series of radiographs is taken. *s.-b.* **meal** (*barium follow-through*) a technique for examining the small bowel in which the patient swallows dilute barium sulphate suspension and then a series of radiographs is taken.

small-cell lung cancer *n. see* oat-cell carcinoma.

small for dates (SFD) *adj. see* intrauterine (growth retardation).

smallpox (smawl-poks) *n.* an acute infectious virus disease causing high fever and a rash that scars the skin. The rash consists of red spots (macules) that appear on the face, spread to the trunk and extremities, and gradually develop into pustules. Most patients recover but serious complications, such as nephritis or pneumonia, may develop. Treatment with thiosemicarbazone is effective. Immunization against smallpox has now totally eradicated the disease. Medical name: **variola**. *See also* alastrim, cowpox.

smear (smeer) *n.* a specimen of tissue or other material taken from part of the body and smeared on a microscope slide for examination. *See* cervical (smear).

smegma (smeg-mă) *n.* the secretion of the glands of the foreskin (prepuce), which accumulates under the foreskin and has a white cheesy appearance.

Smith-Petersen nail (smith-pee-ter-sĕn) *n.* a stainless steel nail used to fix fragments of bone when the neck of the femur is fractured. [M. N. Smith-Petersen (1886–1953), US orthopaedic surgeon]

Smith's fracture *n. see* fracture. [R. W. Smith (1807–73), Irish surgeon]

smooth muscle (involuntary muscle) (smooth) *n.* muscle that produces slow long-term contractions of which the individual is unaware. Smooth muscle occurs in hollow organs, such as the stomach, intestine, blood vessels, and bladder. *Compare* striated muscle.

SNAP *n. see* Schizophrenia Nursing Assessment Protocol.

snare (snair) *n.* an instrument consisting of a wire loop designed to remove polyps, tumours, and other projections of tissue. *See also* diathermy.

A nasal snare

sneeze (sneez) **1.** *n.* an involuntary violent reflex expulsion of air through the nose and mouth provoked by irritation of the mucous membrane lining the nasal cavity. **2.** *vb.* to produce a sneeze.

Snellen chart (snel-ĕn) *n.* the commonest chart used for testing sharpness of distant vision (*see* visual acuity). It consists of rows of capital letters, called *test types*, the letters of each row becoming smaller down the chart. [H. Snellen (1834–1908), Dutch ophthalmologist]

snoring (snor-ing) *n.* noisy breathing while asleep due to vibration of the soft palate, uvula, pharyngeal walls, or epiglottis.

snow blindness (snoh) *n.* a painful disorder of the cornea of the eye due to excessive exposure to ultraviolet light reflected from the snow.

snuffles (snuf-ĕlz) *n.* **1.** partial obstruction of breathing in infants, caused by the common cold. **2.** (formerly) discharge through the nostrils associated with necrosis of the nasal bones: seen in infants with congenital syphilis.

Social Functioning Scale (SFS) (soh-shăl) *n.* a scale to assess the ability of those with mental-health problems to engage in social interactions, interpersonal relationships, and activities of independent living.

socket (sok-it) *n.* (in anatomy) a hollow or depression into which another part fits.

sodium (soh-diŭm) *n.* a mineral element and an important constituent of the human body. The amount of sodium in the body is controlled by the kidneys. An excess of sodium leads to hypernatraemia, which often results in oedema. Sodium is also implicated in hypertension: a high-sodium diet is thought to increase the risk of hypertension in later life. Symbol: Na.

sodium bicarbonate (by-kar-bŏn-ayt) *n.* a salt of sodium that neutralizes acid and is administered by mouth or injection to treat stomach and digestive disorders, acidosis, and sodium deficiency. *See also* antacid.

sodium chloride (klor-ryd) *n.* common salt: a salt of sodium that is an important constituent of the body and is used to replace lost fluids and electrolytes and to irrigate body cavities. Formula: NaCl.

sodium citrate (sit-rayt) *n.* a salt of sodium used in the treatment of cystitis, as an ingredient of oral rehydration therapy, to prevent the clotting of stored blood, and as an osmotic laxative.

sodium fusidate (few-si-dayt) *n.* an antibiotic used mainly to treat infections caused by *Staphylococcus*, including osteomyelitis. It is administered by mouth or injection. Trade name: **Fucidin**.

sodium nitrite (ny-tryt) *n.* a sodium salt administered by injection, with sodium thiosulphate, to treat cyanide poisoning.

sodium thiosulphate (th'y-oh-sul-fayt) *n.* a salt of sodium administered by intravenous injection, with sodium nitrite, to treat cyanide poisoning.

sodium valproate (val-proh-ayt) *n.* an anticonvulsant drug administered by mouth to treat all types of epilepsy. Trade name: **Epilim**.

sodokosis (soh-doh-koh-sis) *n. see* rat-bite fever.

soft sore (chancroid) (soft) *n.* a sexually transmitted disease that is caused by the bacterium *Haemophilus ducreyi*, resulting in enlargement and ulceration of lymph nodes in the groin. Treatment with sulphonamides is effective.

solarium (só-lair-lŭm) *n.* a room in which patients are exposed to either sunlight or artificial sunlight (a blend of visible light and infrared and ultraviolet radiation).

solar plexus (coeliac plexus) (soh-ler pleks-ŭs) *n.* a network of sympathetic nerves and ganglia high in the back of the abdomen.

soleus (soh-li-ŭs) *n.* a broad flat muscle in the calf of the leg. The soleus flexes the foot, so that the toes point downwards.

solution (só-loo-shŏn) *n.* a homogeneous mixture of two or more dissimilar substances, usually of a liquid (the *solvent*) in which a solid (the *solute*) is dissolved.

solvent (sol-věnt) *n. see* solution.

soma (soh-mă) *n.* **1.** the entire body excluding the germ cells. **2.** the body as distinct from the mind.

somat- *prefix denoting* **1.** the body. **2.** somatic.

somatic (sŏ-mat-ik) *adj.* **1.** relating to the nonreproductive parts of the body. **2.** relating to the body wall (i.e. excluding the viscera). *Compare* splanchnic. **3.** relating to the body rather than the mind.

somatization disorder (Briquet's syndrome) (soh-mă-ty-zay-shŏn) *n.* a psychiatric disorder that is characterized by multiple recurrent changing physical symptoms in the absence of physical disorders that could explain them.

somatoform disorders (sŏ-mat-oh-form) *pl. n.* a group of disorders in which there is a history of repeated physical complaints with no physical basis. They include somatization disorder and hypochondriasis.

somatostatin (growth-hormone inhibiting hormone, GHIH) (soh-mă-toh-stay-tin) *n.* a hormone, produced by the hypothalamus and some extraneural tissues, including the gastrointestinal tract and the pancreas (*see* delta cells), that inhibits growth hormone (somatotrophin) release by the pituitary gland. *s. analogue* a drug, such as lanreotide or octreotide, used to treat acromegaly and neuroendocrine tumours.

somatotrophin (soh-mă-toh-troh-fin) *n. see* growth hormone.

somnambulism (noctambulation) (som-nam-bew-lizm) *n.* sleep-walking: walking about and performing other actions in a semi-automatic way during sleep without later memory of doing so. It is common during childhood and can also arise as the result of stress or hypnosis. —**somnambulistic** *adj.*

somnolism (som-noh-lizm) *n.* a hypnotic trance. *See* hypnosis.

Somogyi effect (som-ŏ-gy-i) *n. see* dawn phenomenon. [M. Somogyi (1883–1971), US biochemist]

Sonne dysentery (sonn-i) *n.* bacillary dysentery caused by the species *Shigella sonnei*. [C. Sonne (1882–1948), Danish bacteriologist]

sonography (sonn-og-răfi) *n. see* ultrasonography.

sonoplacentography (soh-noh-plas-en-tog-răfi) *n.* the technique of using ultrasound waves to determine the position of the placenta during pregnancy.

soporific (sop-er-if-ik) *n. see* hypnotic.

sorbitol (sor-bit-ol) *n.* a carbohydrate with a sweet taste, used by diabetics as a substitute for cane sugar. It is also administered by mouth or injection in disorders of carbohydrate metabolism and in drip feeding.

sordes (sor-deez) *pl. n.* the brownish encrustations that form around the mouth and teeth of patients suffering from fevers.

sore (sor) *n.* a lay term for any ulcer or other open wound of the skin or mucous membranes. *See also* bedsore, soft sore.

sore throat *n.* pain at the back of the mouth, commonly due to tonsillitis or pharyngitis. If infection persists the lymph nodes in the neck may become tender and enlarged (cervical adenitis).

sotalol (soh-tă-lol) *n.* a drug (*see*

beta blocker) administered by mouth or injection to treat abnormal heart rhythm. Trade names: **Beta-Cardone, Sotacor**.

souffle (soo-fěl) *n.* a soft blowing sound heard through the stethoscope, usually produced by blood flowing in vessels.

sound (sownd) (in surgery) **1.** *n.* a long rodlike instrument, often with a curved end, used to explore body cavities or to dilate strictures in the urethra or other canals. **2.** *vb.* to explore a cavity using a sound.

Soundbridge (sownd-brij) *n.* trade name for an implantable hearing aid (*see* hearing aid).

Southey's tubes (suth-iz) *pl. n.* fine-calibre tubes for insertion into subcutaneous tissue to drain excess fluid. They are rarely used in practice today. [R. Southey (1835–99), British physician]

Spanish fly (span-ish) *n.* the blister beetle, *Lytta vesicatoria*: source of the irritant and toxic chemical compound cantharidin.

spansule (span-sewl) *n.* a drug in the form of a capsule prepared in such a way that, when taken orally, its contents are released slowly.

spasm (spazm) *n.* a sustained involuntary muscular contraction, which may occur either as part of a generalized disorder or as a local response to an otherwise unconnected painful condition. *carpopedal s.* a spasm that affects the muscles of the hands and feet and is caused by a reduction in the blood calcium level (often transitory), as in hyperventilation.

spasmo- *prefix denoting* spasm.

spasmodic (spaz-mod-ik) *adj.* occurring in spasms or resembling a spasm.

spasmolytic (spaz-moh-**lit**-ik) n. a drug that relieves spasm of smooth muscle. *See also* antispasmodic.

spasmus nutans (spaz-mŭs **new**-tanz) n. a combination of symptoms including a slow nodding movement of the head, nystagmus, and spasm of the neck muscles. It affects infants and it normally disappears within a year or two.

spastic (**spast**-ik) *adj.* characterized by spasms. **s. colon** *see* irritable bowel syndrome. **s. paralysis** weakness of a limb or limbs associated with increased reflex activity. This results in spasticity and is caused by disease affecting the nerve fibres of the corticospinal tract. *See also* cerebral palsy.

spasticity (spas-**tis**-iti) n. resistance to the passive movement of a limb that is maximal at the beginning of the movement and gives way as more pressure is applied. It is a symptom of damage to the corticospinal (pyramidal) tracts in the brain or spinal cord. *Compare* rigidity.

spatula (**spat**-yoo lă) n. an instrument with a blunt blade used to spread ointments or plasters and, particularly in dentistry, to mix materials. A flat spatula is used to depress the tongue during examination of the oropharynx.

special care baby unit (SCBU) (spesh-ăl) n. a unit in a hospital that provides special care for premature, small, and sick babies. Its specialist staff is not equipped to provide intensive care.

special hospital n. a hospital for the care of mentally ill patients who pose a substantial risk to the community and must therefore be kept securely.

special school n. (in Britain) an education establishment for disabled children.

species (**spee**-shiz) n. the smallest unit used in the classification of living organisms. Members of the same species are able to interbreed and to produce fertile offspring. Similar species are grouped together within one genus.

specific (spi-**sif**-ik) **1.** n. a medicine that has properties especially useful for the treatment of a particular disease. **2.** *adj.* (of a disease) caused by a particular microorganism that causes no other disease. **3.** *adj.* of or relating to a species.

specific gravity (**grav**-iti) n. *see* relative density.

spectroscope (**spek**-trŏ-skohp) n. an instrument that is used to split up light or other radiation into components of different wavelengths. The simplest spectroscope uses a prism, which splits white light into the rainbow colours of the visible spectrum.

spectrum (**spek**-trŭm) n. (in pharmacology) the range of effectiveness of an antibiotic. **broad s.** effectiveness against a wide range of microorganisms.

SPECT scanning (single photon emission computing tomography) (spekt) n. (in nuclear medicine) a cross-sectional imaging technique for observing an organ or part of the body using a gamma camera; images are produced after injecting a radioactive tracer. It is used particularly in cardiac nuclear medicine imaging (*see* MUGA scan).

speculum (spek-yoo-lŭm) *n.* (*pl.* **specula**) a metal instrument for inserting into and holding open a cavity of the body, such as the vagina, rectum, or nasal orifice, in order that the interior may be examined.

Vaginal specula

speech therapy (speech) *n.* the rehabilitation of patients who are unable to speak coherently because of congenital causes, accidents, or illness. Speech therapists have special training in this field but are not medically registered.

sperm (sperm) *n.* *see* spermatozoon.

Spermatogenesis

sperm- (**spermi(o)-** **spermo-**) *prefix denoting* sperm or semen.

spermat- (**spermato-**) *prefix denoting* **1.** sperm. **2.** organs or ducts associated with sperm.

spermatic artery (sper-mat-ik) *n.* either of two arteries that originate from the abdominal aorta and travel downwards to supply the testes.

spermatic cord *n.* the cord, consisting of the vas deferens, nerves, and blood vessels, that runs from the abdominal cavity to the testicle in the scrotum.

spermatocele (sperm-ă-toh-seel) *n.* a cystic swelling in the scrotum containing sperm. The cyst arises from the epididymis and can be felt as a lump above the testis. Treatment is by surgical removal.

spermatogenesis (sperm-ă-toh-jen-i-sis) *n.* the process by which mature spermatozoa are produced in the testis. Spermatogonia, in the outermost layer of the seminiferous tubules, multiply throughout reproductive life. Some of them divide by meiosis into spermatocytes, which produce haploid spermatids. These are transformed into mature spermatozoa by the process of *spermiogenesis*. The whole process takes 70–80 days.

spermatorrhoea (sperm-ă-tŏ-ree-ă) *n.* the involuntary discharge of semen without orgasm.

spermatozoon (sperm) (sperm-ă-toh-zoh-ŏn) *n.* (*pl.* **spermatozoa**) a mature male sex cell (*see* gamete). The tail of a sperm enables it to swim, which is important as a means for reaching and fertilizing the ovum. (See illustration.) *See also* acrosome, fertilization.

spermaturia (sperm-ăt-yoor-iă) *n.* the presence of spermatozoa in the urine. Abnormal ejaculation into the bladder on orgasm (retrograde ejaculation) may occur after prostatectomy or other surgical procedures or in certain neurological conditions.

sperm count *n.* an estimate of the total number of spermatozoa in a specimen of ejaculated semen, which is used as a measure of male fertility. Normal values for sperm concentration are 20–200 million spermatozoa per ml ejaculate. *See also* seminal analysis.

spermicide (sperm-i-syd) *n.* an agent that kills spermatozoa. Contraceptive creams and jellies contain chemical spermicides. —**spermicidal** *adj.*

spermiogenesis (sperm-i-oh-jen-i-sis) *n. see* spermatogenesis.

spheno- *prefix denoting* the sphenoid bone.

sphenoid bone (sfee-noid) *n.* a bone forming the base of the cranium behind the eyes. *See* skull.

A spermatozoon

spherocyte (sfeer-oh-syt) *n.* an abnormal form of red blood cell (erythrocyte) that is spherical rather than disc-shaped. They are characteristic of some forms of haemolytic anaemia. Spherocytes tend to be removed from the blood as they pass through the spleen. *See also* spherocytosis.

spherocytosis (sfeer-oh-sy-toh-sis) *n.* the presence in the blood of spherocytes. Spherocytosis may occur as a hereditary disorder (*hereditary s.*) or in certain haemolytic anaemias.

sphincter (sfink-ter) *n.* a specialized ring of muscle that surrounds an orifice. Contractions of the sphincter partly or completely close the orifice. Sphincters are found, for example, around the anus (*anal s.*) and at the openings between the stomach and the oesophagus (*cardiac s.*) and the duodenum (*pyloric s.*).

sphincter- *prefix denoting* a sphincter.

sphincterectomy (sfink-ter-ek-tŏmi) *n.* the surgical division, usually partial, of any sphincter muscle.

sphincterotomy (sfink-ter-ot-ŏmi) *n.* **1.** surgical division of any sphincter muscle. **2.** surgical removal of part of the iris in the eye at the border of the pupil.

sphygmo- *prefix denoting* the pulse.

sphygmocardiograph (sfig-moh-kar-di-ŏ-grahf) *n.* an apparatus for producing a continuous record of both the heartbeat and the subsequent pulse in one of the blood vessels. The recording can be shown on a moving tape or on an electronic screen.

sphygmograph (sfig-moh-grahf) *n.* an apparatus for producing a continuous record of the pulse in one of the blood vessels, showing the strength and rate of the beats.

sphygmomanometer (sfig-moh-mă-nom-it-er) *n.* an instrument for measuring blood pressure in the arteries. It consists of an inflatable cuff connected via a rubber tube to a column of mercury with a graduated scale.

spica (spy-kă) *n.* a bandage wound

Types of spica

repeatedly in a figure-of-eight around an injured limb, forming a series of V-shapes. See illustration.

spicule (spik-yool) *n.* a small splinter of bone.

spigot (spig-ŏt) *n.* a glass or plastic peg used to close the opening of a tube, used in nasogastric tubes and catheters.

spina bifida (rachischisis) (spynǎ bif-id-ǎ) *n.* a developmental defect in which the newborn baby has part of the spinal cord and its coverings exposed through a gap in the backbone (*see* neural tube defects). The symptoms may include paralysis of the legs, incontinence, and mental retardation from the commonly associated brain defect, hydrocephalus. Spina bifida can be diagnosed at about the 16th week of pregnancy by a maternal blood test and confirmed by amniocentesis and ultrasound. *s. b. occulta* a defect in the bony arch of the spine that (unlike spina bifida) has a normal skin covering; there may be an overlying hairy patch. It is not associated with neurological involvement.

spinal accessory nerve (spynǎl) *n. see* accessory nerve

spinal anaesthesia *n.* **1.** suppression of sensation, usually in the lower part of the body, by the injection of a local anaesthetic into the subarachnoid space, most commonly in the lumbar region of the vertebral column. Spinal anaesthesia is useful in patients whose condition makes them unsuitable for a general anaesthetic, to reduce the requirements for general anaesthetic drugs, or in circumstances where a skilled anaesthetist is not available. *See also* epidural (anaesthesia). **2.** loss of sensation in part of the body as a result of injury or disease to the spinal cord.

spinal column *n. see* backbone.

spinal cord *n.* the portion of the central nervous system enclosed in the vertebral column, consisting of nerve cells and bundles of nerves connecting all parts of the body with the brain. It extends from the medulla oblongata in the skull to the level of the second lumbar vertebra.

spinal muscular atrophy (SMA) *n.* a hereditary condition in which cells of the spinal cord die and the muscles in the arms and legs become progressively weaker. It usually develops between the ages of 2 and 12; eventually the respiratory muscles are affected and death usually results from respiratory infection. *infantile s. m. a.* an acute aggressive form of the condition (*see* Werdnig-Hoffmann disease).

spinal nerves *pl. n.* the 31 pairs of nerves that leave the spinal cord and are distributed to the body, passing out from the spinal canal through the spaces between the arches of the vertebrae.

spinal shock *n.* a state of shock accompanied by temporary paralysis of the lower extremities that results from injury to the spine and is often associated with ileus. If the spinal cord is transected, permanent motor paralysis persists below the level of spinal-cord division.

spindle (spin-d'l) *n.* a collection of fibres seen in a cell when it is dividing. It plays an important part in chromosome movement in mitosis and meiosis and is also involved in division of the cytoplasm.

spine (spyn) *n.* **1.** a sharp process on

a bone. **2.** the vertebral column (*see* backbone). —**spinal** *adj.*

spino- *prefix denoting* **1.** the spine. **2.** the spinal cord.

spiral bandage (spyr-ăl) *n.* a bandage wound round a part of the body, overlapping the previous section at each turn.

spiral organ *n. see* organ (of Corti).

Spirillum (spy-ril-ŭm) *n.* a genus of highly motile rigid spiral-shaped bacteria usually found in fresh and salt water containing organic matter. *S. minus* a species that causes rat-bite fever.

spiro- *prefix denoting* **1.** spiral. **2.** respiration.

spirochaetaemia (spy-roh-ki-tee-miă) *n.* the presence of spirochaetes in the bloodstream, occurring in the later stages of syphilis.

spirochaete (spy-roh-keet) *n.* any one of a group of spiral-shaped bacteria that lack a rigid cell wall and move by means of muscular flexions of the cell. The group includes *Borrelia*, *Leptospira*, and *Treponema*.

spirograph (spy-roh-grahf) *n.* an instrument for recording breathing movements. The record obtained is called a *spirogram*. —**spirography** *n.*

spirometer (spy-rom-it-er) *n.* an instrument for measuring the volume of air inhaled and exhaled. It is used in tests of ventilation. —**spirometry** *n.*

spironolactone (spy-rŏ-noh-lak-tohn) *n.* a synthetic corticosteroid that inhibits the activity of the hormone aldosterone and is administered by mouth as a potassium-sparing diuretic to treat heart failure, high blood pressure,

and fluid retention (oedema). Trade name: **Aldactone**.

Spitz-Holter valve (spits-hohl-ter) *n.* a valve used in the treatment of hydrocephalus to drain cerebrospinal fluid from the ventricles of the brain into either the right atrium or the peritoneum.

splanch- (splanchno-) *prefix denoting* the viscera.

splanchnic (splank-nik) *adj.* relating to the viscera. *Compare* somatic. *s. nerves* the series of nerves in the sympathetic system that are distributed to the blood vessels and viscera.

splanchnology (splank-nol-ŏji) *n.* the study of the viscera.

spleen (spleen) *n.* a large dark-red ovoid organ situated on the left side of the body below and behind the stomach. The spongy interior (*pulp*) of the spleen consists of lymphoid tissue within a meshwork of reticular fibres. The spleen is a major component of the reticuloendothelial system, producing lymphocytes in the newborn and containing phagocytes, which remove worn-out red blood cells and other foreign bodies from the bloodstream. Anatomical name: *lien*. —**splenic** (splen-ik) *adj.*

splen- (spleno-) *prefix denoting* the spleen.

splenectomy (spli-nek-tŏmi) *n.* surgical removal of the spleen. This is sometimes necessary in the emergency treatment of bleeding from a ruptured spleen.

splenic anaemia *n.* anaemia associated with portal hypertension and increased destruction of red blood cells by an overactive spleen.

splenitis (spli-ny-tis) *n.* inflammation of the spleen. *See also* peri-splenitis.

splenomegaly (splee-noh-**meg**-ăli) *n.* enlargement of the spleen. It commonly occurs in malaria, blood disorders, leukaemia, and Hodgkin's disease. *See also* hypersplenism.

splenorenal anastomosis (splee-noh-**ree**-năl) *n.* a method of treating portal hypertension by joining the splenic vein to the left renal vein. *Compare* portacaval anastomosis.

splenovenography (splee-noh-vi-**nog**-răfi) *n.* X-ray examination of the spleen and veins associated with it following injection of a radio-paque dye.

splint (splint) *n.* a rigid support to hold broken bones in position until healing has occurred.

splinter haemorrhage (splint-er) *n.* a linear haemorrhage below the nails, usually the result of trauma but also occurring in such conditions as subacute bacterial endocarditis or severe rheumatoid arthritis.

split-skin graft (SSG, Thiersch's graft) (split-skin) *n.* a type of skin graft in which thin partial thicknesses of skin are cut in narrow strips or sheets and placed onto the wound area to be healed.

spondyl- (spondylo-) *prefix denoting* a vertebra or the spine.

spondylitis (spon-di-**ly**-tis) *n.* inflammation of the synovial joints of the backbone. **ankylosing s.** a type of arthritis that predominantly affects young males. The inflammation affects the joint capsules and their attached ligaments and tendons, principally the intervertebral joints and sacroiliac joints (*see*

sacroiliitis). The resultant pain and stiffness are treated by analgesics and regular daily exercises. The disorder can lead to severe deformities of the spine (*see* kyphosis, ankylosis).

spondylolisthesis (spon-di-loh-lis-thi-sis) *n.* a forward shift of one vertebra upon another, due to a defect in the bone or in the joints that normally bind them together. This may be congenital or develop after injury.

spondylosis (spon-di-**loh**-sis) *n.* a spinal condition resulting from degeneration of the intervertebral discs in the cervical, thoracic, or lumbar regions. Symptoms include pain and restriction of movement. Pain is relieved by wearing a collar (when the neck region is affected) or a surgical belt (for the lower spine), which prevents movement. Very severe cases sometimes require surgical fusion.

spondylosyndesis (spon-di-loh-sin-di-sis) *n.* surgical fusion of the intervertebral joints of the backbone.

spongiform encephalopathy (**spunji**-form) *n.* any one of a group of rapidly progressive degenerative neurological diseases that include scrapie in sheep, bovine spongiform encephalopathy (BSE) in cattle, and Creutzfeldt-Jakob disease in humans. Human spongiform encephalopathies are characterized by rapidly progressive dementia associated with myoclonus. The diseases are thought to be caused by abnormal transmissible proteins (*see* prion).

spontaneous (spon-**tay**-niŭs) *adj.* arising without apparent cause or outside aid. The term is applied in medicine to certain conditions, such as pathological fractures, that arise in the absence of outside injury.

sporadic (sper-ad-ik) *adj.* describing a disease that occurs only occasionally or in a few isolated places. *Compare* endemic, epidemic.

spore (spor) *n.* a small reproductive body produced by plants and microorganisms. Some kinds of spores function as dormant stages of the life cycle, enabling the organism to survive adverse conditions. Other spores are the means by which the organism can spread vegetatively. *See also* endospore.

sporicide (spor-i-syd) *n.* an agent that kills spores (e.g. bacterial spores). Most germicides are ineffective since spores are very resistant to chemical action. —**sporicidal** *adj.*

sporotrichosis (spor-oh-trik-oh-sis) *n.* a chronic infection of the skin and superficial lymph nodes that is caused by the fungus *Sporothrix schenckii* and results in the formation of abscesses and ulcers. It occurs mainly in the tropics.

sports injury (sports) *n.* any injury related to the practice of a sport, often resulting from the overuse and stretching of muscles, tendons, and ligaments.

sports medicine *n.* a specialty concerned with the treatment of sports injuries and measures designed to prevent or minimize them.

spotted fever (spot-id) *n. see* Rocky Mountain spotted fever, typhus.

sprain (sprayn) *n.* injury to a ligament, caused by sudden overstretching. Sprains should be treated by cold compresses (icepacks) at the time of injury, and later by restriction of activity.

Sprengel's deformity (spreng-ělz) *n.* a congenital abnormality of the scapula, which is small and positioned high in the shoulder. [O. G. K. Sprengel (1852–1915), German surgeon]

sprue (psilosis) (sproo) *n.* deficient absorption of food due to disease of the small intestine. *tropical s.* sprue that is characterized by diarrhoea (usually steatorrhoea), glossitis, anaemia, and weight loss; the lining of the small intestine is inflamed and atrophied. Treatment with antibiotics and folic acid is usually effective. *See also* coeliac disease (nontropical sprue), malabsorption.

spud (spud) *n.* a blunt needle used for removing foreign bodies embedded in the cornea of the eye.

spur (sper) *n.* a sharp projection, especially one of bone.

sputum (spew-tŭm) *n.* material coughed up from the respiratory tract. Its colour, consistency, and other characteristics often provide important information affecting the diagnosis and the management of respiratory disease. Pathological examination of sputum for microorganisms and abnormal cells may add further information.

squama (skway-mǎ) *n.* (*pl.* **squamae**) **1.** a thin plate of bone. **2.** a scale, such as any of the scales from the cornified layer of the epidermis. —**squamous** *adj.*

squamo- *prefix denoting* **1.** the squamous portion of the temporal bone. **2.** squamous epithelium.

squamous bone (skway-mŭs) *n.* *see* temporal (bone).

squamous cell carcinoma (SCC) *n.* the second commonest form of skin cancer (after basal cell carcinoma), occurring usually in late-middle and old age. Sunlight is the commonest cause: SCC is mainly found on areas exposed to light and is more common in men than in women. It spreads locally at first but later may spread to sites distant from its origin (*see* metastasis). Treatment is usually by surgical excision or radiotherapy.

squamous epithelium *n.* *see* epithelium.

squint (skwint) *n.* *see* strabismus.

SSG *n.* *see* split-skin graft.

SSPE *n.* *see* subacute sclerosing panencephalitis.

SSRI (selective serotonin reuptake inhibitor) *n.* any one of a group of antidepressant drugs that exert their action by blocking the reabsorption of the neurotransmitter serotonin by the nerve endings in the brain. Their effect is to prolong the action of serotonin in the brain. The group includes citolapram, fluoxetine, fluvoxamine, paroxetine, and sertraline. Side-effects include agitation and nausea.

staccato speech (stă-kah-toh) *n.* abnormal speech in which there are pauses between words, sometimes associated with multiple sclerosis.

Stacke's operation (stak-ěz) *n.* an operation in which the bone between the mastoid cells and the middle ear is removed to create a single cavity. It is performed when there is chronic infection of this area. [L. Stacke (1859–1918), German otologist]

stadium (stay-diŭm) *n.* (*pl.* **stadia**) a stage in the course of a disease. **s. invasionis** the period between exposure to infection and the onset of symptoms.

stage (stayj) *vb.* (in oncology) to classify a primary tumour by its size and the presence and site of metastases. In addition to clinical examination, a variety of imaging and surgical techniques provide a more accurate assessment. Staging tumours is important in prognosis and defining appropriate treatment.

staghorn calculus (stag-horn) *n.* a branched stone forming a cast of the collecting system of the kidney and therefore filling and obstructing the calyces and pelvis. It is usually associated with infection and can cause pyonephrosis and, if neglected, a perinephric abscess.

stagnant loop syndrome (stag-nănt) *n.* *see* blind loop syndrome.

stain (stayn) **1.** *n.* a dye used to colour tissues and other specimens for microscopical examination. **2.** *vb.* to treat a specimen for microscopical study with a stain.

Stamey procedure (stay-mee) *n.* an operation devised to cure stress incontinence of urine in women in which the neck of the bladder is stitched to the anterior abdominal wall with unabsorbable suture material. *See also* colposuspension. [T. A. Stamey, US surgeon]

stammering (stuttering) (stam-er-ing) *n.* halting articulation with interruptions to the normal flow of speech and repetition of the initial consonants of words or syllables (*compare* cluttering). The symptoms are most severe when the stammerer is under any psychological

stress. Medical name: **dysphemia**.
—**stammerer** *n.*

stanozolol (stan-oz-ŏ-lol) *n.* an anabolic steroid administered by mouth to treat Behçet's syndrome and hereditary forms of angio-oedema. Trade name: **Stromba**.

St Anthony's fire (sănt ant-ŏ-niz fyr) *n.* an old colloquial name for the inflammation of the skin associated with ergot poisoning. *See* ergotism.

stapedectomy (stay-pi-dek-tŏmi) *n.* surgical removal of the stapes, enabling it to be replaced with a prosthetic bone in the treatment of otosclerosis.

stapediolysis (stă-pee-di-ol-i-sis) *n.* an operation to restore hearing in cases of otosclerosis, in which the stapes is freed from the fenestra ovalis.

stapes (stay-peez) *n.* a stirrup-shaped bone in the middle ear that articulates with the incus and is attached to the membrane of the fenestra ovalis. *See* ossicle.

staphylectomy (staf-i-lek-tŏmi) *n.* *see* uvulectomy.

staphylococcal scalded skin syndrome (Lyell's disease, Ritter's disease) (staf-i-loh-kok-k'l skawl-did) *n.* a potentially serious condition of young infants in which the skin becomes reddened and then peels off. The underlying cause is a staphylococcal infection. Medical name: **toxic epidermal necrolysis**.

Staphylococcus (staf-i-loh-kok-ŭs) *n.* a genus of Gram-positive non-motile spherical bacteria occurring in grapelike clusters. Some species are saprophytes; others parasites. Many species produce exotoxins. More serious infections that are

caused by staphylococci include pneumonia, bacteraemia, osteomyelitis, and enterocolitis. *S. aureus* a species that causes boils and internal abscesses. *See also* MRSA.
—**staphylococcal** *adj.*

staphyloma (staf-i-loh-mă) *n.* abnormal bulging of the cornea or sclera (white) of the eye.

staphylorrhaphy (palatorrhaphy) (staf-il-o-răfi) *n.* surgical suture of a cleft palate.

staple (stay-pŭl) *n.* (in surgery) a piece of metal used to join up pieces of tissue. Staples can be used as an alternative to sutures for an anastomosis; stapling machines have been produced for this purpose. *See also* endostapler.

starch (starch) *n.* the form in which carbohydrates are stored in many plants and a major constituent of the diet. Starch consists of linked glucose units and occurs in two forms, *α-amylose* and *amylopectin*. Starch is digested by means of the enzyme amylase. *See also* dextrin.

startle reflex (star-t'l) *n.* *see* Moro reflex.

starvation (star-vay-shŏn) *n.* *see* malnutrition.

stasis (stay-sis) *n.* stagnation or cessation of flow; for example, of blood or lymph whose flow is obstructed or of the intestinal contents when peristalsis is hindered.

-stasis *suffix denoting* stoppage of a flow of liquid; stagnation.

stat (statim) Latin: at once, used as a direction in prescriptions.

statementing (stayt-měnt-ing) *n.* the provision by a local authority of a statement of special educational needs for children attending school who have mental or physical disabilities severe enough to require extra help at school.

statin (stat-in) *n.* a drug that inhibits the action of an enzyme involved in the liver's production of cholesterol. Statins can lower the levels of low-density lipoproteins (LDLs) by 25–45%; they are used mainly to treat hypercholesterolaemia but also to reduce the risk of coronary heart disease in susceptible patients. *See* atorvastatin, cerivastatin, fluvastatin, pravastatin, simvastatin.

status asthmaticus (stay-tŭs ass-mat-ik-ŭs) *n.* a severe attack of asthma. Patients are very breathless and may die from respiratory failure if not treated with inhaled oxygen, bronchodilators, and corticosteroid therapy; sedatives are absolutely contraindicated

status epilepticus (epi-lep-tik-ŭs) *n.* the occurrence of repeated epileptic seizures without any recovery of consciousness between them. Prolonged status epilepticus may lead to the patient's death or long-term disability.

status lymphaticus (lim-fat-ik-ŭs) *n.* enlargement of the thymus gland and other parts of the lymphatic system, formerly believed to be a predisposing cause to sudden death in infancy and childhood.

STD *n. see* sexually transmitted disease.

steapsin (sti-ap-sin) *n. see* lipase.

stearic acid (sti-a-rik) *n. see* fatty acid.

steat- (steato-) *prefix denoting* fat; fatty tissue.

steatoma (sti-ă-toh-mă) *n.* any cyst or tumour of a sebaceous gland.

steatopygia (sti-ă-toh-pij-iă) *n.* the accumulation of large quantities of fat in the buttocks.

steatorrhoea (sti-ă-tŏ-ree-ă) *n.* the passage of abnormally increased amounts of fat in the faeces due to reduced absorption of fat by the intestine (*see* malabsorption). The faeces are pale and may look greasy.

steatosis (sti-ă-toh-sis) *n.* infiltration of hepatocytes with fat. This may occur in pregnancy, alcoholism, malnutrition, obesity, hepatitis C infection, or with some drugs.

Stein-Leventhal syndrome (styn-lev-ĕn-thal) *n.* secondary amenorrhoea and sterility associated with multiple cysts in both ovaries. [I. F. Stein (20th century) and M. L. Leventhal (1901–71), US gynaecologists]

Steinmann's pin (styn-manz) *n.* a fine metal nail inserted through a fractured bone through which extension is applied to the distal bone fragment. [F. Steinmann (1872–1932), Swiss surgeon]

stellate (stel-ayt) *adj.* star-shaped. **s. fracture** a star-shaped fracture of the kneecap caused by a direct blow. **s. ganglion** a star-shaped collection of sympathetic nerve cell bodies in the root of the neck.

Stellwag's sign (stel-vagz) *n.* apparent widening of the distance between the upper and lower eyelids due to retraction of the upper lid and protrusion of the eyeball. It is a sign of exophthalmic goitre. [C. Stellwag von Carion (1823–1904), Austrian ophthalmologist]

stem cell (stem) *n.* an undifferentiated cell that is able to renew itself and produce all the specialized cells within an organ. *embryonic s. c.*

a cell of the blastocyst from which all the different cell types of the developing embryo are produced. *haemopoietic s. c.* a cell of the bone marrow from which all blood cells are derived.

steno- *prefix denoting* **1.** narrow. **2.** constricted.

stenosis (sti-noh-sis) *n.* the abnormal narrowing of a passage or opening, such as a blood vessel or heart valve. *See* aortic stenosis, carotid-artery stenosis, mitral stenosis, pulmonary (stenosis), pyloric stenosis.

stenostomia (stenostomy) (sten-ŏ-stoh-miă) *n.* the abnormal narrowing of an opening, such as the opening of the bile duct.

Stensen's duct (sten-sĕnz) *n.* the long secretory duct of the parotid salivary gland. [N. Stensen (1638–86), Danish physician]

stent (stent) *n.* a tube placed inside a duct or canal to reopen it or keep it open. Stents may be used at operation to aid healing of an anastomosis, for example of a ureter, or they can be placed across an obstruction to maintain an open lumen, for example in obstruction due to tumour in the oesophagus, stomach, bile ducts, colon, or ureter. In an artery after angioplasty stents help to prevent restenosis.

stepping reflex (step-ing) *n.* a primitive reflex in newborn babies that should disappear by the age of two months. If the baby is held in a 'walking' position with the feet touching the ground, the feet move in a 'stepping' manner. Persistence of this reflex beyond two months is suggestive of cerebral palsy.

sterco- *prefix denoting* faeces.

stercobilin (ster-koh-by-lin) *n.* a brownish-red pigment formed during the metabolism of the bile pigments biliverdin and bilirubin and subsequently excreted in the urine or faeces.

stercolith (ster-koh-lith) *n.* a stone formed of dried compressed faeces.

stercoraceous (ster-ker-ay-shŭs) *adj.* composed of or containing faeces.

stereognosis (ste-ri-og-noh-sis) *n.* the ability to recognize the three-dimensional shape of an object by touch alone. This is a function of the association areas of the parietal lobe of the brain. *See also* agnosia.

stereopsis (ste-ri-op-sis) *n. see* stereoscopic vision.

stereoscopic vision (stereopsis) (ste-ri-ŏ-skop-ik) *n.* perception of the shape, depth, and distance of an object as a result of having binocular vision.

stereotactic (ste-ri-ŏ-tak-tik) *adj.* of or relating to the accurate localization of structures within the body by using three-dimensional measurements. Stereotactic localization enables the accurate positioning within the body of radiotherapy beams or sources for the treatment of tumours and of localizing wires for the biopsy of small tumours. *s. surgery see* stereotaxy.

stereotaxy (stereotactic surgery) (ste-ri-ŏ-taks-i) *n.* a surgical procedure in which a deep-seated area in the brain is operated upon after its position has been accurately established by three-dimensional measurements. The operation may be performed using an electrical current or by heat, cold, or mechanical techniques. *See also* leucotomy.

stereotypy (ste-ri-ŏ-ty-pi) n. the constant repetition of a complex action, which is carried out in the same way each time. It is seen in catatonia and infantile autism; sometimes it is an isolated symptom in mental retardation.

sterile (ste-ryl) adj. **1.** (of a living organism) barren; unable to reproduce its kind (see sterility). **2.** (of inanimate objects) completely free from microorganisms that could cause infection.

sterility (ster-il-itl) n. inability to have children, either due to infertility or (in someone who has been fertile) deliberately induced by surgical procedures as a means of contraception (see sterilization).

sterilization (ste-ri-ly-zay-shŏn) n. **1.** a surgical operation or any other process that induces sterility in men or women. In women this is now usually achieved by tubal occlusion: the permanent closure of the inner (lower) half of the Fallopian tubes through a laparoscope by means of a clip (Hulka-Clemens or Filshie clips) or a small plastic ring (Falope ring) or by introducing a rapid-setting plastic into the tubes through a hysteroscope. Men are usually sterilized by vasectomy. **2.** the process by which all types of microorganisms (including spores) are destroyed. This is achieved by the use of heat, radiation, chemicals, or filtration. See also autoclave.

stern- (sterno-) prefix denoting the sternum.

sternocleidomastoid muscle (ster-noh-kly-doh-mas-toid) n. see sternomastoid muscle.

sternohyoid (ster-noh-hy-oid) n. a muscle in the neck, arising from the sternum and inserted into the hyoid bone. It depresses the hyoid bone.

sternomastoid muscle (sternocleidomastoid muscle) (ster-noh-mas-toid) n. a long muscle in the neck, extending from the mastoid process to the sternum and clavicle. It serves to rotate the neck and flex the head.

sternomastoid tumour n. a small painless nonmalignant swelling in the lower half of the sternomastoid muscle, appearing a few days after birth. It is most common after breech births. The tumour may cause a slight tilt of the head, which can be corrected by physiotherapy.

sternotomy (ster-not-ŏmi) n. surgical division of the sternum, performed to allow access to the heart and its major vessels.

sternum (ster-nŭm) n. (pl. **sterna**) the breastbone: a flat bone extending from the base of the neck to just below the diaphragm and forming the front part of the skeleton of the thorax. The sternum articulates with the collar bones (see clavicle) and the costal cartilages of the first seven pairs of ribs. —**sternal** adj.

steroid (steer-oid) n. one of a group of organic compounds that include the male and female sex hormones (androgens and oestrogens), the hormones of the adrenal cortex (see corticosteroid), progesterone, bile salts, and sterols. Synthetic steroids have been produced for therapeutic purposes.

steroid card n. a card that must be carried by patients taking long-term corticosteroid medication, particularly if high doses are used. The card states that in an emergency treatment with steroids must not be suddenly stopped since this may precipitate an Addisonian crisis.

sterol (steer-ol) *n.* one of a group of steroid alcohols. The most important sterols are cholesterol and ergosterol.

stertor (ster-ter) *n.* a snoring type of noisy breathing heard in deeply unconscious patients.

steth- (stetho-) *prefix denoting* the chest.

stethoscope (steth-ŏ-skohp) *n.* an instrument used for listening to sounds within the body (*see* auscultation). A simple stethoscope usually consists of a diaphragm or an open bell-shaped structure (which is applied to the body) connected by rubber or plastic tubes to shaped earpieces for the examiner.

Stevens-Johnson syndrome (stee-věnz jon-sŏn) *n.* an inflammatory condition characterized by fever, large blisters on the skin, and ulceration of the mucous membranes. It may be a severe allergic reaction to certain drugs or it may follow certain infections. [A. M. Stevens (1884–1945) and F. C. Johnson (1894–1934), US paediatricians]

sthenia (sthee-niă) *n.* a state of normal strength or greater than normal strength. *Compare* asthenia. —**sthenic** (sthen-ik) *adj.*

stigma (stig-mă) *n.* (*pl.* **stigmata**) **1.** a mark that characterizes a particular disease, such as the café au lait spots characteristic of neurofibromatosis. **2.** any spot or lesion on the skin.

stilet (stylet, stylus) (sty-lit) *n.* **1.** a slender probe. **2.** a wire placed in the lumen of a catheter to give it rigidity while the instrument is passed along a body canal.

stillbirth (stil-berth) *n.* birth of a fetus that shows no evidence of life (heartbeat, respiration, or independent movement) at any time later than 24 weeks after conception. A fetus born dead before this time is known as an abortion or miscarriage.

Still's disease (stilz) *n. see* juvenile chronic arthritis. [Sir G. F. Still (1868–1941), British physician]

stimulant (stim-yoo-lănt) *n.* an agent that promotes the activity of a body system or function. Amphetamines and caffeine are stimulants of the central nervous system; doxapram is a respiratory stimulant.

stimulator (stim-yoo-lay-ter) *n.* any apparatus designed to stimulate nerves and muscles for a variety of purposes. It can be used to stimulate particular areas of the brain or to block pain (as in *transcutaneous electrical nerve stimulation, TENS*).

stimulus (stim-yoo-lŭs) *n.* (*pl.* **stimuli**) any agent that provokes a response, or particular form of activity, in a cell, tissue, or other structure.

stirrup (sti-rŭp) *n.* (in anatomy) *see* stapes.

stitch (stich) *n.* **1.** a sharp localized pain, commonly in the abdomen, associated with strenuous physical activity. It is a form of cramp. **2.** *see* suture.

STM *n.* short-term memory.

stock culture *n. see* culture.

Stokes-Adams syndrome (stohks-ad-ămz) *n.* attacks of temporary loss of consciousness that occur when blood flow ceases due to ventricular fibrillation or asystole. This syndrome may complicate heart block. It is treated by means of a battery-operated pacemaker. [W. Stokes (1804–78) and R. Adams (1791–1875), Irish physicians]

stoma (stoh-mă) *n. (pl.* **stomata**) **1.** (in anatomy) the mouth or any mouthlike part. **2.** (in surgery) the artificial opening of a tube that has been brought to the abdominal surface (*see* colostomy, ileostomy). **s. therapist** a nurse specially trained in the care of these openings and the appliances used with them. —**stomal** *adj.*

stomach (stum-ăk) *n.* a distensible saclike organ that forms part of the alimentary canal between the oesophagus and the duodenum. The stomach lies just below the diaphragm, to the right of the spleen. Its function is to continue the process of digestion that begins in the mouth. Gastric juice, secreted by gastric glands in the mucosa, together with the churning action of the muscular layers of the stomach, reduces the food to a semiliquid partly digested mass that passes on to the duodenum.

stomat- (stomato-) *prefix denoting* the mouth.

stomatitis (stoh-mă-ty-tis) *n.* inflammation of the mucous lining of the mouth.

stomatology (stoh-mă-tol-ŏji) *n.* the branch of medicine concerned with diseases of the mouth.

-stomy (-ostomy) *suffix denoting* a surgical opening into an organ or part.

stone (stohn) *n. see* calculus.

stool (stool) *n.* faeces discharged from the anus.

stop needle (stop) *n.* a surgical needle with a shank that has a protruding collar to stop it when the needle has been pushed a prescribed distance into the tissue.

strabismus (heterotropia) (stră-biz-mŭs) *n.* squint: any abnormal alignment of the two eyes. The strabismus is most commonly horizontal (*see* esotropia, exotropia) but it may also be vertical (*see* hypertropia, hypotropia). Double vision is possible, but the image from the deviating eye usually becomes ignored. *See also* heterophoria.

strain (strayn) **1.** *n.* excessive stretching or working of a muscle, resulting in pain and swelling. *Compare* sprain. **2.** *n.* a group of organ-

oesophagus

antrum

pylorus

cardia

fundus

body

greater omentum

Regions of the stomach seen from the front

isms obtained from a particular source or having special properties distinguishing them from other members of the same species. **3.** *vb.* to damage a muscle by overstretching.

strangulated (strang-yoo-layt-id) *adj.* describing a part of the body whose blood supply has been interrupted by compression of a blood vessel. *s. hernia see* hernia.

strangulation (strang-yoo-lay-shŏn) *n.* the closure of a passage, such as the main airway to the lungs (resulting in the cessation of breathing), a blood vessel, or the gastrointestinal tract.

strangury (strang-yoor-i) *n.* severe pain in the urethra associated with an intense desire to pass urine, resulting from irritation of the base of the bladder. It may also occur in such conditions as cancer of the base of the bladder, cystitis, or prostatitis, when it is accompanied by the painful passage of a few drops of urine.

stratified (strat-i-fyd) *adj.* describing tissue consisting of several layers of cells. *See* epithelium.

stratum (strah-tŭm) *n.* a layer of tissue or cells, such as any of the layers of the epidermis. *s. corneum* the outermost layer of the epidermis.

strawberry mark (strawberry naevus) (straw-bě-ri) *n. see* naevus.

streak (streek) *n.* (in anatomy) a line, furrow, or narrow band.

Streptobacillus (strep-toh-bǎ-sil-ŭs) *n.* a genus of Gram-negative aerobic nonmotile rodlike bacteria that tend to form filaments. *S. moniliformis* the cause of rat-bite fever.

streptococcal toxic shock syndrome (strep-tŏ-kok-k'l) *n. see* toxic shock syndrome.

Streptococcus (strep-toh-kok-ŭs) *n.* a genus of Gram-positive nonmotile spherical bacteria occurring in chains. Most species are saprophytes, but some are pathogenic. *Haemolytic streptococci* destroy red blood cells in blood agar and are the cause of many infections, including bacterial endocarditis (α-haemolytic strains) and scarlet fever (β-haemolytic strains). *See also* Lancefield classification, streptokinase. —**streptococcal** *adj.*

streptodornase (strep-toh-dor-nayz) *n.* an enzyme produced by some haemolytic bacteria of the genus *Streptococcus* that is capable of liquefying pus. *See also* streptokinase.

streptokinase (strep-toh-ky-nayz) *n.* an enzyme produced by some haemolytic bacteria of the genus *Streptococcus* that is capable of liquefying blood clots (*see* fibrinolytic). It is injected to treat blockage of blood vessels and is also used in combination with streptodornase, applied topically, to remove slough and blood clot and thus promote healing of ulcers. Trade names: **Kabikinase, Streptase, Varidase Topical**.

streptolysin (strep-tol-i-sin) *n.* an exotoxin that is produced by strains of *Streptococcus* bacteria and destroys red blood cells.

Streptomyces (strep-toh-my-seez) *n.* a genus of aerobic mouldlike bacteria. They are important medically as a source of such antibiotics as streptomycin, dactinomycin, chloramphenicol, and neomycin.

streptomycin (strep-toh-**my**-sin) *n.* an aminoglycoside antibiotic, derived from the bacterium *Streptomyces griseus*, that is used in combination with other drugs for treating tuberculosis and brucellosis. It is administered by intramuscular injection.

stress (stres) *n.* any factor that threatens the health of the body or has an adverse effect on its functioning, such as injury, disease, or worry. Constant stress brings about changes in the balance of hormones in the body.

stretch reflex (myotatic reflex) (strech) *n.* the reflex contraction of a muscle in response to its being stretched.

stria (stry-ă) *n.* (*pl.* **striae**) (in anatomy) a streak, line, or thin band. *striae gravidarum* stretch marks: the lines that appear on the skin of the abdomen of pregnant women, due to excessive stretching of the elastic fibres. Red or purple during pregnancy, they become white after delivery.

striated muscle (stry-**ayt**-id) *n.* a tissue that comprises the bulk of the body's musculature. It is also known as *skeletal muscle*, because it is attached to the skeleton and is responsible for the movement of bones, and *voluntary muscle*, because it is under voluntary control.

stricture (**strik**-cher) *n.* a narrowing of any tubular structure in the body. A stricture may result from inflammation, muscular spasm, growth of a tumour within the affected part, or from pressure on it by neighbouring organs. *urethral s.* a fibrous narrowing of the urethra, usually resulting from injury or inflammation. The patient has increasing difficulty in passing urine and may develop retention.

stricturoplasty (strik-cher-oh-plasti) *n.* an operation in which a stricture (usually in the small intestine) is widened by cutting it.

stridor (**stry**-dor) *n.* the noise heard on breathing in when the trachea or larynx is obstructed. It tends to be louder and harsher than wheeze.

stroke (apoplexy) (strohk) *n.* a sudden attack of weakness affecting one side of the body, resulting from an interruption to the flow of blood to the brain. The flow of blood may be prevented by thrombosis or embolism (*ischaemic s.*) or by haemorrhage (*haemorrhagic s.*). Prolonged reduction of blood pressure may result in more diffuse brain damage, as after a cardiorespiratory arrest. A stroke can vary in severity from a passing weakness or tingling in a limb (*see* transient ischaemic attack) to a profound paralysis, coma, and death. *See also* cerebral haemorrhage.

stroma (stroh-mă) *n.* the connective-tissue basis of an organ, as opposed to the functional tissue (parenchyma). For example, the stroma of the erythrocytes is the spongy framework of protein strands within a red blood cell in which the blood pigment haemoglobin is packed; the stroma of the cornea is the transparent fibrous tissue making up the main body of the cornea.

strongyloidiasis (strongyloidosis) (stron-ji-loi-dy-ă-sis) *n.* an infestation of the small intestine with the parasitic nematode worm *Strongyloides stercoralis*. Larvae enter the body through the skin and migrate to the lungs, where they cause tissue destruction and bleeding. Adult worms burrow into the intestinal wall and may cause ulceration, diarrhoea, abdominal pain, nausea, anaemia, and weakness. Treatment involves use of the drug tiabendazole.

strontium (stron-tiŭm) *n.* a yellow metallic element, absorption of which causes bone damage when its atoms displace calcium in bone. Symbol: Sr. *strontium-90* a radioactive isotope used in radiotherapy for the contact therapy of skin and eye tumours and (given by injection) in the treatment of metastatic prostate cancer.

struma (stroo-mă) *n.* (*pl.* **strumae**) a swelling of the thyroid gland (see goitre). *s. ovarii* a teratoma of the ovary containing thyroid tissue that becomes active and causes thyrotoxicosis. *See also* Riedel's struma.

strychnine (strik-neen) *n.* a poisonous alkaloid produced in the seeds of the East Indian tree *Strychnos nux-vomica*. Poisoning causes painful muscular spasms similar to those of tetanus; death is likely to occur from spasm in the respiratory muscles.

S–T segment *n.* the segment on an electrocardiogram that represents the interval preceding the last phase of the cardiac cycle, when the heart recovers from contraction.

stupe (stewp) *n.* any piece of material, such as a wad of cottonwool, soaked in hot water (with or without medication) and used to apply a poultice.

stupor (stew-per) *n.* a condition of near unconsciousness, with apparent mental inactivity and reduced ability to respond to stimulation.

Sturge-Weber syndrome (sterj-web-er) *n.* angioma of the blood vessels overlying the brain associated with a port-wine stain on the face (*see* naevus). [W. A. Sturge (1850–1919) and F. P. Weber (1863–1962), British physicians]

stuttering (stut-er-ing) *n. see* stammering.

St Vitus' dance (sănt vy-tŭs dahns) *n.* an archaic name for Sydenham's chorea.

stye (sty) *n.* acute inflammation of a gland at the base of an eyelash, caused by bacterial infection. The gland becomes hard and tender and a pus-filled cyst develops at its centre. Medical name: **hordeolum**.

stylet (sty-lit) *n. see* stilet.

stylo- *prefix denoting* the styloid process of the temporal bone.

styloid process (sty-loid) *n.* **1.** a long slender downward-pointing spine projecting from the lower surface of the temporal bone of the skull. It provides attachment for muscles and ligaments of the tongue and hyoid bone. **2.** any of various other spiny projections.

stylus (sty-lŭs) *n.* **1.** a pencil-shaped instrument, commonly used for applying external medication. **2.** *see* stilet.

styptic (stip-tik) *n. see* haemostatic.

sub- *prefix denoting* **1.** below; underlying. **2.** partial or slight.

subacute (sub-ă-kewt) *adj.* describing a disease that progresses more rapidly than a chronic condition but does not become acute.

subacute bacterial endocarditis (SBE) *n.* a form of endocarditis characterized by a slow onset and protracted course. It is usually caused by species of *Streptococcus* or *Staphylococcus*.

subacute combined degeneration of the cord *n*. the neurological disorder complicating a deficiency of vitamin B_{12} and pernicious anaemia. There is selective damage to the motor and sensory nerve fibres in the spinal cord, resulting in spasticity of the limbs and a sensory ataxia.

subacute sclerosing panencephalitis (SSPE) (skleer-ohzing pan-en-sef-ă-ly-tis) *n*. a rare and late complication of measles characterized by a slow progressive neurological deterioration that is usually fatal. It can occur four to ten years after the initial infection.

subarachnoid haemorrhage (SAH) (sub-ă-rak-noid) *n*. sudden bleeding into the subarachnoid space, which causes severe headache with stiffness of the neck. The usual source of such a haemorrhage is a cerebral aneurysm that has burst.

subarachnoid space *n*. the space between the arachnoid and pia meninges of the brain and spinal cord, containing circulating cerebrospinal fluid and large blood vessels.

subclavian artery (sub-klay-viăn) *n*. either of two arteries supplying blood to the neck and arms. The right subclavian artery branches from the innominate artery; the left subclavian arises directly from the aortic arch.

subclavian steal syndrome (steel) *n*. diversion of blood from the vertebral artery to the subclavian

artery when the latter is blocked proximally. It causes attacks of diminished consciousness (syncope).

subclinical (sub-klin-ikăl) *adj*. describing a disease that is suspected but is not sufficiently developed to produce definite signs and symptoms in the patient.

subconscious (sub-kon-shŭs) *adj*. (in psychoanalysis) denoting the part of the mind that includes memories, motives, and intentions that are momentarily not present in consciousness but can more or less readily be recalled to awareness. *Compare* unconscious.

subcutaneous (sub-kew-tay-niŭs) *adj*. beneath the skin. *See also* injection. **s. tissue** loose connective tissue, often fatty, situated under the dermis.

subdural (sub-dewr-ăl) *adj*. below the dura mater; relating to the space between the dura mater and arachnoid. **s. haematoma** *see* haematoma.

subglottis (sub-glot-iss) *n*. that part of the larynx that lies below the vocal folds.

subinvolution (sub-in-vŏ-loo-shŏn) *n*. failure of the uterus to revert to its normal size during the six weeks following childbirth.

subjective (sub-jek-tiv) *adj*. apparent to the affected individual but not to others: applied particularly to symptoms.

sublimation (sub-li-may-shŏn) *n*. the replacement of socially undesirable means of gratifying motives or desires by means that are socially acceptable. *See also* defence mechanism, repression.

subliminal (sub-lim-inăl) *adj*. subconscious: beneath the threshold of conscious perception.

sublingual (sub-ling-wăl) *adj.* beneath the tongue. **s. gland** one of a pair of salivary glands situated in the lower part of the mouth, one on either side of the tongue.

subluxation (sub-luks-ay-shŏn) *n.* partial dislocation of a joint, so that the bone ends are misaligned but still in contact.

submandibular gland (submaxillary gland) (sub-man-dib-yoo-ler) *n.* one of a pair of salivary glands situated below the parotid glands.

submaxillary gland (sub-maks-il-er-i) *n.* see submandibular gland.

submucosa (sub-mew-koh-sa) *n.* the layer of loose connective (areolar) tissue underlying a mucous membrane. —**submucosal** *adj.*

submucous (sub-mew-kŭs) *adj.* beneath a mucous membrane. **s. resection** see resection.

subphrenic abscess (sub-fren-ik) *n.* a collection of pus in the space below the diaphragm, usually on the right side, between the liver and diaphragm. Causes include postoperative infection and perforation of an organ.

substitution (sub-sti-tew-shŏn) *n.* (in psychoanalysis) the replacement of one idea by another: a form of defence mechanism.

substitution therapy *n.* treatment by providing a less harmful alternative to a drug or remedy that a patient has been receiving.

substrate (sub-strayt) *n.* the specific substance or substances on which a given enzyme acts.

subsultus (sub-sul-tus) *n.* abnormal twitching or tremor of muscles, such as may occur in feverish conditions.

subtertian fever (sub-ter-shăn) *n.* a form of malaria resulting from repeated infection by *Plasmodium falciparum* and characterized by continuous fever.

succus (suk-ŭs) *n.* any juice or secretion of animal or plant origin. **s. entericus** (*intestinal juice*) the clear alkaline fluid secreted by the glands of the small intestine. It contains mucus and digestive enzymes.

succussion (suk-ush-ŏn) *n.* a splashing noise heard when a patient who has a large quantity of fluid in a body cavity, such as the pleural cavity, moves suddenly or is deliberately shaken.

sucralfate (sewk-răl-fayt) *n.* an aluminium-containing drug that forms a protective coating over the stomach or duodenal lining. Administered by mouth, sucralfate is used in the treatment of peptic ulcer. Trade name: **Antepsin**.

sucrose (sewk-rohz) *n.* a carbohydrate consisting of glucose and fructose. It is the principal constituent of cane sugar and sugar beet. The increasing consumption of sucrose in the last 50 years has coincided with an increase in the incidence of dental caries, diabetes, coronary heart disease, and obesity.

suction (suk-shŏn) *n.* the use of reduced pressure to remove unwanted fluids or other material through a tube for disposal. During surgery, suction tubes are used to remove blood from the area of operation and to decompress the stomach (*nasogastric s.*) and the pleural space of air and blood (*chest s.*).

sudden infant death syndrome (SIDS) *n.* see cot death.

Sudek's atrophy (soo-deks) *n.*

pain, swelling, stiffness, and skin changes, usually in a hand or foot, sometimes caused by overactivity of the sympathetic nervous system following trauma (often a Colles' fracture) or surgery or occasionally arising spontaneously. [P. H. M. Sudek (1866–1938), German surgeon]

sudor (s'yoo-dor) *n. see* sweat.

sudorific (s'yoo-der-if-ik) *n. see* diaphoretic.

suffocation (suf-ŏ-kay-shŏn) *n.* cessation of breathing as a result of drowning, smothering, etc., leading to unconsciousness or death (*see* asphyxia).

suffusion (sŭ-few-zhŏn) *n.* the spreading of a flush across the skin surface, caused by changes in the local blood supply.

sugar (shuug-er) *n.* any carbohydrate that dissolves in water, is usually crystalline, and has a sweet taste. Sugars are classified chemically as monosaccharides or disaccharides. Table sugar is virtually 100% pure sucrose. *See also* fructose, glucose, lactose.

suggestibility (sŭ-jes-ti-bil-iti) *n.* the state of readily accepting suggestions from others. —**suggestible** *adj.*

suggestion (sŭ-jes-chŏn) *n.* (in psychology) the process of changing people's beliefs, attitudes, or emotions by telling them that they will change. It is sometimes used as a synonym for hypnosis. *See also* autosuggestion.

suicide (soo-i-syd) *n.* self-destruction as a deliberate act. *attempted s.* an attempt at self-destruction in which death is averted although the person concerned intended to kill himself (or herself). *Compare* parasuicide.

sulcus (sul-kŭs) *n.* (*pl.* **sulci**) **1.** one of the many clefts or infoldings of the surface of the brain. **2.** any of the infoldings of soft tissue in the mouth.

sulfadiazine (sulphadiazine) (sul-fă-dy-ă-zeen) *n. see* sulphonamide.

sulfamethoxazole (sulphamethoxazole) (sul-fă-meth-oks-ă-zohl) *n. see* sulphonamide, co-trimoxazole.

sulfametopyrazine (sul-fă-met-oh-py-ră-zeen) *n. see* sulphonamide.

sulfasalazine (sulphasalazine) (sul-fă-sal-ă-zeen) *n.* a drug of the sulphonamide group, used in the treatment of ulcerative colitis, Crohn's disease, and (for its anti-inflammatory action) rheumatoid arthritis. It is given by mouth or in the form of suppositories. Trade name: **Salazopyrin**.

sulfinpyrazone (sulphinpyrazone) (sul-fin-py-ră-zohn) *n.* a uricosuric drug given by mouth for the treatment of chronic gout. It should not be taken by patients with impaired kidney function. Trade name: **Anturan**.

sulpha drug (sul-fă) *n. see* sulphonamide.

sulphonamide (sulpha drug) (sul-fon-ă-myd) *n.* one of a group of drugs, derived from sulphanilamide (a red dye), that prevent the growth of bacteria. Sulphonamides are usually given by mouth and are effective against a variety of infections. Many sulphonamides are rapidly excreted and very soluble in the urine and are therefore used to treat infections of the urinary tract, especially in combination with other drugs. Because of their toxic side-effects, the clinical use of sulphonamides has declined; those still used include *sulfadiazine*, *sulfamethoxazole* (*see* co-trimoxazole), and *sulfametopyrazine*. *See also* sulfasalazine.

sulphone (sul-fohn) *n.* one of a group of drugs closely related to the sulphonamides. Sulphones possess powerful activity against the bacteria that cause leprosy and tuberculosis. The best known sulphone is dapsone.

sulphonylurea (sul-fŏ-nil-yoor-iă) *n.* one of a group of oral hypoglycaemic drugs, derived from a sulphonamide, that are used in the treatment of noninsulin-dependent (type 2) diabetes mellitus. They include chlorpropamide, glibenclamide, and tolbutamide.

sulphur (sul-fer) *n.* a nonmetallic element that is active against fungi and parasites. It is a constituent of ointments and other preparations used in the treatment of skin disorders. Symbol: S.

sulphuric acid (sul-fewr-ik) *n.* a powerful corrosive acid, widely used in industry. Swallowing the acid causes severe burning of the mouth and throat. The patient should drink large quantities of milk or water or white of egg; gastric lavage should not be delayed. Formula: H_2SO_4.

sumatriptan (soo-mă-trip-tan) *n.* *see* $5HT_1$ agonist.

sunburn (sun-bern) *n.* damage to the skin by excessive exposure to the sun's rays, principally UVB (*see* ultraviolet radiation). Sunburn may vary from reddening of the skin to the development of large painful fluid-filled blisters (*see* burn).

sunstroke (sun-strohk) *n.* *see* heatstroke.

super- *prefix denoting* **1.** above; overlying. **2.** extreme or excessive.

superciliary (soo-per-sil-i-er-i) *adj.* of or relating to the eyebrows (*supercilia*).

superego (soo-per-ee-goh) *n.* (in psychoanalysis) the part of the mind that functions as a moral conscience or judge. The superego is the result of the incorporation of parental injunctions into the child's mind.

superfecundation (soo-per-fee-kŭn-day-shŏn) *n.* the fertilization of two or more ova of the same age by spermatozoa from different males. *See* superfetation.

superfetation (soo-per-fee-tay-shŏn) *n.* the fertilization of a second ovum some time after the start of pregnancy, resulting in two fetuses of different maturity in the same uterus.

superficial (soo-per-fish-ăl) *adj.* (in anatomy) situated at or close to a surface. Superficial blood vessels are those close to the surface of the skin.

superinfection (soo-per-in-fek-shŏn) *n.* an infection arising during the course of another infection and caused by a different microorganism, which is usually resistant to the drugs used to treat the primary infection. *See also* MRSA.

superior (soo-peer-i-er) *adj.* (in anatomy) situated uppermost in the body in relation to another structure or surface.

superovulation (soo-per-ov-yoo-lay-shŏn) *n.* **1.** controlled hyperstimulation of the ovary to produce more follicles with oocytes. Usually induced by gonadotrophin preparations, it is performed in in vitro fertilization and other procedures of assisted conception in order to improve the pregnancy rates. **2.** uncontrolled hyperstimulation of the ovary (*ovarian hyperstimulation syndrome*). It may be associated with abdominal pain, ascites, oliguria, or renal failure.

supervisor (soo-per-vy-zer) *n.* an appropriately registered nurse who is accountable for a student's standard of care in a clinical area. The supervisor oversees the student's practice and learning experience during a clinical episode.

supination (soo-pi-**nay**-shŏn) *n.* the act of turning the hand so that the palm is uppermost. *Compare* pronation.

supinator (soo-pi-nay-ter) *n.* a muscle of the forearm that extends from the elbow to the shaft of the radius. It supinates the forearm and hand.

supine (soo-pyn) *adj.* **1.** lying on the back or with the face upwards. **2.** (of the forearm) in the position in which the palm of the hand faces upwards. *Compare* prone.

supportive (sŭ-**port**-iv) *adj.* (of treatment) aimed at reinforcing the patient's own defence mechanisms in overcoming a disease or disorder.

support worker (sŭ-port) *n.* (in the health service) a nursing auxiliary or assistant, physiotherapy helper, occupational therapy helper, speech therapy assistant, foot-care assistant, or ward clerk. Support workers in nursing care work under the supervision of registered practitioners (*see* health-care assistant).

suppository (sŭ-**poz**-it-er-i) *n.* a medicinal preparation in solid form suitable for insertion into a body cavity. *rectal s.* a suppository that is inserted into the rectum. It may contain drugs that act locally in the rectum or anus, drugs that are absorbed and act at other sites, or a simple lubricant. *vaginal s. see* pessary.

suppression (sŭ-**presh**-ŏn) *n.* **1.** the cessation or complete inhibition of any physiological activity. **2.** treatment that removes the outward signs of an illness or prevents its progress. **3.** (in psychology) a defence mechanism by which a person consciously and deliberately ignores an idea that is subjectively unpleasant.

suppuration (sup-yoor-**ay**-shŏn) *n.* the formation of pus.

supra- *prefix denoting* above; over.

supraglottis (soo-prǎ-glot-iss) *n.* that part of the larynx that lies above the vocal folds and includes the epiglottis.

supraorbital (soo-prǎ-or-bit'l) *adj.* of or relating to the area above the eye orbit. *s. reflex* the closing of the eyelids when the supraorbital nerve is struck, due to contraction of the muscle surrounding the orbit.

suprapubic (soo-prǎ-**pew**-bik) *adj.* above the pubic bone. *s. cystotomy see* cystotomy.

suprarenal glands (soo-prǎ-ree-nǎl) *pl. n. see* adrenal glands.

supraventricular tachycardia (SVT) (soo-prǎ-ven-trik-yoo-ler) *n. see* tachycardia.

suramin (s'yoor-ǎ-min) *n.* a nonmetallic drug used in the treatment of trypanosomiasis. It is usually given by slow intravenous injection.

surfactant (ser-**fak**-tǎnt) *n.* a wetting agent. *pulmonary s.* a complex mixture of compounds, secreted by pneumocytes, that prevents the alveoli of the lungs from collapsing by reducing surface tension.

surgeon (serj-ŏn) *n.* a qualified medical practitioner who specializes in surgery.

surgery (serj-er-i) *n.* the branch of medicine that treats injuries, deformities, or disease by operation or manipulation. *See also* cryosurgery, microsurgery. —**surgical** *adj.*

surgical neck (serj-ikăl) *n.* the constriction of the shaft of the humerus, below the head. It is frequently the point at which fracture of the humerus occurs.

surgical spirit *n.* methylated spirit, usually with small amounts of castor oil and oil of wintergreen: used to sterilize the skin before surgery, injections, etc.

surrogate (su-rŏ-găt) *n.* (in psychology) a person or object in someone's life that functions as a substitute for another person. *s. mother* a woman who becomes pregnant (by artificial insemination or embryo insertion) following an arrangement made with another party (usually a couple unable themselves to have children) in which she agrees to hand over the child she carries to that party when it is born.

susceptibility (sŭ-sep-ti-bil-iti) *n.* lack of resistance to disease. It is partly influenced by vaccination or other methods of increasing resistance to specific diseases.

suspensory bandage (su-spen-ser-i) *n.* a bandage arranged to support a hanging part of the body, such as the scrotum.

suspensory ligament *n.* a liga-

ment that serves to support or suspend an organ, such as the lens of the eye, in position.

sustentaculum (sus-ten-**tak**-yoo-lŭm) *n.* any anatomical structure that supports another structure. —**sustentacular** *adj.*

suture (soo-cher) **1.** *n.* (in anatomy) a type of immovable joint, found particularly in the skull, characterized by a minimal amount of connective tissue between the two bones. **2.** *n.* (in surgery) the closure of a wound or incision with any of various materials to facilitate the healing process. *See also* delayed suture. **3.** *n.* the material – silk, nylon,

blanket (skin)

continuous (skin)

vertical mattress (skin)

interrupted (skin)

purse string (intestine)

Types of surgical suture

a polymer, or wire – used to sew up a wound. **4.** *vb.* to close a wound by suture.

suxamethonium (suks-ă-mĕth-**oh**-niŭm) *n.* a drug that relaxes voluntary muscle (*see* muscle relaxant). It is administered by intravenous injection to produce muscle relaxation during surgery. Trade name: **Anectine**.

SVT *n. see* (supraventricular) tachycardia.

swab (swob) *n.* a pad of absorbent material (such as cotton), sometimes attached to a stick or wire, that is used for cleaning out or applying medication to wounds, operation sites, or body cavities.

swallowing (deglutition) (swol-oh-ing) *n.* the process by which food is transferred from the mouth to the oesophagus. Voluntary raising of the tongue forces food backwards towards the pharynx. This stimulates reflex actions in which the larynx and the nasal passages are closed so that food does not enter the trachea.

Swan-Ganz catheter (swon-ganz) *n.* a catheter with an inflatable balloon at its tip, which can be inserted into the pulmonary artery via the right chambers of the heart. Inflation of the balloon enables measurement of pressure in the left atrium and hence pulmonary artery pressure. [H. J. C. Swan (1922–), US cardiologist; W. Ganz (20th century), US engineer]

sweat (swet) *n.* the watery fluid secreted by the sweat glands. Its principal constituents in solution are sodium chloride and urea. The secretion of sweat is a means of excreting nitrogenous waste; it also has a cooling effect as the sweat evaporates from the surface of the skin. Anatomical name: **sudor**. **s. gland** a simple coiled tubular exocrine gland that lies in the dermis of the skin. Sweat glands occur over most of the surface of the body; they are particularly abundant in the armpits, on the soles of the feet and palms of the hands, and on the forehead.

sycosis (sy-koh-sis) *n.* inflammation of the hair follicles caused by infection with *Staphylococcus aureus.* It commonly affects the beard area (*s. barbae*) of men in their thirties or forties.

Sydenham's chorea (sid-ĕn-ămz) *n. see* chorea. [T. Sydenham (1624– 89), English physician]

symbiosis (sim-by-oh-sis) *n.* an intimate and obligatory association between two different species of organism (*symbionts*) in which there is mutual aid and benefit. *Compare* commensal, parasite.

symblepharon (sim-blef-er-on) *n.* a condition in which the eyelid adheres to the eyeball. It is usually the result of chemical (especially alkali) burns to the conjunctiva.

symbolism (sim-bŏl-izm) *n.* (in psychology) the process of representing an object or an idea by something else. Psychoanalytic theorists hold that conscious ideas frequently act as symbols for unconscious thoughts and that this is particularly evident in dreaming, in free association, and in the formation of psychological symptoms. —**symbolic** (sim-bol-ik) *adj.*

Syme's amputation (symz) *n.* amputation of the foot just above the ankle joint. [J. Syme (1799–1870), British surgeon]

symmetry (sim-it-ri) *n.* (in anatomy) the state of opposite parts of an organ or parts at opposite sides of the body corresponding to each other.

sympathectomy (sim-pă-**thek**-tŏmi) *n.* the surgical division of sympathetic nerve fibres. It is done to minimize the effects of normal or excessive sympathetic activity.

sympathetic nervous system (sim-pă-**thet**-ik) *n.* one of the two divisions of the autonomic nervous system, having fibres that leave the central nervous system in the thoracic and lumbar regions and are distributed to the blood vessels, sweat glands, salivary glands, heart, lungs, intestines, and other abdominal organs. It is responsible for increasing the heart rate and dilating the pupil, among other effects.

sympathin (sim-pă-thin) *n.* the name given by early physiologists to the substances released from sympathetic nerve endings, now known to be a mixture of adrenaline and noradrenaline.

sympatholytic (sim-pă-thoh-**lit**-ik) *adj.* opposing the effects of the sympathetic nervous system. Sympatholytic drugs include guanethidine, alpha blockers, and beta blockers.

sympathomimetic (sim-pă-thoh-mi-**met**-ik) *adj.* having the effect of stimulating the sympathetic nervous system. The actions of sympathomimetic drugs are adrenergic (resembling those of noradrenaline). These drugs include *alpha-adrenergic stimulants* (or *alpha agonists*), such as ephedrine, phenylephrine, metaraminol, apraclonidine, and brimonidine; and

beta-adrenergic stimulants (*beta agonists*), such as salbutamol, salmeterol, and terbutaline.

sympathy (sim-pă-thi) *n.* (in physiology) a reciprocal influence exercised by different parts of the body on one another.

symphysiotomy (sim-fizi-**ot**-ŏmi) *n.* the operation of cutting through the front of the pelvis at the pubic symphysis in order to enlarge the diameter of the pelvis and aid delivery of a fetus whose head is too large to pass through the pelvic opening. This procedure is now rarely employed.

symphysis (sim-fi-sis) *n.* **1.** a joint in which the bones are separated by fibrocartilage, which minimizes movement and makes the bony structure rigid. Examples are the pubic symphysis (*see* pubis) and the joints of the backbone, which are separated by intervertebral discs. **2.** the line that marks the fusion of two bones that were separate at an early stage of development.

symptom (simp-tŏm) *n.* an indication of a disease or disorder noticed by the patient himself. *Compare* sign.

symptomatology (semeiology) (simp-tŏm-ă-**tol**-ŏji) *n.* **1.** the branch of medicine concerned with the study of symptoms of disease. **2.** the symptoms of a disease, collectively.

syn- (sym-) *prefix denoting* union or fusion.

synaesthesia (sin-is-**theez**-iă) *n.* a condition in which a secondary subjective sensation (often colour) is experienced at the same time as the sensory response normally evoked by the stimulus. For example, the sound of the word 'cat' might evoke the colour purple.

synalgia (sin-al-jiă) *n. see* referred pain.

synapse (sy-naps) *n.* the minute gap across which nerve impulses pass from one neurone to the next, at the end of a nerve fibre. Reaching a synapse, an impulse causes the release of a neurotransmitter, which diffuses across the gap and triggers an electrical impulse in the next neurone. *See also* neuromuscular junction.

synarthrosis (sin-arth-roh-sis) *n.* an immovable joint in which the bones are united by fibrous tissue. Examples are the cranial sutures. *See also* gomphosis, schindylesis.

synchondrosis (sin-kon-droh-sis) *n.* a slightly movable joint (*see* amphiarthrosis) in which the surfaces of the bones are separated by hyaline cartilage, as occurs between the ribs and sternum.

synchronized intermittent mandatory ventilation (SIMV) (sin-krŏ-nyzd) *n. see* intermittent mandatory ventilation.

synchysis (sink-i-sis) *n.* softening of the vitreous humour of the eye. *s. scintillans* tiny refractile crystals of cholesterol suspended in the vitreous humour. They usually cause no symptoms.

syncope (fainting) (sink-ŏ-pi) *n.* loss of consciousness induced by a temporarily insufficient flow of blood to the brain. It commonly occurs in otherwise healthy people and may be caused by an emotional shock, by standing for prolonged periods, or by injury and profuse bleeding.

syncytium (sin-sit-ium) *n.* (*pl.*

syncytia) a mass of protoplasm containing several nuclei. Muscle fibres are syncytia. —**syncytial** *adj.*

syndactyly (dactylion) (sin-daktili) *n.* congenital webbing of the fingers, which are joined along part or all of their length. Adjacent fingers may be joined only by skin, or the bones of the fingers may be joined.

syndesm- (syndesmo-) *prefix denoting* connective tissue, particularly ligaments.

syndesmology (sin-des-mol-ŏji) *n.* the branch of anatomy dealing with joints and their components.

syndesmosis (sin-des-moh-sis) *n.* an immovable joint in which the bones are separated by connective tissue. An example is the articulation between the bases of the tibia and fibula.

syndrome (sin-drohm) *n.* a combination of signs and/or symptoms that forms a distinct clinical picture indicative of a particular disorder.

syndrome of inappropriate secretion of antidiuretic hormone (SIADH) *n.* a condition of inappropriately high plasma levels of ADH (*see* vasopressin) with associated water retention, dilutional hyponatraemia, and the production of highly concentrated urine. Renal, adrenal, thyroid, and hepatic function are normal, as is the volume of circulating blood (euvolaemia). It is caused by a variety of pathological conditions and also by a number of drugs.

synechia (sin-ek-iă) *n.* an adhesion between the iris and another part of the eye. *anterior s.* synechia between the iris and the cornea. *posterior s.* synechia between the iris and the lens.

syneresis (sin-eer-i-sis) *n.* **1.** contraction of a blood clot to produce a firm mass that seals the damaged blood vessels. **2.** the degenerative shrinkage of the vitreous humour due to ageing.

synergist (sin-er-jist) *n.* **1.** a drug that interacts with another to produce increased activity, which is greater than the sum of the effects of the two drugs given separately. **2.** a muscle that acts with a prime mover (agonist) in making a particular movement. —**synergism, synergy** *n.* —**synergistic** (sin-er-jist-ik) *adj.*

synergistic gangrene *n.* gangrene of tissues produced by different bacteria acting together, usually a mixture of aerobic and anaerobic organisms. Synergistic gangrene has a pronounced tendency to spread along fascial planes, causing necrotizing fasciitis.

syngeneic (sin-jĕn-ay-ik) *adj.* describing grafted tissue that is genetically identical to the recipient's tissue, as when the donor and recipient are identical twins.

synoptophore (sin-op-toh-for) *n.* see amblyoscope.

synostosis (sin-os-toh-sis) *n.* the joining by ossification of two adjacent bones. It occurs, for example, at the cranial sutures.

synovectomy (sy-noh-vek-tŏmi) *n.* surgical removal of the synovium of a joint. This is performed in cases of chronic synovitis (such as rheumatoid arthritis), when other measures have been ineffective.

synovia (synovial fluid) (sy-noh-vi-ă) *n.* the thick colourless lubricating fluid that surrounds a joint or a bursa and fills a tendon sheath.

It is secreted by the synovial membrane.

synovial joint (sy-noh-vi-ăl) *n.* see diarthrosis.

synovial membrane (synovium) *n.* the membrane that forms the sac enclosing a freely movable joint (*see* diarthrosis). It secretes the lubricating synovial fluid.

synovioma (sy-noh-vi-oh-mă) *n.* a benign or malignant tumour of the synovial membrane.

synovitis (sy-noh-vy-tis) *n.* inflammation of the synovial membrane, resulting in pain and swelling (arthritis). It is caused by injury, infection, or rheumatic disease.

synovium (sy-**noh**-vi-ŭm) *n.* see synovial membrane.

synthesis (sin-thi-sis) *n.* the formation of complex substances from simple constituents. —**synthesize** *vb.* —**synthetic** (sin-thet-ik) *adj.*

syphilide (syphilid) (sif-i-lyd) *n.* the skin rash that appears in the second stage of syphilis. Syphilides occur in crops that may last from a few days to several months. They denote a highly infectious stage of the disease.

syphilis (sif-i-lis) *n.* a chronic sexually transmitted disease caused by the bacterium *Treponema pallidum*. Bacteria usually enter the body during sexual intercourse; they may also pass from an infected pregnant woman across the placenta to the developing fetus, resulting in the disease being present at birth (*congenital s.*). The primary symptom is a hard ulcer (chancre) at the site of infection. Secondary stage symptoms include fever, malaise, general enlargement of lymph nodes, and a faint red rash on the chest. After months, or even years, the disease enters its tertiary stage with widespread formation of tumour-like masses (gummas). Tertiary syphilis may cause serious damage to the heart and blood vessels (*cardiovascular s.*) or to the brain and spinal cord (*neurosyphilis*), resulting in tabes dorsalis, blindness, and general paralysis of the insane. *See also* bejel. —**syphilitic** (sif-i-**lit**-ik) *adj.*

syring- (syringo-) *prefix denoting* a tube or long cavity, especially the central canal of the spinal cord.

syringe (si-**rinj**) *n.* an instrument consisting of a piston in a tight-fitting tube that is attached to a hollow needle or thin tube. A syringe is used to give injections, remove material from a part of the body, or to wash out a cavity.

syringobulbia (si-ring-oh-**bulb**-iă) *n. see* syringomyelia.

syringoma (si-ring-oh-**mă**) *n.* multiple benign tumours of the sweat glands, which show as small hard swellings usually on the face, neck, or chest.

syringomyelia (si-ring-oh-my-ee-liă) *n.* a disease of the spinal cord in which longitudinal cavities form within the cord in the cervical (neck) region. Characteristically there is weakness and wasting of the muscles in the hands with a loss of awareness of pain and temperature.

An extension of the cavitation into the lower brainstem is called *syringobulbia*. Cerebellar ataxia, a partial loss of pain sensation in the face, and weakness of the tongue and palate may occur.

syringomyelocele (si-ring-oh-my-**ĕl**-oh-seel) *n.* protrusion of the spinal cord through a defect in the spine together with a fluid-filled sac continuous with the central canal of the cord.

system (**sis**-tĕm) *n.* (in anatomy) a group of organs and tissues associated with a particular physiological function, such as the nervous system or respiratory system.

systemic (sis-**tem**-ik) *adj.* relating to or affecting the body as a whole, rather than individual parts and organs. *s. circulation see* circulation. *s. sclerosis* a rare multisystem connective-tissue disease in which scleroderma may be associated with pulmonary fibrosis, renal failure, and gastrointestinal and myocardial disease. Genetic and autoimmune factors may be implicated. *See also* CREST syndrome.

systole (**sis**-tŏ-li) *n.* the period of the cardiac cycle during which the heart contracts. —**systolic** (sis-**tol**-ik) *adj.*

systolic pressure *n. see* blood pressure.

Tt

T₃ *n.* triiodothyronine (*see* thyroid hormone).

T₄ *n.* thyroxine (*see* thyroid hormone).

tabes dorsalis (locomotor ataxia) (tay-beez dor-sah-lis) *n.* a form of neurosyphilis occurring 5–20 years after the original sexually transmitted infection. The infecting organisms progressively destroy the sensory nerves. Severe stabbing pains in the legs and trunk, an unsteady gait, and loss of bladder control are common. *See also* syphilis, general paralysis of the insane.

tablet (tab-lit) *n.* (in pharmacy) a small disc containing one or more drugs, made by compressing a powdered form of the drug(s). It is usually taken by mouth.

tabo-paresis (tay-boh-pă-ree-sis) *n.* a late effect of syphilitic infection of the nervous system in which the patient shows features of tabes dorsalis and general paralysis of the insane.

TAB vaccine *n.* a combined vaccine used to produce immunity against the diseases typhoid, paratyphoid A, and paratyphoid B.

tachy- *prefix denoting* fast; rapid.

tachycardia (tak-i-kar-diă) *n.* an increase in the heart rate above normal. **sinus t.** tachycardia that may occur normally with exercise or excitement. It may also be due to illness, such as fever. *supraventricu-* *lar t.* (*SVT*) tachycardia, often benign, stemming from an abnormal area in the atria. *ventricular t.* (*VT*) tachycardia stemming from an abnormal focus of electrical activity in the ventricles, which can result in a sudden drop in blood pressure or cardiac arrest. *See also* paroxysmal tachycardia.

tachypnoea (tak-ip-nee-ă) *n.* rapid breathing.

tacrolimus (tak-rŏ-ly-mŭs) *n.* a powerful immunosuppressant drug administered orally or by intravenous infusion to prevent rejection of transplanted organs. It is also used, in the form of an ointment, to treat atopic eczema. Side-effects include damage to the kidneys, tremor, headache, and gastrointestinal upsets. Trade name: **Prograf**.

tactile (tak-tyl) *adj.* relating to or affecting the sense of touch.

taenia (tee-niă) *n.* (*pl.* **taeniae**) a flat ribbon-like anatomical structure. *taeniae coli* the longitudinal ribbon-like muscles of the colon.

Taenia *n.* a genus of large tapeworms, some of which are parasites of the human intestine. *T. saginata* the beef tapeworm: the most common tapeworm parasite of humans. *See* taeniasis. *T. solium* the pork tapeworm. Its larval stage may develop in humans, in whom it may cause cysticercosis.

taeniacide (taenicide) (tee-niă-syd) *n.* an agent that kills tapeworms.

taeniafuge (tee-niă-fewj) *n.* an agent, such as niclosamide, that eliminates tapeworms from the body of their host.

taeniasis (tee-ny-ă-sis) *n.* an infestation with tapeworms of the genus *Taenia*, resulting from ingestion of raw or undercooked meat containing the larval stage of the parasite. Symptoms include increased appetite, hunger pains, weakness, and weight loss. *See also* cysticercosis.

Tagamet (tag-ă-met) *n. see* cimetidine.

Takayasu's disease (pulseless disease) (tak-ă-yas-ooz) *n.* progressive occlusion of the arteries arising from the arch of the aorta (including those to the arms and neck), resulting in the absence of pulses in the arms and neck. Symptoms include attacks of unconsciousness (syncope), paralysis of facial muscles, and transient blindness, due to an inadequate supply of blood to the head. [M. Takayasu (1860–1938), Japanese ophthalmologist]

tal- (talo-) *prefix denoting* the ankle bone (talus).

talc (tal'k) *n.* a soft white powder consisting of magnesium silicate, used as a dusting powder.

talipes (tal-i-peez) *n.* club-foot: a congenital deformity of one or both feet in which the patient cannot stand with the sole of the foot flat on the ground. *t. equinovarus* the most common variety of talipes, in which the foot points downwards, the heel is inverted, and the forefoot twisted. *t. valgus* talipes in which the hind foot is twisted outwards. *t.*

varus talipes in which the hind foot is turned inwards.

talus (astragalus) (tay-lŭs) *n.* the ankle bone. It forms part of the tarsus, articulating with the tibia above, the fibula to the side, and the calcaneus below.

tamoxifen (tam-oks-i-fen) *n.* a drug used in the treatment of breast cancer: it combines with hormone receptors in the tumour to inhibit the effect of oestrogens (*see* anti-oestrogen). Trade name: **Nolvadex**.

tampon (tam pon) *n.* a pack of gauze, cotton wool, or other absorbent material used to plug a cavity or canal in order to absorb blood or secretions.

tamponade (tam-pon-ayd) *n.* **1.** the insertion of a tampon. **2.** abnormal pressure on a part of the body. *cardiac t.* a build-up of fluid around the heart within the pericardium, causing compression of the heart. This results in heart failure, a drop in blood pressure, or cardiac arrest and requires drainage of the fluid.

tamsulosin (tam-soo-lŏ-sin) *n.* a highly selective alpha blocker taken by mouth to treat lower urinary tract symptoms thought to be due to benign prostatic hyperplasia (*see* prostate gland). Trade name: **Flomax**.

tantalum (tant-ă-lŭm) *n.* a rare heavy metal used in surgery. Tantalum sutures and plates are used for repair of defects in the bones of the skull. Symbol: Ta.

tapeworm (cestode) (tayp-werm) *n.* any of a group of flatworms that have a long thin ribbonlike body and live as parasites in the intestines of humans and other vertebrates. The body of a tapeworm consists of a head (*see* scolex), a short neck, and a chain of separate segments (*see* proglottis). Humans are the primary hosts for some tapeworms (*see* Taenia). However, other genera are also medically important (*see* Echinococcus).

tapotement (ta-poht-**mahn**) *n*. a technique used in massage in which a part of the body is struck rapidly and repeatedly with the hands.

tapping (tap-ing) *n*. *see* paracentesis.

tar (tar) *n*. a blackish viscous liquid produced by the destructive distillation of pine wood (*pine t.*) or coal (*coal t.*), used in skin preparations to treat eczema and psoriasis. As a constituent of cigarettes, tar is known to have carcinogenic properties.

tardive dyskinesia (tard-iv) *n*. *see* dyskinesia.

tars- (**tarso-**) *prefix denoting* **1.** the ankle; tarsal bones. **2.** the edge of the eyelid.

tarsal (tar-săl) **1.** *adj*. relating to the bones of the ankle and foot (tarsus). **2.** *adj*. relating to the eyelid, especially to its supporting tissue (tarsus). *t. glands see* meibomian glands. **3.** *n*. any of the bones forming the tarsus.

tarsalgia (tar-sal-jiă) *n*. aching pain arising from the tarsus in the foot.

tarsectomy (tar-sek-tŏmi) *n*. **1.** surgical excision of the tarsal bones of the foot. **2.** surgical removal of a section of the tarsus of the eyelid.

tarsitis (tar-sy-tis) *n*. inflammation of the eyelid.

tarsorrhaphy (tars-o-răfi) *n*. an operation in which the upper and lower eyelids are joined together. It

is performed to protect the cornea or to allow a corneal injury to heal.

tarsus (tar-sŭs) *n*. (*pl*. **tarsi**) **1.** the seven bones of the ankle and proximal part of the foot (see illustration). The tarsus articulates with the metatarsals distally and with the tibia and fibula proximally. **2.** the firm fibrous connective tissue that forms the basis of each eyelid.

Bones of the right ankle and foot

tartar (tar-ter) *n*. an obsolete name for calculus, the hard deposit that forms on the teeth.

task allocation (tahsk al-ŏ-kay-shŏn) *n*. a method of organizing nursing care in which patient care is divided into a number of tasks and a series of nurses is allocated to perform these tasks, on the basis of seniority. The patient thus receives fragmented care in which the emphasis is on the tasks (rather than the patient), which prevents holistic care and the development of a therapeutic relationship between patient and nurse. *Compare* patient allocation.

taste (tayst) *n.* the sense for the appreciation of the flavour of substances in the mouth. There are four basic taste sensations – sweet, bitter, sour, and salt. *t.* **buds** the sensory receptors concerned with the sense of taste. They are located in the epithelium that covers the surface of the tongue and in the soft palate, the epiglottis, and parts of the pharynx. When a taste cell is stimulated by the presence of a dissolved substance impulses are sent via nerve fibres to the brain.

taurine (tor-een) *n.* an amino acid that is a constituent of the bile salt sodium taurocholate and also functions as a neurotransmitter in the central nervous system.

taurocholic acid (tor-oh-koh-lik) *n. see* bile acids.

taxane (taks-ayn) *n.* a cytotoxic drug that interferes with a protein involved in cell division and exercises control on the growth of certain cancers. *See* docetaxel, paclitaxel.

taxis (tak-sis) *n.* (in surgery) the returning to a normal position of displaced bones, organs, or other parts by manipulation only.

Taxol (taks-ol) *n. see* paclitaxel.

Tay-Sachs disease (amaurotic familial idiocy) (tay-saks) *n.* an inherited disorder of lipid metabolism (*see* lipidosis) in which abnormal accumulation of lipid in the brain leads to blindness, mental retardation, and death in infancy. [W. Tay (1843–1927), British physician; B. Sachs (1858–1944), US neurologist]

TB *n. see* tuberculosis.

T bandage *n.* a T-shaped bandage used for the perineum and sometimes the head.

TBI *n. see* total body irradiation.

TBW *n.* total body water.

TCA *n. see* (tricyclic) antidepressant.

T-cell *n.* a type of lymphocyte that matures in the thymus and is primarily responsible for cell-mediated immunity. *cytotoxic T-c.* a T-cell that destroys cancerous cells, virus-infected cells, and allografts. *helper T-c.* a T-cell that stimulates the production of cytotoxic T-cells. *suppressor T-c.* a T-cell that prevents an immune response by other T-cells or B-cells to an antigen.

TCP *n.* **1.** *Trade name.* a solution of halogenated phenols: an effective antiseptic for minor skin injuries and irritations. It may also be used as a gargle for colds and sore throats. **2.** *see* thrombocytopenia.

t.d.s. (ter die sumendus) Latin: three times a day, used as a direction in prescriptions.

team nursing (teem) *n.* a method of organizing nursing care in which a team of nurses is responsible for the assessment, planning, implementation, and evaluation of a patient's hospital stay and subsequent discharge from the hospital.

tears (teerz) *pl. n.* the fluid secreted by the lacrimal glands to keep the front of the eyeballs moist and clean. Tears contain lysozyme, an enzyme that destroys bacteria.

technetium-99m (tek-nee-shi-ŭm) *n.* an isotope of the artificial radioactive element technetium. It emits gamma radiation and is widely used in nuclear medicine as a tracer for the examination of many organs.

tectospinal tract (tek-toh-**spy**-năl) *n.* a tract that conveys nerve impulses from the midbrain to the spinal cord in the cervical (neck) region.

tectum (tek-tŭm) *n.* the roof of the midbrain, behind and above the cerebral aqueduct.

TEDs *pl. n. see* thromboembolic deterrents.

teeth (teeth) *pl. n. see* tooth.

tegmen (teg-měn) *n.* (*pl.* **tegmina**) a structure that covers an organ or part of an organ.

tegmentum (teg-men-tŭm) *n.* the region of the midbrain below and in front of the cerebral aqueduct.

tel- (**tele-, telo-**) *prefix denoting* **1.** end or ending. **2.** distance.

tela (tee-lă) *n.* any thin weblike tissue. *t. choroidea* a folded double layer of pia mater containing numerous small blood vessels that extends into several of the ventricles of the brain.

telangiectasis (til-an-ji-ek-tă-sis) *n.* (*pl.* **telangiectases**) a localized collection of distended blood capillary vessels. It is recognized as a red spot, sometimes spidery in appearance, that blanches on pressure. Telangiectases may be found in the skin or the lining of the mouth, gastrointestinal, respiratory, and urinary passages.

teleceptor (tel-i-sep-ter) *n.* a sensory receptor that is capable of responding to distant stimuli.

telemedicine (tel-i-med-sin) *n.* the use of the telephone or the Internet in the diagnosis and treatment of patients by seeking the advice, or a second opinion, from experts at a distant hospital.

telencephalon (tel-en-sef-ă-lon) *n. see* cerebrum.

teleradiology (tel-i-ray-di-ol-ŏji) *n.* the process of transmitting and receiving medical images, to and from distant sites, using the telephone (or cable or satellite) network. This requires a dedicated broad-band link, such as an ISDN line, that has greater capacity for data transfer than standard telephone lines.

teletherapy (tel-i-th'e-ră-pi) *n.* a form of radiotherapy in which penetrating radiation is directed at a patient from a distance.

telmisartan (tel-miss-ar-tan) *n. see* angiotensin II antagonist.

telogen (tel-oh-jěn) *n. see* anagen.

temazepam (te-maz-ĕ-pam) *n.* a benzodiazepine given by mouth in the treatment of insomnia associated with difficulty falling asleep, frequent nocturnal awakenings, or early morning awakening.

temple (tem-pŭl) *n.* the region of the head in front of and above each ear.

temporal (temp-er-ăl) *adj.* of or relating to the temple. *t. arteritis see* arteritis. *t. artery* a branch of the external carotid artery that supplies blood mainly to the temple and scalp. *t. bone* either of a pair of bones of the cranium. The *squamous* portion forms part of the side of the cranium. The *petrous* part contributes to the base of the skull and contains the middle and inner ears. *See also* skull. *t. lobe* one of the main divisions of the cerebral cortex in each hemisphere of the brain, lying at the side within the temple. Areas of the cortex in this lobe are concerned with the appreciation of sound and spoken language. *t. lobe epilepsy see* epilepsy.

temporalis (tem-per-**ay**-lis) *n.* a fan-shaped muscle at the side of the head, extending from the temporal fossa to the mandible. This muscle lifts the lower jaw.

temporo- *prefix denoting* **1.** the temple. **2.** the temporal lobe of the brain.

temporomandibular joint (TMJ) (tem-per-oh-man-**dib**-yoo-ler) *n.* the articulation between the mandible and the temporal bone. *t. j. syndrome* a condition in which the patient has painful temporomandibular joints, tenderness in the muscles that move the jaw, clicking of the joints, and limitation of jaw movement.

tenaculum (tin-**ak**-yoo-lŭm) *n.* **1.** a sharp wire hook with a handle, used in surgical operations to pick up pieces of tissue or the cut end of an artery. **2.** a band of fibrous tissue that holds a part of the body in place.

tendinitis (ten-di-**ny**-tis) *n.* inflammation of a tendon. It occurs most commonly after excessive overuse but is sometimes due to bacterial infection (e.g. gonorrhoea) or a generalized rheumatic disease (e.g. rheumatoid arthritis, ankylosing spondylitis). *See also* jumper's knee, tennis elbow. *Compare* tenosynovitis.

tendon (ten-dŏn) *n.* a tough whitish cord, consisting of numerous parallel bundles of collagen fibres, that serves to attach a muscle to a bone. Tendons assist in concentrating the pull of the muscle on a small area of bone. *t. sheath* a tubular sac, lined with synovial membrane and con-taining synovial fluid, that surrounds some tendons. *See also* aponeurosis. *t. transfer* plastic surgery in which the tendon from an unimportant muscle is used to replace the damaged tendon of an important muscle. —**tendinous** (ten-din-ŭs) *adj.*

tendovaginitis (tenovaginitis) (ten-doh-vaj-i-**ny**-tis) *n.* inflammatory thickening of the fibrous sheath containing one or more tendons, usually caused by repeated minor injury. It usually occurs at the back of the thumb (*de Quervain's t.*) and results in pain on using the wrists.

tenesmus (tin-**ez**-mŭs) *n.* a sensation of the desire to defecate, which is continuous or recurs frequently, without the production of significant amounts of faeces. It may be due to proctitis, prolapse of the rectum, rectal tumour, or irritable bowel syndrome.

tennis elbow (ten-iss) *n.* a painful inflammation of the origin of the common extensor tendon on the lateral epicondyle of the humerus, caused by overuse of the forearm muscles. *See also* tendinitis. *Compare* golfer's elbow.

teno- *prefix denoting* a tendon.

tenonectomy (ten-ŏn-**ek**-tŏmi) *n.* surgical removal of a portion of Tenon's capsule.

tenonotomy (ten-ŏn-ot-ŏmi) *n.* a surgical incision made into Tenon's capsule.

Tenon's capsule (tĕ-nonz) *n.* the fibrous tissue that lines the orbit and surrounds the eyeball. [J. R. Tenon (1724–1816), French surgeon]

tenoplasty (ten-oh-plasti) *n.* surgical repair of a ruptured or severed tendon.

tenorrhaphy (tĕn-o-răfi) *n.* the surgical operation of uniting the ends of divided tendons by suture.

tenosynovitis (peritendinitis) (ten-oh-sy-noh-vy-tis) *n.* inflammation of a tendon sheath, producing pain, swelling, and an audible creaking on movement. It may result from a bacterial infection or occur as part of a rheumatic disease.

tenotomy (tĕ-not-ŏmi) *n.* surgical division of a tendon. This may be necessary to correct a joint deformity caused by tendon shortening.

tenovaginitis (ten-oh-vaj-i-ny-tis) *n. see* tendovaginitis.

TENS *n.* transcutaneous electrical nerve stimulation: *see* stimulator.

tensor (ten-ser) *n.* any muscle that causes stretching or tensing of a part of the body.

tent (tent) *n.* **1.** an enclosure of material (usually transparent plastic) around a patient in bed, into which a gas or vapour can be passed as part of treatment. *oxygen t.* a tent into which oxygen is passed. **2.** a piece of dried vegetable material, usually a seaweed stem, shaped to fit into an orifice, such as the cervical canal. As it absorbs moisture it expands, dilating the orifice.

tentorium (ten-tor-iŭm) *n.* a curved infolded sheet of dura mater that separates the cerebellum below from the occipital lobes of the cerebral hemispheres above.

terat- (terato-) *prefix denoting* a monster or congenital abnormality.

teratogen (te-ră-toh-jen) *n.* any substance, agent, or process that induces the formation of developmental abnormalities in a fetus. Known

teratogens include the drug thalidomide, German measles, and irradiation with X-rays. —**teratogenic** *adj.*

teratogenesis (te-ra-toh-jen-i-sis) *n.* the process leading to developmental abnormalities in the fetus.

teratology (te-ră-tol-ŏji) *n.* the study of developmental abnormalities and their causes.

teratoma (te-ră-toh-mă) *n.* a tumour composed of a number of tissues not usually found at that site. Teratomas most frequently occur in the testis and ovary, possibly derived from remnants of embryological cells. *malignant t. of the testis* a teratoma occurring in young men, frequently as a painless swelling of one testis. Treatment is by orchidectomy.

teratospermia (te-ră-toh-sper-miă) *n.* the presence in the semen of many bizarre or immature forms of spermatozoa, revealed by seminal analysis.

terbinafine (ter-bin-ă-feen) *n.* an antifungal drug used to treat severe ringworm (*see* tinea). It is administered by mouth or topically. Trade name: **Lamisil**.

terbutaline (ter-bew-tă-leen) *n.* a bronchodilator drug (*see* sympathomimetic) administered by mouth, injection, or inhalation in the treatment of asthma, bronchitis, and other respiratory disorders. Trade names: **Bricanyl**, **Monovent**.

teres (te-reez) *n.* either of two muscles of the shoulder, extending from the scapula to the humerus. *t. major* the muscle that rotates the arm inwards. *t. minor* the muscle that rotates the arm outwards.

terfenadine (ter-fen-ă-deen) *n.* an

antihistamine used for the treatment of the symptoms of hay fever and urticaria. It is administered by mouth.

terlipressin (ter-li-pres-in) *n.* a drug that releases vasopressin over a period of hours. It is administered by injection to control bleeding from oesophageal varices. Trade name: **Glypressin**.

terminal dribble (term-in-ăl drib-ĕl) *n.* a lower urinary tract symptom in which the flow of urine does not end quickly, but dribbles slowly towards an end. *Compare* postmicturition dribble.

Terramycin (te-ră-my-sin) *n. see* oxytetracycline.

tertian fever (ter-shăn) *n.* a type of malaria, caused by *Plasmodium ovale* or *P. vivax*, in which there is a two-day interval between fever attacks.

tertiary care (ter-sher-i) *n.* the services provided by specialized hospitals equipped with diagnostic and treatment facilities not available at general hospitals or by doctors who are uniquely qualified to treat unusual disorders that do not respond to therapy that is available at secondary care centres. *Compare* primary care, secondary care.

test (test) *n.* a laboratory examination or chemical analysis to determine the presence of a specific substance, microorganism, disease, etc. (See individual entries for named tests.)

testicle (test-ikŭl) *n.* either of the pair of male sex organs within the scrotum. It consists of the testis and its system of ducts (the vasa efferentia and epididymis).

testis (tes-tis) *n.* (*pl.* **testes**) either of the pair of male sex organs that produce spermatozoa and secrete the male sex hormone androgen under the control of gonadotrophins from the pituitary gland. The testes are contained within the scrotum (*see* reproductive system). *See also* spermatogenesis.

test meal *n.* a standard meal given to stimulate secretion of digestive juices, which can then be withdrawn by tube and measured as a test of digestive function.

testosterone (test-ost-er-ohn) *n.* the principal male sex hormone (*see* androgen).

test-tube baby (test-tewb) *n. see* in vitro fertilization.

tetan- (tetano-) *prefix denoting* **1.** tetanus. **2.** tetany.

tetanus (lockjaw) (tet-ăn-ŭs) *n.* an acute infectious disease, affecting the nervous system, caused by the bacterium *Clostridium tetani*. Infection occurs by contamination of wounds by bacterial spores. Symptoms consist of muscle stiffness, spasm, and subsequent rigidity, first in the jaw and neck then in the back, chest, abdomen, and limbs; in severe cases the spasm may affect the whole body, which is arched backwards (*see* opisthotonos). Prompt treatment with penicillin and antitoxin is effective; immunization against tetanus is effective but temporary. —**tetanic** (tě-tan-ik) *adj.*

tetanus toxoid (TT) *n.* a vaccine used in active immunization against tetanus. *See* DPT vaccine.

tetany (tet-ăn-i) *n.* spasm and twitching of the muscles, particularly those of the face, hands, and feet. Tetany is caused by a reduction in the blood calcium level, which may be due to underactive parathyroid glands, rickets, or alkalosis.

tetra- *prefix denoting* four.

tetracaine (amethocaine) (tet-ră-kayn) *n.* a potent local anaesthetic applied as a gel to the skin before intravenous injections or the insertion of a cannula. It is also applied as eye drops before eye operations and as a cream for the relief of local pain. Trade name: **Ametop**.

tetracosactide (tetracosactin) (tet-ră-kohz-**ak**-tyd) *n. see* short Synacthen test.

tetracycline (tet-ră-**sy**-kleen) *n.* **1.** one of a group of antibiotic compounds derived from cultures of *Streptomyces* bacteria. These drugs, including chlortetracycline, oxytetracycline, and tetracycline, are effective against a wide range of bacterial infections, including respiratory tract infections, syphilis, and acne. They are usually given by mouth. **2.** a particular antibiotic of the tetracycline group. Trade name: **Achromycin**.

tetradactyly (tet-ră-**dak**-tili) *n.* a congenital abnormality in which there are only four digits on a hand or foot. —**tetradactylous** *adj.*

tetrahydrocannabinol (tet-ră-hydroh-kan-**ab**-in-ol) *n.* a derivative of marijuana that has antiemetic activity and also produces euphoria. These two properties are utilized in the prevention of chemotherapy-induced sickness.

tetralogy of Fallot (te-tral-ŏji ŏv fa-loh) *n.* a form of congenital heart disease in which there is pulmonary stenosis, enlargement of the right ventricle, and a ventricular septal defect over which the origin of the

aorta lies. The affected child is blue (cyanosed). [E. L. A. Fallot (1850–1911), French physician]

tetraplegia (tet-ră-**plee**-jiă) *n. see* quadriplegia.

thalam- (thalamo-) *prefix denoting* the thalamus.

thalamencephalon (thal-ăm-en-**sef**-ă-lon) *n.* the structures, collectively, at the anterior end of the brainstem, comprising the epithalamus, thalamus, hypothalamus, and subthalamus.

thalamic syndrome (thă-**lam**-ik) *n.* a condition resulting from damage to the thalamus, often by a stroke, that is characterized by severe intractable pain and hypersensitivity in the area of the body served by the damaged brain region.

thalamotomy (thal-ă-**mot**-ŏmi) *n.* an operation on the brain in which a lesion is made in a precise part of the thalamus. It has been used to control psychiatric symptoms of severe anxiety and distress. *See also* psychosurgery.

thalamus (thal-ă-mŭs) *n. (pl.* **thalami**) one of two egg-shaped masses of grey matter that lie deep in the cerebral hemispheres in each side of the forebrain. The thalami are relay stations for all the sensory messages that enter the brain, before they are transmitted to the cortex.

thalassaemia (Cooley's anaemia) (thal-ă-**see**-miă) *n.* a hereditary blood disease, widespread in the Mediterranean countries, Asia, and Africa, in which there is an abnormality in the protein part of the haemoglobin molecule. Symptoms include anaemia, enlargement of the spleen, and abnormalities of the bone marrow. Individuals inheriting the disease from both parents are severely affected (*t. major*), but those inheriting it from only one parent are usually symptom-free.

thalidomide (thă-lid-ŏ-myd) *n.* a drug that was formerly used as a sedative. If taken during the first three months of pregnancy, it was found to cause fetal abnormalities involving limb malformation. Recently it has been found to be effective in treating certain cancers and other disorders (including Behçet's syndrome).

thallium scan (thal-iŭm) *n.* a method of studying blood flow through the heart muscle (myocardium) and diagnosing myocardial ischaemia using an injection of the radioisotope thallium-201. Defects of perfusion, such as a recent infarct, emit little or no radioactivity and are seen as 'cold spots' when an image is formed using a gamma camera and computer. Exercise may be used to provoke 'cold spots' in the diagnosis of ischaemic heart disease.

theca (th'ee-kă) *n.* a sheathlike surrounding tissue.

theine (th'ee-een) *n.* the active volatile principle found in tea (*see* caffeine).

thelarche (th'ee-lar-ki) *n.* the process of breast development, which occurs as a normal part of puberty. Isolated premature breast development in girls is not uncommon and is almost always benign.

thenar (th'oo-nar) *n.* **1.** the palm of the hand. **2.** the fleshy prominent part of the hand at the base of the thumb. *Compare* hypothenar. —**thenar** *adj.*

theobromine (thi-ŏ-broh-meen) *n.* an alkaloid, occurring in cocoa, coffee, and tea, that has a weak diuretic action and dilates coronary and other arteries.

theophylline (thi-off-i-leen) *n.* an alkaloid, occurring in the leaves of the tea plant, that has a diuretic effect and relaxes smooth muscles. Theophylline preparations, particularly aminophylline, are used mainly to control bronchial asthma. Trade names: **Nuelin, Slo-Phyllin, Theo-Dur, Uniphyllin Continus**.

therapeutic index (th'e-ră-pew-tik) *n.* the ratio of a dose of a therapeutic agent that produces damage to normal cells to the dose necessary to have a defined level of anticancer activity. It indicates the relative efficacy of a treatment against tumours.

therapeutics (th'e ră-pew-tiks) *n.* the branch of medicine that deals with different methods of treatment and healing (*therapy*), particularly the use of drugs in the cure of disease.

therm (therm) *n.* a unit of heat equal to 100,000 British thermal units. 1 therm = 1.055×10^8 joules.

therm- (thermo-) *prefix denoting* **1.** heat. **2.** temperature.

thermoanaesthesia (therm-oh-anis-theez-iă) *n.* absence of the ability to recognize the sensations of heat and coldness. It may indicate damage to the spinothalamic tract in the spinal cord.

thermocautery (therm-oh-kaw-ter-i) *n.* the destruction of unwanted tissues by heat (*see* cauterize).

thermocoagulation (therm-oh-koh-ag-yoo-lay-shŏn) *n.* the coagulation and destruction of tissues by cautery.

thermography (ther-mog-răfi) *n.* a technique for measuring and recording the heat produced by different parts of the body, by using photographic film sensitive to infrared radiation. The picture produced is called a *thermogram*. A tumour with an abnormally increased blood supply may be revealed on the thermogram as a 'hot spot'.

thermokeratoplasty (therm-oh-ke-ră-toh-plasti) *n.* the application of heat to the periphery of the cornea in order to shrink the cornea and hence change its refractive power: used to correct long-sightedness (hypermetropia) and presbyopia.

thermolysis (ther-mol-i-sis) *n.* (in physiology) the dissipation of body heat by such processes as the evaporation of sweat from the skin surface.

thermometer (ther-mom-i-ter) *n.* a device for registering temperature. *clinical t.* a sealed narrow-bore glass tube containing mercury, which expands when heated and rises up the tube. The tube is designed to register body temperatures between 35°C (95°F) and 43.5°C (110°F).

thermophilic (therm-oh-fil-ik) *adj.* describing organisms, especially bacteria, that grow best at temperatures of 48–85°C.

thermoreceptor (therm-oh-ri-septer) *n.* a sensory nerve ending that responds to heat or to cold.

thermotaxis (therm-moh-tak-sis) *n.* the physiological process of regulating or adjusting body temperature.

thermotherapy (therm-oh-th'e-ră-pi) *n.* the use of heat to alleviate pain and stiffness in joints and muscles and to promote an increase in circulation.

thiabendazole (th'y-ă-ben-dă-zohl) *n. see* tiabendazole.

thiamin (vitamin B₁) (th'y-ă-min) *n. see* vitamin B.

thiazide diuretic (th'y-ă-zyd) *n. see* diuretic.

thiazolidinediones (th'y-ă-zol-i-deen-dy-ohnz) *pl. n. see* oral hypoglycaemic drug.

Thiersch's graft (teer-shĕz) *n. see* split-skin graft. [K. Thiersch (1822–95), German surgeon]

thigh (th'y) *n.* the upper part of the lower limb, between the hip and the knee. *t. bone see* femur.

thioguanine (th'y-oh-gwah-neen) *n. see* tioguanine.

thiopental (thiopentone) (th'y-oh-pen-tal) *n.* a short-acting barbiturate. It is given by intravenous injection to produce general anaesthesia or as a premedication prior to surgery.

thioridazine (th'y-oh-rid-ă-zeen) *n.* a phenothiazine antipsychotic drug administered by mouth in the treatment of a range of mental, behavioural, and emotional disturbances, including schizophrenia. Trade name: **Melleril**.

Thomas's splint (tom-ă-siz) *n.* a metal splint used for immobilizing a fractured lower limb, especially the femur. There is a ring at the hip, a cross-piece at the foot, and sidepieces for the attachment of material to support the leg. [H. O. Thomas (1834–1891), British orthopaedic surgeon]

thorac- (thoraco-) *prefix denoting* the thorax or chest.

thoracentesis (thor-ă-sen-tee-sis) *n. see* pleurocentesis.

thoracic cavity (thor-ass-ik) *n.* the chest cavity. *See* thorax.

thoracic duct *n.* one of the two main trunks of the lymphatic system. It receives lymph from both legs, the lower abdomen, left thorax, left side of the head, and left arm and drains into the left innominate vein.

thoracic vertebrae *pl. n.* the 12 bones of the backbone to which the ribs are attached. *See also* vertebra.

thoracocentesis (thor-ă-koh-sen-tee-sis) *n. see* pleurocentesis.

thoracoplasty (thor-ă-koh-plasti) *n.* a former treatment for pulmonary tuberculosis involving surgical removal of parts of the ribs, thus allowing the chest wall to fall in and collapse the affected lung.

thoracoscope (thor-ă-koh-skohp) *n.* an instrument used to inspect the pleural cavity. —**thoracoscopy** (thor-ă-kosk-ŏpi) *n.*

thoracotomy (thor-ă-kot-ŏmi) *n.* surgical opening of the chest cavity to inspect or operate on the heart, lungs, or other structures within.

thorax (thor-aks) *n.* the chest: the part of the body cavity between the neck and the diaphragm. The skeleton of the thorax is formed by the sternum, costal cartilages, ribs, and thoracic vertebrae. It encloses the lungs, heart, oesophagus, and associated structures. *Compare* abdomen. —**thoracic** *adj.*

threadworm (pinworm) (thred-werm) *n.* a parasitic nematode worm of the genus *Enteroblus* (*Oxyuris*), which lives in the upper part of the human large intestine. Threadworms cause enterobiasis, a disease common in children throughout the world.

threonine (three-ŏ-neen) *n.* an essential amino acid. *See also* amino acid.

threshold (thresh-ohld) *n.* (in neurology) the point at which a stimulus begins to evoke a response, and therefore a measure of the sensitivity of a system under particular conditions.

thrill (thril) *n.* a vibration felt on placing the hand on the body.

-thrix *suffix denoting* a hair or hair-like structure.

thromb- (thrombo-) *prefix denoting* **1.** a blood clot (thrombus). **2.** thrombosis. **3.** blood platelets.

thrombectomy (throm-bek-tŏmi) *n.* a surgical procedure in which a blood clot (thrombus) is removed from an artery or a vein (*see* endarterectomy, phlebothrombosis).

thrombin (throm-bin) *n.* a substance (coagulation factor) that acts as an enzyme, converting the soluble protein fibrinogen to the insoluble protein fibrin in the final stage of blood coagulation. Thrombin is derived from the inactive substance prothrombin.

thromboangiitis obliterans (throm-boh-an-ji-I-tis ŏ-blit-er-anz) *n. see* Buerger's disease.

thromboarteritis (throm-boh-ar-ter-I-tis) *n.* inflammation of an artery (*see* arteritis) associated with thrombosis.

thrombocyte (throm-boh-syt) *n. see* platelet.

thrombocythaemia (throm-boh-si-th'ee-miă) *n.* a disease in which there is an abnormal proliferation of megakaryocytes, leading to an increased number of platelets in the blood.

thrombocytopenia (TCP) (throm-boh-sy-toh-**pee**-niă) *n.* a reduction in the number of platelets in the blood. This results in bleeding into the skin (*see* purpura), spontaneous bruising, and prolonged bleeding after injury. —**thrombocytopenic** *adj.*

thrombocytosis (throm-boh-sy-**toh**-sis) *n.* an increase in the number of platelets in the blood. It may occur in a variety of diseases, including cancers and certain blood diseases, and is likely to cause an increased tendency to thrombosis.

thromboembolic deterrents (TEDs) (throm-boh-em-**bol**-ik) *pl. n.* stockings worn to reduce the risk of deep vein thrombosis, especially after surgery.

thromboembolism (throm-boh-em-bŏ-lizm) *n.* the condition in which a blood clot (thrombus), formed at one point in the circulation, becomes detached and lodges at another point.

thromboendarterectomy (throm-boh-end-ar-ter-**ek**-tŏmi) *n. see* endarterectomy.

thromboendarteritis (throm-boh-end-ar-ter-**I**-tis) *n.* thrombosis complicating endarteritis, seen in temporal arteritis, polyarteritis nodosa, and syphilis.

thrombokinase (throm-boh-**ky**-nayz) *n. see* thromboplastin.

thrombolysis (throm-**bol**-i-sis) *n.* the dissolution of a blood clot (thrombus) by the infusion of a fibrinolytic agent into the blood.

thrombolytic (throm-boh-**lit**-ik) *adj.* describing an agent that breaks up blood clots (thrombi). *See* fibrinolytic, tissue-type plasminogen activator.

thrombophilia (throm-boh-**fil**-iă) *n.* an inherited or acquired condition that predisposes individuals to thrombosis.

thrombophlebitis (throm-boh-fli-by-tis) *n.* inflammation of the wall of a vein (*see* phlebitis) with secondary thrombosis occurring within the affected segment of vein. Pregnant women are more prone to thrombophlebitis because of physiological changes in the blood and the effects of pressure within the abdomen. It may involve superficial or deep veins of the legs (the latter being less common in pregnancy than the former).

thromboplastin (thrombokinase) (throm-boh-**plast**-in) *n.* a substance formed during the earlier stages of blood coagulation. It acts as an enzyme, converting the inactive substance prothrombin to the enzyme thrombin.

thrombopoiesis (throm-boh-poi-**ee**-sis) *n.* the process of blood platelet production. Platelets are formed as fragments of cytoplasm shed from giant cells (megakaryocytes) in the bone marrow by a budding process.

thrombosis (throm-**boh**-sis) *n.* a condition in which the blood changes from a liquid to a solid state and produces a blood clot (*thrombus*). Thrombosis in an artery obstructs the blood flow to the tissue it supplies (*see* coronary thrombosis, stroke). Thrombosis can also occur in a vein (*deep vein t.; see* phlebothrombosis), and it may be associated with inflammation (*see* thrombophlebitis).

thrombus (throm-bŭs) *n.* a blood clot (*see* thrombosis).

thrush (thrush) *n.* see candidosis.

thumb (thum) *n.* the first digit on the radial side of the hand. It can oppose the other four fingers of the hand.

thym- (thymo-) *prefix denoting* the thymus.

thymectomy (th'y-**mek**-tŏmi) *n.* surgical removal of the thymus.

-thymia *suffix denoting* a condition of the mind.

thymine (th'y-meen) *n.* one of the nitrogen-containing bases (*see* pyrimidine) occurring in the nucleic acid DNA.

thymitis (th'y-**my**-tis) *n.* inflammation of the thymus.

thymocyte (th'y-moh-syt) *n.* a lymphocyte within the thymus.

thymol (th'y-mol) *n.* an antiseptic active against bacteria and fungi, used in mouthwashes, gargles, and skin preparations.

thymoma (th'y-moh-mă) *n.* a benign or malignant tumour of the thymus. It is sometimes associated with myasthenia gravis.

thymoxamine (th'y-**moks**-ă-meen) *n.* see moxisylyte.

thymus (th'y-mŭs) *n.* a bilobed organ in the root of the neck, above and in front of the heart. In relation to body size the thymus is largest at birth. It doubles in size by puberty, after which it gradually shrinks, its functional tissue being replaced by fatty tissue. In infancy the thymus controls the development of lymphoid tissue and immune response to microbes and foreign proteins. Its

function in the adult is unclear. —**thymic** *adj.*

thyro- *prefix denoting* the thyroid gland.

thyrocalcitonin (th'y-roh-kal-si-toh-nin) *n.* see calcitonin.

thyrocele (th'y-roh-seel) *n.* a swelling of the thyroid gland. See goitre.

thyroglobulin (th'y-roh-**glob**-yoo-lin) *n.* a protein in the thyroid gland from which the thyroid hormones are synthesized.

thyroglossal (th'y-roh-**glos**-ăl) *adj.* relating to the thyroid gland and the tongue. *t.* **duct** a duct in the embryo between the thyroid and the back of the tongue.

thyroid cartilage (th'y-roid) *n.* the main cartilage of the larynx, consisting of two broad plates that join at the front. *See also* Adam's apple.

thyroidectomy (th'y-roid-**ek**-tŏmi) *n.* surgical removal of the thyroid gland. *partial t.* thyroidectomy in which only the diseased part of the gland is removed. *subtotal t.* a method of treating thyrotoxicosis, in which the surgeon removes 90% of the gland.

thyroid gland *n.* a large endocrine gland situated in the base of the neck. It consists of two lobes, one on either side of the trachea, that are joined by an isthmus. The thyroid gland is concerned with regulation of the metabolic rate by the secretion of thyroid hormone. The C cells of the thyroid gland secrete calcitonin. See illustration.

thyroid hormone *n.* an iodine-containing substance, synthesized and secreted by the thyroid gland, that is essential for normal metahyoid bone

thyroid cartilage

cricoid cartilage

left lobe of thyroid gland

isthmus

right lobe of thyroid gland

trachea

Position of the thyroid gland

bolic processes and mental and physical development. There are two thyroid hormones, *triiodothyronine* (T_3) and *thyroxine* (T_4). Lack of these hormones gives rise to cretinism in infants and myxoedema in adults. Excessive production of thyroid hormones gives rise to thyrotoxicosis.

thyroiditis (th'y-roid-I-tis) *n.* inflammation of the thyroid gland. *acute t.* thyroiditis due to bacterial infection. *chronic t.* thyroiditis that is commonly caused by an abnormal immune response (*see* autoimmunity) in which lymphocytes invade the tissues of the gland. *See* Hashimoto's disease.

thyroid-stimulating hormone (TSH, thyrotrophin) *n.* a hormone, synthesized and secreted by the anterior pituitary gland under the control of thyrotrophin-releasing hormone, that stimulates activity of the thyroid gland.

thyroid storm *n.* a life-threatening condition due to a severe worsening of thyrotoxicosis that is previously

undiagnosed or inadequately treated. It often follows infections, childbirth, nonthyroid surgery, or trauma and presents as fever, severe agitation, nausea and vomiting, diarrhoea, abdominal pains, an accelerated heart rate and irregularity of the heart rhythm.

thyroplasty (th'y-roh-plasti) *n.* a surgical procedure performed on the thyroid cartilage of the larynx to alter the characteristics of the voice.

thyrotomy (th'y-**rot**-ŏmi) *n.* surgical incision of either the thyroid cartilage or the thyroid gland itself.

thyrotoxicosis (th'y-roh-toks-i-koh-sis) *n.* the syndrome due to excessive amounts of thyroid hormones in the bloodstream, causing a rapid heartbeat, sweating, tremor, anxiety, increased appetite, loss of weight, and intolerance of heat. Causes include simple overactivity of the gland, a hormone-secreting tumour, and Graves' disease (*exophthalmic goitre*), in which there are additional symptoms including swelling of the neck (goitre) and protrusion of the eyes (exophthalmos). —**thyrotoxic** (th'y-roh-**toks**-ik) *adj.*

thyrotoxic periodic paralysis *n.* a condition in which attacks of sudden weakness and flaccidity occur in patients with thyrotoxicosis, seen most often in Asian males.

thyrotrophin (th'y-roh-**troh**-fin) *n. see* thyroid-stimulating hormone.

thyrotrophin-releasing hormone (TRH) *n.* a hormone that is secreted from the hypothalamus (in the brain) and acts on the anterior pituitary gland to stimulate the release of thyroid-stimulating hormone.

thyroxine (th'y-roks-een) *n.* *see* thyroid hormone.

TIA *n.* *see* transient ischaemic attack.

tiabendazole (thiabendazole) (ty-ă-ben-dă-zohl) *n.* an anthelmintic administered orally to treat infestations of threadworms and other intestinal worms. Trade name: **Mintezol**.

TIBC *n.* total iron-binding capacity (of blood serum).

tibia (tib-iă) *n.* the shin bone: the inner and larger bone of the lower leg. It articulates with the femur above, with the talus below, and with the fibula to the side. —**tibial** (tib-iăl) *adj.*

tibialis (tib-i-ay-lis) *n.* either of two muscles in the leg, extending from the tibia to the metatarsal bones of the foot. *t. anterior* the muscle that turns the foot inwards and flexes the toes backwards. *t. posterior* the muscle that extends the toes and inverts the foot.

tibial torsion *n.* a normal variation in posture in which there is an in-toe gait due to mild internal rotation of the tibia. The condition is often apparent in infancy when the child starts walking and resolves spontaneously with time.

tibio- *prefix denoting* the tibia.

tic (tik) *n.* a repeated and largely involuntary movement varying in complexity from the twitch of a muscle to elaborate well-coordinated actions. Simple tics occur in about a quarter of children and usually disappear within a year. *See also* Gilles de la Tourette syndrome. *t. douloureux see* neuralgia.

ticarcillin (tik-ar-sil-in) *n.* a penicillin type antibiotic used in combination with clavulanic acid (as *Timentin*) to treat infections caused by *Pseudomonas* and *Proteus* bacteria.

tick (tik) *n.* a bloodsucking parasite belonging to the order of arthropods (Acarina) that also includes the mites. Tick bites can cause serious skin lesions and occasionally paralysis, and certain tick species transmit typhus, Lyme disease, and relapsing fever. Dimethyl phthalate is used as a tick repellent. *t. fever* any infectious disease transmitted by ticks, especially Rocky Mountain spotted fever.

tidal volume (TV) (ty-d'l) *n.* the volume of air that is taken into the lungs and exhaled in normal quiet breathing.

timolol (tim-ō-lol) *n.* a beta blocker used in the treatment of high blood pressure (hypertension), long-term prophylaxis after an acute myocardial infarction, and glaucoma. It is administered by mouth or in solution as eye drops. Trade names: **Betim, Blocadren, Timoptol**.

tincture (tink-cher) *n.* an alcoholic extract of a drug derived from a plant.

tinea (ringworm) (tin-iă) *n.* a fungus infection of the skin, scalp, or nails. It is caused by the dermatophyte fungi – *Microsporum*, *Trichophyton*, and *Epidermophyton* – and can be spread by direct contact or via infected materials. The lesions of ringworm may form partial or complete rings and may cause intense itching. The disease is treated with antifungal agents taken by mouth (such as itraconazole or terbinafine) or applied locally. *t. barbae* ringworm of the skin under a beard. *t. capitis* ringworm of the scalp, of which favus is a severe form. *t. cruris see* dhobie itch. *t. pedis see* athlete's foot.

Tinel's sign (ti-nelz) *n.* a method for checking the regeneration of a nerve, usually in patients with carpal tunnel syndrome. Direct tapping over the sheath of the nerve elicits a distal tingling sensation (*see* paraesthesiae), which indicates the beginning of regeneration. [J. Tinel (1879–1952), French neurologist]

tinnitus (ti-ny-tŭs) *n.* the sensation of sounds in the ears, head, or around the head in the absence of an external sound source. It can occur with any form of hearing loss or with normal hearing and is thought to be due to a misinterpretation of signals in the central auditory pathways in the brain. *t. retraining therapy (TRT)* a unified method of treating tinnitus, including explanation, counselling, relaxation techniques, and sound therapy (*see* white noise instrument).

tintometer (tin-tom-it-er) *n.* an instrument for measuring the depth of colour in a liquid. The colour can then be compared with those from standard charts so that the concentration of a particular compound in solution can be estimated.

tioguanine (thioguamine) (ty-oh-gwah-neen) *n.* a drug that prevents the growth of cancer cells (*see* antimetabolite) and is administered by mouth in the treatment of leukaemia. Trade name: **Lanvis**.

tissue (tis-yoo) *n.* a collection of cells specialized to perform a particular function. Aggregations of tissues constitute organs. *t. culture* the culture of living tissues, removed from the body, in a suitable medium supplied with nutrients and oxygen. *t. typing* determination of the HLA profiles of tissues (*see* HLA system) to assess their compatibility. It is the most important predictor of success or failure of a transplant operation.

tissue-type plasminogen activator (tPA, TPA) *n.* a natural protein, found in the body and now able to be manufactured by genetic engineering, that can break up a thrombus (*see* thrombolysis). It requires the presence of fibrin as a cofactor and capable of activating plasminogen on the fibrin surface, which distinguishes it from the other plasminogen activators streptokinase and urokinase.

titration (ty-tray-shŏn) *n.* a method of determining the concentration of a substance in solution. A measured volume of a reagent of known concentration is added to a known volume of the test solution until the end point of the reaction has occurred.

titre (ty-ter) *n.* (in immunology) the extent to which a sample of blood serum containing antibody can be diluted before losing its ability to cause agglutination of the relevant antigen. It is used as a measure of the amount of antibody in the serum.

TLC *n. see* total lung capacity.

T-lymphocyte *n. see* lymphocyte, T-cell.

TMJ *n. see* temporomandibular joint.

TNF *n. see* tumour necrosis factor.

TNM classification *n.* a classification defined by the UICC (Union International Contre le Cancer) for the extent of spread of a cancer. T refers to the size of the tumour, N the presence and extent of lymph node involvement, and M the presence of distant spread (metastasis).

tobacco (tŏ-bak-oh) *n.* the dried leaves of the plant *Nicotiana tabacum* or related species, used in smoking and as snuff. Tobacco contains the stimulant but poisonous alkaloid nicotine, which enters the bloodstream during smoking. The volatile tarry material released during smoking contains carcinogenic chemicals.

tobramycin (toh-bră-my-sin) *n.* an antibiotic used to treat septicaemia, external eye infections, and lower respiratory, urinary, skin, abdominal, and central nervous system infections. It is administered by intravenous or intramuscular injection or by inhalation. Trade names: **Nebcin, Tobri**.

toco- (toko-) *prefix denoting* childbirth or labour.

tocography (tok-og-răfi) *n.* the measuring and recording of the force and frequency of uterine contractions during labour using an instrument called a *tocodynamometer*.

tocopherol (tok-off-er-ol) *n. see* vitamin E.

toddler's diarrhoea (tod-lerz) *n.* a disorder of young children characterized by the passage of frequent loose, offensive, and bulky stools in which partially digested or undigested food may be visible (the 'peas and carrot' stool). It resolves by school age.

Todd's paralysis (Todd's palsy) (todz) *n.* transient paralysis of a part of the body that has previously been involved in a focal epileptic seizure (*see* epilepsy). [R. B. Todd (1809–60), British physician]

toko- *see* toco-.

tokophobia (tocophobia) (tok-ŏ-foh-bia) *n.* a profound fear of childbirth. *primary t.* tokophobia that develops in adolescence and causes many women to avoid childbirth altogether. *secondary t.* tokophobia that occurs after a traumatic delivery and can stop a woman having another child.

tolbutamide (tol-bew-tă-myd) *n.* a drug taken by mouth in the treatment of noninsulin-dependent diabetes mellitus. It acts directly on the pancreas to stimulate insulin production and is particularly effective in elderly patients with mild diabetes. *See also* sulphonylurea.

tolerance (tol-er-ăns) *n.* the reduction or loss of the normal response to a substance that usually provokes a reaction in the body. *drug t.* tolerance that may develop after taking a particular drug over a long period of time. In such cases increased doses are necessary to produce the desired effect. *See also* glucose tolerance test, immunological tolerance.

tolnaftate (tol-naf-tayt) *n.* an antifungal drug applied topically as a cream, powder, or solution in the treatment of various fungal infections of the skin, including ringworm. Trade name: **Mycil**.

tolterodine (tol-te-rŏ-deen) *n.* an anticholinergic drug used to treat detrusor overactivity giving rise to the lower urinary tract symptoms of frequency, urgency, or urge incontinence. Trade name: **Detrusitol**.

-tome *suffix denoting* a cutting instrument.

tomo- *prefix denoting* **1.** section or sections. **2.** surgical operation.

tomography (tŏ-mog-răfi) *n.* the technique of rotating a radiation detector around the patient so that the image obtained gives additional three-dimensional information. In plain film tomography this produces an image of structures at a particular depth within the body, bringing them into sharp focus, while deliberately blurring structures above and below them. The visual record of this technique is called a *tomogram. See also* computerized tomography, positron emission tomography, SPECT scanning.

-tomy (-otomy) *suffix denoting* a surgical incision into an organ or part.

tone (tohn) *n. see* tonus.

tongue (tung) *n.* a muscular organ attached to the floor of the mouth. It is covered by mucous membrane and its surface is raised in minute projections (papillae), which give it a furred appearance. Taste buds are arranged in grooves around the papillae. The tongue helps in manipulating food during mastication and swallowing; it is the main organ of taste; and it plays an important role in the production of articulate speech. Anatomical name: **glossa**.

tongue-tie (tung-ty) *n.* a disorder of young children in which the tongue is anchored in the floor of the mouth more firmly than usual. No treatment is required unless the condition is extreme and associated with forking of the tongue, in which case surgery may be necessary.

tonic (ton-ik) **1.** *adj. a.* relating to normal muscle tone. *b.* marked by continuous tension (contraction),

e.g. a tonic muscle spasm. *t. pupil* (*Adie's pupil*) a pupil that is dilated as a result of damage to the nerves supplying the ciliary muscle and iris. **2.** *n.* a medicinal substance purporting to increase vigour and liveliness and produce a feeling of wellbeing: beneficial effects of tonics are probably due to their placebo action.

tonicity (toh-nis-iti) *n.* **1.** the normal state of slight contraction, or readiness to contract, of healthy muscle fibres. **2.** the effective osmotic pressure of a solution. *See* hypertonic, hypotonic, osmosis.

tono- *prefix denoting* **1.** tone or tension. **2.** pressure.

tonography (toh-nog-răfi) *n.* measurement of the pressure within the eyeball in such a way as to record variations in pressure over a period of several minutes.

tonometer (toh-nom-it-er) *n.* **1.** (**ophthalmotonometer**) an instrument for measuring pressure inside the eye. *Goldman applanation t.* a tonometer that measures the force required to flatten an area of cornea $3\,mm^2$. A greater force is required when the pressure inside the eye is increased. **2.** an instrument for measuring pressure in any other part of the body. —**tonometry** *n.*

tonsil (ton-sil) *n.* a mass of lymphoid tissue on either side of the back of the mouth, between the anterior and posterior pillars of the fauces. The tonsils are concerned with protection against infection. *See also* adenoids (nasopharyngeal tonsil).

tonsillectomy (ton-sil-ek-tŏmi) *n.* surgical removal of the tonsils.

tonsillitis (ton-sil-I-tis) *n.* inflammation of the tonsils due to bacterial or viral infection, causing a sore throat, fever, and difficulty in swallowing.

tonsillotome (ton-**sil**-ŏ-tohm) *n.* a surgical knife used for cutting into or removing a tonsil.

tonus (tone) (toh-nŭs) *n.* the normal state of partial contraction of a resting muscle.

tooth (tooth) *n.* (*pl.* **teeth**) one of the hard structures in the mouth used for cutting and chewing food. Each tooth is embedded in a socket in the jawbone, to which it is attached by the periodontal membrane. The exposed part of the tooth (*crown*) is covered with enamel and the part

within the bone (*root*) is coated with cementum; the bulk of the tooth consists of dentine enclosing the pulp. There are four different types of teeth (*see* canine, incisor, premolar, molar). See illustration. *See also* dentition.

toothpaste (tooth-payst) *n. see* dentifrice.

TOP *n.* termination of pregnancy. *See* (induced) abortion.

topagnosis (top-ag-**noh**-sis) *n.* inability to identify a part of the body that has been touched. It is a symptom of disease in the parietal lobes of the brain.

tophus (toh-fŭs) *n.* (*pl.* **tophi**) a hard deposit of crystalline uric acid

enamel

neck

gum (gingiva)

pulp cavity

nerves and blood vessels

dentine

periodontal membrane

root canal

alveolar bone

cementum

apical foramen

crown

root

Section of a molar tooth

and its salts in the skin, cartilage (especially of the ears), or joints: a feature of gout.

topical (top-ikăl) *adj.* local: used for the route of administration of a drug that is applied directly to the part being treated.

topo- *prefix denoting* place; position; location.

topography (tŏ-pog-răfi) *n.* the study of the different regions of the body, including the description of its parts in relation to the surrounding structures. **corneal t.** (*videokeratography*) a technique in which an image projected onto the cornea is analysed by computer to produce a representation of the shape and refractive power of the corneal surface. —**topographical** (top-ŏ-graf-ikăl) *adj.*

topotecan (top-oh-tee-kăn) *n.* a cytotoxic drug administered by intravenous infusion for treating advanced ovarian cancer. Trade name: **Hycamtin.**

tormina (tor-min-ă) *n. see* colic.

torpor (tor-per) *n.* a state of sluggishness and diminished responsiveness: a characteristic of certain mental disorders and a symptom of certain forms of poisoning or metabolic disorder.

torsion (tor-shŏn) *n.* twisting. *See also* tibial torsion.

torticollis (wryneck) (tor-ti-kol-iss) *n.* an irresistible turning movement of the head that becomes more persistent, so that eventually the head is held continually to one side. A form of dystonia, it may be caused by a birth injury to the sternomastoid muscle (*see* sternomastoid tumour).

total body irradiation (TBI)

(toh-t'l) *n.* exposure of the whole of the patient's body to radiotherapy. It is used in certain forms of cancer, such as cancers of the blood-forming tissues, prior to a bone marrow transplant.

total lung capacity (TLC) *n.* the volume of air held by the lungs after a deep inspiration.

total quality management (TQM) *n.* an approach to management that aims to ensure quality, effectiveness, and flexibility throughout an organization, with all individuals in the organization contributing to achieve this.

Tourette syndrome (toor-et) *n. see* Gilles de la Tourette disease.

tourniquet (toor-ni-kay) *n.* a device to press upon an artery and prevent flow of blood through it, usually a cord, rubber tube, or tight bandage. Tourniquets are no longer recommended as a first-aid measure to stop bleeding from a wound; direct pressure on the wound itself is considered less harmful.

tow (toh) *n.* the teased-out short fibres of flax, hemp, or jute, used in swabs, stupes, and for a variety of other purposes.

tox- (toxi-, toxo-, toxic(o)-) *prefix denoting* **1.** poisonous; toxic. **2.** toxins or poisoning.

toxaemia (toks-eem-iă) *n.* blood poisoning that is caused by toxins formed by bacteria growing in a local site of infection. *Compare* pyaemia, sapraemia, septicaemia.

toxic (toks-ik) *adj.* having a poisonous effect; potentially lethal.

toxicity (toks-iss-iti) *n.* the degree to which a substance is poisonous.

toxicology (toks-i-kol-ŏji) *n.* the study of poisonous materials and

their effects upon living organisms.
—**toxicologist** n.

toxicosis (toks-i-**koh**-sis) n. the deleterious effects of a toxin; poisoning.

toxic shock syndrome (TSS) n. a state of acute shock due to septicaemia. The commonest cause is a retained foreign body (e.g. a tampon or IUCD) combined with the presence of staphylococci. The condition can be life-threatening if not treated aggressively with appropriate antibiotics and supportive care (including fluid and electrolyte replacement). **streptococcal t. s. s.** a similar condition caused by Type A streptococci. *See also* necrotizing fasciitis.

toxin (toks-in) n. a poison produced by a living organism, especially by a bacterium (*see* endotoxin, exotoxin). In the body toxins act as antigens (*see* antitoxin).

toxocariasis (visceral larva migrans) (toks-oh-kair-**I**-a-sis) n. an infestation with the larvae of the dog and cat roundworms, *Toxocara canis* and *T. cati*. It is characterized by enlargement of the liver, pneumonitis, fever, joint and muscle pains, vomiting, an irritating rash, and convulsions.

toxoid (toks-oid) n. a preparation of a toxin that has been rendered harmless by chemical treatment while retaining its antigenic activity. Toxoids are used in vaccines.

toxoid-antitoxin n. a mixture of a toxoid and its antitoxin used as a vaccine to produce active immunity.

toxoplasmosis (toks-oh-plaz-**moh**-sis) n. a disease of mammals and birds due to the protozoan *Toxo-*

plasma gondii, which may be transmitted to humans (usually by eating undercooked infected meat or by contact with cat faeces). Generally symptoms are mild (swollen lymph nodes and an influenza-like illness), but the disease can be serious in immunocompromised patients. **congenital t.** toxoplasmosis transmitted by a woman infected during pregnancy to her fetus. It may produce severe malformations of the skull and eyes or active liver infection in the newborn.

tPA (TPA) n. *see* tissue-type plasminogen activator.

TPN n. *see* (total parenteral) nutrition.

TPR temperature, pulse, respiration.

TQM n. *see* total quality management.

trabecula (trǎ-bek-yoo-lǎ) n. (*pl.* **trabeculae**) **1.** any of the bands of tissue that pass from the outer part of an organ to its interior, dividing it into separate chambers. **2.** any of the thin bars of bony tissue in spongy bone. —**trabecular** adj.

trabeculectomy (trǎ-bek-yoo-lek-tŏmi) n. an operation for glaucoma, one part of which is the removal of a small segment of tissue from part of the wall of Schlemm's canal. This area is known as the *trabecular meshwork*. Trabeculectomy allows aqueous fluid to filter out of the eye under the conjunctiva, thus reducing the pressure inside the eye.

trabeculoplasty (trǎ-bek-yoo-loh-plasti) n. a method used to selectively destroy parts of the trabecular meshwork (*see* trabeculectomy) and hence reduce intraocular pressure in the treatment of glaucoma.

This may be achieved by means of a laser (*argon laser t.*).

trace element (trayss) *n.* an element required in minute amounts for the normal functioning of the body. Examples are copper, cobalt, and manganese.

tracer (tray-ser) *n.* a substance that is introduced into the body and whose progress can subsequently be followed so that information is gained about metabolic processes. Radioactive tracers, which are substances labelled with radionuclides, are used for a variety of purposes in nuclear medicine.

trache- (tracheo-) *prefix denoting* the trachea.

trachea (tray-kiă) *n.* the windpipe: the part of the air passage between the larynx and the main bronchi. —**tracheal** (tray-ki-ăl) *adj.*

tracheal tugging *n.* a sign indicative of an aneurysm of the aortic arch: a downward tug is felt on the windpipe when the finger is placed in the midline at the root of the neck.

tracheitis (tray-ki-I-tis) *n.* inflammation of the trachea, usually secondary to bacterial or viral infection in the nose or throat. Tracheitis causes soreness in the chest and a painful cough and is often associated with bronchitis.

trachelorrhaphy (tray-kĕl-o-răfi) *n.* an operation for suturing tears in the cervix of the uterus.

tracheobronchitis (tray-ki-oh-brong-ky-tis) *n.* inflammation of the trachea and bronchi.

tracheostomy (tracheotomy) (tray-ki-ost-ŏmi) *n.* a surgical operation in which a hole is made into the trachea through the neck to relieve obstruction to breathing, as in diphtheria. A curved metal, plastic, or rubber tube is usually inserted through the hole and held in position by tapes tied round the neck. *See also* minitracheostomy.

tracheotomy (tray-ki-ot-ŏmi) *n. see* tracheostomy.

trachoma (tră-koh-mă) *n.* a chronic contagious eye disease – a severe form of conjunctivitis caused by the bacterium *Chlamydia trachomatis* – that is common in some hot countries. If untreated, the conjunctiva becomes scarred and shrinks, causing trichiasis; blindness can be a late complication. Treatment with tetracyclines is effective in the early stages of the disease.

tract (trakt) *n.* **1.** a group of nerve fibres passing from one part of the brain or spinal cord to another, forming a distinct pathway. **2.** an organ or collection of organs providing for the passage of something, e.g. the digestive tract.

traction (trak-shŏn) *n.* the application of a pulling force, especially as a means of counteracting the natural tension in the tissues surrounding a broken bone, to produce correct alignment of the fragments. Considerable force, exerted with weights, ropes, and pulleys, may be necessary to ensure that a broken femur is kept correctly positioned during the early stages of healing. Traction is also used by physiotherapists for the treatment of back pain.

tractotomy (trak-tot-ŏmi) *n.* a neurosurgical operation for the relief of intractable pain, in which the nerve fibres that carry painful sensation to consciousness are severed within the medulla oblongata. *See also* cordotomy.

tragus (tray-gŭs) *n.* the projection of cartilage in the pinna of the outer ear that extends back over the opening of the external auditory meatus.

TRAM flap (tram) *n.* transverse rectus *abdominis myocutaneous* flap: a piece of tissue (skin, muscle, and fat) dissected from the abdomen and used to reconstruct the breast after mastectomy.

trance (trahns) *n.* a state in which reaction to the environment is diminished although awareness is not impaired. It may be caused by hypnosis, meditation, catatonia, conversion disorder, or drugs.

tranexamic acid (tran-eks-am-ik) *n.* an antifibrinolytic drug administered by mouth as an antidote to overdosage with fibrinolytic drugs and to control severe bleeding, for example after surgery or to treat menorrhagia. Trade name: **Cyklokapron**.

tranquillizer (trank-wi-ly-zer) *n.* a drug that produces a calming effect, relieving anxiety and tension. **major t.** *see* antipsychotic. **minor t.** *see* anxiolytic.

trans- *prefix denoting* through or across.

transaminase (trans-am-in-ayz) *n.* an enzyme that is involved in the process of transamination. Examples are aspartate aminotransaminase (AST) and alanine aminotransaminase (ALT).

transamination (trans-am-i-nay-shŏn) *n.* a process involved in the metabolism of amino acids in which amino groups (–NH$_2$) are transferred from amino acids to certain

α-keto acids, with the production of a second keto acid and amino acid. The reaction is catalysed by transaminases.

transcription (tran-skrip-shŏn) *n.* the process in which the information contained in the genetic code is transferred from DNA to RNA: the first step in the manufacture of proteins in cells. *See* messenger RNA, translation.

transcultural nursing (trans-kul-cher-ăl) *n.* a major area of nursing that focuses on the comparative study and analysis of different cultures and subcultures in the world with respect to their caring values, perceptions of health and illness, and patterns of behaviour, with the aim of developing knowledge to provide culture-specific practice. The concept of transcultural nursing was developed by US nursing theorist M. Leininger (1924–).

transcutaneous electrical nerve stimulation (TENS) (trans kew-tay-niŭs) *n. see* stimulator.

transdermal (trans-der-măl) *adj.* through the skin: applied to the route of administration of drugs that are absorbed through the skin.

transducer (trans-dew-ser) *n.* a device used to convert one form of signal into another, allowing its measurement or display to be made appropriately. For example, an ultrasound probe converts reflected ultrasound waves into electronic impulses, which can be displayed on a TV monitor.

transection (tran-sek-shŏn) *n.* **1.** a cross section of a piece of tissue. **2.** cutting across the tissue of an organ (*see also* section).

transferase (trans-fer-ayz) *n.* an enzyme that catalyses the transfer of a group (other than hydrogen) between a pair of substrates.

transference (trans-fer-ĕns) *n.* (in psychoanalysis) the process by which a patient comes to feel and act towards the therapist as though he or she were somebody from the patient's past life, especially a powerful parent. The patient's transference feelings may be of love or of hatred.

transferrin (siderophilin) (transfer-in) *n.* a glycoprotein, found in the blood plasma, that acts as a carrier for iron in the bloodstream.

transfer RNA (trans-fer) *n.* a type of RNA whose function is to attach the correct amino acid to the protein chain being synthesized at a ribosome. *See also* translation.

transfusion (trans-few-zhŏn) *n.* **1.** the injection of a volume of blood obtained from a healthy person into the circulation of a patient whose blood is deficient in quantity or quality, through accident or disease. The blood is allowed to drip, under gravity, through a needle inserted into one of the patient's veins. Blood transfusion is routine during major surgical operations in which much blood is likely to be lost. **2.** the administration of any fluid, such as plasma or saline solution, into a patient's vein by means of a drip.

transient ischaemic attack (TIA) (tran-zi-ĕnt isk-ee-mik) *n.* the result of temporary disruption of the circulation to part of the brain due to embolism, thrombosis to brain arteries, or spasm of the vessel walls. The symptoms may be similar to those of a stroke but patients recover within 24 hours.

transillumination (tranz-i-loo-mi-nay-shŏn) *n.* the technique of shining a bright light through part of the body to examine its structure. Transillumination of the paranasal sinuses is a means of detecting abnormalities.

transitional cell carcinoma (tran-si-zhŏn-ăl) *n.* a form of cancer that affects the urothelium, which lines the urinary collecting system of the kidney, ureters, bladder, and most of the urethra. It is the most common type of bladder cancer.

translation (tranz-lay-shŏn) *n.* (in cell biology) the manufacture of proteins in a cell, which takes place at the ribosomes. *See* messenger RNA, transfer RNA.

translocation (tranz-loh-kay-shŏn) *n.* (in genetics) a type of chromosome mutation in which part of a chromosome is transferred to another part of the same chromosome or to a different chromosome. This can lead to serious genetic disorders, e.g. chronic myeloid leukaemia.

translumbar (tranz-lum-ber) *adj.* through the lumbar region: describing the route for injecting the aorta for aortography.

transmigration (tranz-my-gray-shŏn) *n.* the act of passing through or across, e.g. the passage of blood cells through the intact walls of capillaries and venules (*see* diapedesis).

transoesophageal echocardiography (tranz-ee-sof-ă-jee-ăl) *n.* *see* echocardiography.

transplacental (trans-plă-sen-t'l) *adj.* across the placenta: describing the transport of substances, etc., between mother and fetus.

transplantation (trans-plahn-**tay**-shŏn) *n.* the implantation of an organ or tissue from one part of the body to another, as in skin or bone grafting, or from one person to another, as in kidney or heart transplants. Transplanting organs or tissues between individuals is a difficult procedure because of the natural rejection processes in the recipient of the graft. Special treatment (e.g. with immunosuppressant drugs) is needed to prevent graft rejection.

transposition (trans-pŏ-**zish**-ŏn) *n.* the abnormal positioning of a part of the body such that it is on the opposite side to its normal site in the body. *t. of the great vessels* a congenital abnormality of the heart in which the aorta arises from the right ventricle and the pulmonary artery from the left ventricle.

transrectal ultrasonography (TRUS) (trans-**rek**-tăl) *n. see* ultrasonography.

transsexualism (tranz-**seks**-yoo-ăl-izm) *n.* the condition of one who firmly believes that he (or she) belongs to the sex opposite to his (or her) biological gender. In adults surgical sex reassignment is sometimes justifiable, to make the externals of the body conform to the individual's view of himself (or herself). —**transsexual** *adj., n.*

transudation (trans-yoo-**day**-shŏn) *n.* the passage of a liquid through a membrane, especially of blood through the wall of a capillary vessel. The liquid is called the *transudate*.

transuretero-ureterostomy

(trans-yoor-ee-ter-oh-yoor-i-ter-**ost**-ŏmi) *n.* the operation of connecting one ureter to the other in the abdomen. The damaged or obstructed ureter is cut above the diseased or damaged segment and joined end-to-side to the other ureter.

transurethral (trans-yoor-ee-**thrăl**) *adj.* through the urethra. *t. resection of the prostate see* resection. *t. vaporization of the prostate* (TUVP) a technique in which the prostate is vaporized: used to treat lower urinary tract symptoms due to benign prostatic hyperplasia and urinary retention.

transvaginal (tranz-vă-**jy**-năl) *adj.* through or across the vagina. *t. ultrasonography see* ultrasonography.

transverse (tranz-**vers**) *adj.* (in anatomy) situated at right angles to the long axis of the body or an organ. *t. process* the long projection from the base of the neural arch of a vertebra.

transvestism (cross-dressing) (tranz-**vest**-izm) *n.* dressing in clothes normally associated with the opposite sex, which may occur in both heterosexual and homosexual people. Cross-dressing may be practised by transsexuals (*see* transsexualism), in whom it is not sexually arousing. In fetishistic transvestites (*see* fetishism) cross-dressing is sexually arousing. —**transvestite** *n.*

tranylcypromine (tran-il-**sy**-prohmeen) *n.* an antidepressant drug – one of the MAO inhibitors – given by mouth for the treatment of severe mental depressive states. Trade name: **Parnate**.

trapezium (tră-**pee**-ziŭm) *n.* a bone

of the wrist (*see* carpus). It articulates with the scaphoid bone behind, with the first metacarpal in front, and with the trapezoid and second metatarsal on either side.

trapezius (trǎ-pee-zi-ǔs) *n.* a flat triangular muscle covering the back of the neck and shoulder. It moves the scapula and draws the head backwards to either side.

trapezoid bone (tras-pee-zoid) *n.* a bone of the wrist (*see* carpus). It articulates with the second metatarsal bone in front, with the scaphoid bone behind, and with the trapezium and capitate bones on either side.

trastuzumab (tras-too-zoo-mab) *n.* a monoclonal antibody used to treat certain types of highly malignant breast cancer. It is administered by intravenous infusion. Trade name: **Herceptin**.

trauma (traw-mǎ) *n.* **1.** a physical wound or injury. *t. scores* numerical systems for assessing the severity and prognosis of serious injuries. **2.** (in psychology) an emotionally painful and harmful event, which may lead to neurosis. *See* post-traumatic stress disorder. —**traumatic** (traw-mat-ik) *adj.*

traumatic fever *n.* a fever resulting from a serious injury.

traumatology (traw-mǎ-tol-ǒji) *n.* accident surgery: the branch of surgery that deals with wounds and disabilities arising from injuries.

travel sickness (trav-ěl) *n. see* motion sickness.

trazodone (traz-oh-dohn) *n.* a drug administered by mouth in the treatment of depression with and without anxiety. Trade name: **Molipaxin**.

Treacher Collins syndrome (Treacher Collins deformity) (tree-cher kol-inz) *n.* a hereditary disorder of facial development. The lower jaw and zygomatic (cheek) bones are underdeveloped and the precursors of the ear fail to develop, which results in a variety of ear and facial malformations. [E. Treacher Collins (1862–1919), British ophthalmologist]

treatment field (treet-měnt) *n.* (in radiotherapy) an area of the body selected for treatment with radiotherapy. Radiation is administered to the field by focusing the beam of particles emitted by the radiotherapy machine and shielding the surrounding area of the body. *mantle f.* the neck, armpits, and central chest.

trematode (trem-ǎ-tohd) *n. see* fluke.

tremor (trem-er) *n.* a rhythmical alternating movement that may affect any part of the body. *essential t.* a slow tremor that particularly affects the hands and arms when held out. *intention t.* tremor that occurs when a patient with disease of the cerebellum tries to touch an object. *physiological t.* a feature of the normal mechanism for maintaining posture. It may be more apparent in states of fatigue or anxiety or in people with an overactive thyroid gland. *resting t.* tremor that occurs only when the patient is at rest and disappears when movement is attempted. It is a prominent symptom of parkinsonism.

trench foot (immersion foot) (trench) *n.* blackening of the toes and the skin of the foot due to death of the superficial tissues and caused by prolonged immersion in cold water or exposure to damp and cold.

Trendelenburg position (tren-del-ĕn-berg) *n.* a special operating-table posture for patients undergoing surgery of the pelvis or suffering from shock or to reduce blood loss in operations on the legs. The patient is laid on his back with the pelvis higher than the head, inclined at an angle of about 45°. *See* position. [F. Trendelenburg (1844–1924), German surgeon]

Trendelenburg's operation *n.* ligation of the long saphenous vein at the groin: performed to remove weakened portions of varicose veins.

Trendelenburg's sign *n.* a sign indicating congenital dislocation of the hip: when the patient stands on the affected leg with the other leg flexed, the pelvis is lower on the side of the flexed leg.

trephine (trif-een) *n.* a surgical instrument used to remove a circular area of tissue, usually from the cornea of the eye or from bone.

Treponema (trep-ŏ-nee-mă) *n.* a genus of anaerobic spirochaete bacteria. All species are parasitic; some cause disease, such as *T. carateum* (pinta), *T. pallidum* (syphilis), and *T. pertenue* (yaws).

treponematosis (trep-ŏ-nee-mă-toh-sis) *n.* any infection caused by spirochaete bacteria of the genus *Treponema*.

tretinoin (tre-tin-oh-in) *n.* a drug (*see* retinoid) used in the treatment of acne. It is administered topically as a cream, gel, or liquid. Trade name: **Retin-A**.

TRH *n. see* thyrotrophin-releasing hormone.

triad (try-ad) *n.* (in medicine) a group of three united or closely associated structures or three symptoms or effects that occur together.

triage (tree-ahzh) *n.* a system whereby a group of casualties or other patients is sorted according to the seriousness of their injuries or illnesses so that treatment priorities can be allocated between them. In emergency situations it is designed to maximize the number of survivors.

triamcinolone (try-am-sin-ŏ-lohn) *n.* a synthetic corticosteroid hormone that reduces inflammation but does not cause salt and water retention. Administered by mouth, injection, nasal spray, or topically, it is used for treating a wide range of inflammatory and allergic conditions. Trade names: **Adcortyl, Kenalog, Lederspan, Nasacort**.

triamterene (try-am-ter-een) *n.* a potassium-sparing diuretic that causes the loss of sodium and chloride from the kidneys and is administered by mouth in the treatment of various forms of fluid retention (oedema).

triangle (try-ang-ŭl) *n.* (in anatomy) a three-sided structure or area; for example, the femoral triangle.

triangular bandage (try-ang-yoo-ler) *n.* a piece of material cut or folded into a triangular shape and used for making an arm sling or holding dressings in position.

triceps (try-seps) *n.* a muscle with three heads of origin. *t. brachii* the muscle that is situated on the back of the upper arm and contracts to extend the forearm. It is the antagonist of the brachialis.

trich- (tricho-) *prefix denoting* hair or hairlike structures.

trichiasis (trik-I-ă-sis) *n.* a condition in which the eyelashes rub against the eyeball, producing discomfort and sometimes ulceration of the cornea. It accompanies all forms of entropion.

trichinosis (trichiniasis) (triki-**noh**-sis) *n.* a disease caused by larvae of the nematode worm *Trichinella spiralis*, contracted by eating imperfectly cooked infected meat. Symptoms include diarrhoea, nausea, fever, vertigo, delirium, and pains in the limbs. The larvae eventually settle within cysts in the muscles, which may result in pain and stiffness.

trichloracetic acid (try-klor-ă-**see**-tik) *n.* an astringent used in solution for a variety of skin conditions. It is also applied topically to produce sloughing, especially for the removal of warts.

trichobezoar (trik-oh-**bee**-zor) *n.* hairball: a mass of swallowed hair in the stomach. *See* bezoar.

Trichocephalus (trik-oh-**sef**-ă-lŭs) *n. see* whipworm.

trichology (trik-ol-ŏji) *n.* the study of hair.

Trichomonas (trik-oh-**moh**-năs) *n.* a genus of parasitic flagellate protozoans. *T. hominis* a species that lives in the large intestine. *T. vaginalis see* trichomoniasis.

trichomoniasis (trik-oh-mŏ-**ny**-ă-sis) *n.* **1.** an infection of the digestive system by the protozoan *Trichomonas hominis*, causing dysentery. **2.** an infection of the vagina due to the protozoan *Trichomonas vaginalis*, causing inflammation of genital tissues with vaginal discharge. It can be transmitted to males in whom it causes urethral discharge. Treatment with metronidazole is effective.

trichomycosis (trik-oh-my-**koh**-sis) *n.* any hair disease caused by infection with a fungus.

Trichophyton (trik-oh-**fy**-tŏn) *n.* a genus of fungi, parasitic in humans, that frequently infect the skin, nails, and hair and cause tinea (ringworm). *See also* dermatophyte.

trichophytosis (trik-oh-fy-**toh**-sis) *n.* a fungal infection caused by species of *Trichophyton*.

trichromatic (try-kroh-**mat**-ik) *adj.* describing or relating to the normal state of colour vision, in which a person is sensitive to all three of the primary colours. *Compare* dichromatic.

trichuriasis (trik-yoor-I-ă-sis) *n.* an infestation of the large intestine by the whipworm, *Trichuris trichiura*. Symptoms, including bloody diarrhoea, anaemia, weakness, and abdominal pain, are evident only in heavy infestations. Trichuriasis can be treated with various anthelmintics, including tiabendazole and piperazine salts.

Trichuris (trik-**yoor**-iss) *n. see* whipworm.

tricuspid valve (try-**kusp**-id) *n.* the valve in the heart between the right atrium and right ventricle. It consists of three cusps that channel the flow of blood from the atrium to the ventricle and prevent any backflow.

tricyclic antidepressant (try-sy-klik) *n. see* antidepressant.

tridactyly (try-**dak**-tili) *n.* a congenital abnormality in which there are only three digits on a hand or foot.

trifluoperazine (try-floo-oh-**pair**-ă-zeen) *n.* a phenothiazine antipsychotic drug with uses and effects similar to those of chlorpromazine. Trade name: **Stelazine**.

trigeminal nerve (try-jem-in-ăl) *n.* the fifth and largest cranial nerve (V), which is split into the ophthalmic, maxillary, and mandibular nerves. The motor fibres are responsible for controlling the muscles involved in chewing, while the sensory fibres relay information from the front of the head and from the meninges.

trigeminal neuralgia (tic douloureux) *n. see* neuralgia.

trigeminy (try-jem-in-i) *n.* a condition in which the heartbeats can be subdivided into groups of three. The first beat is normal, but the second and third are premature beats (*see* ectopic beat).

trigger finger (trig-er) *n.* an impairment in the ability to extend a finger, resulting either from a nodular thickening in the flexor tendon or a narrowing of the flexor tendon sheath. On unclenching the fist, the affected finger at first remains bent then suddenly straightens.

triglyceride (try-glis-eryd) *n.* a lipid or neutral fat consisting of glycerol combined with three fatty-acid molecules. Triglycerides are the form in which fat is stored in the body.

trigone (try-gohn) *n.* a triangular region of tissue, such as the triangular region of the wall of the bladder that lies between the openings of the two ureters and the urethra.

trigonitis (try-goh-ny-tis) *n.* inflammation of the trigone (base) of the urinary bladder. This can occur as part of a generalized cystitis or it can be associated with inflammation in the urethra, prostate, or neck (cervix) of the uterus.

trigonocephaly (try-gŏ-noh-**sef**-ăli) *n.* a deformity of the skull in which the vault of the skull is sharply angled just in front of the ears, giving the skull a triangular shape. —**trigonocephalic** (try-gŏ-noh-si-fal-ik) *adj.*

trihexyphenidyl (benzhexol) (try-hek-si-fen-i-dil) *n.* an anticholinergic drug used mainly to reduce muscle spasm in parkinsonism. It is taken by mouth. Trade name: **Broflex**.

triiodothyronine (try-I-oh-doh-th'y-rŏ-neen) *n. see* thyroid hormone.

trimeprazine (try-mep-ră-zeen) *n. see* alimemazine.

trimester (try-mest-er) *n.* (in obstetrics) any one of the three successive three-month periods into which a pregnancy may be divided.

trimethoprim (try-meth-oh-prim) *n.* an antibacterial drug that is active against a range of microorganisms. Administered by mouth or injection, it is used mainly in the treatment of chronic urinary-tract infections and respiratory-tract infections. Trade names: **Monotrim**, **Trimopan**. *See also* co-trimoxazole.

trimipramine (try-mip-ră-meen) *n.* a tricyclic antidepressant drug that also possesses sedative properties. It is given by mouth or by injection for the treatment of acute or chronic mental depression. Trade name: **Surmontil**.

trinitrophenol (try-ny-troh-**fee**-nol) *n. see* picric acid.

triple marker test (trip-ŭl **mark**-er) *n.* a blood test used in the prenatal diagnosis of Down's syndrome, which can be performed at about the 16th week of pregnancy. It measures levels of alpha-fetoprotein (afp), unconjugated oestriol (uE₃), and human chorionic gonadotrophin in maternal serum.

triploid (**trip**-loid) *adj.* describing cells, tissues, or individuals in which there are three complete chromosome sets. *Compare* haploid, diploid. —**triploid** *n.*

triprolidine (try-**proh**-li-deen) *n.* an antihistamine drug used to treat hay fever and, in combination with other drugs (e.g. dextromethorphan), to relieve the symptoms of colds. Trade name: **Actidil**.

triquetrum (triquetral bone) (try-**kwee**-trŭm) *n.* a bone of the wrist (*see* carpus). It articulates with the ulna behind and with the pisiform, hamate, and lunate bones in the carpus.

trismus (**triz**-mŭs) *n.* spasm of the jaw muscles, keeping the jaw tightly closed. This is the characteristic symptom of tetanus but it also occurs as a sensitivity reaction to certain drugs and in disorders of the basal ganglia.

trisomy (**try**-soh-mi) *n.* a condition in which there is one extra chromosome present in each cell in addition to the normal (diploid) chromosome set; the cause of such disorders as Down's syndrome. —**trisomic** (try-**soh**-mik) *adj.*

tritanopia (try-tă-noh-piă) *n.* a rare defect of colour vision in which affected persons are insensitive to blue light and confuse blues and greens. *Compare* deuteranopia, Daltonism.

trocar (**troh**-kar) *n.* an instrument used in combination with a cannula to draw off fluids from a body cavity. It comprises a metal tube containing a removable shaft with a sharp three-cornered point.

trochanter (troh-**kant**-er) *n.* either of the two protuberances that occur below the neck of the femur.

troche (trohsh) *n.* a medicinal lozenge, taken by mouth, used to treat conditions of the mouth, throat, or alimentary canal.

trochlea (**trok**-li-ă) *n.* an anatomical part having the structure or function of a pulley; for example the fibrocartilaginous ring in the frontal bone through which the tendon of the superior oblique eye muscle passes. —**trochlear** (**trok**-li-er) *adj.*

trochlear nerve *n.* the fourth cranial nerve (IV), which supplies the superior oblique eye muscle.

trochoid joint (pivot joint) (**troh**-koid) *n.* a form of diarthrosis (freely movable joint) in which a bone moves round a central axis, allowing rotational movement.

troph- (tropho-) *prefix denoting* nourishment or nutrition.

trophic (**trof**-ik) *adj.* relating to nutrition or to the supply of nutrients, etc., to a part of the body. *t. ulcer* an ulcer due to insufficient supply of blood or nutrients to the affected part.

trophoblast (**trof**-ŏ-blast) *n.* the tissue that forms the wall of the blastocyst.

-trophy *suffix denoting* nourishment, development, or growth.

-tropic *suffix denoting* **1.** turning towards. **2.** having an affinity for; influencing.

tropical medicine (trop-ikăl) *n.* the study of diseases more commonly found in tropical regions than elsewhere, such as malaria, leprosy, trypanosomiasis, schistosomiasis, and leishmaniasis.

tropical ulcer (Naga sore) *n.* a skin disease prevalent in wet tropical regions. A large open sloughing sore usually develops at the site of a wound or abrasion. The ulcer is often infected with spirochaetes and bacteria and may extend deeply and cause destruction of muscles and bones.

tropicamide (trŏ-pik-ă-myd) *n.* a drug used in the form of eye drops to dilate the pupil so that the inside of the eye can more easily be examined or operated upon. Trade name: **Mydriacyl**.

Trousseau's sign (troo-sohz) *n.* spasmodic contractions of muscles, especially the muscles of mastication, in response to nerve stimulation (e.g. by tapping). It is a characteristic sign of hypocalcaemia (*see* tetany). [A. Trousseau (1801–67), French physician]

TRT *n. see* tinnitus (retraining therapy).

truncus (trunk-ŭs) *n.* a trunk: a main vessel or other tubular organ from which subsidiary branches arise. ***t. arteriosus*** the main arterial trunk arising from the fetal heart. It develops into the aorta and pulmonary artery.

trunk (trunk) *n.* **1.** *see* truncus. **2.** the body excluding the head and limbs.

TRUS *n. see* (transrectal) ultrasonography.

truss (trus) *n.* a device for applying pressure to a hernia to prevent it from protruding. It usually consists of a pad attached to a belt worn under the clothing.

trust (trust) *n.* (in the NHS) a self-governing body that provides any of a range of health-care services, including hospital services, community health services, and services for the mentally ill and other groups.

trypanocide (trip-an-ŏ-syd) *n.* an agent that kills trypanosomes. The main trypanocides are arsenic-containing compounds.

Trypanosoma (trip-ă-nŏ-soh-mă) *n. see* trypanosomiasis.

trypanosomiasis (trip-ă-nŏ-sŏ-my-ă-sis) *n.* any disease caused by the presence of parasitic protozoans of the genus *Trypanosoma*. The two most important diseases are Chagas' disease (*South American t.*), caused by *T. cruzi*, and sleeping sickness (*African t.*), caused by *T. rhodesiense* or *T. gambiense*.

tryparsamide (trip-ar-să-myd) *n.* a drug used in the treatment of trypanosomiasis (sleeping sickness). Usually given by injection, it penetrates the cerebrospinal fluid and is highly active against the infective organism.

trypsin (trip-sin) *n.* an enzyme that continues the digestion of proteins by breaking down peptones into smaller peptide chains (*see* peptidase). It is secreted by the pancreas in an inactive form, *trypsinogen*, which is converted in the duodenum to trypsin by the action of the enzyme enteropeptidase.

trypsinogen (trip-sin-ŏ-jĭn) *n. see* trypsin.

tryptophan (trip-tŏ-fan) *n.* an essential amino acid. *See also* amino acid.

tsetse (tet-si) *n.* a large bloodsucking fly of tropical Africa belonging to the genus *Glossina*. Tsetse flies transmit the blood parasites that cause sleeping sickness, *Trypanosoma gambiense* and *T. rhodesiense*.

TSH *n. see* thyroid-stimulating hormone.

TSS *n. see* toxic shock syndrome.

tsutsugamushi disease (tsoo-tsoo-gă-**moo**-shi) *n. see* scrub typhus.

TT *n. see* tetanus toxoid.

tubal occlusion (tew-bal) *n.* blocking of the Fallopian tubes. This is achieved by surgery as a means of sterilization; it is also a result of pelvic inflammatory disease.

tubal pregnancy (oviducal pregnancy) *n. see* ectopic pregnancy.

tube (tewb) *n.* (in anatomy) a long hollow cylindrical structure, e.g. a Fallopian tube.

tuber (tew-ber) *n.* (in anatomy) a thickened or swollen part.

tubercle (tew-ber-kŭl) *n.* **1.** (in anatomy) a small rounded protuberance on a bone. **2.** the specific nodular lesion of tuberculosis.

tubercular (tew-ber-kew-ler) *adj.* having small rounded swellings or nodules, not necessarily caused by tuberculosis.

tuberculide (tew-ber-kew-lyd) *n.* an eruption of the skin that arises in response to an internal focus of tuberculosis.

tuberculin (tew-ber-kew-lin) *n.* a protein extract from cultures of tubercle bacilli, used to test whether a person has suffered from or been in contact with tuberculosis (*see* Mantoux test).

tuberculoma (tew-ber-kew-loh-mă) *n.* a mass of cheeselike material resembling a tumour, seen in some cases of tuberculosis. Tuberculomas are found in a variety of sites, including the lung or brain.

tuberculosis (TB) (tew-ber-kew-loh-sis) *n.* an infectious disease caused by the bacillus *Mycobacterium tuberculosis* and characterized by the formation of nodular lesions (tubercles) in the tissues. In the most common form of the disease (*pulmonary t.*) the bacillus is inhaled into the lungs where it sets up a primary tubercle and spreads to the nearest lymph nodes (the *primary complex*). Many people become infected but show no symptoms. Others develop a chronic infection and can transmit the bacillus by coughing and sneezing. Symptoms of the active disease include fever, night sweats, weight loss, and the spitting of blood. In some cases the bacilli spread from the lungs to the bloodstream, setting up millions of tiny tubercles throughout the body (*miliary t.*). Bacilli entering by the mouth, usually in infected cows' milk, set up a primary complex in abdominal lymph nodes, leading to peritonitis, and sometimes spread to other organs, joints, and bones (*see* Pott's disease).

Tuberculosis is curable by various combinations of the antibiotics streptomycin, ethambutol, isoniazid (INH), rifampicin, and pyrazinamide. Preventive measures in the

UK include the detection of cases by X-ray screening of vulnerable populations and inoculation with BCG vaccine. *See also* direct observed therapy.

tuberculous (tew-ber-kew-lŭs) *adj.* relating to or affected with tuberculosis.

tuberose (tew-ber-ohz) *adj.* *see* tuberous.

tuberosity (tew-ber-os-iti) *n.* a large rounded protuberance on a bone.

tuberous (tuberose) (tew-ber-ŭs) *adj.* knobbed; having nodules or rounded swellings. *t. sclerosis* (*epiloia*, *Bourneville's disease*) a hereditary disorder in which the brain, eyes, skin, and other organs are studded with small plaques or tumours. Symptoms include epilepsy, mental retardation, and behavioural disorders.

tubo- *prefix denoting* a tube, especially a Fallopian tube or the Eustachian tube.

tuboabdominal (tew-boh-ab-dom-inăl) *adj.* relating to or occurring in a Fallopian tube and the abdomen.

tubo-ovarian (tew-boh-oh-vair-iăn) *adj.* relating to or occurring in a Fallopian tube and an ovary.

tubotympanal (tew-boh-timp-ăn-ăl) *adj.* relating to the tympanic cavity and the Eustachian tube.

tubular necrosis *n.* localized death of renal tubules. *acute t. n.* (*ATN*) tubular necrosis, usually as a result of ischaemia, in which urine flow is reduced and renal failure can develop.

tubule (tew-bewl) *n.* (in anatomy) a small cylindrical hollow structure. *See also* renal (tubule), seminiferous tubule. —**tubular** (tew-bew-ler) *adj.*

tularaemia (rabbit fever) (tew-lă-ree-miă) *n.* a disease of rodents and rabbits, caused by the bacterium *Francisella tularensis*, that may be transmitted to humans. Symptoms include an ulcer at the site of infection, inflamed and ulcerating lymph nodes, headache, aching pains, loss of weight, and a fever lasting several weeks. Treatment with chloramphenicol, streptomycin, or tetracycline is effective.

tulle gras (tewl grah) *n.* a soft dressing consisting of open-woven silk (or other material) impregnated with a waterproof soft paraffin wax.

tumefaction (tew-mi-fak-shŏn) *n.* the process in which a tissue becomes swollen and tense by accumulation within it of fluid under pressure.

tumescence (tew-mes-ĕns) *n.* a swelling, or the process of becoming swollen, usually because of an accumulation of blood or other fluid within the tissues.

tumid (tew-mid) *adj.* swollen.

tumor (tew-mer) *n.* swelling: one of the four classical signs of inflammation in a tissue. *See also* calor, dolor, rubor.

tumour (tew-mer) *n.* any abnormal swelling in or on a part of the body. The term is usually applied to an abnormal growth of tissue, which may be benign or malignant. *Compare* cyst.

tumour necrosis factor (TNF) either of two proteins, TNF-α (produced mainly by monocytes and macrophages) or TNF-β (produced by lymphoid cells), that act as mediators for immune responses. Among their many actions is destruction of tumour cells.

tunica (tew-nik-ă) *n.* a covering or

layer of an organ or part; for example, a layer of the wall of a blood vessel (*see* adventitia, intima, media).

tunnel (tun-ĕl) *n.* (in anatomy) a canal or hollow groove.

tunnel vision *n.* a visual-field defect in which only the central area of the visual field remains. It occurs in advanced glaucoma.

TUR (TURP) *n.* transurethral resection of the prostate: *see* resection.

turbinate bone (ter-bin-ayt) *n. see* nasal (concha).

turbinectomy (ter-bin-ek-tŏmi) *n.* the surgical removal of one of the turbinate bones.

turgescence (ter-jes-ĕns) *n.* a swelling, or the process by which a swelling arises in tissues, usually by the accumulation of blood or other fluid under pressure.

turgid (ter-jid) *adj.* swollen and congested, especially with blood.

turgor (ter-ger) *n.* a state of being swollen or distended.

Turner's syndrome (ter-nerz) *n.* a genetic defect in women in which there is only one X chromosome instead of the usual two. Affected women are infertile: they have female external genitalia but no ovaries. Characteristically they are short and have variable developmental defects. [H. H. Turner (1892–1970), US endocrinologist]

turricephaly (tu-ri-sef-ăli) *n. see* oxycephaly.

tussis (tus-iss) *n. see* coughing.

TUVP *n. see* transurethral (vaporization of the prostate).

TV *n. see* tidal volume.

twilight state (twy-lyt) *n.* a condition of disturbed consciousness in which the individual can still carry out some normal activities but has impaired awareness and no memory of what he or she has done. It is encountered after epileptic attacks, in alcoholism, and in organic states of confusion.

twins (twinz) *pl. n.* two individuals who are born at the same time and of the same parents. *fraternal* (or *dizygotic*) *t.* twins resulting from the simultaneous fertilization of two egg cells; they may be of different sexes and are no more alike than ordinary siblings. *identical* (or *monozygotic*) *t.* twins resulting from the fertilization of a single egg cell that subsequently divides to give two separate fetuses. They are of the same sex and otherwise genetically identical. *See also* Siamese twins.

tylosis (ty-loh-sis) *n.* focal keratosis occurring especially on the palms and soles. It occurs early in life and is inherited as an autosomal dominant.

tympan- (tympano-) *prefix denoting* **1.** the eardrum. **2.** the middle ear.

tympanic cavity (tim-pan-ik) *n. see* middle ear.

tympanic membrane (eardrum) *n.* the membrane at the inner end of the external auditory meatus, separating the outer and middle ears. When sound waves reach the ear the tympanum vibrates, transmitting these vibrations to the malleus.

tympanites (meteorism) (timpă-ny-teez) *n.* distension of the abdomen with air or gas: the abdomen is resonant on percussion. Causes include intestinal obstruction, irritable bowel syndrome, and aerophagy.

tympanoplasty   (timp-ă-noh-plasti) *n.* surgical repair of defects of the eardrum and middle ear ossicles. *See* myringoplasty.

tympanotomy (timp-ă-not-ŏmi) *n.* a surgical operation to expose the middle ear and allow access to the ossicles.

tympanum (timp-ă-nŭm) *n.* the middle ear (tympanic cavity) and/ or the eardrum (tympanic membrane).

typho- *prefix denoting* **1.** typhoid fever. **2.** typhus.

typhoid fever (ty-foid) *n.* an infection of the digestive system by the bacterium *Salmonella typhi*, causing general weakness, high fever, a rash of red spots on the chest and abdomen, chills, sweating, and in serious cases inflammation of the spleen and bones, delirium, and erosion of the intestinal wall leading to haemorrhage. It is transmitted through contaminated food or drinking water. Treatment with such antibiotics as ciprofloxacin or chloramphenicol reduces the severity of symptoms. Vaccination with TAB provides temporary immunity. *Compare* paratyphoid fever.

typhus (spotted fever) (ty-fŭs) *n.* any one of a group of infections caused by rickettsiae and characterized by severe headache, a widespread rash, prolonged high fever, and delirium. They all respond to treatment with chloramphenicol or tetracyclines. The rickettsiae may be transmitted by lice (*epidemic*, *classical*, or *louse-borne t.*); rat fleas (*endemic*, *murine*, or *flea-borne t.*); ticks (*see* Rocky Mountain spotted fever); or mites (*see* rickettsial pox, scrub typhus).

tyramine (ty-ră-meen) *n.* an amine naturally occurring in cheese. It has a similar effect in the body to that of adrenaline. This effect can be dangerous in patients taking MAO inhibitors (antidepressants), in whom blood pressure may become very high.

tyrosine (ty-roh-seen) *n. see* amino acid.

tyrosinosis (ty-roh-si-noh-sis) *n.* an inborn defect of metabolism of the amino acid tyrosine causing excess excretion of parahydroxyphenylpyruvic acid in the urine.

Uu

UC *n. see* (ulcerative) colitis.

UKCC *n.* United Kingdom Central Council for Nursing, Midwifery, and Health Visiting: a statutory body, established by the Nurses, Midwives and Health Visitors Act (1979), that regulated the nursing, midwifery, and health visiting professions in the public interest. The UKCC took over the roles of the General Nursing Councils in England and Wales, Scotland, and Northern Ireland. It was superseded in 2002 by the Nursing and Midwifery Council.

ulcer (ul-ser) *n.* a break in the skin or in the mucous membrane lining the alimentary tract that fails to heal and is often accompanied by inflammation. *decubitus u. see* bedsore. *rodent u. see* basal cell carcinoma. *venous* (or *hypostatic* or *varicose*) *u.* the most common type of skin ulcer, occurring on the legs and caused by increased venous pressure. It most commonly affects older women. *See also* aphthous ulcer, dendritic ulcer, duodenal ulcer, gastric (ulcer), peptic (ulcer).

ulcerative colitis (ul-ser-ay-tiv) *n. see* colitis.

ulcerative gingivitis (Vincent's angina) *n.* acute painful inflammation and ulceration of the gums associated with infection by the microorganisms *Fusobacterium* and *Bacteroides*.

ule- (ulo-) *prefix denoting* **1.** scars; scar tissue. **2.** the gums.

ulna (ul-nă) *n.* the inner and longer bone of the forearm. It articulates with the humerus and radius above and with the radius and indirectly with the wrist bones below. —**ulnar** (ul-ner) *adj.*

ulnar artery *n.* a branch of the brachial artery arising at the elbow and running deep within the muscles of the medial side of the forearm to the palm of the hand.

ulnar nerve *n.* one of the major nerves of the arm. It originates in the neck and runs down the inner side of the upper arm to behind the elbow. It supplies the muscles of the forearm and the skin of the palm and fourth and fifth fingers.

ultra- *prefix denoting* **1.** beyond. **2.** an extreme degree (e.g. of large or small size).

ultradian (ul-tray-diăn) *adj.* denoting a biological rhythm or cycle that occurs more frequently than once in 24 hours.

ultrafiltration (ultră-fil-tray-shŏn) *n.* filtration under pressure. In the kidney, blood is subjected to ultrafiltration to remove the waste material that goes to make up urine.

ultramicroscopic (ultră-my-krŏ-skop-ik) *adj.* too small to be seen by means of an ordinary light microscope.

ultrasonics (ultră-sonn-iks) *n.* the

study of the uses and properties of ultrasound. —**ultrasonic** *adj.*

ultrasonography (sonography) (ultră-sonn-og-răfi) *n.* the use of ultrasound to produce images of structures in the human body. The ultrasound probe sends out a short pulse of high-frequency sound and detects the reflected waves (echoes) occurring at interfaces within the organs. The direction of the pulse can then be moved across the area of interest with each pulse to build up a complete image. As far as is known, there are no adverse effects from the use of ultrasound used at diagnostic energies. Ultrasonography is used extensively in obstetrics and also to examine the abdominal organs, urinary tract, blood vessels, muscles, and tendons. *transrectal u.* (*TRUS*) ultrasonography for examination of the prostate gland and seminal vesicle, in which the ultrasound probe is placed through the anus to lie directly behind these structures. *transvaginal u.* ultrasonography using a vaginal probe, which provides a detailed anatomy of the female pelvis and early accurate identification of fetal structures.

ultrasound (ultrasonic waves) (ul-tră-sownd) *n.* sound waves of extremely high frequency (above 20,000 Hz), inaudible to the human ear. Ultrasound, usually in the range 2–20 MHz, can be used to examine the structure of the inside of the body (*see* ultrasonography); the vibratory effect of ultrasound can also be used to break up stones (*see* lithotripsy) and cataracts (*see* phacoemulsification) and in the treatment of rheumatic conditions.

ultrasound marker (mark-er) *n.* the appearance, on ultrasound examination, of a particular physical abnormality in the fetus at a specific stage in fetal development. Such markers suggest the presence of specific chromosomal or developmental abnormalities. *See also* nuchal (thickness scanning).

ultraviolet radiation (UV) *n.* (ultră-vy-ŏ-lit) invisible short-wavelength radiation beyond the violet end of the visible spectrum, which is emitted by the sun. *UVA* UV radiation in the range 310–400 nm, which is not filtered by the atmosphere and penetrates deeply into the skin, causing age-related wrinkling and drug-induced photosensitivity reactions and contributing to the development of skin cancer. *UVB* UV radiation in the range 280–310 nm, which is largely filtered by the atmosphere. Depending on its strength, it causes suntan and sunburn and contributes to the development of skin cancer.

umbilical cord (um-bil-ikăl) *n.* the strand of tissue connecting the fetus to the placenta. It contains two arteries that carry blood to the placenta and one vein that returns it to the fetus.

umbilicated (um-bil-i-kayt-id) *adj.* having a navel-like depression.

umbilicus (omphalus) (um-bil-ikŭs) *n.* the navel: a circular depression in the centre of the abdomen marking the site of attachment of the umbilical cord in the fetus. —**umbilical** *adj.*

umbo (um-boh) *n.* a projecting centre of a round surface, especially the projection of the inner surface of the eardrum to which the malleus is attached.

unciform bone (un-si-form) *n. see* hamate bone.

uncinate fits (un-sin-ayt) *pl. n.* a form of temporal lobe epilepsy in which hallucinations of taste and smell and inappropriate chewing movements are prominent features.

unconscious (un-kon-shŭs) *adj.* **1.** in a state of unconsciousness. **2.** (in psychoanalysis) denoting the part of the mind that includes memories, motives, and intentions that are not accessible to awareness and cannot be made conscious without overcoming resistances. *Compare* subconscious.

unconsciousness (un-kon-shŭs-nis) *n.* a condition of being unaware of one's surroundings, as in sleep, or of being unresponsive to stimulation. An unnatural state of unconsciousness may be caused by factors that produce reduced brain activity, such as lack of oxygen or head injuries, or it may be brought about deliberately during general anaesthesia. *See also* coma.

uncus (unk-ŭs) *n.* any hook-shaped structure, especially a projection of the lower surface of the cerebral hemisphere.

undecenoic acid (un-des-i-noh-ik) *n.* an antifungal agent, applied to the skin in the form of powder, ointment, lotion, or aerosol spray for the treatment of such infections as athlete's foot. Trade name: **Mycota**.

undine (un-deen) *n.* a small rounded container, usually made of glass, for solutions used to wash out the eye. It has a small neck for filling and a long tapering spout with a narrow outlet.

undulant fever (un-dew-lănt) *n. see* brucellosis.

ungual (ung-wăl) *adj.* relating to the fingernails or toenails (ungues).

unguentum (ung-wen-tŭm) *n.* (in pharmacy) an ointment.

unguis (ung-wis) *n.* a fingernail or toenail. *See* nail.

uni- *prefix denoting* one.

unicellular (yoo-ni-sel-yoo-ler) *adj.* describing organisms or tissues that consist of a single cell.

unilateral (yoo-ni-lat-erăl) *adj.* (in anatomy) relating to or affecting one side of the body or one side of an organ or other part.

union (yoon-yŏn) *n.* (in a fractured bone) the successful result of healing of a fracture, in which the bone ends have become firmly united by newly formed bone. *Compare* malunion.

uniovular (yoo-ni-ov-yoo-ler) *adj.* derived from a single ovum, as in identical twins. *Compare* binovular.

unipolar (yoo-ni-poh-ler) *adj.* (in neurology) describing a neurone that has one main process extending from the cell body. *Compare* bipolar. Visiting

United Kingdom Central Council for Nursing, Midwifery, and Health Visiting (yoo-ny-tid) *n. see* UKCC.

Unna's paste (oo-năz) *n.* a dressing for varicose ulcers consisting of a mixture of zinc oxide, gelatin, and glycerine, applied between layers of a spiral bandage. [P. G. Unna (1850–1929), German dermatologist]

UPPP *n. see* uvulopalatopharyngoplasty.

urachus (yoor-ă-kŭs) *n.* the remains of the cavity of the allantois. It usually disappears during embryonic development, leaving a solid fibrous cord connecting the bladder with the umbilicus. —**urachal** *adj.*

uracil (yoor-ă-sil) *n.* one of the nitrogen-containing bases (*see* pyrimidine) occurring in the nucleic acid RNA.

uraemia (yoor-ee-miă) *n.* the presence of excessive amounts of urea and other nitrogenous waste compounds in the blood. This occurs in kidney failure and results in nausea, vomiting, lethargy, drowsiness, and eventually (if untreated) death. Treatment may require haemodialysis. —**uraemic** *adj.*

uran- (urano-) *prefix denoting* the palate.

urataemia (yoor-ă-tee-miă) *n.* the presence in the blood of sodium urate and other urates, formed by the reaction of uric acid with bases. *See also* gout.

urate (yoor-ayt) *n.* a salt of uric acid, normally present in the urine. Excess amounts occur in the joints in gout.

uraturia (yoor-ăt-yoor-iă) *n.* the presence in the urine of urates. Abnormally high concentrations of urates in urine occur in gout.

urea (yoor-ee-ă) *n.* the main breakdown product of protein metabolism. It is the chemical form in which unrequired nitrogen is excreted by the body in the urine. Urea is formed in the liver from ammonia and carbon dioxide.

urease (yoor-i-ayz) *n.* an enzyme that catalyses the hydrolysis of urea to ammonia and carbon dioxide.

urecchysis (yoor-ek-i-sis) *n.* the

escape of uric acid from the blood into spaces in the connective tissue.

uresis (yoor-ee-sis) *n. see* urination.

ureter (yoor-ee-ter) *n.* either of a pair of tubes, 25–30 cm long, that conduct urine from the pelvis of kidneys to the bladder. —**ureteral**, **ureteric** (yoor-i-te-rik) *adj.*

ureter- (uretero-) *prefix denoting* the ureter(s).

ureterectomy (yoor-i-ter-ek-tŏmi) *n.* surgical removal of a ureter. This usually includes removal of the associated kidney as well (*see* nephroureterectomy).

ureteritis (yoor-i-ter-I-tis) *n.* inflammation of the ureter. This usually occurs in association with cystitis, particularly if caused by vesicoureteric reflux.

ureterocele (yoor-ee-ter-oh-seel) *n.* a cystic swelling of the wall of the ureter at the point where it passes into the bladder. It is associated with stenosis of the opening of the ureter and it may cause impaired drainage of the kidney with dilatation of the ureter and hydronephrosis.

ureteroenterostomy (yoor-ee-ter-oh-en-ter-ost-ŏmi) *n.* an artificial communication that is surgically created between the ureter and the bowel. *See also* ureterosigmoidostomy.

ureterolith (yoor-ee-ter-oh-lith) *n.* a stone in the ureter. *See* calculus, ureterolithotomy.

ureterolithotomy (yoor-ee-ter-oh-lith-ot-ŏmi) *n.* the surgical removal of a stone (calculus) from the ureter. If the stone occupies the lower portion of the ureter, it may be extracted by cystoscopy, thus avoiding open surgery.

ureterolysis (yoor-i-ter-ol-i-sis) *n.* an operation to free one or both ureters from surrounding fibrous tissue causing an obstruction.

ureteroneocystostomy (yoor-ee-ter-oh-nee-oh-sist-ost-ŏmi) *n.* the surgical reimplantation of a ureter into the bladder. This is most commonly performed to cure vesico-ureteric reflux.

ureteronephrectomy (yoor-ee-ter-oh-ni-frek-tŏmi) *n. see* nephro-ureterectomy.

ureteroplasty (yoor-ee-ter-oh-plasti) *n.* surgical reconstruction of the ureter using a segment of bowel or a tube of bladder.

ureteropyelonephritis (yoor-ee-ter-oh-py-ĕ-loh-ni-fry-tis) *n.* inflammation involving both the ureter and the renal pelvis (*see* ureteritis, pyelitis).

ureteroscope (yoor-ee-ter-ŏ-skohp) *n.* a rigid or flexible instrument that can be passed into the ureter and up into the pelvis of the kidney. It is most commonly used to visualize a stone in the ureter and remove it safely under direct vision with a stone basket or forceps. Larger stones need to be fragmented before removal with an ultrasound or electrohydraulic lithotripsy probe, lithoclast, or lasers.

ureteroscopy (yoor-i-ter-ŏs-kŏ-pi) *n.* inspection of the lumen of the ureter with a ureteroscope.

ureterosigmoidostomy (yoor-ee-ter-oh-sig-moid-ost-ŏmi) *n.* the operation of implanting the ureters into the sigmoid colon. This method of permanent urinary diversion may be used after cystectomy or to bypass a diseased or damaged bladder. The urine is passed together with the faeces, avoiding the need for an external opening and appliance to collect the urine.

ureterostomy (yoor-i-ter-ost-ŏmi) *n.* the surgical creation of an external opening into the ureter. This usually involves bringing the ureter to the skin surface so that the urine can drain into a suitable appliance (*cutaneous u.*).

ureterotomy (yoor-i-ter-ot-ŏmi) *n.* surgical incision into the ureter, most commonly performed in ureterolithotomy.

ureterovaginal (yoor-ee-ter-oh-vă-jy-năl) *adj.* relating to or between the ureter and vagina.

urethr- (**urethro-**) *prefix denoting* the urethra.

urethra (yoor-ee-thră) *n.* the tube that conducts urine from the bladder to the exterior. The female urethra is quite short (about 3.5 cm) and opens just within the vulva, between the clitoris and vagina. The male urethra is longer (about 20 cm) and runs through the penis. It also serves as the ejaculatory duct. —**urethral** *adj.*

urethritis (yoor-i-thry-tis) *n.* inflammation of the urethra, due either to infection or to the presence of a catheter in the urethra. The symptoms are those of urethral discharge with painful or difficult urination (dysuria). *nongonococcal* (or *nonspecific*) *u.* (NGU, NSU) urethritis due to a sexually transmitted infection other than gonorrhoea, often infection with *Chlamydia trachomatis*. *specific u.* urethritis due to gonorrhoea.

urethrocele (yoor-ee-throh-seel) *n.* prolapse of the urethra into the vaginal wall causing a bulbous swelling to appear in the vagina, particularly on straining. The condition is associated with previous childbirth. Treatment usually involves surgical repair of the lax tissues.

urethrography (yoor-i-**throg**-răfi) *n.* X-ray examination of the urethra, after introduction of a contrast medium, so that its outline and any narrowing or other abnormalities may be observed in X-ray images (*urethrograms*).

urethroplasty (yoor-ee-**throh**-plasti) *n.* surgical repair of the urethra, especially a urethral stricture. The operation entails the insertion of a flap or patch of skin from the scrotum or perineum into the urethra at the site of the stricture, which is laid widely open. *transpubic u.* surgical repair of a ruptured posterior urethra following a fractured pelvis. Access to the damaged urethra is achieved by partial removal of the pubic bone.

urethrorrhaphy (yoor-i-**thro**-răfi) *n.* surgical restoration of the continuity of the urethra. This may be required following laceration of the urethra.

urethrorrhoea (yoor-ee-thrŏ-**ree**-ă) *n.* a discharge from the urethra. This is a symptom of urethritis.

urethroscope (yoor-ee-thrŏ-skohp) *n.* an endoscope, consisting of a fine tube fitted with a light and lenses, used for examination of the interior of the male urethra. —**urethroscopy** (yoor-i-**throsk**-ŏpi) *n.*

urethrostenosis (yoor-ee-throh-sti-**noh**-sis) *n.* a stricture of the urethra.

urethrostomy (yoor-i-**throst**-ŏmi) *n.* the operation of creating an open-ing of the urethra in the perineum in men. This can be permanent, to bypass a severe stricture of the urethra in the penis, or it can form the first stage of a urethroplasty.

urethrotomy (yoor-i-**throt**-ŏmi) *n.* the operation of cutting a stricture in the urethra. It is usually performed with a *urethrotome*: a type of endoscope that consists of a sheath down which is passed a fine knife.

urgency (er-jĕn-si) *n.* (in urology) a desire to pass urine urgently; this may or may not be associated with incontinence (urge incontinence). *See* lower urinary tract symptoms.

-uria *suffix denoting* **1.** a condition of urine or urination. **2.** the presence of a specified substance in the urine.

uric acid (yoor-ik) *n.* a nitrogenous organic acid that is the end-product of nucleic acid metabolism and is a component of the urine. Excess uric acid is present in the blood of people suffering from gout.

uricosuric drug (yoor-i-koh-**sewr**-ik) *n.* a drug, such as probenecid or sulfinpyrazone, that increases the amount of uric acid excreted in the urine. Uricosuric drugs are used to treat gout and other conditions in which the levels of uric acid in the blood are increased.

uridrosis (yoor-i-**droh**-sis) *n.* the presence of excessive amounts of urea in the sweat; when the sweat dries, a white flaky deposit of urea may remain on the skin. The phenomenon occurs in uraemia.

urin- (urino-, uro-) *prefix denoting* urine or the urinary system.

urinalysis (yoor-in-al-i-sis) *n.* the analysis of urine, using physical, chemical and microscopical tests, to determine the proportions of its normal constituents and to detect alcohol, drugs, sugar, or other abnormal constituents.

urinary bladder (yoor-in-er-i) *n.* see bladder.

urinary diversion (dy-ver-shŏn) *n.* any of various techniques for the collection and diversion of urine away from its usual excretory channels, after the bladder has been removed (see cystectomy) or bypassed. These techniques include ureterosigmoidostomy and the construction of an ileal conduit. *See also* continent diversion.

urinary tract *n.* the entire system of ducts and channels that conduct urine from the kidneys to the exterior. It includes the ureters, the bladder, and the urethra.

urination (micturition) (yoor-in-ay-shŏn) *n.* the periodic discharge of urine from the bladder through the urethra.

urine (yoor-in) *n.* the fluid excreted by the kidneys, which contains many of the body's waste products. It is the major route by which the end-products of nitrogen metabolism – urea, uric acid, and creatinine – are excreted. The other major constituent is sodium chloride. Biochemical analysis of urine (see urinalysis) is commonly used in the diagnosis of diseases; immunological analysis of urine is the basis of most pregnancy tests.

uriniferous tubule (yoor-in-if-er-ŭs) *n.* see renal (tubule).

urinogenital (urogenital) (yoor-in-oh-jen-it'l) *adj.* of or relating to the organs and tissues concerned with excretion and reproduction.

urinometer (yoor-in-om-it-er) *n.* a

hydrometer for measuring the specific gravity of urine.

urobilin (yoor-oh-by-lin) *n.* see urobilinogen.

urobilinogen (yoor-oh-by-lin-ŏ-jin) *n.* a colourless product of the reduction of the bile pigment bilirubin. Urobilinogen is formed from bilirubin in the intestine by bacterial action. Part of it is reabsorbed and returned to the liver; part of it is excreted. When exposed to air, urobilinogen is oxidized to a brown pigment, *urobilin*.

urocele (yoor-oh-seel) *n.* a cystic swelling in the scrotum, containing urine that has escaped from the urethra. This may arise following urethral injury.

urochesia (yoor-oh-kee-ziă) *n.* the passage of urine through the rectum. This may follow a penetrating injury involving both the lower urinary tract and the bowel.

urochrome (yoor-oh-krohm) *n.* the pigment responsible for the colour of urine.

urodynamics (yoor-oh-dy-nam-iks) *n.* the recording of pressures within the bladder by the use of special equipment that can also record urethral sphincter pressures. It is an essential investigation in the study of urinary incontinence.

urogenital (yoor-oh-jen-it'l) *adj.* see urinogenital.

urogram (yoor-oh-gram) *n.* an X-ray of the urinary tract or any part of it. It is usually obtained after the intravenous injection of a radiopaque substance, as in an *intravenous u.* (*IVU*), which reveals the outline of the kidneys, ureters, and bladder, but the contrast medium can also be introduced percutaneously or, in the case of the bladder, transurethrally (for a *cystogram*; *see* cystography.

urography (yoor-og-răfi) *n.* X-ray examination of any part of the urinary tract after the introduction of a contrast medium. *intravenous* (or *excretion*) *u.* urography in which the contrast medium is injected into a vein and concentrated and excreted by the kidneys. *See* cystography, urethrography.

urokinase (yoor-oh-**ky**-nayz) *n.* an enzyme, produced by the kidney and also present in blood and urine, that activates the system involved in dissolving blood clots. *See* plasminogen (activator).

urolith (yoor-oh-lith) *n.* a stone in the urinary tract. *See* calculus.

urology (yoor-ol-ŏji) *n.* the branch of medicine concerned with the study and treatment of diseases of the urinary tract. —**urological** (yoor-ŏ-loj-ikăl) *adj.* —**urologist** *n.*

ursodeoxycholic acid (er-soh-dee-oks-i-**koh**-lik) *n.* a drug (a bile acid) used to dissolve cholesterol gallstones; it is administered by mouth. Trade names: **Destolit, Ursofalk**.

URT *n.* upper respiratory tract.

URTI *n.* upper respiratory tract infection.

urticaria (nettle rash, hives) (er-ti-**kair**-iă) *n.* an itchy rash resulting from the release of histamine by mast cells. Individual swellings (weals) appear rapidly and resolve spontaneously within hours. *Angio-oedema* occurs when the weals involve the lips, eyes, or tongue, which may swell alarmingly and constitute a medical emergency. *acute u.* a common and immediate response to such allergens as seafood or strawberries. *cholinergic u.* a condition in which very small weals are brought on by heat, exercise, or emotion. *chronic u.* a condition that is not allergic and may persist for years.

US *n.* ultrasound scan. *See* ultrasonography.

uter- (utero-) *prefix denoting the* uterus.

uterine (yoo-teryn) *adj.* of or relating to the uterus.

uterography (yoo-ter-og-răfi) *n.* radiography of the uterus.

uterosalpingography (hysterosalpingography) (yoo-ter-oh-sal-ping-og-răfi) *n.* radiography of the interior of the uterus and the Fallopian tubes following injection of a radiopaque fluid.

uterovesical (yoo-ter-oh-**ves**-ikăl) *adj.* relating to the uterus and bladder.

uterus (womb) (yoo-ter-ŭs) *n.* the part of the female reproductive tract that is specialized to allow the embryo to become implanted in its inner wall and to nourish the growing fetus from the maternal blood. The nonpregnant uterus is a pear-shaped organ, about 7.5 cm long, suspended in the pelvic cavity. The upper part is connected to the two Fallopian tubes and the lower part joins the vagina at the cervix. *u. didelphys* double uterus: a congenital condition resulting from incomplete midline fusion of the two paramesonephric (Müllerian) ducts during early embryonic development. The usual result is a double uterus with one or two cervices and a single vagina. Complete failure of fusion results in a double uterus with double cervices and two separate vaginae.

UTI *n.* urinary tract infection.

utilitarianism (yoo-til-i-**tair**-iăn-izm) *n.* an ethical theory that bases moral judgments or policies on their usefulness or practical value in adding to the sum total of human happiness.

utricle (utriculus) (yoo-**trik**-ŭl) *n.* **1.** the larger of the two membranous sacs within the vestibule of the ear. It contains a macula, which responds to gravity and relays information to the brain about the position of the head. **2.** a small sac (the *prostatic u.*) extending out of the urethra of the male into the substance of the prostate gland.

UVA *n. see* ultraviolet radiation.

UVB *n. see* ultraviolet radiation.

uvea (uveal tract) (yoo-vi-ă) *n.* the vascular pigmented layer of the eye, which lies beneath the outer layer (sclera). It consists of the choroid, ciliary body, and iris. —**uveal** *adj.*

uveitis (yoo-vi-I-tis) *n.* inflammation of any part of the uveal tract of the eye, either the iris (*iritis*), ciliary body (*cyclitis*), or choroid (*choroiditis*). All types may lead to visual impairment, and uveitis is an important cause of blindness.

uveoparotitis (uveoparotid fever) (yoo-vi-oh-pa-rŏ-ty-tis) *n.* inflammation of the uvea and swelling of the parotid salivary gland: one of the manifestations of the chronic disease sarcoidosis.

UVPP *n. see* uvulopalatopharyngoplasty.

uvula (yoov-yoo-lă) *n.* a small soft extension of the soft palate that hangs from the roof of the mouth above the root of the tongue. It is composed of muscle, connective tissue, and mucous membrane.

uvulectomy (staphylectomy) (yoov-yoo-lek-tŏmi) *n.* surgical removal of the uvula.

uvulitis (yoov-yoo-ly-tis) *n.* inflammation of the uvula.

uvulopalatopharyngoplasty (uvulopharyngopalatoplasty, UPPP, UVPP) (yoov-yoo-loh-pal-ă-toh-fă-ring-oh-plasti) *n.* a surgical operation to remove the uvula, part of the soft palate, and the tonsils in the treatment of snoring and obstructive sleep apnoea.

Vv

vaccination (vak-si-nay-shŏn) n. a means of producing immunity to a disease by using a vaccine. The name was applied originally only to treatment with vaccinia (cowpox) virus, which gives protection against cowpox and smallpox. However, it is now used synonymously with inoculation as a method of immunization against any disease.

vaccine (vak-seen) n. a special preparation of antigenic material that can be used to stimulate the development of antibodies and thus confer active immunity against a specific disease or number of diseases. It is usually given by injection but may be introduced into the skin through light scratches; for some diseases (e.g. polio), oral vaccines are available. Many vaccines are produced by culturing bacteria or viruses under conditions that lead to a loss of their virulence but not of their antigenic nature. Other vaccines consist of specially treated toxins (toxoids) or of dead bacteria that are still antigenic. *See* immunization.

vaccinia (vak-sin-iă) n. *see* cowpox.

vaccinotherapy (vak-sin-oh-th'e-ră-pi) n. the treatment of disease by the use of vaccines.

vacuole (vak-yoo-ohl) n. a space within the cytoplasm of a cell, formed by infolding of the cell membrane, that contains material taken in by the cell.

vacuum extractor (ventouse) (vak-yoo ŭm) n. a device to assist delivery consisting of a suction cup that is attached to the head of the fetus: traction is then applied slowly. It has now virtually replaced rotational obstetric forceps.

vagal (vay-găl) adj. relating to the vagus nerve.

vagin- (vagino-) prefix denoting the vagina.

vagina (vă-jy-nă) n. the lower part of the female reproductive tract: a muscular tube, lined with mucous membrane, connecting the cervix of the uterus to the exterior. It receives the erect penis during coitus. —**vaginal** adj.

vaginismus (vaj-i-niz-mŭs) n. sudden and painful contraction of the muscles surrounding the vagina, usually in response to the vulva or vagina being touched. The condition may be associated with fear of or aversion to coitus; other causative factors include vaginal injury and dryness of the lining membrane of the vagina. *See also* dyspareunia.

vaginitis (vaj-i-ny-tis) n. inflammation of the vagina, which may be caused by infection (commonly with *Trichomonas vaginalis*), dietary deficiency, or poor hygiene. There is often itching (see pruritus), increased vaginal discharge, and pain on passing urine. *postmenopausal* (or *atrophic*) v. vaginitis caused by a deficiency of female sex hormones.

vaginoplasty (colpoplasty) (vă-jy-noh-plasti) n. **1.** a tissue-grafting operation on the vagina. **2.** surgical construction of a vagina, as performed in some intersex conditions.

vaginoscope (vaj-in-oh-skohp) n. see colposcope.

vago- *prefix denoting* the vagus nerve.

vagotomy (vag-ot-ŏmi) n. the surgical cutting of any of the branches of the vagus nerve. This is usually performed to reduce secretion of acid and pepsin by the stomach in order to cure a peptic ulcer.

vagus nerve (vay-gŭs) n. the tenth cranial nerve (X), which supplies motor nerve fibres to the muscles of swallowing and parasympathetic fibres to the heart and organs of the chest cavity and abdomen. Sensory branches carry impulses from the viscera and the sensation of taste from the mouth.

valaciclovir (val-ă-sik-lŏ-veer) n. an antiviral drug, similar to aciclovir, used to treat genital herpes and shingles. Trade name: **Valtrex**.

valgus (val-gŭs) adj. describing any deformity that displaces the distal end of a limb away from the midline. See hallux (valgus), knock-knee (genu valgum), talipes (valgus).

valine (vay-leen) n. an essential amino acid. See also amino acid.

Valium (val-iŭm) n. see diazepam.

valsartan (val-sar-tan) n. see angiotensin II antagonist.

valve (valv) n. a structure found in some tubular organs or parts that restricts the flow of fluid within them to one direction only (see cusp). Valves are important structures in the heart, veins, and lymphatic vessels (see illustration). See also mitral valve, tricuspid valve, semilunar valve.

valvoplasty (valvuloplasty) (val-voh-plasti) n. the surgical reconstruction of a heart valve affected by stenosis or incompetence.

valvotomy (valvulotomy) (val-vot-ŏmi) n. surgical cutting through a valve. The term is usually used to describe the operation to relieve obstruction caused by stenosed valves in the heart (e.g. mitral v.). **percutaneous balloon v.** balloon dilatation of narrowed valves after introduction of a balloon via a catheter passed up a great vessel.

valvula (val-vew-lă) n. (pl. **valvulae**) a small valve. *valvulae conniventes* circular folds of mucous membrane in the small intestine.

valvulitis (val-vew-ly-tis) n. inflammation of one or more valves, particularly the heart valves. This is most often due to rheumatic fever (see endocarditis).

vancomycin (vank-oh-my-sin) n. an antibiotic, derived from the bacterium *Streptomyces orientalis*, that is effective against most Gram-positive organisms. It is given by intravenous infusion for serious infections due to strains that are resistant to other antibiotics. Trade name: **Vancocin**.

van den Bergh's test (van-den-bergz) n. a test to determine whether jaundice in a patient is due to haemolysis or to disease of the liver or bile duct. [A. A. H. van den Bergh (1869–1943), Dutch physician]

vanillylmandelic acid (VMA) (van-i-lil-man-del-ik) n. a metabolite of catecholamines excreted in abnormal amounts in the urine in conditions of excess catecholamine production, such as phaeochromocytoma. Measurement of VMA levels can be used as a screening test for phaeochromocytoma.

vaporizer (vay-per-I-zer) *n.* a piece of equipment for producing an extremely fine mist of liquid droplets by forcing a jet of liquid through a narrow nozzle with a jet of air. *See also* aerosol.

Vaquez-Osler disease (vak-ay ohs-ler) *n. see* polycythaemia (vera). [L. H. Vaquez (1860–1936), French physician; Sir W. Osler (1849–1919), Canadian physician]

varicectomy (va-ri-sek-tŏmi) *n. see* phlebectomy.

varicella (va-ri-sel-ă) *n. see* chickenpox.

varices (va-ri-seez) *pl. n. see* varicose veins.

varicocele (va-ri-koh-seel) *n.* a collection of dilated veins in the spermatic cord. It usually produces no symptoms apart from occasional aching discomfort. In some cases varicocele is associated with oligospermia, which can be improved by surgical correction or radiological embolization of the varicocele (*varicocelectomy*).

varicose veins (va-ri-kohs) *pl. n.* veins that are distended, lengthened, and tortuous. The superficial veins of the legs are most commonly affected; other sites include the oesophagus (*see* oesophageal varices) and testes (*see* varicocele). There is an inherited tendency to varicose veins but obstruction to blood flow is responsible in some cases. Treatment includes elastic support and sclerotherapy, but

stripping or excision is required in some cases. Medical name: **varices**.

varicotomy (va-ri-kot-ŏmi) *n.* incision into a varicose vein (*see* phlebectomy).

variola (vă-ry-ŏ-lă) *n. see* smallpox.

varioloid (vair-i-ŏ-loid) **1.** *n.* a mild form of smallpox in people who have previously had smallpox or have been vaccinated against it. **2.** *adj.* resembling smallpox.

varix (vair-iks) *n.* (*pl.* **varices**) a single varicose vein.

varus (vair-ŭs) *adj.* describing any deformity that displaces the distal end of a limb towards the midline. *See* bow-legs (genu varum), hallux (varus), talipes (varus).

vas- (vaso-) *prefix denoting* **1.** vessels, especially blood vessels. **2.** the vas deferens.

vasa efferentia (vay-să ef-er-en-shiă) *pl. n.* (*sing.* **vas efferens**) the many small tubes that conduct spermatozoa from the testis to the epididymis.

vasa vasorum (vas-or-ŭm) *pl. n.* the tiny arteries and veins that supply the walls of blood vessels.

vascular (vas-kew-ler) *adj.* relating to or supplied with blood vessels. *v. system see* cardiovascular system.

vascularization (vas-kew-ler-I-zay-shŏn) *n.* the development of blood vessels (usually capillaries) within a tissue.

vasculitis (vas-kew-ly-tis) *n. see* angiitis.

vas deferens (vas def-er-ĕnz) *n.* (*pl.* **vasa deferentia**) either of a pair of ducts that conduct spermatozoa from the epididymis to the urethra on ejaculation.

vasectomy (vă-sek-tŏmi) *n.* the surgical operation of severing the vas deferens. Bilateral vasectomy causes sterility and is an increasingly popular means of birth control.

vaso- *prefix. see* vas-.

vasoactive (vay-zoh-**ak**-tiv) *adj.* affecting the diameter of blood vessels, especially arteries. Examples of vasoactive agents are emotion, pressure, carbon dioxide, and temperature. *v. intestinal peptide see* VIP.

vasoconstriction (vay-zoh-kŏn-**strik**-shŏn) *n.* a decrease in the diameter of blood vessels, especially arteries.

vasoconstrictor (vay-zoh-kŏn-**strik**-ter) *n.* an agent that causes narrowing of the blood vessels and therefore a decrease in blood flow. Examples are metaraminol and methoxamine. Vasoconstrictors are used to raise the blood pressure in disorders of the circulation, shock, or severe bleeding and to maintain blood pressure during surgery. Some (e.g. phenylephrine) are used to treat nasal congestion.

vasodilatation (vay-zoh-dy-lă-**tay**-shŏn) *n.* an increase in the diameter of blood vessels, especially arteries.

vasodilator (vay-zoh-dy-**lay**-ter) *n.* a drug that causes widening of the blood vessels and therefore an increase in blood flow. Vasodilators are used to lower blood pressure in cases of hypertension. *coronary v.* a drug, such as glyceryl trinitrate, that increases the blood flow through the heart and is used to relieve and prevent angina. *peripheral v.* a drug, such as an alpha blocker or moxisylyte, that affects the blood

vessels of the limbs and is used to treat conditions of poor circulation.

vaso-epididymostomy (vay-zoh-epi-did-i-**mos**-tŏmi) *n.* the operation of joining the vas deferens to the epididymis in a side-to-side manner in order to bypass an obstruction in the epididymis to the passage of sperm from the testis.

vasography (vayz-**og**-răfi) *n.* X-ray imaging of the vas deferens. A contrast medium is injected either into the exposed vas deferens at surgery, using a fine needle, or by inserting a catheter into the ejaculatory duct (which discharges semen from the vesicle into the vas deferens) via an endoscope.

vasoligation (vay-zoh-ly-**gay**-shŏn) *n.* the surgical tying of the vas deferens. This is performed to prevent infection spreading from the urinary tract causing recurrent epididymitis.

vasomotion (vay-zoh-**moh**-shŏn) *n.* an increase or decrease in the diameter of blood vessels, particularly the arteries. *See* vasoconstriction, vasodilatation.

vasomotor (vay-zoh-**moh**-ter) *adj.* controlling the muscular walls of blood vessels, especially arteries, and therefore their diameter. *v. centre* a collection of nerve cells in the medulla oblongata that brings about reflex changes in the rate of the heartbeat and in the diameter of blood vessels, so that the blood pressure can be adjusted. *v. nerve* any nerve, usually belonging to the autonomic nervous system, that controls the circulation of blood through blood vessels by its action on the muscle fibres within their walls or its action on the heartbeat.

v. **symptoms** subjective sensations experienced by women around the time of the menopause, often described as explosions of heat, mostly followed by profuse sweating. Physiological changes include peripheral vasodilatation, tachycardia with normal blood pressure, and raised skin temperature with normal body temperature.

vasopressin (antidiuretic hormone, ADH) (vay-zoh-press-in) *n.* a hormone, released by the pituitary gland, that increases the reabsorption of water by the kidney and causes constriction of blood vessels. It is administered by injection to treat diabetes insipidus and to control bleeding from oesophageal varices.

vasopressor (vay-zoh-press-er) *adj.* stimulating the contraction of blood vessels and therefore bringing about an increase in blood pressure.

vasospasm (vay-zoh-spazm) *n. see* Raynaud's disease.

vasovagal (vay-zoh-vay-găl) *adj.* relating to the action of impulses in the vagus nerve on the circulation. The vagus reduces the rate at which the heart beats, and so lowers its output. *v.* **attack** excessive activity of the vagus nerve, causing slowing of the heart and a fall in blood pressure, which leads to fainting. *See* syncope.

vasovasostomy (vay-zoh-vă-sos-tŏmi) *n.* the surgical operation of re-anastomosing the vas deferens after previous vasectomy: the reversal of vasectomy, undertaken to restore fertility.

vasovesiculitis (vay-zoh-ve-sik-yoo-ly-tis) *n.* inflammation of the seminal vesicles and vas deferens. This usually occurs in association with prostatitis and causes pain in the perineum, groin, and scrotum and a high temperature.

vector (vek-ter) *n.* an animal, usually an insect or a tick, that transmits parasitic microorganisms – and therefore the diseases they cause – from person to person or from infected animals to human beings.

vectorcardiography (vek-ter-kar-di-og-răfi) *n. see* electrocardiography.

vegetation (vej-i-tay-shŏn) *n.* (in pathology) an abnormal outgrowth from a membrane. In ulcerative endocarditis, outgrowths consisting of fibrin with enmeshed blood cells are found on the membrane lining the heart valves.

vegetative (vej-i-tă-tiv) *adj.* **1.** relating to growth and nutrition rather than to reproduction. **2.** functioning unconsciously; autonomic.

vehicle (vee-ikŭl) *n.* (in pharmacy) any substance, such as sterile water or dextrose solution, that acts as the medium in which a drug is administered.

vein (vayn) *n.* a blood vessel conveying blood towards the heart. All veins except the pulmonary vein carry deoxygenated blood from the tissues to the vena cava. Veins contain valves that assist the flow of blood back to the heart. (See illustrations.) Anatomical name: **vena**. —**venous** (vee-nŭs) *adj.*

vena cava (vee-nă kay-vă) *n.* (*pl.* **venae cavae**) either of the two main veins, conveying deoxygenated blood from the other veins to the right atrium of the heart. *in-*

(A)

(B)

valve open

direction of
blood flow

blood pressure
closes valve so
preventing
backflow

(A) cut vein showing the two
cusps of a valve; (B) action of a
venous valve

ferior v. c. (IVC) the vein that receives blood from parts of the body
below the diaphragm. *superior v. c.*
the vein that drains blood from the
head, neck, thorax, and arms.

vene- (veno-) *prefix denoting*
veins.

venene (ven-een) *n.* a mixture of
two or more venoms: used to produce antiserum against venoms
(antivenene).

venepuncture (venipuncture)
(ven-i-punk-cher) *n.* the puncture of
a vein for any therapeutic purpose;
for example, to extract blood for laboratory tests. *See also* phlebotomy.

venereal disease (VD) (vin-eer-
iǎl) *n. see* sexually transmitted disease.

venesection (ven-i-sek-shŏn) *n. see*
phlebotomy.

veno- *prefix. see* vene-.

venoclysis (vi-nok-li-sis) *n.* the
continuous infusion into a vein of
saline or other solution.

venography (phlebography) (vi-
nog-rǎfi) *n.* imaging of the anatomy
of veins in a particular region of the
body, commonly to demonstrate
deep vein thrombosis in the legs.
Traditionally, a radiopaque contrast
medium is injected into a vein and
X-ray photographs (*venograms*) are
taken as the medium flows towards
the heart. *compression v.* an ultrasound technique to look for block-
ages in leg veins. Pressing a healthy
vein with the ultrasound probe usually causes it to empty and flatten,
which does not occur if there is
thrombus in the lumen. *See also* angiography.

venom (ven-ŏm) *n.* the poisonous
material produced by snakes, scor-
pions, etc. Some venoms produce no
more than local pain and swelling;
others can prove lethal.

ventilation (ven-ti-lay-shŏn) *n.* the
passage of air into and out of the respiratory tract. In the alveoli of the
lungs gas exchange is most efficient
when matched by an adequate blood
flow (perfusion). Ventilation/perfu-
sion imbalance is an important
cause of anoxia and cyanosis.

**ventilation-perfusion scanning
(V/Q scanning)** *n.* a nuclear med-

internal jugular
external jugular
superior
vena cava
subclavian
cephalic
axillary
hepatic
brachial
suprarenal
inferior vena cava
renal
median cubital
testicular
(ovarian)
common iliac
basilic
external iliac
femoral
superficial
palmar
network
great
saphenous
popliteal
small saphenous
anterior tibial
dorsal
venous arch

The principal veins of the body

icine technique in which two different isotopes are used, one inhaled, to examine lung ventilation, and one injected, to examine lung perfusion. It is used to detect pulmonary embolism, in which the area of lung supplied by the blocked artery is not being perfused with blood but has normal ventilation.

ventilator (ven-ti-lay-ter) *n.* **1.** a device used to ensure a supply of fresh air. **2.** equipment that is manually or mechanically operated to maintain a flow of air into and out of the lungs of a patient who is unable to breathe normally. *See also* respirator.

ventouse (von-**toos**) *n. see* vacuum extractor.

ventral (ven-trăl) *adj.* relating to or situated at or close to the front of the body or to the anterior part of an organ.

ventricle (ven-trik-ŭl) *n.* **1.** either of the two lower chambers of the heart. The left ventricle receives blood from the pulmonary vein and pumps it into the aorta. The right ventricle pumps blood from the venae cavae into the pulmonary artery. **2.** one of the four fluid-filled cavities within the brain. The paired first and second ventricles (lateral ventricles) communicate with the third ventricle. This leads to the fourth ventricle in the hindbrain, which is continuous with the spinal canal. Cerebrospinal fluid circulates through all the cavities. —**ventricular** (ven-trik-yoo-ler) *adj.*

ventricul- (ventriculo-) *prefix denoting* a ventricle (of the brain or heart).

ventricular folds *pl. n. see* vocal folds.

ventricular septal defect *n. see* septal defect.

ventricular tachycardia (VT) *n. see* tachycardia.

ventriculitis (ven-trik-yoo-ly-tis) *n.* inflammation in the ventricles of the brain, usually caused by infection.

ventriculoatriostomy (ven-trik-yoo-loh-ay-tri-ost-ŏmi) *n.* an operation for the relief of raised pressure due to the build-up of cerebrospinal fluid that occurs in hydrocephalus.

ventriculography (ven-trik-yoo-log-răfi) *n.* X-ray examination of the ventricles of the brain after the introduction of a contrast medium. This procedure has been largely made redundant by CT and MRI scanning.

ventriculoscopy (ven-trik-yoo-losk-ŏpi) *n.* observation of the ventricles of the brain through a fibre-optic instrument. *See* endoscope, fibre optics.

ventriculostomy (ven-trik-yoo-lost-ŏmi) *n.* an operation to introduce a hollow needle (cannula) into one of the lateral ventricles of the brain. This may be done to relieve raised intracranial pressure, to obtain cerebrospinal fluid for examination, or to introduce antibiotics or contrast material for X-ray examination.

ventro- *prefix denoting* **1.** ventral. **2.** the abdomen.

ventrofixation (ven-troh-fiks-ay-shŏn) *n. see* ventrosuspension.

ventrosuspension (ventrofixation) (ven-troh-sus-pen-shŏn) *n.* surgical fixation of a displaced uterus to the anterior abdominal wall. This may be achieved by shortening the round ligaments at their attachment either to the uterus or to the abdominal wall.

venule (ven-yool) *n.* a minute vessel that drains blood from the capillaries.

verapamil (ve-rap-ă-mil) *n.* a calcium antagonist administered by mouth in the treatment of essential hypertension, angina, and arrhythmia. Trade names: **Cordilox, Securon, Univer**.

verbigeration (ver-bij-er-ay-shŏn) *n.* repetitive utterances of the same words over and over again. It is most common in institutionalized schizophrenics.

vermicide (verm-i-syd) *n.* a chemical agent used to destroy parasitic worms living in the intestine. *Compare* vermifuge.

vermiform appendix (verm-i-form) *n. see* appendix.

vermifuge (verm-i-fewj) *n.* any drug or chemical agent used to expel worms from the intestine. *See also* anthelmintic.

vermix (ver-miks) *n.* the vermiform appendix.

vernal conjunctivitis (ver-năl) *n. see* conjunctivitis.

Verner-Morrison syndrome (ver-ner mo-ri-sŏn) *n. see* VIPoma. [J. V. Verner (1927–), US physician; A. B. Morrison (1922–), Irish pathologist]

vernix caseosa (ver-niks kay-si-oh-să) *n.* the layer of greasy material that covers the skin of a fetus or newborn baby. It is produced by the sebaceous glands and contains skin scales and fine hairs.

verruca (plantar wart) (ver-oo-kă) *n.* (*pl.* **verrucae**) *see* wart.

verrucous carcinoma (ver-oo-kŭs) *n.* an indolent preinvasive wartlike carcinoma of the oral cavity, which is associated with chewing tobacco.

version (ver-shŏn) *n.* a manoeuvre to alter the position of a fetus in the uterus to facilitate delivery. For example, the fetus may be turned from a transverse to a longitudinal position or from a buttocks-first to a head-first presentation. *See also* cephalic version.

vertebra (ver-tib-ră) *n* (*pl.* **vertebrae**) one of the 33 bones of which the backbone is composed. Each vertebra typically consists of a *body*, from the back of which arises an arch of bone (the *neural arch*) enclosing a cavity through which the spinal cord passes. Individual vertebrae are bound together by liga-

- spine
- articulating process
- transverse process
- vertebral canal
- intervertebral disc
- body
- facets for articulation with ribs

A typical thoracic vertebra
(from above)

ments and intervertebral discs. —**vertebral** (ver-tib-răl) *adj.*

vertebral column *n. see* backbone.

vertex (ver-teks) *n.* the crown of the head.

vertigo (vert-i-goh) *n.* a disabling sensation in which affected individuals feel that either they themselves or their surroundings are in a state of constant movement. It is a symptom of disease either in the labyrinth of the inner ear or in the vestibular nerve or its nuclei in the brainstem. *See also* benign paroxysmal positional vertigo.

vesical (ves-ikăl) *adj.* relating to or affecting a bladder, especially the urinary bladder.

vesicant (ves-i-kănt) *n.* an agent that causes blistering of the skin.

vesicle (ves-ikŭl) *n.* **1.** a very small blister in the skin that contains serum. Vesicles occur in a variety of skin disorders, including eczema and herpes. **2.** (in anatomy) any small bladder, especially one filled with fluid. —**vesicular** (ves-ik-yoo-ler) *adj.*

vesico- *prefix denoting* the urinary bladder.

vesicofixation (ves-i-koh-fiks-ay-shŏn) *n. see* cystopexy.

vesicostomy (ves-i-kos-tŏmi) *n.* the surgical creation of an artificial channel between the bladder and the skin surface for the passage of urine. It is sometimes combined with closure of the urethra.

vesicoureteric reflux (VUR) (ves-i-koh-yoor-i-te-rik) *n.* the backflow of urine from the bladder into the ureters, due to defective valves. Infection is conveyed to the kidneys, causing recurrent attacks of acute pyelonephritis and scarring of the kidneys in childhood.

vesicovaginal (ves-i-koh-vă-jy-năl) *adj.* relating to the bladder and vagina.

vesicular breath sounds *pl. n.* normal breath sounds, which may be increased or decreased in disease states.

vesicular mole *n. see* hydatidiform mole.

vesiculitis (ve-sik-yoo-ly-tis) *n.* inflammation of the seminal vesicles. *See* vasovesiculitis.

vesiculography (ve-sik-yoo-log-răfi) *n.* any technique for imaging the seminal vesicles. This is now usually performed either by injecting a contrast medium into the vas deferens during transrectal ultrasonography or by magnetic resonance imaging. Both these techniques are useful for investigation of patients with azoospermia.

vessel (ves-ĕl) *n.* a tube conveying a body fluid, especially a blood vessel or a lymphatic vessel.

vestibular glands (ves-tib-yoo-ler) *pl. n.* the two pairs of glands that open at the junction of the vagina and vulva. Their function is to lubricate the entrance to the vagina during coitus.

vestibular nerve *n.* the division of the vestibulocochlear nerve that carries impulses from the semicircular canals, utricle, and saccule of the inner ear, conveying information about posture, movement, and balance.

vestibule (vest-i-bewl) *n.* (in anatomy) a cavity situated at the entrance to a hollow part. The vestibule of the ear is the cavity of the bony labyrinth that contains the saccule and utricle.

vestibulocochlear nerve (acoustic nerve, auditory nerve) (ves-tib-yoo-loh-**kok**-li-er) *n.* the eighth cranial nerve (VIII), responsible for carrying sensory impulses from the inner ear to the brain. It has two branches (*see* cochlear nerve, vestibular nerve).

vestigial (ves-**tij**-iăl) *adj.* existing only in a rudimentary form. The term is applied to organs whose structure and function have been diminished during the course of evolution.

VF *n. see* (ventricular) fibrillation.

viable (vy-ăbŭl) *adj.* capable of living a separate existence. The legal age of viability of a fetus is 24 weeks, but some fetuses now survive birth at an even earlier age.

Viagra (vy-ag-ră) *n. see* sildenafil.

Vibramycin (vy-bră-**my**-sin) *n. see* doxycycline.

Vibrio (vib-ri-oh) *n.* a genus of Gram-negative motile comma-shaped bacteria widely distributed in soil and water. *V. cholerae* is the species that causes cholera.

vicarious (vik-**air**-iŭs) *adj.* describing an action or function performed by an organ not normally involved in the function. *v. menstruation* a rare disorder in which monthly bleeding occurs from places other than the vagina, such as the sweat glands, breasts, nose, or eyes.

videofluoroscopy (vid-i-oh-floo-er-os-kŏ-pi) *n.* the technique of viewing and recording real time X-ray investigation using a video camera (*see* real-time imaging). This enables the moving images to be reviewed at a later time, by individual frames or in slow motion.

videokeratography (vid-i-oh-ke-ră-**tog**-răfi) *n. see* (corneal) topography.

videokymography (vid-i-oh-ky-**mog**-răfi) *n.* a method of studying the vibration of the vocal folds of the larynx using high-speed digital photography. *See* laryngeal (stroboscopy).

video-otoscope (vid-i-oh-**oh**-toh-skohp) *n.* a small endoscope connected to a digital camera for examining the outer ear and eardrum.

villus (**vil**-ŭs) *n.* (*pl.* **villi**) one of many short finger-like processes that project from the surfaces of some membranes. *arachnoid v.* any of arachnoid. *chorionic v.* any of the folds of the chorion from which the fetal part of the placenta is formed. They provide an extensive area for the exchange of oxygen, nutrients, etc., between maternal and fetal blood. *intestinal v.* any of numerous projections that line the small intestine. Each contains a network of blood capillaries and a lacteal. Their function is to absorb the products of digestion and they greatly increase the surface area over which this can take place.

vinblastine (vin-**blas**-teen) *n.* a vinca alkaloid that is given by intravascular injection mainly in the treatment of cancers of the lymphatic system, such as Hodgkin's disease. It is highly toxic. Trade name: **Velbe**.

vinca alkaloid (ving-kă) *n.* one of a group of antimitotic drugs (*see* cytotoxic drug) derived from the periwinkle (*Vinca rosea*). Vinca alkaloids, usually administered intravenously, are used especially to treat leukaemias and lymphomas; they include vinblastine, vincristine, and vindesine.

Vincent's angina (vin-sĕnts) *n. see* ulcerative gingivitis. [H. Vincent (1862–1950), French physician]

vincristine (vin-**kris**-teen) *n.* a vinca alkaloid with uses similar to those of vinblastine. Trade name: **Oncovin**.

vindesine (vin-dĕ-seen) *n.* a vinca alkaloid with similarities to vinblastine. Trade name: **Eldisine**.

VIP (vasoactive intestinal peptide) *n.* a peptide hormone produced by cells of the pancreas. Large amounts cause severe diarrhoea (*see* VIPoma).

VIPoma (vy-**poh**-mă) *n.* a usually malignant tumour of islet cells of the pancreas that secrete excess VIP, resulting in severe diarrhoea ('pancreatic cholera' or the *Verner-Morrison syndrome*), with loss of potassium and bicarbonate and a low level of stomach acid.

viraemia (vyr-ee-miă) *n.* the presence in the blood of virus particles.

viral pneumonia (vy-răl) *n.* an acute infection of the lung caused by a virus, such as respiratory syncytial virus, adenovirus, influenza and parainfluenza viruses, or an enterovirus. It is characterized by headache, fever, muscle pain, and a cough that produces a thick sputum. The pneumonia often occurs with or subsequent to a systemic viral infection.

virilism (vi-ril-izm) *n.* the development in a female of increased body hair, muscle bulk, deepening of the voice, and male psychological characteristics.

virilization (vi-ri-ly-**zay**-shŏn) *n.* the most extreme result of excessive androgen production (hyperandrogenism) in women. It is characterized by temporal balding, a male body form, muscle bulk, deepening of the voice, enlargement of the clitoris, and hirsutism. Virilization in prepubertal boys may be caused by some tumours (*see* Leydig tumour) or the adrenogenital syndrome.

virology (vyr-ol-ŏji) *n.* the science of viruses. *See also* microbiology.

virulence (vi-rew-lĕns) *n.* the disease-producing (pathogenic) ability of a microorganism. *See also* attenuation.

virus (vy-rŭs) *n.* a minute particle that is capable of replication but only within living cells. Viruses are too small to be visible with a light microscope or to be trapped by filters. They infect animals, plants, and microorganisms. Viruses cause many diseases, including herpes, influenza, mumps, polio, AIDS, and rabies. Antiviral drugs are effective against some of them, and many viral diseases are controlled by means of vaccines. —**viral** *adj.*

viscera (vis-er-ă) *pl. n.* (*sing.* **viscus**) the organs within the body cavities, especially the organs of the abdominal cavities. —**visceral** (vis-er-ăl) *adj.*

visceral pouch *n. see* pharyngeal (pouch).

viscero- *prefix denoting* the viscera.

visceroptosis (vis-er-op-toh-sis) *n.* downward displacement of the abdominal organs.

viscid (vis-id) *adj.* glutinous and sticky.

viscoelastic material (vis-koh-i-lasst-ik) *n.* any gel-like material used in ophthalmic surgery (such as cataract surgery) to help maintain the shape of ocular tissues as well as lubricate and minimize trauma.

viscus (vis-kŭs) n. see viscera.

visual acuity (vizh-yoo-ăl) n. sharpness of vision. Acuity of distant vision is often expressed as a Snellen score (see Snellen chart).

visual field n. the area in front of the eye in any part of which an object can be seen without moving the eye.

visual purple n. see rhodopsin.

vital capacity (vy-t'l) n. the maximum volume of air that a person can exhale after maximum inspiration. *forced v. c.* (FVC) the maximum volume of air that the lungs can expel in a forced expiration after the deepest possible inspiration.

vital centre n. any of the collections of nerve cells in the brain that act as governing centres for different vital body functions, such as breathing, blood pressure, etc.

Vitallium (vy-tal-iŭm) n. *Trademark.* an alloy of chromium and cobalt that is used in instruments, prostheses, surgical appliances, and dentures.

vital statistics pl. n. statistics relating to the births, marriages, deaths, and incidence of disease within a population.

vitamin (vit-ă-min) n. any of a group of substances that are required, in very small amounts, for healthy growth and development: they cannot be synthesized by the body and are therefore essential constituents of the diet. Vitamins are divided into two groups, according to whether they are soluble in water or fat.

vitamin A (retinol) n. a fat-soluble vitamin that occurs preformed in foods of animal origin (especially milk products, egg yolk, and liver) and is formed in the body from the pigment β-carotene, present in some vegetable foods (for example cabbage, lettuce, and carrots). Retinol is essential for growth, vision in dim light, and the maintenance of soft mucous tissue. A deficiency causes stunted growth, night blindness, xerophthalmia, keratomalacia, and eventual blindness. Recommended daily intake: 750 µg retinol equivalents.

vitamin B n. any one of a group of water-soluble vitamins that are often found together in the same kinds of food, such as liver, yeast, and eggs, and all function as coenzymes. B_1 (*thiamin*, *aneurine*) a vitamin deficiency of which leads to beriberi. Recommended daily intake: 1 mg. B_2 (*riboflavin*) a vitamin important in tissue respiration. A deficiency causes ariboflavinosis. Recommended daily intake: 1.7 mg. B_6 (*pyridoxine*) a vitamin from which the coenzyme pyridoxal phosphate is formed. Deficiency is very rare. B_{12} (*cyanocobalamin*) a vitamin that can be absorbed only in the presence of intrinsic factor, secreted in the stomach. A deficiency can lead to pernicious anaemia and degeneration of the nervous system. Recommended daily intake: 3–4 µg. *See also* biotin, folic acid, nicotinic acid, pantothenic acid.

vitamin C (ascorbic acid) n. a water-soluble vitamin with antioxidant properties that is essential in maintaining healthy connective tissues. A deficiency of vitamin C leads to scurvy. Recommended daily intake: 30 mg; rich sources are citrus fruits and vegetables.

vitamin D *n.* a fat-soluble vitamin that enhances the absorption of calcium and phosphorus from the intestine and promotes their deposition in the bone. *D₂* (*ergocalciferol, calciferol*) a form obtained from the diet; good sources are fatty fish, eggs, and margarine. *D₃* (*cholecalciferol*) a form manufactured in the skin in the presence of sunlight. A deficiency of vitamin D leads to rickets and osteomalacia. Recommended daily intake: 10 µg (for a child up to five years); 2.5 µg (thereafter).

vitamin E *n.* any of a group of chemically related fat-soluble compounds (*tocopherols* and *tocotrienols*) that have antioxidant properties and are thought to stabilize cell membranes. Good sources of the vitamin are vegetable oils, eggs, butter, and wholemeal cereals. It is fairly widely distributed in the diet and a deficiency is therefore unlikely.

vitamin K *n.* a fat-soluble vitamin occurring in two main forms – *phytomenadione* and *menaquinone* – essential for the normal clotting of blood. A dietary deficiency does not often occur as the vitamin is synthesized by bacteria in the large intestine and is widely distributed in green leafy vegetables and meat.

vitelliform degeneration (Best's disease) (vy-tel-i-form) *n.* degeneration of the macula of the eye that is inherited as a dominant characteristic and usually starts in childhood. There is widespread abnormality of retinal pigment epithelium (*see* retina) with the accumulation of a yellowish material, especially in the macular area.

vitellus (vi-tel-ŭs) *n.* the yolk of an ovum.

vitiligo (vit-i-ly-goh) *n.* a common disorder in which symmetrical white or pale macules appear on the skin. It affects all races, but is more conspicuous in dark-skinned races. Vitiligo is an autoimmune disease and is usually progressive, although spontaneous repigmentation may occur.

vitrectomy (vi-trek-tŏmi) *n.* the removal of all or part of the vitreous humour of the eye, including vitreous haemorrhage. It is often necessary in surgery to repair a detached retina.

vitreous detachment (vit-ri-ŭs) *n.* the separation of the vitreous humour from the underlying retina. This is a normal ageing process, but it is also more common in such conditions as diabetes and severe myopia. It can sometimes cause a tear in the retina and lead to retinal detachment.

vitreous humour (vitreous body) *n.* the transparent jelly-like material that fills the chamber behind the lens of the eye.

vitritis (vi-try-tis) *n.* inflammation within the vitreous humour of the eye.

vivisection (viv-i-sek-shŏn) *n.* a surgical operation on a living animal for experimental purposes.

VMA *n. see* vanillylmandelic acid.

vocal folds (vocal cords) (vohkăl) *pl. n.* the two folds of tissue protruding from the sides of the larynx to form a narrow slit (glottis) across

root of the tongue
epiglottis
vocal fold (true vocal cord)
ventricular fold (false vocal cord)
glottis
larynx

The vocal folds

the air passage (see illustration). Their controlled interference with the expiratory air flow produces audible vibrations that make up speech, song, and all other vocal noises.

vocal fremitus *n. see* fremitus.

vocal resonance *n.* the sounds heard through the stethoscope when the patient speaks. These are normally just audible but they become much louder (*bronchophony*) if the lung under the stethoscope is consolidated. Vocal resonance is lost over pleural fluid except at its upper surface, when it has a bleating quality (*aegophony*). *See also* pectoriloquy.

volar (voh-ler) *adj.* relating to the palm of the hand or the sole of the foot (the *vola*).

volatile (vol-ă-tyl) *adj.* describing a liquid that evaporates at room temperature.

volition (vŏl-ish-ŏn) *n.* the act of or capacity for exercising the will.

Volkmann's contracture (fohlk-mahnz) *n.* shrinkage and shortening of muscles due to inadequate blood supply. This arises if the blood supply is interrupted by pressure on the blood vessels from a fracture fragment, or from raised pressure due to compartment syndrome, or by pressure from constricting bandages or plaster casts. [R. von Volkmann (1830–89), German surgeon]

volsellum (vulsellum) (vol-sel-ŭm) *n.* surgical forceps with claw-like hooks at the ends of both blades.

volt (vohlt) *n.* the SI unit of electric potential. Symbol: V.

voluntary admission (vol-ŭn-ter-i) *n.* entry of a patient into a psychiatric hospital with his (or her) agreement. *Compare* compulsory admission.

voluntary muscle *n. see* striated muscle.

volvulus (vol-vew-lŭs) *n.* twisting of part of the digestive tract, usually leading to partial or complete obstruction and sometimes reducing the blood supply, causing gangrene.

vomer (voh-mer) *n.* a thin plate of bone that forms part of the nasal septum.

vomica (vom-ik-ă) *n.* **1.** an abnormal cavity in an organ, usually a lung, sometimes containing pus. **2.** the abrupt expulsion from the mouth of a large quantity of pus or decaying matter originating in the throat or lungs.

vomit (vom-it) **1.** *vb.* to eject the contents of the stomach through the mouth (*see* vomiting). **2.** *n.* the contents of the stomach ejected during vomiting. Medical name: **vomitus**.

vomiting (vom-it-ing) *n.* the reflex action of ejecting the contents of the stomach through the mouth. Vomiting is controlled by a special centre in the brain that may be stimulated by drugs acting directly on it or by impulses transmitted from the stomach (e.g. after ingesting irritating substances), the intestine (e.g. in intestinal obstruction), or from the inner ear (in motion sickness). Medical name: **emesis**.

von Recklinghausen's disease (von **rek**-ling-how-zĕnz) *n.* **1.** a syndrome due to hyperparathyroidism, characterized by loss of mineral from bones, which become weakened and fracture easily, and formation of kidney stones. Medical name: **osteitis fibrosa**. **2.** *see* neurofibromatosis. [F. D. von Recklinghausen (1833–1910), German pathologist]

von Willebrand's disease (von **wil**-i-brandz) *n.* an inherited disorder of the blood characterized by episodes of spontaneous bleeding similar to haemophilia. It is due to abnormalities in the von Willebrand factor, a glycoprotein necessary for normal platelet function. [A. von Willebrand (1870–1949), Swedish physician]

voxel (voks-ĕl) *n.* short for 'volume element', the volume of tissue in a body that is represented by a pixel in a cross-sectional image.

VSD *n. see* (ventricular) septal defect.

VT *n. see* (ventricular) tachycardia.

vulsellum (vul-**sel**-ŭm) *n. see* volsellum.

vulv- (vulvo-) *prefix denoting* the vulva.

vulva (**vul**-vă) *n.* the female external genitalia. Two pairs of fleshy folds (*see* labium) surround the openings of the vagina and urethra and extend forward to the clitoris. *See also* vestibular glands.

vulvectomy (vul-**vek**-tŏmi) *n.* surgical removal of the vulva. *simple v.* excision of the labia majora, labia minora, and clitoris to eradicate a nonmalignant growth. *radical v.* excision of the labia majora and minora, the clitoris, and all regional lymph nodes on both sides, together with the skin covering these areas. It is carried out for a malignant growth.

vulvitis (vul-**vy**-tis) *n.* inflammation of the vulva, which is often accompanied by intense itching (*see* pruritus).

vulvovaginitis (vul-voh-vaj-i-ny-tis) *n.* inflammation of the vulva and vagina (*see* pruritus, vaginitis).

VUR *n. see* vesicoureteric reflux.

Waardenburg's syndrome (vah-den-bergz) *n.* an inherited form of deafness accompanied by a characteristic white forelock of hair and multiple colours within the irises of the eyes. It is inherited as an autosomal dominant disease, although severity is variable. [P. J. Waardenburg (1886–1979), Dutch ophthalmologist]

wafer (way-fer) *n.* a thin sheet made from moistened flour, formerly used to enclose a powdered medicine that is taken by mouth.

waiting list (wayt-ing) *n.* a list of the names of patients who are awaiting admission to hospital after having been assessed either as an out-patient or on a domiciliary consultation involving a specialist. In general the patients are offered places in the order in which their names were placed on the list.

Waldeyer's ring (vahl-dy-erz) *n.* the ring of lymphoid tissue formed by the tonsils. [H. W. G. von Waldeyer (1836–1921), German anatomist]

walking distance (wawk-ing) *n.* the measured distance that a patient can walk before he or she is stopped by pain in the muscles, usually the calf muscles. It is a useful estimate of the degree of impairment of the blood supply. *See* claudication.

Wallerian degeneration (wol-eer-iăn) *n.* degeneration of a ruptured nerve fibre that occurs within the nerve sheath distal to the point of severance. [A. V. Waller (1816–70), British physician]

Wangensteen tube (wang-ĕn-steen) *n.* a tube with a suction apparatus that is passed into the stomach through the nose and is used to drain the contents of the stomach and duodenum to relieve abdominal distention. [O. H. Wangensteen (1898–1980), US surgeon]

ward manager (wawd man-ă-jer) *n.* a person responsible for the management of a hospital ward. The ward manager may be a non-nurse administrator with management training or the position can be (or be combined with) a nursing post.

warfarin (wor-fer-in) *n.* an anticoagulant used mainly in the treatment of coronary or venous thrombosis to reduce the risk of embolism. It is given by mouth. Trade name: **Marevan**.

wart (wort) *n.* a benign growth on the skin caused by infection with human papillomavirus. Treatment of warts is with over-the-counter remedies, such as lactic and salicylic acids, but cryotherapy with liquid nitrogen is probably more effective. *common w.* a firm horny papule found mainly on the hands. Most will clear spontaneously within two years. *genital w.* a wart that is frequently associated with other genital infections; affected woman have an increased risk of developing cervical cancer. *plane w.* a flat skin-coloured wart usually found on the face; it may be present in very large numbers. *plantar w.* (*verruca*) a wart occurring on the sole of the foot. Plantar warts are often tender.

Warthin's tumour (adenolymphoma) (wor-thinz) *n.* a tumour of the parotid salivary glands, containing epithelial and lymphoid tissues with cystic spaces. [A. S. Warthin (1866–1931), US pathologist]

Wassermann reaction (wass-er-măn) *n.* formerly, the most commonly used test for the diagnosis of syphilis. A sample of the patient's blood is examined for the presence of antibodies to *Treponema pallidum.* [A. P. von Wassermann (1866–1925), German bacteriologist]

water bed (waw-ter) *n.* a bed with a flexible water-containing mattress. The surface of the bed adapts itself to the patient's posture, which leads to greater comfort and fewer bedsores.

waterbrash (waw-ter-brash) *n.* a sudden filling of the mouth with dilute saliva. This often accompanies dyspepsia, particularly if there is nausea.

water-deprivation test *n.* a test for diabetes insipidus in which fluid and food intake is withheld completely for (usually) 24 hours, with regular measurement of plasma and urinary osmolality and body weight. In a patient with diabetes insipidus the urine osmolality will remain low and of high volume while the patient steadily dehydrates.

water-hammer pulse *n.* see Corrigan's pulse.

Waterhouse-Friderichsen syndrome (waw-ter-howss frid-er-ik-sĕn) *n.* fever, cyanosis, and bleeding into the skin resulting from haemorrhage of both adrenal glands, caused by septicaemia resulting from bacterial meningitis. [R. Waterhouse (1873–1958), British physician; C. Friderichsen (20th century), Danish physician]

Waterston's operation (waw-ter-stŏnz) *n.* the operation of joining the right pulmonary artery to the ascending aorta, performed to relieve tetralogy of Fallot. [D. Waterston (1910–), British surgeon]

watt (wot) *n.* the SI unit of power, equal to 1 joule per second. Symbol: W.

WBC *n.* white blood cell (*see* leucocyte).

weal (weel) *n.* a transient swelling, confined to a small area of the skin, that is characteristic of urticaria and occurs following dermographism.

Weber-Christian disease (web-er **kris**-chăn) *n.* a form of panniculitis in which there is fever and enlargement of the liver and spleen. [F. P. Weber (1863–1962), British physician; H. A. Christian (1876–1951), US physician]

Weber's test (vay-berz) *n.* a hearing test in which a vibrating tuning fork is placed at the midpoint of the forehead. If one ear is affected by conductive deafness the sound appears louder in the affected ear; if one ear has sensorineural deafness the sound appears louder in the unaffected ear. [F. E. Weber (1832–91), German otologist]

web space (web spays) *n.* the soft

tissue between the bases of the fingers and toes.

Wechsler scales (weks-ler) *pl. n.* standardized scales for the measurement of intelligence quotient (IQ) in adults and children. They are administered by a chartered psychologist. *See* intelligence test. [D. Wechsler (1896–1981), US psychologist]

Wegener's granulomatosis (vay-gĕ-nerz) *n.* an autoimmune disease predominantly affecting the nasal passages, lungs, and kidneys, characterized by granuloma formation in addition to arteritis. It is usually fatal but can be controlled (sometimes for years) with steroids, cyclophosphamide, and azathioprine. [F. Wegener (1907–90), German pathologist]

Weil-Felix reaction (vyl fay-liks) *n.* a diagnostic test for typhus. A sample of the patient's serum is tested for the presence of antibodies against the organism *Proteus vulgaris*. [E. Weil (1880–1922), German physician; A. Felix (1887–1956), Czech bacteriologist]

Weil's disease (vylz) *n. see* leptospirosis. [A. Weil (1848–1916), German physician]

Welch's bacillus (welch-ŭz) *n. see* Clostridium. [W. H. Welch (1850–1934), US pathologist]

wen (wen) *n. see* sebaceous cyst.

Werdnig-Hoffmann disease (verd-nig hof-man) *n.* a hereditary disorder that is a severe form of spinal muscular atrophy affecting infants. It causes a symmetrical muscle weakness that eventually affects respiratory and facial muscles. Children usually die by the age of 20 months. [G. Werdnig (1844–1919),

Austrian neurologist; J. Hoffmann (1857–1919), German neurologist]

Wermer's syndrome (werm-erz) *n. see* MENS. [P. Wermer, US physician]

Werner's syndrome (vair-nerz) *n.* a rare genetic disorder resulting in premature ageing that starts at adolescence. Growth may be retarded and affected individuals may suffer from a thin skin, arterial disease, leg ulcers, and diabetes. [C. W. O. Werner (1879–1936), German physician]

Wernicke's encephalopathy (ver-nik-ĕz) *n.* mental confusion or delirium occurring in combination with paralysis of the eye muscles, nystagmus, and an unsteady gait. It is caused by a deficiency of vitamin B_1 and is most commonly seen in alcoholics and in patients with persistent vomiting or an unbalanced diet. [K. Wernicke (1848–1905), German neurologist]

Wertheim's hysterectomy (vertymz) *n.* a radical operation performed for cervical cancer, involving removal of the entire uterus, the connective tissue and lymph nodes close to it, Fallopian tubes, ovaries, and the upper part of the vagina. [E. Wertheim (1864–1920), Austrian gynaecologist]

West Nile fever (west nyl) *n.* a viral disease spread by the *Culex pipiens* mosquito. It causes encephalitis, with influenza-like symptoms, enlarged lymph nodes, and a bright red rash on the chest and abdomen. In patients with a weakened immune system (such as the elderly) it can progress to convulsions, coma, and paralysis.

Wharton's duct (wor-t'nz) *n.* the

secretory duct of the submandibular salivary gland. [T. Wharton (1614–73), English physician]

Wharton's jelly *n.* the mesoderm tissue of the umbilical cord, which becomes converted to a loose jelly-like mesenchyme surrounding the umbilical blood vessels.

Wheelhouse's operation (weel-howss-ŭz) *n.* an operation to relieve urethral stricture in which the incision is made through the perineum. [G. Wheelhouse (1826–1909), British surgeon]

wheeze (weez) *n.* an abnormal high-pitched (sibilant) or low-pitched sound that is heard mainly during expiration. Wheezes occur as a result of narrowing of the airways, such as results from bronchospasm or increased secretion and retention of sputum; they are commonly heard in patients with asthma or chronic bronchitis. *Compare* stridor.

whiplash injury (wip-lash) *n.* damage to the ligaments, vertebrae, or spinal cord caused by sudden jerking back of the head and neck, often in occupants of a car hit from behind. It causes pain and stiffness in the neck; symptoms may last for months or even years.

Whipple's disease (wip-ŭlz) *n.* a rare disease, occurring only in males, in which there is malabsorption, usually accompanied by skin pigmentation and arthritis. [G. H. Whipple (1878–1976), US pathologist]

Whipple's operation *n.* see pancreatectomy. [A. O. Whipple (1881–1963), US surgeon]

Whipple's triad *n.* a combination of three clinical features that indicate the presence of an insulinoma: (1) attacks of fainting, dizziness, and sweating on fasting; (2) severe hypoglycaemia present during the attacks; (3) relief from the attacks achieved by administering glucose. [A. O. Whipple]

whipworm (wip-werm) *n.* a small parasitic whiplike nematode worm, *Trichuris trichiura* (*Trichocephalus dispar*), that lives in the large intestine. Human infection (*see* trichuriasis) results from the consumption of water or food contaminated with faecal material.

white blood cell (wyt) *n.* see leucocyte.

white finger *n.* the appearance of a finger resulting from spasm of the vessels of the finger. It occurs in Raynaud's disease but can also be attributed to the long-term use of percussion implements.

white leg *n.* inflammation of the femoral vein of the leg, with secondary thrombosis: the leg becomes pale, swollen, tense, and painful. It commonly accompanied puerperal fever (now rare) in women after childbirth. Medical name: **phlegmasia alba dolens**.

white matter *n.* nerve tissue of the central nervous system that is paler in colour than the associated grey matter because it contains more nerve fibres and thus larger amounts of myelin.

white noise instrument *n.* a device, resembling a small hearing aid, that produces sounds of many frequencies at equal intensities and is used in the treatment of tinnitus. It was formerly known as a *tinnitus masker*.

Whitfield's ointment (wit-feeldz) *n.* an ointment containing benzoic and salicylic acids, used to treat fungal infections of the skin. [A. Whitfield (1868–1947), British dermatologist]

whitlow (wit-loh) n. see paronychia.

WHO n. see World Health Organization.

whoop (hoop) n. see whooping cough.

whooping cough (hoop-ing) n. an acute infectious disease, primarily affecting infants, due to infection of the respiratory tract by the bacterium Bordetella pertussis. It is characterized by an increasingly severe cough that is accompanied by a noisy involuntary drawing in of the breath (whoop). The child can become exhausted and may stop breathing. The most common complication is pneumonia. Immunization, usually given in the form of the DPT vaccine (see Appendix 8), offers protection; an attack usually confers lifelong immunity. Medical name: **pertussis**.

Widal reaction (vi-dahl) n. an agglutination test for the presence of antibodies against the Salmonella organisms that cause typhoid fever. [G. F. I. Widal (1862–1929), French physician]

Williams syndrome (wil-yǎmz) n. a hereditary condition marked by a characteristic 'elfin' facial appearance, hypercalcaemia, short stature, mental retardation, and aortic stenosis. Most affected children are highly sociable and have unusual conversational ability, using a rich and complex vocabulary. [J. C. P. Williams (20th century), British cardiologist]

Wilms' tumour (vilmz) n. see nephroblastoma. [M. Wilms (1867–1918), German surgeon]

Wilson's disease (wil-sǒnz) n. an inborn defect of copper metabolism in which there is a deficiency of caeruloplasmin (which normally forms a nontoxic complex with copper). The free copper may be deposited in the liver, causing jaundice and cirrhosis, or in the brain, causing mental retardation and symptoms resembling parkinsonism. Medical name: **hepatolenticular degeneration**. [S. A. K. Wilson (1878–1936), British neurologist]

windpipe (wind-pyp) n. see trachea.

wisdom tooth (wiz-dǒm) n. the third molar tooth on each side of either jaw, which erupts normally around the age of 20.

witch hazel (hamamelis) (wich hay-zěl) n. a preparation made from the leaves and bark of the tree Hamamelis virginiana. It is used as an astringent, especially for the treatment of sprains and bruises.

withdrawal (with-draw-ǎl) n. **1.** (in psychology) the removal of one's interest from one's surroundings. **2.** see coitus (interruptus).

withdrawal symptoms pl. n. see dependence.

Wolffian body (vol-fi-ǎn) n. see mesonephros. [K. F. Wolff (1733–94), German anatomist]

Wolffian duct n. the mesonephric duct (see mesonephros).

Wolff-Parkinson-White syndrome (WPW syndrome) (wuulf par-kin-sǒn wyt) n. a congenital abnormality of heart rhythm caused by the presence of an accessory conduction pathway between the atria and ventricles (see atrioventricular bundle). It results in premature excitation of one ventricle and is characterized by an abnormal wave (delta wave) at the start of the QRS complex on the electrocardiogram. [L. Wolff (1898–1972, US cardiologist; Sir J. Parkinson (1885–1976), British physician; P. D. White (1886–1973), US cardiologist]

womb (woom) *n. see* uterus.

Wood's glass (wuudz) *n.* a nickel-oxide filter that holds back all but a few rays projected from an ultraviolet light source. These rays (*W. light*) cause fluorescence in hair and skin affected by some fungal and bacterial infections and are therefore useful in diagnosis. [R. W. Wood (1868–1955), US physician]

woolsorter's disease (wuul-sor-terz) *n. see* anthrax.

word blindness (werd) *n. see* alexia.

World Health Organization (WHO) (werld) *n.* an international organization in which health issues are discussed and policies evolved mainly through working groups, including acknowledged authorities, and published reports. WHO handles information on internationally notifiable diseases and publishes the International Classification of Diseases.

worm (werm) *n.* any of various soft-bodied legless animals, including flatworms, nematode worms, earthworms, and leeches.

wound (woond) *n.* a break in the structure of an organ or tissue caused by an external agent; for example, a bruise, cut, or burn.

WPW syndrome *n. see* Wolff-Parkinson-White syndrome.

wrist (rist) *n.* **1.** the joint between the forearm and hand. It consists of the proximal bones of the carpus, which articulate with the radius and ulna. **2.** the whole region of the wrist joint, including the carpus and lower parts of the radius and ulna.

wrist drop *n.* paralysis of the muscles that raise the wrist, which is caused by damage to the radial nerve.

wryneck (ry-nek) *n. see* torticollis.

Wuchereria (voo-ker-eer-iă) *n.* a genus of white threadlike parasitic worms (*see* filaria) that live in the lymphatic vessels. *W. bancrofti* the species that causes elephantiasis.

Xx Yy Zz

xanthaemia (carotenaemia)
(zanth-ee-mia) *n.* the presence in
the blood of the yellow pigment
carotene, from excessive intake of
carrots, tomatoes, or other vegetables containing the pigment.

xanthelasma (zanth-ĕ-laz-mă) *n.*
yellow plaques occurring symmetrically around the eyelids.

xanthine (zanth-een) *n.* a nitrogenous breakdown product of the
purines adenosine and guanine.
Xanthine is an intermediate product of the breakdown of nucleic
acids to uric acid.

xantho- *prefix denoting* yellow colour.

xanthochromia (zanth-oh-kroh-
miă) *n.* yellow discoloration, such
as may affect the skin in jaundice
or the cerebrospinal fluid when it
contains the breakdown products of
haemoglobin from red blood cells
that have entered it.

xanthoma (zanth-oh-mă) *n.* (*pl.*
xanthomata) a yellowish skin lesion associated with any of various
disorders of lipid metabolism.
Tuberous xanthomata are found on
the knees and elbows; *tendon xanthomata* involve the extensor tendons of the hands and feet and the
Achilles tendon. Crops of small yellow papules at any site are known as
eruptive xanthomata, while larger
flat lesions are called *plane xanthomata*.

xanthomatosis (zanth-oh-mă-toh-

sis) *n.* the presence of multiple xanthomata in the skin. *See* xanthoma.

xanthopsia (zanth-op-siă) *n.* yellow vision: the condition in which
all objects appear to have a yellowish tinge. It is sometimes experienced in digitalis poisoning.

X chromosome *n.* the sex chromosome present in both sexes.
Women have two X chromosomes
and men one. Genes for some important genetic disorders, including
haemophilia, are carried on the X
chromosomes. *See* sex-linked. *Compare* Y chromosome.

xeno- *prefix denoting* different; foreign; alien.

xenogeneic (zen-oh-ji-nay-ik) *adj.*
describing grafted tissue derived
from a donor of a different species.

xenograft (heterograft) (zen-oh-
grahft) *n.* a living tissue graft that is
made from an animal of one species
to another of a different species.

xenon-133 (zen-on) *n.* a radioactive isotope that has a half-life of
about five days and is used in ventilation scanning of the lungs in
nuclear medicine (*see* ventilation-
perfusion scanning). Symbol: Xe-
133.

Xenopsylla (zen-op-sil-ă) *n.* a genus
of tropical and subtropical fleas. *X.
cheopis* the rat flea, which occasionally attacks humans and can transmit plague; it also transmits murine
typhus and two tapeworms.

xenotransplantation (zen-oh-trans-plahn-**tay**-shŏn) *n.* the transplantation of organs from one species into another.

xero- *prefix denoting* a dry condition.

xeroderma (zeer-oh-**der**-mǎ) *n.* a mild form of the hereditary disorder ichthyosis, in which the skin develops slight dryness and forms branlike scales. It is common in the elderly. *x. pigmentosum* a rare genetically determined skin disorder in which there is an inherited defect in DNA repair following damage from ultraviolet radiation. This leads to multiple skin cancers.

xerophthalmia (zeer-off-**thal**-miǎ) *n.* a progressive nutritional disease of the eye due to deficiency of vitamin A. The cornea and conjunctiva become dry, thickened, and wrinkled. This may progress to keratomalacia and eventual blindness.

xerosis (zeer-**oh**-sis) *n.* abnormal dryness of the conjunctiva, the skin, or the mucous membranes. In xerosis of the conjunctiva, the membrane becomes thickened and grey in the area exposed when the eyelids are open.

xerostomia (zeer-oh-**stoh**-miǎ) *n. see* dry mouth *Compare* ptyalism.

xiphi- (xipho-) *prefix denoting* the xiphoid process of the sternum.

xiphisternum (zif-i-**ster**-nǔm) *n. see* xiphoid process.

xiphoid process (xiphoid cartilage) (zif-oid) *n.* the lowermost section of the breastbone (*see* sternum): a flat pointed cartilage that gradually ossifies until it is completely replaced by bone, a process not completed until after middle age. It does not articulate with any ribs. Also called: **ensiform**

process or **cartilage, xiphisternum.**

X-linked disease (eks-linkt) *n. see* sex-linked.

X-linked lymphoproliferative syndrome (XLP syndrome, Duncan's disease) (lim-foh-prŏ-lif-er-ǎ-tiv) *n.* a hereditary disorder of the immune system caused by a defective sex-linked gene carried on an X-chromosome. There is uncontrolled proliferation of B-lymphocytes in response to infection by the Epstein-Barr virus, which can lead to fulminating hepatitis or lymphoma.

XLP syndrome *n. see* X-linked lymphoproliferative syndrome.

X-rays *pl. n.* electromagnetic radiation of extremely short wavelength (beyond the ultraviolet), which passes through matter to varying degrees depending on its density. X-rays are used in diagnostic radiology (*see* radiography, nuclear medicine) and in radiotherapy. Great care is needed to avoid unnecessary exposure, because the radiation is harmful (*see* radiation (sickness)).

X-ray screening *n.* the use of an image intensifier to produce real-time imaging during an X-ray examination on a TV monitor. It is widely used in angiography and interventional radiology to guide procedures. *See* videofluoroscopy.

xylene (dimethylbenzene) (zy-leen) *n.* a liquid used for increasing the transparency of tissues prepared for microscopic examination after they have been dehydrated.

xylometazoline (zy-loh-mi-**taz**-oh-leen) *n.* a sympathomimetic drug that constricts blood vessels (*see* vasoconstrictor). It is applied topically as a nasal decongestant in the relief of the common cold and sinusitis. Trade name: **Otrivine**.

xylose (zy-lohz) *n.* a pentose sugar that is involved in carbohydrate interconversions within cells. It is used as a diagnostic aid for intestinal function.

YAG laser (yag) *n.* yttrium–aluminium–garnet laser: *see* laser.

yawning (yawn-ing) *n.* a reflex action in which the mouth is opened wide and air is drawn into the lungs then slowly released. It is a result of drowsiness, fatigue, or boredom.

yaws (pian, framboesia) (yawz) *n.* a tropical infectious disease caused by the presence of the spirochaete *Treponema pertenue* in the skin and its underlying tissues. Yaws occurs chiefly in conditions of poor hygiene. It is characterized by small tumours, each covered by a yellow crust of dried serum, on the hands, face, legs, and feet. These tumours may deteriorate into deep ulcers. The disease responds well to treatment with antibiotics.

Y chromosome *n.* a sex chromosome present in men but not in women; it is believed to carry the genes for maleness. *Compare* X chromosome.

yeast (yeest) *n.* any of a group of fungi in which the body consists of individual cells, which may occur singly, in groups of two or three, or in chains. Baker's yeast (*Saccharomyces*) ferments carbohydrates to produce alcohol and carbon dioxide and is important in brewing and breadmaking. Some yeasts are a commercial source of proteins and of vitamins of the B complex; others

(e.g. *Candida*, *Cryptococcus*, *Pityrosporum*) cause disease.

yellow fever (yel-oh) *n.* an infectious disease, caused by an arbovirus, occurring in tropical Africa and South America. It is transmitted by mosquitoes, principally *Aëdes aegypti*. The virus causes degeneration of the tissues of the liver and kidneys. Symptoms include chill, headache, pains in the back and limbs, fever, vomiting, constipation, a reduced flow of urine (which contains high levels of albumin), and jaundice. Yellow fever often proves fatal.

yellow spot *n. see* macula (lutea).

Yersinia (yer-sin-iă) *n.* a genus of aerobic or facultatively anaerobic Gram-negative bacteria that are parasites of animals and humans. *Y. pestis* the cause of bubonic plague. *Y. enterocolitica* a cause of intestinal infections.

yolk sac (vitelline sac) (yohk) *n.* the membranous sac that lies ventral to the embryo. One of the extraembryonic membranes, it probably assists in transporting nutrients to the early embryo and is one of the first sites where blood cells are formed.

yttrium-90 (it-riŭm) *n.* an artificial radioactive isotope of the element yttrium, used in radiotherapy.

zafirlukast (zaf-eer-loo-kăst) *n. see* leukotriene receptor antagonist.

zalcitabine (ddC) (zal-sy-tă-been) *n.* a drug, similar to didanosine, that is used to prolong the lives of patients with AIDS and HIV infection. It is administered by mouth. Trade name: **Hivid**.

zanamivir (ză-nam-i-veer) *n.* an

antiviral drug used for the treatment of influenza A and B. It is administered by inhalation. Trade name: **Relenza**.

Zantac (zan-tak) *n. see* ranitidine.

zein (zee-in) *n.* a protein found in maize.

zidovudine (AZT) (zy-dov-yoo-deen) *n.* an antiviral drug used in the treatment of AIDS and HIV infection. The drug slows the growth of HIV infection in the body, but is not curative. It is administered by mouth and intravenously; the most common side-effects are nausea, headache, and insomnia, and it may damage the blood-forming tissues of the bone marrow. Trade name: **Retrovir**.

Zieve's syndrome (zee-věz) *n.* a combination of severe hyperlipidaemia, haemolytic anaemia, and jaundice seen in susceptible individuals taking alcohol to excess. [L. Zieve (1915–), US physician]

ZIFT *n.* zygote intrafallopian transfer: *see* gamete intrafallopian transfer.

zinc (zink) *n.* a trace element that is a cofactor of many enzymes. Deficiency is rare with a balanced diet but may occur in alcoholics and those with kidney disease; symptoms include lesions of the skin, oesophagus, and cornea and (in children) retarded growth. Symbol: Zn.

zinc oxide *n.* a mild astringent used in various skin conditions, usually mixed with other substances. It is applied as a cream, ointment, dusting powder, or as a paste.

zinc sulphate *n.* a preparation that is used in the treatment of proven zinc deficiency. It is administered

by mouth. Trade names: **Solvazinc**, **Z Span Spansule**.

zinc undecenoate (zinc undecylenate) *n.* an antifungal agent with uses similar to those of undecenoic acid.

Zollinger-Ellison syndrome (zol-inj-er el-i-sŏn) *n.* a rare disorder in which there is excessive secretion of gastric juice due to high levels of circulating gastrin, which is produced by a pancreatic tumour (*see* gastrinoma) or an enlarged pancreas. The high levels of stomach acid cause diarrhoea and peptic ulcers. [R. M. Zollinger (1903–92) and E. H. Ellison (1918–70), US physicians]

zolmitriptan (zol-mi-**trip**-tan) *n. see* $5HT_1$ agonist.

zona pellucida (zoh-nǎ pel-oo-sid-a) *n.* the thick membrane that develops around the mammalian oocyte within the ovarian follicle. *See* ovum.

zonula (zon-yoo-lǎ) *n. see* zonule.

zonule (zonula) (zon-yool) *n.* (in anatomy) a small band or zone. *z. of Zinn (zonula ciliaris)* the suspensory ligament of the lens of the eye. —**zonular** *adj.*

zonulolysis (zon-yoo-lol-i-sis) *n.* dissolution of the zonule of Zinn, which facilitates removal of the lens in cases of cataract. This technique is not used for modern cataract surgery.

zoo- *prefix denoting* animals.

zoonosis (zoh-ŏ-noh-sis) *n.* any infectious disease of animals that can be transmitted to humans, such as anthrax or rabies.

zygoma (zy-goh-mǎ) *n. see* zygomatic arch, zygomatic bone.

zygomatic arch (zygoma) (zy-goh-**mat**-ik) *n.* the horizontal arch of bone on either side of the face, just below the eyes, formed by connected processes of the zygomatic and temporal bones. *See* skull.

zygomatic bone (zygoma, malar bone) *n.* either of a pair of bones that form the prominent part of the cheeks and contribute to the orbits. *See* skull.

zygote (zy-goht) *n.* the fertilized ovum before cleavage begins. *z. intrafallopian transfer (ZIFT) see* gamete intrafallopian transfer.

zym- (zymo-) *prefix denoting* **1.** an enzyme. **2.** fermentation.

zymogen (zy-moh-jen) *n. see* pro-enzyme.

zymosis (zy-moh-sis) *n.* **1.** the process of fermentation, brought about by yeast organisms. **2.** the changes in the body that occur in certain infectious diseases, once thought to be the result of a process similar to fermentation. —**zymotic** (zy-**mot**-ik) *adj.*

zymotic disease *n.* an old name for a contagious disease.

Appendix 1 Biochemical Reference Values for Blood

(B = whole blood; P = plasma; S = serum)

Table 1.1 Everyday tests

Determination	Sample	Reference range
Alcohol		
legal limit (UK)	B or P	<17.4 mmol/l
Albumin	P	35–50 g/l
in pregnancy	P	25–38 g/l
Ammonia	B	<40 μmol/l
α-Amylase	P	25–180 somogyi units/dl
Anion gap $(Na^+ + K^+) - (HCO_3^- + Cl^-)$	P	12–16 mmol/l
Bilirubin	P	3–17 μmol/l
Bicarbonate (see also Table 1.2)	P	22–28 mmol/l
Calcium		
ionized	P	1.0–1.25 mmol/l
total	P	2.12–2.65 mmol/l
total in pregnancy	P	1.95–2.35 mmol/l
Chloride	P	95–105 mmol/l
Cholesterol (see also Table 1.6)	P	3.9–7.8 mmol/l
Copper	P	12–26 μmol/l
Creatinine	P	70–150 μmol/l
in pregnancy	P	24–68 μmol/l
Digoxin		
children	P	2.0–3.0 nmol/l
adults	P	1.0–2.0 nmol/l
Glucose (fasting)	P	3.0–5.0 mmol/l
Glycated haemoglobin (HbA$_{1C}$)	B	5–8%

Table 1.1 (cont.)

Determination	Sample	Reference range
Iron		
male	S	14–31 µmol/l
female	S	11–30 µmol/l
total iron-binding capacity (TIBC)	S	45–75 µmol/l
Lactate		
venous	B	0.5–2.2 mmol/l
arterial	B	0.5–1.6 mmol/l
Magnesium	P	0.75–1.05 mmol/l
Osmolality	P	278–305 mosm/kg
Phosphate (inorganic)	P	0.8–1.45 mmol/l
Potassium	P	3.5–5.0 mmol/l
Protein (total)	P	60–80 g/l
Sodium	P	135–145 mmol/l
Urea	P	2.5–6.7 mmol/l
in pregnancy	P	2.0–4.2 mmol/l
Urea nitrogen (BUN)	P	1.16–3.12 mmol/l
Uric acid		
male	P	210 480 µmol/l
female	P	150–390 µmol/l
in pregnancy	P	100–270 µmol/l
Zinc	P	6–25 µmol/l

Table 1.2 Blood gases

Measurement	Reference range
Arterial CO_2 ($Pa CO_2$)	4.7–6.0 kPa
Mixed venous CO_2 ($Pv CO_2$)	5.5–6.8 kPa
Arterial oxygen ($Pa O_2$)	12.0–14.5 kPa
Mixed venous oxygen ($Pv O_2$)	4.0–6.0 kPa
Newborn arterial oxygen	5.3–8.0 kPa
H^+ ion activity	36–44 nmol/l

Table 1.2 (cont.)

Measurement	Reference range
Arterial pH	7.35–7.45 pH units
Bicarbonate	
arterial – whole blood	19–24 mmol/l
venous – plasma	22–28 mmol/l
cord blood	14–22 mmol/l
Base excess	± 2 mmol/l
Carboxyhaemoglobin	
non-smoker	<2%
smoker	3–15%
toxic at:	>15%
coma at:	>50%

Table 1.3 Diagnostic enzymes

Enzyme	Sample	Reference range
Acid phosphatase		
total	S	1–5 U/l
prostatic	S	0–1 U/l
Alkaline phosphatase	P	80–250 U/l
Alanine aminotransferase (ALT)	P	5–35U/l
α-Amylase	P	25–180 somogyi units/dl
Angiotensin-converting enzyme (ACE)	S	21–54 U/l
Aspartate aminotransferase (AST)	P	15–42 U/l
Creatine kinase (CK)		
male	P	24–195 U/l
female	P	24–170 U/l
Gamma-glutamyl transferase (GGT)		
male	P	11–51 U/l
female	P	7–35 U/l
Lactate dehydrogenase (total)	P	240–525 U/l

Table 1.4 Hormones

Hormone	Sample	Reference range
Adrenaline (epinephrine)	P	0.03–1.31 nmol/l
ACTH	P	3.3–15.4 pmol/l
Aldosterone		
recumbent	P	100–450 pmol/l
midday	p	2-fold increase of recumbent level
Angiotensin II	P	5–35 pmol/l
Antidiuretic hormone (ADH)	P	0.9–4.6 pmol/l
Calcitonin		
male	P	<100 nmol/l
female	P	<30 nmol/l
Cortisol		
00.00 h	P	80–280 nmol/l
09.00 h	P	280–700 nmol/l
Follicle-stimulating hormone (FSH)		
follicular phase	P or S	0.5–5.0 U/l
ovulatory peak	P or S	8–15 U/l
luteal phase	P or S	2–8 U/l
postmenopause	P or S	> 30 U/l
male	P or S	0.5–5.0 U/l
Gastrin		
male + female (>60 yr)	P	<50 pmol/l
female (16–60 yr)	P	<38 pmol/l
Glucagon	P	<50 pmol/l
Growth hormone	P	<20 mU/l
Human chorionic gonadotrophin	S	<5 U/l
Insulin (fasting)	P	<15 mU/l
Insulin C-peptide (fasting)	P	<0.4 nmol/l (undetectable in hypoglycaemia)
Insulin-like growth factor-1 (IGF-1)	P	0.52–3.4 kU/l
Luteinizing hormone		
premenopausal	P or S	6–13 U/l
follicular phase	P or S	3–12 U/l

Table 1.4 (*cont.*)

Hormone	Sample	Reference range
ovulatory peak	P or S	20–80 U/l
luteal phase	P or S	3–16 U/l
postmenopause	P or S	>30 U/l
male	P or S	3–8 U/l
Noradrenaline	P	0.47–4.14 mmol/l
17-β-oestradiol		
follicular phase	P	75–260 pmol/l
mid-cycle	P	370–1470 pmol/l
luteal phase	P	180–1100 pmol/l
male	P	<220 pmol/l
Parathyroid hormone (intact)	P	0.9–5.4 pmol/l
Pancreatic polypeptide	P	<200 pmol/l
Progesterone		
male	P	<5 nmol/l
female postovulation	P	15–77nmol/l
follicular (newborn)	P	<3 nmol/l
17-Hydroxyprogesterone	P	7–16 nmol/l
Prolactin		
male	P	<450 U/l
female	P	<600 U/l
Renin activity	P	
recumbent		1.1–2.7 pmol/ml per hr
erect after 30 min		3.0–4.3 pmol/ml per hr
Somatostatin	P	30–166 pmol/l
Testosterone		
male	P or S	9–42 nmol/l
female	P or S	1–2.5 nmol/l
Thyroid-stimulating hormone	P	0.5–5.5 mU/l
Thyroid-binding globulin	P	13–28 mg/l
Tri-iodothyronine (T₃)	P	1–3 nmol/l
Free T₃	P	3.3–8.2 pmol/l
Thyroxine (T₄)	P	70–140 nmol/l
Free T₄	P	9–25 pmol/l
Vasoactive intestinal peptide (VIP)	P	<30 pmol/l

Table 1.5 Proteins and immunoproteins

Protein/immunoprotein	Sample	Reference range
Albumin	P	35–50 g/l
α₁-Antitrypsin	S	107–209 mg/l
Complement		
C3		65–190 mg/dl
C4		15–50 mg/dl
Caeruloplasmin	S	16–60 mg/dl
C1 esterase inhibitor	S	15–35 mg/dl
C-reactive protein (CRP)	S	<10 mg/l
Ferritin	S	14–200 µg/l
Fibrinogen	P	2–4 g/l
D-dimer	S	<500 µg/l
Haptoglobins	S	0.6–2.6 g/l
Immunoglobulins		
IgG	S	6.0–13.0 g/l
IgA	S	0.8–3.0 g/l
IgM	S	0.4–2.5 g/l
IgE	S	<120 kU/l
β₂-Microglobulin	S	<3 mg/l
Thyroid microsomal antibodies		
male	S	<1/400
female (<44 yr)	S	<1/400
female (>44 yr)	S	<1/6400
Total protein	P	60–80 g/l
β₁-Transferrin	S	1.2–2.0 g/l

Table 1.6 Lipids and lipoproteins

Lipid/lipoprotein	Sample	Reference range
Cholesterol	P	3.9–7.8 mmol/l
ideal upper limit		5.2 mmol/l
acceptable upper limit		6.5 mmol/l
Triglyceride (fasting)	P	0.55–1.90 mmol/l

Table 1.6 (*cont.*)

Lipid/lipoprotein	Sample	Reference range
Nonesterified (free)	S	
fatty acids (NEFA)		
male		0.19–0.78 mmol/l
female		0.06–0.9 mmol/l
Lipoproteins (as cholesterol)		
low-density (LDL)	S	1.55–4.4 mmol/l
ideal upper limit		3.4 mmol/l
acceptable upper limit		4.2 mmol/l
high density (HDL)	S	0.8–2.0 mmol/l
ideal (male)		>0.9 mmol/l
ideal (female)		>1.2 mmol/l
Total cholesterol/HDL	S	
ideal		<5

Table 1.7 Vitamins

Vitamin	Sample	Reference range
Vitamin A		
retinol	S	
male		1.06–3.35 µmol/l
female		0.84–2.95 µmol/l
β-carotene	S	
male		0.01–6.52 µmol/l
female		0.019–2.93 µmol/l
Vitamin B		
Thiamin (B_1)	P	>40 nmol/l
Riboflavin (B_2)	S	100–630 nmol/l
Pyridoxine (B_6)	P (EDTA)	20–120 nmol/l
Vitamin B_{12}	S	138–780 nmol/l
Folate	S	12–33 µmol/l
red blood cell folate	B	500–1300 µmol/l
Vitamin D metabolites		
25-(OH) D	S	17–125 nmol/l
1,25-(OH)$_2$ D_3	S	50–120 pmol/l
Vitamin E (α–tocopherol)	S	11.5–35 µmol/l

Table 1.8 Paediatric reference values

Determination	Sample	Reference range
Alkaline phosphatase	P	
<1 year		30–250 IU/l
1–14 years		150–570 IU/l
>14 years		80–250 IU/l
Ammonia	P	
newborn		64–107 µmol/l
0–2 weeks		56–92 µmol/l
>1 month		21–50 µmol/l
Aspartate aminotransferase	P	
1–3 years		20–60 IU/l
4–6 years		15–50 IU/l
Bicarbonate	P	
infants		18–22 mmol/l
older children		20–26 mmol/l
Bilirubin	P	
first week of life		100–200 µmol/l (total)
after first week of life		2–14 µmol/l (total)
and throughout childhood		0–0.4 µmol/l (direct)
Calcium	P	
1–3 weeks		1.9–2.85 mmol/l
3 weeks and above		2.12–2.65 mmol/l
β-Carotene	S	
<1 year (upper limit falls with age up to 3½ years)		1.3–6.3 µmol/l
3½ years onwards		1.9–2.8 µmol/l
Creatinine	P	
cord blood		57–100 µmol/l
2 weeks–6 years		33–61 µmol/l
6 years–10 years		39–70 µmol/l
>12 years		49–81 µmol/l
Creatinine clearance	P	
3–13 years		94–142 ml/min per 1.73m²
Creatine kinase (CK)	P	
neonates		75–400 U/l
infants 3–12 months		10–145 U/l
children 1–15 years		15–130 U/l
Glucose (fasting)	S	
cord		2.5–5.3 mmol/l

Table 1.8 (*cont.*)

Determination	Sample	Reference range
premature/low birth wt		1.1–3.3 mmol/l
neonates		1.67–3.3 mmol/l
1 day		2.2–3.3 mmol/l
1–7 days		2.8–4.6 mmol/l
>7 days		3.3–5.5 mmol/l
Total protein	P	
1st month		51 g/l (mean)
1st year		61 g/l (mean)
1–6 years		61–78 g/l
7–16 years		66–82 g/l
Immunoglobulins		
IgG	S	
cord		5.2–18.0 g/l
0–2 weeks		5.0–17.0 g/l
2–6 weeks		3.9–13.0 g/l
6–12 weeks		2.1–7.7 g/l
3–6 months		2.4–8.8 g/l
6–9 months		3.0–9.0 g/l
9–12 months		3.0–10.9 g/l
1–2 years		3.1–13.8 g/l
2–3 years		3.7–15.8 g/l
3–6 years		4.9–16.1 g/l
6–9 years		5.4–16.1 g/l
9–12 years		5.4–16.1 g/l
12–15 years		5.4–16.1 g/l
IgA	S	
cord		0.00–0.02 g/l
0–2 weeks		0.01–0.08 g/l
2–6 weeks		0.02–0.15 g/l
6–12 weeks		0.05–0.4 g/l
3–6 months		0.1–0.5 g/l
6–9 months		0.15–0.7 g/l
9–12 months		0.20–0.7 g/l
1–2 years		0.3–1.2 g/l
2–3 years		0.3–1.3 g/l
3–6 years		0.4–2.0 g/l
6–9 years		0.5–2.4 g/l
9–12 years		0.8–2.8 g/l
12–15 years		0.8–2.8 g/l

Table 1.8 (*cont.*)

Determination	Sample	Reference range
IgM	S	
cord		0.02–0.2 g/l
0–2 weeks		0.05–0.2 g/l
2–6 weeks		0.08–0.4 g/l
6–12 weeks		0.15–0.7 g/l
3–6 months		0.20–1.0 g/l
6–9 months		0.40–1.6 g/l
9–12 months		0.60–2.1 g/l
1–2 years		0.50–2.2 g/l
2–3 years		0.50–2.2 g/l
3–6 years		0.50–2.0 g/l
6–9 years		0.50–1.8 g/l
9–12 years		0.50–1.9 g/l
12–15 years		0.50–1.9 g/l
Lactate	P (venous)	0.5–2.2 mmol/l
	P (arterial)	0.5–1.6 mmol/l
	B	0.5–1.7 mmol/l
Phosphate (inorganic)	P	
newborn		1.20–2.78 mmol/l
young children		1.29–1.78 mmol/l
girls 15 years		0.9–1.38 mmol/l
boys 17 years		0.83–1.49 mmol/l
Potassium	P	
newborn		up to 6.6 mmol/l
>1 month–6 years		4.1–5.6 mmol/l
boys 7–16 years		3.3–4.7 mmol/l
girls 7–16 years		3.4–4.5 mmol/l
Sweat sodium		10–40 mmol/l
Sweat chloride		0–50 mmol/l
Thyroid-stimulating hormone (TSH) (outside neonatal period)	S	0.5–5.0 mU/l
Uric acid	P	
childhood		0.06–0.24 mmol/l
boys 16 years		0.23–0.46 mmol/l
girls 16 years		0.19–0.36 mmol/l

Appendix 2 Biochemical Reference Values for Urine

Determination	Reference range
Aldosterone	10–50 nmol/24 h
Albumin	<80 mg/24 h
α-Aminolaevulinic acid	9.9–53.4 µmol/24 h
Amylase	
secretion rate	1–17 somogyi U/h
clearance	0.01–0.04 of creatinine clearance value
Arginine	1.3–6.5 µmol/mol creat
Ascorbic acid	34–68 µmol/l
Calcium	2.5–7.5 mmol/24 h
Catecholamines	<2.6 µmol/24 h
Chloride	110–250 mmol/24 h
Copper	0.47–0.55 µmol/l
Cortisol	60–1500 nmol/l
	<280 nmol/24 h
Creatinine	
male	9.0–17.0 mmol/24 h
female	7.5–12.5 mmol/24 h
pregnancy	8.0–13.5 mmol/24 h
Glucose	0.06–0.84 mmol/l
Homovanillic acid (HVA) – adults	<43 µmol/24 h
Hydroxyindoleacetic acid (5-HIAA)	16–73 µmol/24 h
Hydroxymethylmandelic acid (HMMA)	16–48 µmol/24 h
Iron	<1.8 µmol/24 h
Lead	<0.4 µmol/l
β_2-Microglobulin	4–370 µg/l
Magnesium	3.3–4.9 mmol/24 h
Osmolality	350–1000 mosm/kg
Oxalate	<450 µmol/24 h
Phosphate (inorganic)	15–50 mmol/24 h
Porphyrins	
coproporphyrin	50–350 nmol/24 h
porphobilinogen	0.9–8.8 µmol/24 h
uroporphyrin	0–49 nmol/24 h

Appendix 2 (*cont.*)

Determination	Reference range
Potassium	20–60 mmol/l
	40–120 mmol/24 h
Protein	<120 mg/24 h
pregnancy	<300 mg/24 h
Sodium	50–125 mmol/l
	100–250 mmol/24 h
Urea	250–500 mmol/24 h
Uric acid	<5.0 mmol/24 h
pregnancy (except late)	<7.0 mmol/24 h
Urobilinogen	<6.7 mmol/24 h
Vanillylmandelic acid (VMA)	<35 µmol/24 h
Zinc	2.1–11.0 µmol/24 h

Appendix 3 Biochemical Reference Values for Faeces

Determination	Reference range
Fat (on normal diet)	<7 g/24 h
Nitrogen	70–140 mmol/24 h
Urobilinogen	67–473 µmol/24 h
Coproporphyrin	<0.46 nmol/g dry weight
Protoporphyrin	<2.67 µmol/24 h
Protoporphyrin	≤0.11 nmol/kg dry weight
Total porphyrin	
(ether soluble)	10–200 nmol/g dry weight
(ether insoluble)	0–24 nmol/g dry weight

Appendix 4 Haematological Reference Values

Measurement	Reference range
haemoglobin	(male) 13.5–18.0 g/dl
	(female) 11.5–16.0 g/dl
packed red cell volume of haematocrit (PCV)	(male) 0.40–0.54 l/l
	(female) 0.37–0.47 l/l
red cell count	(male) 4.5–6.5×10^{12}/l
	(female) 3.9–5.6×10^{12}/l
mean cell volume (MCV)	81–100 fl
mean cell haemoglobin (MCH)	27–32 pg
mean cell haemoglobin concentration (MCHC)	32–36 g/dl
reticulocyte count	0.8–2.0 per cent
absolute count	25–100×10^{9}/l
total blood volume	70 ± 10 ml/kg
plasma volume	45 ± 5 ml/kg
red cell volume	(male) 30 ± 5 ml/kg
	(female) 25 ± 5 ml/kg
white cell count	4.0–11.0×10^{9}/l
neutrophils	2.0–7.5×10^{9}/l
lymphocytes	1.3–3.5×10^{9}/l
eosinophils	0–0.44×10^{9}/l
basophils	0–0.10×10^{9}/l
monocytes	0.2–0.8×10^{9}/l
platelet count	150–400×10^{9}/l
bleeding time	1–9 min
coagulation time	5–11 min
thrombin time	10–15 s
prothrombin time	10–14 s
activated partial thromboplastin time	35–45 s
fibrinogen concentration	1.6–4.2 g/l
fibrinogen titre	normal – up to 1/128
erythrocyte sedimentation rate	(male) 0–10 mm
	(female) 0–15 mm
cold agglutinin titre at 4°C	less than 64

Appendix 5 Standard Values for Body Weight

Table 5.1 Appropriate body weight and lower limits for defining overweight and obesity in adults

Men

Height (cm)	Average (kg)	Acceptable range (kg)	Overweight (kg)	Obese (kg)
158	55.8	44–64	70	77
160	57.6	44–65	72	78
162	58.6	46–66	73	79
164	59.6	47–67	74	80
166	60.6	48–69	76	83
168	61.7	49–71	78	85
170	63.5	51–73	80	88
172	65.0	52–74	81	89
174	66.5	53–75	83	90
176	68.0	54–77	85	92
178	69.4	55–79	87	95
180	71.0	58–80	88	96
182	72.6	59–82	90	98
184	74.2	60–84	92	101
186	75.8	62–86	95	103
188	77.6	64–88	97	106
190	79.3	66–90	99	108
192	81.0	68–93	102	112

Table 5.1 (cont.)

Women

Height (cm)	Average (kg)	Acceptable range (kg)	Overweight (kg)	Obese (kg)
146	46.0	37–53	58	64
148	46.5	37–54	59	65
150	47.0	38–55	61	66
152	48.5	39–57	63	68
156	49.5	39–58	64	70
158	50.4	40–58	64	70
160	51.3	41–59	65	71
162	52.6	42–61	67	73
164	54.0	43–62	68	74
166	55.4	44–64	70	77
168	56.8	45–65	72	78
170	58.1	45–66	73	79
172	60.0	46–67	74	80
174	61.3	48–69	76	83
176	62.6	49–70	77	84
178	64.0	51–72	79	86
180	65.3	52–74	81	89

Table 5.2 Median and range of standard values for weight for height of children

Boys

Height (cm)	Weight (kg) Median	Range	Height (cm)	Weight (kg) Median	Range
50	3.3	2.5–4.4	98	14.9	12.8–17.1
52	3.7	2.8–4.8	100	15.5	13.3–17.7
54	4.1	3.1–5.3	102	16.3	13.4–19.6
56	4.6	3.4–5.9	104	16.8	13.9–20.2
58	5.1	3.9–6.4	106	17.4	14.4–20.8
60	5.7	4.4–7.1	108	18.1	14.9–21.5
62	6.2	4.9–7.7	110	18.7	15.5–22.2
64	6.8	5.4–8.7	112	19.4	16.1 23.0
66	7.4	6.0–9.0	114	20.0	16.7–23.9
68	8.0	6.5–9.6	116	20.7	17.3–24.8
70	8.5	7.0–10.2	118	21.5	17.9–25.8
72	9.1	7.5–10.8	120	22.2	18.6–26.9
74	9.6	8.0–11.4	122	23.0	19.3–28.2
76	10.0	8.4–11.9	124	23.9	20.0–29.5
78	10.5	8.8–12.4	126	24.8	20.7–30.9
80	10.9	9.2–12.9	128	25.7	21.5–32.3
82	11.3	9.6–13.3	130	26.7	22.3–33.9
84	11.7	9.9–13.8	132	27.8	23.1–35.6
86	12.1	10.3–14.2	134	29.0	23.9–37.4
88	12.5	10.6–14.7	136	30.2	24.8–39.3
90	13.0	11.0–15.1	138	31.5	25.7–41.3
92	13.4	11.4–15.6	140	33.0	26.6–43.4
94	13.9	11.9–16.1	142	34.5	27.5–45.5
96	14.4	12.3–16.6	144	36.1	28.4–47.8

Table 5.2 (cont.)

Girls

Height (cm)	Weight (kg) Median	Weight (kg) Range	Height (cm)	Weight (kg) Median	Weight (kg) Range
50	3.4	2.6–4.2	94	13.5	11.5–15.6
52	3.7	2.8–4.7	96	14.0	12.0–16.1
54	4.1	3.1–5.2	98	14.6	12.5–16.8
56	4.5	3.5–5.7	100	15.4	12.7–18.8
58	5.0	3.9–6.3	102	15.9	13.1–19.4
60	5.5	4.3–6.9	104	16.5	13.6–20.0
62	6.1	4.8–7.5	106	17.0	14.0–20.6
64	6.7	5.3–8.1	108	17.6	14.5–21.3
66	7.3	5.8–8.7	110	18.2	15.0–22.0
68	7.8	6.3–9.3	112	18.9	15.6–22.8
70	8.4	6.8–9.9	114	19.6	16.2–23.7
72	8.9	7.2–10.5	116	20.3	16.8–24.7
74	9.4	7.7–11.0	118	21.0	17.4–25.8
76	9.8	8.1–11.4	120	21.8	18.1–27.0
78	10.2	8.5–11.9	122	22.7	18.8–28.3
80	10.6	8.8–12.3	124	23.6	19.5–29.8
82	11.1	9.3–12.9	126	24.6	20.3–31.4
84	11.4	9.6–13.2	128	25.7	21.0–33.2
86	11.8	9.9–13.6	130	26.8	21.9–35.1
88	12.2	10.3–14.1	132	28.0	22.7–37.3
90	12.6	10.7–14.5	134	29.4	23.6–39.6
92	13.0	11.1–15.0	136	30.8	24.5–42.2

Appendix 6 Nutrition and Energy

Table 6.1 Normal body compositon (of a 70 kg man)

	kg
water	42
intracellular	28
extracellular	14
solids	
fat	12.6
protein	11.2
intracellular (muscle)	8.4
extracellular (collagen)	2.8
minerals	3.8
carbohydrate	0.4

Table 6.2 Daily requirements for energy

	Age	Energy	
		kcal/kg	kJ/kg
infant	3 months	120	500
child	4–6 years	90	380
adolescent			
male	13–25 years	57	240
female	13–25 years	50	210
adult			
male		46	190
female		40	170

Table 6.3 Energy expenditure of a normal adult

	Time	kcal	kJ	Total range kcal (kJ)
male				
bed	8 h	500	2100	
non-occupational activities	8 h	700–1500	3000–6300	
work	8 h			
light		1100	4600	2300–3100 (9660–13 000)
very heavy		2400	10 100	3600–4400 (15 100–18 500)
female				
bed	8 h	420	1760	
non-occupational activities	8 h	580–980	2430–4120	
work	8 h			
light		800	3360	1800–2200 (7560–9240)
heavy		1400	5880	2400–2700 (10 100–11 340)

Table 6.4 Macronutrient stores in relation to daily intake

Macronutrient	Total amount in body	Energy equivalent	Days' supply if the only energy source	Daily intake g	% of store
Carbohydrate	0.6 kg	8.5 MJ	<1	300	60
free glucose	12 g				
liver glycogen	100 g				
muscle glycogen	500 g				
Fat (triacylglycerol)	12–18 kg	550 MJ	56	100	0.7
circulating in plasma	5 g				
stored in adipocytes	12–18 kg				
Protein and amino acids	12 kg	200 MJ		100	0.8
free amino acids	100 g				
protein	12 kg				

Table 6.5 Recommended daily amounts of some nutrients for population groups

Age range (years)	Occupational category	Thiamin (mg)	Riboflavin (mg)	Nicotinic acid equivalents[a] (mg)	Total folate (µg)	Ascorbic acid (mg)	Vitamin A retinol equivalents[b] (µg)	Vitamin D cholecalciferol (µg)	Calcium (mg)	Iron (mg)
boys										
under 1		0.3	0.4	5	50	20	450	7.5	600	6
1		0.5	0.6	7	100	20	300	10	600	7
2		0.6	0.7	8	100	20	300	10	600	7
3-4		0.6	0.8	9	100	20	300	10	600	8
5-6		0.7	0.9	10	200	20	300	†	600	10
7-8		0.8	1.0	11	200	20	400	†	600	10
9-11		0.9	1.2	14	200	25	575	†	700	12
12-14		1.1	1.4	16	300	25	725	†	700	12
15-17		1.2	1.7	19	300	30	750	†	600	12
girls										
under 1		0.3	0.4	5	50	20	450	7.5	600	6
1		0.4	0.6	7	100	20	300	10	600	7
2		0.5	0.7	8	100	20	300	10	600	7
3-4		0.6	0.8	9	100	20	300	10	600	8
5-6		0.7	0.9	10	200	20	300	†	600	10
7-8		0.8	1.0	11	200	20	400	†	600	10
9-11		0.8	1.2	14	300	25	575	†	700	12‡
12-14		0.9	1.4	16	300	25	725	†	700	12‡
15-17		0.9	1.7	19	300	30	750	†	600	12‡

Table 6.5 (cont.)

Age range (years)	Occupational category	Thiamin (mg)	Riboflavin (mg)	Nicotinic acid equivalents[a] (mg)	Total folate (μg)	Ascorbic acid (mg)	Vitamin A retinol equivalents[b] (μg)	Vitamin D cholecalciferol (μg)	Calcium (mg)	Iron (mg)
men										
18–34	sedentary	1.0	1.6	18	300	30	750	†	500	10
	moderately active	1.2	1.6	18	300	30	750	†	500	10
	very active	1.3	1.6	18	300	30	750	†	500	10
35–64	sedentary	1.0	1.6	18	300	30	750	†	500	10
	moderately active	1.1	1.5	18	300	30	750	†	500	10
	very active	1.3	1.5	18	300	30	750	†	500	10
65+	sedentary	0.9–1.0	1.5	18	300	30	750	†	500	10
women										
18–54	most occupations	0.9	1.3	15	300	30	750	†	500	12‡
55+	sedentary	0.7–0.8	1.3	15	300	30	750	†	500	10
pregnancy		1.0	1.6	18	500	60	750	10	1200*	13
lactation		1.1	1.8	21	400	60	1200	10	1200	15

Notes

a 1 nicotinic acid equivalent = 1 mg available nicotinic acid or 60 mg tryptophan.

b 1 retinol equivalent = 1 μg retinol or 6 μg β-carotene or 12 μg other biologically active carotenoids.

† No dietary sources may be necessary for children and adults who are sufficiently exposed to sunlight but during the winter children and adolescents should receive 10 μg (400 i.u.) daily by supplementation.

‡ This intake may not be sufficient for 10% of girls and women with large menstrual losses.

* For the third trimester only.

Appendix 7 Formulae for Calculating Drug Doses

solid drugs	amount of stock	$=$	$\dfrac{\text{strength required}}{\text{stock strength}}$	
liquid drugs	amount of stock	$=$	$\dfrac{\text{strength required}}{\text{stock strength}}$	$\times$ volume of stock strength
drugs measured in units	amount of stock	$=$	$\dfrac{\text{no. units required}}{\text{no. units in stock strength}}$	$\times$ volume of stock strength
preparation of solutions	amount of stock	$=$	$\dfrac{\text{strength required}}{\text{stock strength}}$	$\times$ final total volume

children's dose

(1) Clarke's body surface weight rule	child's dose	$=$	adult dose	$\times$	$\dfrac{\text{weight of child (kg)}}{\text{average adult weight (70 kg)}}$
(2) Clarke's body surface area rule	child's dose	$=$	adult dose	$\times$	$\dfrac{\text{surface area of child}}{\text{surface area of adult}}$
drip flow rate	rate (drops/ minute)	$=$			$\dfrac{\text{volume of solution (ml)} \times \text{no. drops/ml}}{\text{time (minutes)}}$

Note: macrodrop delivers 15 drops/ml
microdrop delivers 60 drops/ml

Appendix 8 Immunization Schedule

Children

Vaccine	Age
DPT vaccine (diphtheria, pertussis, tetanus), polio, Hib vaccine, meningitis C	2 months (1st dose) 3 months (2nd dose) 4 months (3rd dose)
MMR vaccine (measles, mumps, rubella)	12–15 months
booster diphtheria, tetanus, polio, and MMR	3–5 years
BCG	10–14 years (or infancy)
booster tetanus, diphtheria, and polio	13–18 years

Adults

Vaccine	Subjects
rubella	women sero-negative for rubella
polio, tetanus, and diphtheria	previously unimmunized individuals
hepatitis B, hepatitis A, and pneumococcal vaccine	individuals in high-risk groups

Appendix 9 Health Care Web Site Addresses

Appendix 9.1 Organizations and associations

General sites

Age Concern   www.ace.org.uk
Alcoholic Anonymous   www.alcoholics-anonymous.org.uk
Alzheimer's Disease Education and Referral Center
   www.alzheimers.org
Audit Commission   www.audit-commission.gov.uk
British Deaf Association   www.bda.org.uk
British Epilepsy Association   www.epilepsy.org.uk
Coeliac Society   www.coeliac.co.uk
Department of Heath   www.doh.gov.uk
Diabetes UK   www.diabetes.org.uk
Emedicine – an information site   www.emedicine.com
Health Authorities in the UK   www.nhs.uk/organisations/ha
Health Education Authority   www.hea.org.uk
International Council of Nurses   www.icn.ch
King's Fund   www.kingsfund.org.uk
Multiple Sclerosis Society   www.mssociety.org.uk
National Institute for Clinical Excellence   www.nice.org.uk
National Institutes of Health   www.nih.gov
Nursing & Midwifery Admissions Service   www.nmas.ac.uk
Nursing and Midwifery Council   www.nmc-uk.org
OMNI – internet resources in health and medicine   www.omni.ac.uk
Royal National Institute for the Deaf   www.rnid.org.uk
Tissue Viability Society   www.tvs.org.uk
UK Thalassaemia Society   www.ukts.org
World Health Organization   www.who.org

Infection Control Sites

Association for Professionals in Infection Control and Epidemiology
   www.apic.org/educ/
Hospital Infection Society   www.his.org.uk
Infection Control Nurses Association   www.icna.co.uk
Public Health Laboratory Service Network   www.phls.co.uk

Appendix 9.1 (*cont.*)

Continence
Association for Continence Advice   www.aca.uk.com
Continence Foundation For People with Bladder and Bowel Problems
   www.continence-foundation.org .uk
Institute of Urology and Nephrology   www.ucl.ac.uk/uro-neph

Child Health
Action for Sick Children   www.actionforsickchildren.org
Association for Spina Bifida and Hydrocephalus   www.asbah.org
Association of Pediatric Oncology Nursing   www.apon.org
Child Bereavement Trust   www.childbereavement.org.uk
Childline   www.childline.org.uk
Cystic Fibrosis Trust   www.cftrust.org.uk
Down's Syndrome Association   www.downs-syndrome.org.uk
Foundation for the Study of Infant Deaths   www.sids.org.uk
Great Ormond Street Hospital   www.gosh.nhs.uk
Institute of Child Health – Centre for Evidence Based Child Health
   www.ich.ucl.ac.uk
International Paediatric Nursing Research Network
   www.man.ac.uk/rcn/international/ipnrn.html
Kid's Health Organisation   www.kidshealth.org
National Association of Pediatric Nurse Practitioners   www.napnap.org
National Children's Bureau   www.ncb.org.uk
Paediatric Nursing Forum – archives
   www.jiscmail.ac.uk/lists.paediatric-nursing-forum.html
Stillbirth and Neonatal Death Society   www.uk-sands.org

Mental Health
International Society of Psychiatric Mental Health Nurses   www.ispn-psych.org
Internet Mental Health   www.mentalhealth.com
Mental Health Charity   www.mind.org.uk
Mental Health Foundation   www.mentalhealth.org.uk
Mentalwellness – a resource for schizophrenia and other mental health
   information   www.mentalwellness.com
National Institute of Mental Health – a US government-funded site
   www.nimh.nih.gov
Psychomatic Medicine   www.pychosomaticmedicine.org

Appendix 9.1 (*cont.*)

Rethink (formerly National Schizophrenia Fellowship)   www.nsf.org.uk
UK psychiatric nursing mail base   www.jiscmail.ac.uk/lists/psychiatric-nursing.html
University of Adelaide Library – generalized search reviews of areas in mental health   www.library.adelaide.edu.au/guide/med/menthealth/bibl.html/html

Women's Health
Gender and Women's Health Department (WHO)   www.who.int/frh-whd
Menopause Facts   www.menopausefacts.co.uk
Obgyn – an information site   www.obgyn.net
Women's Health Information   www.womens-health .co.uk

Transcultural Nursing
Transcultural Nursing: Basic Concepts & Case Studies   www.culturediversity.org
Transcultural Nursing Society   www.tcns.org

Learning Disability Care
British Institute for Learning Disabilities   www.bild.org.uk/information/index
Manchester Learning Disability Partnership   www.ld-research-nw.org.uk
Mencap   www.mencap.org.uk
National Autistic Society   www.nas.org.uk
National Network for Learning Disability Nurses   www.fons.org/networks/nnidn
Royal National Institute for the Blind multiple disability   www.rnib.org.uk/multdis/welcome.html
Scope (formerly Spastics Society)   www.scope.org.uk

Cancer
British Association of Cancer United Patients   www.cancerbacup.org.uk
Cancersource – a US site for health-care professionals   www.cancersource.com
Imperial Cancer Research Fund   www.icnet.uk
Oncology Nursing Society   www.ons.org
Terence Higgins Trust   www.tht.org.uk

Ostomy Care
British Colostomy Association   www.bcass.org.uk
Living With a Colostomy   www.ostomy.fsnet.co.uk

Appendix 9.1 (cont.)

Dermatology

British Association of Dermatologists and the British Dermatology
Nursing Group   www.bad.org.uk

Dermatology – a general site   www.dermatology.co.uk

Critical Care

American Association of Critical Care Nurses   www.aacn.org

British Association of Critical Care Nurses   www.baccn.org.uk

Emergency Care

British Trauma Society   www.trauma.org

Emergency-nurse   www.emergency-nurse.com

Royal Society for the Prevention of Accidents   www.rospa.co.uk

Research Sites

International Centre for Nursing Ethics   www.freedomtocare.org.iane

Nursing ethics   www.nursingethics.ca

RCN Research Society   www.man.ac.uk/rcn/rs/index

UK Centre for the History of Nursing   www.qmuc.ac.uk/hn/history

UK Foundation of Nursing Studies   www.fons.org.uk

University of York, Dept of Health Sciences – centre for evidence-based
nursing   www.york.ac.uk/healthsciences

Operating Department Care

National Association of Theatre Nurses   www.natn.org.uk

Association of Operating Department Professionals   www.aodp.org

British Anaesthetic and Recovery Nurses Association
www.barna.org.uk

Medical Devices Agency   www.medical-devices.gov.uk

Nutrition

British Nutrition Foundation   www.nutrition.org.uk

British Pharmaceutical Nutrition Group   www.bpng.co.uk

Medical Research Council Dunn Nutrition Unit
www.mrc.dunn.cam.ac.uk

British Association for Parenteral and Enteral Nutrition
www.bapen.org.uk

British Dietetic Association   www.bda.com.uk

Appendix 9.2 Poison information centres

United Kingdom

TOXBASE	NPIS clinical toxicology database www.spib.axl.co.uk	
London	National Poisons Information Service New Cross Hospital Avonley Road London SE14 5ER	0207 635 9191
Birmingham	Poisons Information Service City Hospital Dudley Road Birmingham B18 7QH	0121 507 5588/9
Newcastle	Poisons Information Service Wolfson Unit Claremont Place Newcastle-upon-Tyne NE2 4HH	01912 820300
Edinburgh	Scottish Poisons Information Bureau The Royal Infirmary Lauriston Place Edinburgh 3	0131 536 2300
Cardiff	Poisons Information Service Cardiff Royal Infirmary Cardiff CF2 1SZ	0292 070 9901
Belfast	Poisons Information Service Royal Victoria Hospital Grosvenor Road Belfast BT12 6BB	02890 240503

Republic of Ireland

Dublin	Poisons Information Centre Beaumont Hospital Beaumont Road Dublin 9	00 353 1 8379964/6

Appendix 10 Degrees and Diplomas

BA	Bachelor of Arts
BEd	Bachelor of Education
BN	Bachelor of Nursing
BSc	Bachelor of Science
CMT	Clinical Midwife Teacher
CPH	Certificate of Public Health
DCD	Diploma of Child Development
DCH	Diploma in Child Health
DipNEd	Diploma in Nursing Education
DipHE	Diploma in Higher Education
DN	Diploma in Nursing
DPH	Diploma in Public Health
DPhil	Doctor of Philosophy
DPM	Diploma in Psychological Medicine
DTM&H	Diploma in Tropical Medicine and Hygiene
EN(G)	Enrolled Nurse (General)
EN(M)	Enrolled Nurse (Mental)
EN(MH)	Enrolled Nurse (Mental Handicap)
FETC	Further Education Teaching Certificate
FRcn	Fellow of the Royal College of Nursing
FRSH	Fellow of the Royal Society of Health
HV	Health Visitor
MA	Master of Arts
MBA	Master of Business Administration
MBIM	Member of the British Institute of Management
MEd	Master of Education
MSc	Master of Science
MTD	Midwife Teachers' Diploma
NVQ	National Vocational Qualification
OHNC	Occupational Health Nursing Certificate
ONC	Orthopaedic Nurses' Certificate
OND	Ophthalmic Nursing Diploma
PhD	Doctor of Philosophy

Appendix 10 (*cont.*)

RCNT	Registered Clinical Nurse Tutor
RGN	Registered General Nurse
RM	Registered Midwife
RMN	Registered Mental Nurse
RN	Registered Nurse
RNMH	Registered Nurse for the Mentally Handicapped
RNT	Registered Nurse Teacher
RSCN	Registered Sick Children's Nurse
SCM	State Certified Midwife
SEN	State Enrolled Nurse
SRN	State Registered Nurse

Appendix 11 SI Units

Table 11.1 Base and supplementary SI units

Physical quantity	Name	Symbol
length	metre	m
mass	kilogram	kg
time	second	s
electric current	ampere	A
thermodynamic temperature	kelvin	K
luminous intensity	candela	cd
amount of substance	mole	mol
*plane angle	radian	rad
*solid angle	steradian	sr

*supplementary units

Table 11.2 Decimal multiples and submultiples to be used with SI units

Submultiple	Prefix	Symbol	Multiple	Prefix	Symbol
10^{-1}	deci	d	10^{1}	deca	da
10^{-2}	centi	c	10^{2}	hecto	h
10^{-3}	milli	m	10^{3}	kilo	k
10^{-6}	micro	μ	10^{6}	mega	M
10^{-9}	nano	n	10^{9}	giga	G
10^{-12}	pico	p	10^{12}	tera	T
10^{-15}	femto	f	10^{15}	peta	P
10^{-16}	atto	a	10^{16}	exa	E
10^{-21}	zepto	z	10^{21}	zetta	Z
10^{-24}	yocto	y	10^{24}	yotta	Y

Table 11.3 Conversion of units to and from SI units

From	To	Multiply by
in	m	0.0254
ft	m	0.3048
sq in	m^{2}	0.00064516
sq ft	m^{2}	0.092903
cu in	m^{3}	0.0000164
cu ft	m^{3}	0.0283168
l(itre)	m^{3}	0.001
gal(lon)	m^{3}	0.0045609
gal(lon)	litres	4.5609
lb	kg	0.453592
g cm^{-3}	kg m^{-3}	1000
lb/in^{3}	kg m^{-3}	27679.9
mmHg	Pa	133.322
cal	J	4.1868
m	in	39.3701

Table 11.3 (cont.)

From	To	Multiply by
cm	in	0.393701
cm^2	sq in	0.155
m^2	sq in	1550
m^2	sq ft	10.7639
m^3	cu in	61023.6
m^3	cu ft	35.3146
m^3	l(itre)	1000
m^3	gal(lon)	219.969
kg	lb	2.20462
kg m^{-3}	g cm^{-3}	0.001
kg m^{-3}	lb/in^3	0.0000363
Pa	mmHg	0.0075006
J	cal	0.238846

Temperature conversion

°C (Celsius) $= 5/9(°F - 32)$

°F (Fahrenheit) $= (9/5 \times °C) + 32$

Appendix 12 Code of Professional Conduct
(Nursing and Midwifery Council, April 2002)

As a registered nurse or midwife, you must:

Protect and support the health of individual patients and clients

Protect and support the health of the wider community

Act in such a way that justifies the trust and confidence the public have in you

Uphold and enhance the good reputation of the professions

As a registered nurse or midwife, you must respect the patient or client as an individual. You must recognise and respect the role of patients and clients as partners in their care and recognise the contribution they can make to it. This involves identifying their preferences regarding care and respecting these within the limits of professional practice, existing legislation, resources and the goals of the therapeutic relationship. You are personally accountable for ensuring that you promote and protect the interests and dignity of patients and clients, irrespective of gender, age, race, ability, sexuality, economic status, lifestyle, culture and religious or political beliefs. You must at all times maintain appropriate professional boundaries in the relationships you have with patients and clients. You must ensure that all aspects of the relationship focus exclusively upon the needs of the patient or the client. You must promote the interests of patients and clients. This includes helping individuals and groups to gain access to health and social care, information and support relevant to their needs. You must report to a relevant person or authority, at the earliest possible time, any conscientious objection that may be relevant to your professional practice. You must continue to provide care to the best of your ability until alternative arrangements are implemented.

As a registered nurse or midwife, you must obtain consent before you give any treatment or care. All patients have the right to receive information about their condition. You must be sensitive to their needs and respect the wishes of those who refuse or are unable to receive information about their condition. Information should be accurate, truthful and presented in such a way as to make it easily understood. You may need to seek legal or professional advice or guidance from your employer, in relation to the giving or withholding of consent. You must respect patients' and clients' autonomy – their right to decide whether or not to undergo any health intervention – even where a refusal may result in harm or death to themselves or a foetus, unless a court of law orders to the contrary. This right is protected in law, although in circumstances where the health of the foetus would be severely compromised by any refusal to give consent, it would be appropriate to discuss this matter fully within the team, and possibly seek external advice and guidance. When obtaining valid consent, you must ensure that it is given by a legally competent person, given voluntarily and it is informed. You should presume that every patient and client is legally competent unless otherwise assessed by a suitably qualified practitioner. A patient or client who is legally competent can understand and retain treatment information and can retain it to make an informed choice. Those who are legally competent may give consent in writing, orally or by cooperation. They may also refuse consent. You must ensure that all your discussions and associated decisions relating to obtaining consent are documented in the patients' or clients' health care records. When patients or clients are no longer legally competent and thus have lost the capacity to consent to or refuse treatment and care, you should try to find out whether they have previously indicated preferences in an advance statement. You must respect any refusal of treatment or care given when they legally competent, provided that the decision is clearly applicable to the present circumstances and that there is no reason to believe that they have changed their minds. When such a statement is not available, the patient's or client's wishes, if known, should be taken into account. If these wishes are not known, the criteria for treatment must be that it is in their best interests. The principles of obtaining consent apply equally to those people who have a mental illness. Whilst you should be involved in their assessment, it will also be necessary to involve relevant people close to them; this may include a psychiatrist. When patients and clients are detained under statutory powers, you must ensure that you know the circumstances and safeguards needed for providing treatment and care without consent. In emergencies where treatment is necessary to preserve life, you may provide care without patients' or clients' consent, if they are unable to give it, provided you can demonstrate that you are acting in their best interests. No one has the right to give consent on the behalf of another competent adult. In relation to obtaining consent for a child, the involvement of those with parental responsibility in the consent procedure is usually necessary, but will depend on the age and understanding of the child. If the child is under 16 in England and Wales, 12 in Scotland and 17 in Northern Ireland, you must be aware of legislation and local protocols relating to consent. Usually the individual performing the procedure should be the person to obtain the patient's or client's consent. In certain circumstances, you may seek consent on the behalf of colleagues if you have been specially trained for that specific area of practice. You must ensure that the use of complementary or alternative therapies is safe and in the interests of patients and clients. This must be discussed with the team as part of the therapeutic process and the patient or client must consent to their use.

Appendix 12 *(cont.)*

As a registered nurse or midwife, you must protect confidential information. You must treat information about patients and clients as confidential and use it only for the purposes for which it was given. As it is impractical to obtain consent every time you need to share information with others, you should ensure that patients and clients understand that some information may be made available to other members of the team involved in the delivery of care. You must guard against breaches of confidentiality by protecting information from improper disclosure at all times. You should seek patients' and clients' wishes regarding the sharing of information with their family and others. When a patient or client is considered incapable of giving permission, you should consult relevant colleagues. If you are required to disclose information outside the team that will have personal consequences for patients or clients, you must obtain their consent. If the patient or client withholds consent, or if consent cannot be obtained for whatever reason, disclosures may be made only where they can be justified in the public interest (usually where disclosure is essential to protect the patient or client or someone else from the risk of significant harm) or if they are required by law or by order of a court. Where there is an issue of child protection, you must act at all times in accordance with national and local policies.

As a registered nurse or midwife, you must maintain your professional knowledge and competence. You must keep your skills and knowledge up to date throughout your working life. In particular, you should take part regularly in learning activities that develop your competence and performance. To practice competently, you must possess the knowledge, skills and abilities required for lawful, safe and effective practice without direct supervision. You must acknowledge the limits of your professional competence and only undertake practice and accept responsibilities for those activities in which you are competent. If the aspect of practice is beyond your level of competence or outside your area of registration, you must obtain help and supervision from a competent practitioner until you and your employer consider that you have acquired the requisite knowledge and skill. You have a duty to facilitate students of nursing and midwifery and others to develop their competence. You have a responsibility to deliver care based on current evidence, best practice and, where acceptable, validated research when it is available.

As a registered nurse or midwife, you must be trustworthy. You must behave in such a way that upholds the reputation of the professions. Behaviour that compromises this reputation may call your registration into question even if it is not directly connected to your professional practice.

Appendix 12 *(cont.)*

You must ensure that your registration status is not used in the promotion of commercial products or services declare any financial or other interests in relevant organisations providing such goods or services, and ensure that your professional judgement is not influenced by any financial considerations. When providing advice regarding any product or service relating to your professional role or area of practice, you must be aware of the risk that, on account of your professional title or qualification, you could be perceived by the patient or the client as endorsing the product. You should fully explain the advantages and disadvantages of alternative products so that the patient or client can make an informed choice. Where you recommend a specific product, you must ensure that your advice is based on evidence and is not for your own commercial gain. You must refuse any gift, favour or hospitality that may be interpreted, now or in the future, as an attempt to obtain preferential consideration. You must neither ask for nor accept loans from patients, clients or their relatives and friends.

As a registered nurse or midwife, you must act to identify and minimise the risk to patients and clients. You must work with other members of the team to promote health care environments that are conducive to safe, therapeutic and ethical practice. You must act quickly to protect patients and clients from risk if you have good reason to believe that you or a colleague, from your own or another profession, may not be fit to practice for reasons of conduct, health or competence. You should be aware of the terms of legislation that offer protection for people who raise concerns about health and safety issues. Where you cannot remedy circumstances in the environment of care that jeopardise standards of practice, you must report them to a senior person with sufficient authority to manage them and also, in the case of midwifery, to the supervisor of midwives. This must be supported by a written record. When working as a manager, you have a duty towards patients and clients, colleagues, the wider community and the organisation in which you and your colleagues work. When facing professional dilemmas, your first consideration in all activities must be the interests and safety of patients and clients. In an emergency, in or outside the work setting, you have a professional duty to provide care. The care provided would be judged against what would be reasonably expected from someone with your knowledge, skills and abilities when placed in those particular circumstances.

Appendix 12 *(cont.)*

The Scope of Professional Practice

The Code of Professional Conduct provides a firm bedrock upon which decisions about the scope of professional practice can be made. Practice must remain dynamic, sensitive, relevant and responsive to the changing needs of patients and clients and so must education for practice. The registered nurse, midwife or health visitor:

- must be satisfied that each aspect of practice is directed to meeting the needs and serving the interests of the patient or client;
- must endeavour always to achieve, maintain and develop knowledge, skill and competence to respond to those needs and interests;
- must honestly acknowledge any limits of personal knowledge and skill and take steps to remedy any relevant deficits effectively and appropriately in order to meet the needs of patients and clients;
- must ensure that any enlargement or adjustment of the scope of personal professional practice must be achieved without compromising or fragmenting existing aspects of professional practice and care and that the requirements of the Council's Code of Professional Conduct are satisfied throughout the whole area of practice;
- must recognise and honour the direct or indirect personal accountability born for all aspects of professional practice and
- must, in serving the interests of patients and clients and the wider interests of society, avoid any inappropriate delegation to others which compromises those interests.